Care of the
Critically Ill Child

Important notice

Every effort has been made to check the drug dosages given in this book. However, as it is possible that dosage schedules have been revised, the reader is strongly urged to consult the drug companies' literature before administering any of the drugs listed.

Commissioning Editor: Maria Khan
Project Editor: Rachel Robson
Project Supervisor: Mark Sanderson

Typeset by Saxon Graphics Ltd, Derby
Printed in China
NPCC/01

Care of the Critically Ill Child

EDITED BY

Andrew J. Macnab MD (London) FRCPC

Professor and Director Post Graduate Education, Department of Pediatrics,
University of British Columbia
Director, Pediatric Transport Program, Division of Critical Care,
British Columbia's Children's Hospital, Vancouver, Canada

Duncan J. Macrae MBBS FRCA FRCPCH

Consultant in Paediatric Intensive Care, Department of Intensive Care,
Great Ormond Street Hospital for Children, London, UK

Robert Henning FRCA FFICANZCA DCH

Staff Specialist, Paediatric Intensive Care Unit, Royal Children's Hospital,
Melbourne, Australia

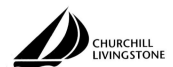

**CHURCHILL
LIVINGSTONE**

LONDON EDINBURGH NEW YORK PHILADELPHIA SYDNEY TORONTO

CHURCHILL LIVINGSTONE
An Division of Harcourt Publishers Limited

© Harcourt Brace and Company 1999. All rights reserved.
© Harcourt Publishers Limited 2001. All rights reserved.

 is a registered trademark of Harcourt Publishers
Limited

ISBN 0-4430-5394-4

British Library Cataloguing in Publication Data
A catalogue record for this book is available from the
British Library

Library of Congress Cataloging in Publication Data
A catalog record for this book is available from the Library
of Congress

Medical knowledge is constantly changing. As new
information becomes available, changes in treatment,
procedures, equipment and the use of drugs become
necessary. The authors and publishers have, as far as it is
possible, taken care to ensure that the information given
in this text is accurate and up to date. However, readers
are strongly advised to confirm that the information,
especially with regard to drug usage, complies with latest
legislation and standards of practice.

The
publisher's
policy is to use
**paper manufactured
from sustainable forests**

Contents

PART 4: ENVIRONMENTAL EMERGENCIES

PART 5: THERAPEUTIC PRINCIPLES AND PRACTICE GUIDELINES FOR CRITICAL CARE

PART 6: PROCEDURES

Contributors

Robert J Adderley MD, FRCPC
Intensive Care Unit, Paediatric Special Needs Unit, British Columbia's Children's Hospital, Vancouver, Canada

John Alexander MBChB, MCRP, FRCPCh
Consultant, Paediatric Intensive Care Unit, City General Hospital, Stoke-on-Trent, UK

Shirley M Alexander MBChB (Edin), MRCP, DCH
ECMO Fellow, Great Ormond Street Hospital for Children, London, UK

Helen Anthony BSc (Hons), M Hum Nutr, APD
Clinical Specialist Dietitian, Royal Children's Hospital, Melbourne, Australia

Claire Aston BSc (Pharm)
Clinical Pharmacist, British Columbia's Children's Hospital, Vancouver, Canada

Jennifer Balfour MD
Fellow, Infectious Diseases, British Columbia's Children's Hospital, Vancouver, Canada

Mary M Bennett MD, FRCPC
Division of Critical Care, British Columbia's Children's Hospital, Vancouver, Canada

Robert Bingham MBBS, MRCS, FRCA
Consultant Anaesthetist, Department of Anaesthesia, Great Ormond Street Hospital for Children, London UK

Aileen Britton RN, RSCN, BA, MPH
Unit Manager, Paediatric Intensive Care Unit, Royal Children's Hospital, Melbourne, Australia

Warwick Butt FRACP
Paediatric Intensive Care Unit, Royal Children's Hospital, Melbourne, Australia

John Christodoulou PhD, FRACP, CGHGSA
Associate Professor, Director, Western Sydney Genetics Program, The Children's Hospital, Westmead, Australia

Arthur F Cogswell MBBS, B Med Sc, Dip Obs RACOG, DCH, FRACP, FRCPC
Staff Physician, Division of Critical Care, British Columbia's Children's Hospital, Vancouver, Canada

R Gregory Delbridge FRACP, MBBS
Staff Specialist, Paediatric Intensive Care Unit, Royal Children's Hospital, Herston, Brisbane, Australia

Michael J Dillon MB, FRCP, FRCPCH, DCH
Professor of Paediatric Nephrology, Great Ormond Street Hospital for Children, London, UK

Simon Dobson MD, FRCPC
Infectious Diseases, British Columbia's Children's Hospital, Vancouver, Canada

Michael Fairley MBBS, FRANZCP
Senior Staff Specialist, Department of Psychological Medicine, The Children's Hospital, Westmead, Australia

David Field MBBS, DCN, FRCP (Edin), DM, FRCP
Professor of Neonatal Medicine, Department of Paediatrics, University of Leicester, Leicester, UK

Reinoud JBJ Gemke MD, PhD
Senior Lecturer in Paediatric Critical Care, Department of Paediatrics, Free University Hospital, Amsterdam, The Netherlands

Victoria Gilmore B Health Admin, RN
Nurse Manager, Haematology, Oncology and Bone Marrow Transplant Unit, Sydney Children's Hospital, Sydney, Australia

Allan P Goldman MBBCh
Consultant in Pediatric Intensive Care, Cardiac Intensive Care Unit, Great Ormond Street Hospital for Children, London, UK

Chula DA Goonasekera MD, PhD, MBBS, MCRP, FFARCSI
Research Fellow and Honorary Senior Registrar in Paediatric Nephrology, Nephrology Unit, Institute of Child Health and Great Ormond Street Hospital for Children, London

Tom Grattan-Smith FRACP
Director, Department of Paediatrics, St. George Hospital, Kogarah, Australia

Gordon Green MD, FRCPC
CMAC, Charleston, West Virginia, USA

Robert Henning FRCA FFICANZCA DCH
Staff Specialist, Paediatric Intensive Care Unit, Royal Children's Hospital, Melbourne, Australia

Henry Hui MBBS, MRCP (UK), FRCPC
Fellow, Division of Critical Care, British Columbia's Children's Hospital, Vancouver, Canada

Ian G James MBChB, FFA
Director, Paediatric Intensive Care Unit, Great Ormond Street Hospital for Children, London, UK

Stephen Keeley FRACP
Specialist in Paediatric Intensive Care, Adelaide Women's and Children's Hospital, Adelaide, Australia

Nigel Klein BSc, MRCP, PhD
Senior Lecturer in Immunology and Infectious Diseases, Great Ormond Street Hospital for Children, London, UK

Bruce Lister MBBS, FANZCA, FFICANZCA
Director, Paediatric Intensive Care Unit, Mater Children's Hospital, Brisbane, Australia

Duncan J Macrae MBBS, FRCA, FRCPCH
Department of Intensive Care, Great Ormond Street Hospital for Children, London, UK

John J Macready BSc, Phm, PharmD
Clinical Specialist, Pharmacy, British Columbia's Children's Hospital, Vancouver, Canada

Andrew J Macnab MD (London), FRCPC
Professor and Director Post Graduate Education, Department of Pediatrics, University of British Columbia
Director, Pediatric Transport Program, Division of Critical Care, British Columbia's Children's Hospital, Vancouver, Canada

Neil T Matthews FFICANZA
Director, Paediatric Intensive Care Unit, Adelaide Women's and Children's Hospital, Adelaide, Australia

Rebecca J Mawer BMBS, BMedSci, FRCA, DCH
Specialist Registrar, Department of Anaesthetists, Great Ormond Street Hospital for Children, London, UK

Fiona JC Maxton MN, RSCN, RGN
Clinical Nurse Consultant, Paediatric Intensive Care Unit, The New Children's Hospital, Westmead, Australia

Julie McEniery MBBS, FRACP
Director, Paediatric Intensive Care, Royal Children's Hospital, Herston, Brisbane, Australia

Quen Q Mok MBBS, DCH, MRCP, MRCPI
Consultant Intensivist, Paediatric Intensive Care Unit, Great Ormond Street Hospital for Children, London, UK

Vas Novelli FRACP, FCP, FRCPCH
Consultant in Infectious Diseases, Great Ormond Street Hospital for Children, London, UK

Mark J Peters MBChB
Great Ormond Street Hospital for Children, London, UK

Glynis Price MBBCh, DHC, FCP
Staff Specialist in Endocrinology, Department of Endocrinology and Diabetes, Royal Children's Hospital, Melbourne, Australia

Robert I Ross Russell MD, FRCP
Consultant in Paediatric Intensive Care, Addenbrookes Hospital, Cambridge, UK

Karen Ryall RN, BSN
Patient Services Director, Critical Care, British Columbia's Children's Hospital, Vancouver, Canada

Frédéric Sage MD, FRCA
Consultant Paediatric Anaesthetist, East Surrey Hospital, Redhill, UK

Margrid Schindler MBBS, FANZCA
Consultant Intensivist, Great Ormond Street Hospital
for Children, London, UK

Steven Scuplak MBBS
Consultant Anaesthetist, Great Ormond Street Hospital
for Children, London, UK

Michael D Seear MD, FRCPC
Division of Critical Care, British Columbia's Children's
Hospital, Vancouver, Canada

Elizabeth Segedin FRACP
Director, Paediatric Intensive Care, Starship Children's
Hospital, Auckland, New Zealand

Peter W Skippen MD, FRCPC
Division of Critical Care, British Columbia's Children's
Hospital, Vancouver, Canada

Anthony Slater FRACP
Specialist in Paediatric Intensive Care, Adelaide
Women's and Children's Hospital, Adelaide, Australia

Liz Smith MSc, RGN, RSCN
ECMO Co-ordinator, Cardiac Intensive Care
Unit/ECMO, Great Ormond Street Hospital for
Children, London, UK

Michael South MD, MRCP, FRACP
Associate Professor, Department of Paediatrics,
University of Melbourne, Specialist in Paediatric Care,
Royal Children's Hospital, Melbourne, Australia

Robert C Tasker MBBS, MA, MRCP, DCH
University Lecturer, Paediatric Intensive Care,
Addenbrookes Hospital, Cambridge, UK

Russell Taylor FRACS
Department of Surgery, Royal Children's Hospital,
Melbourne, Australia

Adrianus J van Vught MD PhD
Professor of Pediatric Critical Care and Intensive Care,
Wilhemina Children's Hospital, Utrecht, Netherlands

Theo van Willigenburg MD
Professor of Ethics, Erasmus University, Rotterdam and
Professor of Medical Ethics, Amsterdam Medical
School, Netherlands

David Wensley MBBS, FRCPC
Director of Paediatric Intensive Care, British Columbia's
Children's Hospital, Vancouver, Canada

Barry Wilkins MD, MRCP (UK), FRACP, FRCPCH, DCH (Lond)
Senior Specialist in Paediatric Intensive Care, The New
Children's Hospital, Parramatta, Australia

Simon Young MBBS, Dip Crim, FACEM
Director of Emergency Services, Royal Children's
Hospital, Melbourne, Australia

Michael Yung MD, FRACP
Paediatric Intensive Care Unit, Royal Victoria Infirmary,
Newcastle upon Tyne, UK

Foreword

Paediatric intensive care is a new specialty. Although its origins may lie in the 'Department of Weaklings' that Stephanie Tarnier established at the Paris maternity hospital in 1893, intensive care units for older children did not develop until the 1950s, when they were started in Sweden and the United States to provide postoperative care. At that time, endotracheal tubes were made from metal or rubber, and there was a very high incidence of subglottic stenosis. In the early 1960s, the introduction of polyvinyl chloride tubes, which soften at body temperature, enabled children to be intubated more safely – and this allowed paediatric intensive care to develop rapidly.

The technical problems involved in looking after very ill children took many years to overcome, but it has taken even longer to define the best way to organise paediatric intensive care: it is only in the last decade that evidence has been accumulated that very ill children are best looked after in specialist paediatric intensive care units by doctors and nurses who practise paediatric intensive care full-time. It is also only recently that attempts have been made to collate our knowledge about the treatment of very sick children: the first textbook of paediatric intensive care was not published until 1988.

Although there are now five large textbooks of paediatric intensive care, these have all originated in the United States of America. *Care of the Critically Ill Child* has been written by paediatric intensivisits from Canada, the United Kingdom and Australia, where there are important differences from the United States in the care of very ill children. The book is therefore a very welcome addition to the literature. It provides didactic practical advice about many aspects of paediatric intensive care, as well as a brief physiological background. The highlighted lists of key points and common errors at the end of many sections are particularly useful – 'The Golden Rules' of paediatric intensive care. Although the text is not referenced, most chapters provide an annotated list of suggestions for further reading – a valuable resource.

This book provides a sensible compromise between a lengthy discussion of basic sciences on the one hand, and a didactic handbook on the other. It will be an excellent source of information for doctors and nurses learning about the care of very ill children, and a useful reference for experienced paediatric intensivists.

Frank Shann
Director of Intensive Care,
Royal Children's Hospital, Melbourne

Professor of Critical Care Medicine,
University of Melbourne, Australia

Preface

Children sweeten labours; but make misfortune the more bitter

Francis Bacon (1561–1626), *Of Parents and Children*

It is encouraging that in spite of the pace of life today and the world's materialism, a critically ill child remains a sight to which every human being responds. None the less, few situations make physicians more uneasy than being called on to take responsibility for the care of such a child. The recent advances in pediatric care provide us with many more things to do constructively, but also an intimate awareness of the perils of error or omission. When striving to resuscitate a child, all that matters is the individual life at hand. Temporarily we suppress thoughts of the population explosion, the potential misery of long-term handicap, or of children being kept alive only to die later from nutritional or emotional starvation.

Pediatric intensive care is the interface between the magic and promise of childhood and the anguish and uncertainty of critical illness and/or injury. Today dedicated units provide intensive care for this remarkable and distressing population. These units centralize human and technical expertise in the management of critical illnesses which are specific to children, and provide an environment that is sensitive to children's special needs and those of their families. Intensive care involves prompt action to deal with emergencies, anticipation of potential deterioration, prevention of secondary problems, meticulous attention to detail, competence with procedural skills, familiarity with monitoring technology, awareness of the possibilities of definitive care and appropriate triage. However, immediate care of critical illness and injury in childhood often requires management of these issues in environments other than a pediatric intensive care unit. Intensive care can and should be offered immediately and as comprehensively as possible wherever it is required under such circumstances.

Confronting a critically ill child is immensely demanding for all involved. The harsh realities are hard for the child and family to bear. The practical necessities are hard for the care givers. Prioritization, attention to detail and expertise are required for care to be optimal. This applies equally to the physical, mental and biochemical status of the child, the technical elements of care and the dynamics of the family if a thorough knowledge of each child's pathological problems, immediate and long-term needs, and the family's response to the child's need for care, are to be understood. Many small hospitals, emergency rooms and adult intensive care units do manage to look after critically ill children skillfully in the initial stages of illness, but limited pediatric expertise and the lack of a child- and family-oriented environment will, in the long term, prove detrimental to their patients' physical and emotional wellbeing.

The purpose of this book is to extend the skills of pediatric intensive care physicians beyond the intensive care unit into the community. It is intended to be a primer of the principles underlying modern intensive care. The emphasis of the book is on practical advice based on the experience of intensive care pediatricians. Background physiology and epidemiology are provided to assist the process of understanding and diagnosing childhood critical illness and injury. This is more than a handbook for emergency physicians, but it is not intended to be an all-encompassing text on pediatric intensive care. The authors hope that the didactic nature of the text will enable physicians less familiar with managing critically ill and injured children to act appropriately in emergencies: dealing with the priorities of care, initiating effective treatment, beginning the process of investigation and definitive diagnosis, triaging appropriately, and transferring each patient safely for ongoing intensive care. The text deliberately includes sections on controversial care and stresses in each chapter the key points in the management of the conditions discussed or failure of the systems described. Errors in management commonly seen by intensive care pediatricians in cases referred to them are included, with the aim of reducing the incidence of secondary problems and avoidable errors which can contribute to deterioration or death.

This book sets out the principles and practice of modern pediatric intensive care to help physicians and other health care professionals to act effectively when they find themselves providing for the immediate needs of critically ill children and their families. The book is written primarily by practicing pediatric intensive care physicians and nurses, with contributions from physiologists and biochemists, and the authors combine their experience from British Columbia's Children's Hospital, Vancouver, Canada; Great Ormond Street Children's Hospital, London, England; the Royal Children's Hospital, Melbourne, Australia, and allied units.

Andrew J. Macnab
amacnab@cw.bc.ca
Duncan Macrae
Robert Henning

Acknowledgments

Few care concepts are wholly original and the authors acknowledge the influence of their colleagues' practice, teaching and writing on the content style and views expressed in this book.

This book came about because of the special talents of Lucy Gardner, Inta Ozols and Dinah Thom at Harcourt Brace. The manuscript was prepared by Leatha Semrick with editorial assistance from Damian Duffy, Faith Gagnon, Cathy Halstead, Gundy Macnab and Janet Witheridge.

Dedication

This book is for all those who care for children,
and for:
Magnus, Camilla, Julia, Duncan, Christopher,
and
Alice, Catriona and Jenny.

List of drugs with UK/US alternative names

UK name	US name
adrenaline	epinephrine
amethocaine	tetracaine
benzylpenicillin	penicillin G
co-trimoxazole	trimethoprim and sulfamethoxazole
desferrioxamine	deferoxamine
dicoumarol	dicumarol
frusemide	furosemide
glyceryl trinitrate	nitroglycerin
isoprenaline	isoproterenol
lignocaine	lidocaine
mepacrine	quinacrine
noradrenaline	norepinephrine
paracetamol	acetaminophen
pethidine	meperidine
phenobarbitone	phenobarbital
phenoxymethylpenicillin	penicillin V
phytomenadione	phytonadione
suxamethonium	succinylcholine
thiopentone	thiopental

Abbreviations

AA amino acids
AAP American Academy of Pediatrics
ABC airway, breathing, circulation (basic life support)
ABG arterial blood gases
ACE angiotensin converting enzyme
ACT activated clotting time
ACTH adrenocorticotropic hormone
ADH antidiuretic hormone
AIDS acquired immune deficiency syndrome
ALT alanine aminotransferase
ALTE apparent life-threatening episode
AMP adenosine monophosphate
ANA antinuclear antibodies
ANCA antineutrophil cytoplasmic autoantibodies
AP anteroposterior
APLS advanced pediatric life support
APRV airway pressure release ventilation
APTT activated partial thromboplastin time
ARDS acute respiratory distress syndrome
ARF acute renal failure
ASA acetylsalicylic acid; American Society of Anesthesiologists
ASD atrial septal defect
ASOT antistreptolysin O titre
AST aspartate aminotransferase
ATLS advanced trauma life support
ATN acute tubular necrosis
AV atrioventricular
AVM arteriovenous malformation
AVP arginine vasopressin
AVSD atrioventricular septal defect
AXR abdominal X-ray
BAL bronchoalveolar lavage; British antiLewisite
BCAA branched-chain amino acids
BiPAP Bilevel positive airway pressure ventilation

BMT bone marrow transplant
BP blood pressure
BPD bronchopulmonary dysplasia
BSA body surface area
BT Blalock-Taussig (shunt)
BUN blood urea nitrogen
CAA coronary artery aneurysms
CAVH continuous arteriovenous hemofiltration
CAVHD continuous arteriovenous hemodialysis
CBC complete blood count
CBF cerebral blood flow
CCF congestive cardiac failure
CDC Centers for Disease Control
CDH congenital diaphragmatic hernia
CHF congestive heart failure
CIP critical illness polyneuropathy
CK creatine kinase
CMRO$_2$ cerebral metabolic rate for oxygen
CMV cytomegalovirus
CNS central nervous system
COHb carboxyhemoglobin
CPAP continuous positive airway pressure
CPB cardiopulmonary bypass
CPK creatine phosphokinase (= CK)
CPP cerebral perfusion pressure
CPR cardiopulmonary resuscitation
CRIB clinical risk index for babies
CSF cerebrospinal fluid
CT computed tomography
CV controlled ventilation
CVP central venous pressure
CVVH continuous venovenous hemofiltration
CVVHDF continuous venovenous hemodiafiltration
CXR chest X-ray
DDAVP deamino-D-arginine vasopressin (desmopressin)

DC direct current
D+ (D–) HUS hemolytic–uremic syndrome with (without) diarrhea
DI diabetes insipidus
DIC disseminated intravascular coagulation
DKA diabetic ketoacidosis
DNR do not resuscitate
DPG diphosphoglycerate
DPT diphtheria, pertussis and tetanus
DSVNI distress scale for ventilated newborn infants
DTPA diethylenetriaminepentaacetic acid
EBM expressed breast milk
ECF extracellular fluid
ECG electrocardiogram
ECLS extracorporeal life support
ECMO extracorporeal membrane oxygenation
ECV extracellular volume
EDTA ethylenediaminetetraacetic acid
EEG electroencephalogram
ELAM endothelial leukocyte adhesion molecule
ELSO Extracorporeal Life Support Organization
EMG electromyogram
EN enteral nutrition
ENT ear, nose and throat
EP evoked potential
EPO emergency protection order
ER emergency room
ESR erythrocyte sedimentation rate
ET endotracheal
ETT endotracheal tube
FAO Food and Agriculture Organization
FB foreign body
FDP fibrin degradation products
FEV$_1$ forced expiratory volume in 1 minute
FFA free fatty acids
FFP fresh frozen plasma
FG French gauge
FIO$_2$ fractional inspired oxygen concentration
FRC functional residual capacity
FUO fever of unknown origin
GBM glomerular basement membrane
GCS Glasgow coma scale
GFR glomerular filtration rate
GI gastrointestinal
G6PD glucose 6-phosphate deficiency
GMP guanosine monophosphate
GVHD graft-versus-host disease
Hb hemoglobin

Hct hematocrit (packed cell volume)
HD hemodialysis
HEPA high efficiency particulate airflow
HFJV high-frequency jet ventilation
HFO high-frequency oscillation
HFOV high-frequency oscillatory ventilation
HFPPV high-frequency positive pressure ventilation
HFV high-frequency ventilation
Hib *Haemophilus influenzae* b
HIE hypoxic ischemic encephalopathy
HITTS heparin-induced thrombosis-thrombocytopenia syndrome
HIV human immunodeficiency virus
HLHS hypoplastic left heart syndrome
HMD hyaline membrane disease
HOCM hypertrophic obstructive cardiomyopathy
HSW herpes simplex virus
HR heart rate
HUI health utility index
HUS hemolytic–uremic syndrome
ICP intracranial pressure
ICU intensive care unit
IDDM insulin-dependent diabetes mellitus
IE infective endocarditis
I:E inspiratory:expiratory
Ig immunoglobulin
IGF insulin-like growth factor
IL interleukin
i.m., IM intramuscular
IMV intermittent mandatory ventilation
INR International Normalized Ratio
IO intraosseous
IPPV intermittent positive pressure ventilation
IRV inverse ratio ventilation
ITP idiopathic thrombocytopenic purpura
i.v., IV intravenous
IVC inferior vena cava
IVI intravenous infusion
IVIG IV immunoglobulin
JET junctional ectopic tachycardia
LA left atrium
LAP left atrial pressure
LCT long-chain triacylglycerol
LDH lactate dehydrogenase
LIP lymphocytic interstitial pneumonitis
LP lumbar puncture
MAP mean arterial pressure
MBT modified Blalock–Taussig (shunt)

MCAD medium-chain acyl-CoA dehydrogenase
MCV mean corpuscular volume
MDI metered dose inhaler
MEN multiple endocrine neoplasia
MI myocardial infarction
MMR measles, mumps and rubella
MODS multiple organ dysfunction syndrome
MRI magnetic resonance imaging
MRSA methicillin resistant *Staphylococcus aureus*
MSUD maple syrup urine disease
NAI nonaccidental injury
NCA nurse-controlled analgesia
NEC necrotizing entercolitis
NG nasogastric
NIAV noninvasive assisted ventilation
NIRS near infrared spectroscopy
NKH nonketotic hyperglycinemia
NMDA *N*-methyl-D-aspartate
NPA nasopharyngeal aspirate
NPE nonprotein energy
NRTI nucleoside reverse transcriptase inhibitor
NSAID nonsteroidal antiinflammatory drug
NTD neural tube defect
OER oxygen extraction ratio
OHP hydroxyprogesterone
OI oxygenation index
PAF platelet activating factor
PALS pediatric advanced life support
PAP pulmonary artery pressure
PCA patient-controlled analgesia
PChE plasma cholinesterase
PCP *Pneumocystis carinii* pneumonia
PCR polymerase chain reaction
PCV packed cell volume
PD peritoneal dialysis
PDA patent ductus arteriosus
PEEP positive end-expiratory pressure
PEFR peak expiratory flow rate
PEM protein–energy malnutrition
PFO patent foramen ovale
PG prostaglandin
PI protease inhibitor
PICU pediatric intensive care unit
PIM pediatric index of mortality
PIP peak inflation pressure
PN parenteral nutrition
PO per os (by mouth)
PPHN primary pulmonary hypertension of the newborn

PR per rectum
PRA plasma renin activity
PRISM pediatric risk of mortality score
PT prothrombin time
PTT partial thromboplastin time
PVC polyvinyl chloride
PVL periventricular leukomalacia
PVR pulmonary vascular resistance
QALY quality-adjusted life year
RA right atrium
RBC red blood cell
RBF renal blood flow
RDI recommended daily intake
REM rapid eye movement
RMSF Rocky Mountain spotted fever
RR respiratory rate
RSI rapid sequence induction
RSV respiratory syncytial virus
RVOT right ventricular outflow tract
SC subcutaneous
SCD sickle cell disease
SCID severe combined immunodeficiency
SIADH syndrome of inappropriate antidiuretic hormone secretion
SID strong ion difference
SIDS sudden infant death syndrome
SIMV synchronized intermittent mandatory ventilation
SLE systemic lupus erythematosus
SMR standardized mortality rate
SSPE subacute sclerosing pan encephalitis
SVC superior vena cava
SVR systemic vascular resistance
SVT supraventricular tachycardia
SWI sterile water for injection
TB tuberculosis
TCPC total cavopulmonary connection
TDU technology-dependent unit
TGA transposition of the great arteries
THAM tris(hydroxymethyl)aminomethane or tromethamine
THAN transient hyperammonemia of the newborn
TISS therapeutic intervention scoring system
TNF tumor necrosis factor
TPA tissue plasminogen activator
TPN total parenteral nutrition
TTP thrombotic thrombocytopenic purpura
TSS toxic shock syndrome

URTI upper respiratory tract infection

V-A ECLS venoarterial extracorporeal life support

VSD ventricular septal defect

VT ventricular tachycardia

V-V ELCS venovenous extracorporeal life support

vWF von Willebrand factor

VZIG varicella-zoster immune globulin

WBL whole bowel lavage

WBC white blood cells

WHO World Health Organization

Emergency drugs

Drug	Dose	How Supplied	Remarks
Oxygen		Via nasal prongs/ mask/bag valve mask/ET tube/ ventilator	
Volume (isotonic fluid)	10–20 ml/kg IV or IO		– Repeat bolus if circulation remains poor
Adrenalin/Epinephrine		1:10 000 (0.1 mg/ml) OR	– Most useful drug in cardiac arrest; 1:1000 must be diluted
	Bradycardia: –0.01 mg/kg (0.1 ml/kg of 1:10 000)	1:1000 (1.0 mg/ml)	
	Asystolic or pulseless arrest: *First dose* 0.01 mg/kg IV/IO 0.1 mg/kg ET Doses as high as 0.2 mg/kg may be effective *Subsequent doses* IV/IO/ET: 0.1 mg/kg Doses as high as 0.2 mg/kg may be effective		
Atropine sulfate	0.02 mg/kg IV (0.2 ml/kg)	0.1 mg/ml	*Minimum dose:* 0.1 mg (1 ml): use for bradycardia after assessing ventilation *Maximum dose:* infants and children – up to 0.5 mg; adolescents – up to 1.0 mg
Adenosine	0.1–0.2 mg/kg		Rapid IV bolus (maximum dose 12 mg)
Lidocaine/Lignocaine	1 mg/kg IV infusion: 20–50 μg/kg·min	10 mg/ml (1% solution) 20 mg/ml (2% solution)	– Use for ventricular arrhythmias *only* – Via ET tube dilute with saline to a volume of 2–3 cc. Follow with IPPV
Bretylium	5 mg/kg IV	50 mg/ml	– Use if lidocaine is not effective; repeat dose with 10 mg/kg if first dose is not effective
Sodium bicarbonate	1mEq/kg IV (1 ml/kg) 0.3 × kg × base deficit	1mEq.ml (8.4% solution)	– Infuse slowly and only when ventilation is adequate
Calcium chloride	20 mg/kg IV (0.2 ml/kg)	100 mg/ml (10% solution)	– Use only for hypocalcemia, calcium channel blocker overdose, hyperkalemia, or hypermagnesemia; give slowly
Dopamine	5–20 μg/kg·min IV		– Titrate to desired effect
Glucose	0.25 g/kg (2.5 ml/kg $D_{10}W$)		– Give slowly IV hypertonic
Diazepam	0.2 mg/kg·dose IV		– Give slowly. May ↓ respiratory effort and/or BP. Irritant to veins (not compatible dextrose)

Drug	Dose	How Supplied	Remarks
Midazolam	0.1 mg/kg·dose IV		– Give slowly for sedation. May ↓ respiratory effort and/or BP
Phenytoin	15–20 mg/kg IV		– Give as loading dose over 20 minutes. May ↓ BP
Furosemide	1 mg/kg IV (0.1 ml/kg)	10 mg/ml	– Give slowly over 5 minutes
Diazoxide	1–3 mg/kg IV	15 mg/ml	– Rapid IV bolus for hypertensive crisis. – Keep child lying down (risk of postural hypotension). May be repeated once

Introduction

1.1 Introduction: the rationale for, and provision of, pediatric intensive care

Andrew J. Macnab and David F. Wensley

INTRODUCTION AND DEFINITIONS

Illness or injury becomes critical when one or more organ systems are in danger of failing or begin to fail, raising the possibility of death or incomplete recovery. Intensive care provides the necessary support, interventions and treatment entities for systems in failure. At its most basic level, intensive care consists of resuscitation or recognition of the impending need for resuscitation, while attending to the 'big picture' of a child's condition. However, the needs of critically ill children change dramatically over time, and progressively smaller issues can become increasingly important as intensive care progresses. Ongoing intensive care necessitates vigilance, monitoring and continuous reevaluation, anticipation of change, inquiry as to causation, and seeking appropriate advice and assistance. As the physiologic disturbance caused by a child's illness progresses or becomes prolonged, the risk of death or incomplete recovery increases. At its most complex level, intensive care involves balancing the needs of multiple systems in failure to ensure maximal physiologic benefit from therapy, while minimizing the adverse consequences of treatment. Intensive care at this level is provided in a regionalized pediatric intensive care unit (PICU) which is able to provide sophisticated state-of-the-art care, monitoring, diagnostic investigation, and technological support for the special needs of the child and the family.

Intensive care for the critically ill child is particularly challenging because of the many different illnesses potentially involved at different ages, the difficulty of performing procedures on small patients, and the range of physiologic values that constitute 'normal' in relation to different ages and the fact that a sick child often compensates well in the initial stages of illness but can then go on to decompensate abruptly. These facts underlie the recognition that children cannot be treated as 'small adults,' and that comprehensive care of a critically ill or injured child requires provision of intensive care specifically tailored to the needs of that individual child.

Intensive care relies on a team approach by trained people acting logically to anticipate and manage a series of urgent or emergent priorities. In addition, these caregivers must collaborate with other professionals who have additional expertise or resources that are considered necessary. Intensive care combines acute therapeutic interventions with ongoing meticulous attention to detail, and an open mind prepared to investigate further whenever the child's clinical condition and/or the data from investigations 'don't add up.'

When death is inevitable, intensive care extends to include compassionate and comprehensive support of the child and family through the process of dying.

WHERE DOES INTENSIVE CARE HAPPEN?

Ongoing intensive care requires committed experienced staff, technical expertise, and modern technology and equipment. Children who require this level of care have a better chance of intact survival in a dedicated tertiary PICU. The literature indicates that a substantial reduction in mortality rate could be achieved if children requiring care as basic as endotracheal intubation for more than 12–24 hours were transferred to regional tertiary PICUs for care.

However, common sense and research also indicate that basic intensive care begins for the critically ill child wherever resuscitation occurs, and ideally whenever a child's condition is such that caregivers anticipate that the need for advanced care is imminent. Thus, children must have their initial intensive care needs met in a variety of settings: prehospital scenes (even doctors' offices), small community hospitals, emergency rooms, interfacility transport vehicles, and general wards of large tertiary medical centers. Resources available at each of these healthcare sites obviously vary. Optimum care relies upon full use being made of whatever facilities and expertise are available and an established network providing local and regional prehospital, interhospital, and hospital resources. How this care is delivered has a significant bearing on outcome.

Guidelines for development of such a regionalized structure exist to ensure that the intensive care needs of an individual community are met.

If, at the basic intensive care level, anticipation and timely, appropriate intervention occur, deterioration to cardiorespiratory arrest (with its bleak prognosis) can often be prevented, and the incidence of secondary physiologic insults (particularly to the brain) can be reduced. These secondary insults are often common sequelae of failing to anticipate and address basic elements of care (e.g. hypoxia, hypotension, seizures, raised intracranial pressure, fever, or hypoglycemia). Importantly, in the context of critical illness, these elements can, singly or particularly in combination, have profoundly detrimental physiologic effects which reduce a child's chances of intact survival and increase the risk of death.

This means that staff in any hospital, emergency room, or adult ICU who may have to manage the initial care of a critically ill child, and those responsible for transporting such children between hospitals, must be able to:

- recognize the potential for impending physiologic deterioration in a child's condition
- intervene to provide comprehensive support for compromised vital organ function
- obtain all necessary advice and assistance (local and regional) for resuscitation, stabilization, and to begin definitive care, and for the decision to be made regarding the optimal location for further care, and organize safe, timely transport to a regional PICU
- anticipate and intervene to avoid additional secondary insults to organs with compromised function
- avoid the errors often made inadvertently in the management of pediatric critical illness or injury

Nevertheless, the majority of critically ill or injured children will ultimately need care in a regionalized unit (PICU) with the resources to provide everything required by a critically ill child and the family.

Thus there are two separate elements to the care of the critically ill child:

- provision of intensive care outside a PICU
- provision of care once the PICU is reached

ESSENTIAL ELEMENTS FOR PROVISION OF INTENSIVE CARE OUTSIDE A PICU

- Recognize the special needs of the critically ill child and the family
- Designate an area for managing a critically ill child where the necessary equipment can be assembled or held in readiness (e.g. the trauma/resuscitation room in an emergency room, or a treatment or admission room on a children's ward)
- Have charts and tapes for age, weight, drug dosages, equipment size, vital sign ranges, and treatment algorithms prominently displayed or readily available for reference
- Have phone and pager numbers listed for useful emergency contacts, both internal and external (e.g. other physicians, surgeons, anesthetists, regional PICU, poison center, regional transport team)
- Hold practice management scenarios for the staff who will be involved with children who have potentially critical conditions. Such scenarios should address clinical emergencies (e.g. progressive respiratory failure, coma, persistent shock) rather than just the traditional 'code' for cardiorespiratory arrest
- Consider forming a team that will review any child in the hospital whose symptoms or signs are of concern, rather than using respiratory or cardiac arrest as the endpoint for calling for assistance. Protocols for such a review can be developed, defining criteria by age (e.g. respiratory rate/ effort, temperature, pulse, blood pressure/perfusion, central nervous system status/ Glasgow Coma Score, abnormal laboratory data). The specific criteria can be developed to reflect local expertise and resources
- Establish criteria for timely transfer for PICU care (i.e. before the abilities of the local center are exceeded)
- Organize pediatric continuing medical education

ESSENTIAL ELEMENTS FOR PROVISION OF CARE IN A PICU

Blending the art and science of medicine in a PICU is an ongoing challenge. There must be balance between the technologic advances, costs, need for evidence-based direction to care, and continued efforts to involve families appropriately. Care must be taken to maintain the interprofessional dialog, educational initiatives, administrative and problem-solving processes necessary for a PICU to function effectively. It is also clear that care can be enhanced with research and continuous quality improvement initiatives.

ORGANIZATION

- Recognize the special needs of the critically ill child and the family
- Have the necessary physical structure, space, bed number, and support services
- Have adequate numbers of full-time, specially trained pediatric intensive care physicians, nurses, and support staff dedicated to the unit to ensure seamless provision of care, assumption of responsibility, timely decision-making, and ongoing communication
- Have appropriate access to anesthesia, surgery, subspecialty, and imaging expertise
- Have the necessary technology and technologic expertise to provide state-of-the-art care

FUNCTIONAL ROLE

- Play a regional role in the provision of intensive care. Provide telephone consultation for other physicians
- Organize, train, and coordinate a transport team
- Have a clear and transparent admission policy which:
  - (a) meets the needs of the population served in the context of the resources available
  - (b) provides admission for children needing or likely to need intensive care to support organ function (e.g. assisted ventilation or inotropic drug support)

    (c) provides admission for children needing comprehensive monitoring or medical/nursing observation

    (d) provides admission when the presumptive diagnosis places a child at particular risk for critical deterioration, although the child currently appears 'stable'

- Identify the physician with overall responsibility for decision-making and communication for each child

COMMUNICATION

- Recognize the importance of different elements of effective communication:
  1. *interprofessional*
  2. *internal*: communication with families
  3. *external:* communication with those seeking advice, admission, and/or transport
- Accept that involvement with the PICU organization can be intimidating. Units must combine professionalism with being 'user friendly'

CARE

- Cultivate a medical and nursing team that diagnose and treat skillfully and with empathy, yet with appropriate detachment and without undue grief
- Establish a pattern of care that incorporates continuous attention to all relevant details and clear identification of management priorities. Retain focused direction and a sense of the 'big picture' of the child's illness while processing the large volume of clinical and laboratory data accumulating on the child
- Organize rounds with senior and multidisciplinary staff to ensure that a variety of expertise is brought to bear on each complex patient and that different approaches to management are considered and taught
- Use a system that ensures patient care and medication orders are written only by PICU staff

FAMILY

- Generate an atmosphere that fosters confidentiality and respect, and demonstrates professionalism and approachability
- Recognize that each child is part of a family that also has needs for information, communication, involvement, empathy, and care throughout and sometimes beyond the PICU admission
- Provide comprehensive, compassionate, supportive care of the child and family prior to death, and during death, and provide appropriate follow-up

ADMINISTRATION

- Establish a management structure to facilitate care, plan change, set priorities, address problems, define protocols, identify equipment needs, support educational goals, review mortality rates regularly, coordinate research, and promote interprofessional relations
- Provide advocacy and leadership concerning the prioritization and allocation of critical care resources for children

EDUCATION AND RESEARCH

- Initiate and deliver outreach education and feedback to referring centers as a courtesy and quality improvement measure
- Conduct research and carry out quality assurance/continuous quality improvement reviews. Know the literature

ABOUT THIS BOOK

This text addresses the provision of the immediate intensive care needs of the critically ill or injured child, focusing particularly on the need to anticipate problems, intervene expeditiously, obtain advice, and avoid commonly made errors. The book is intended to help physicians to be more proactive and effective earlier in the course of an illness, to initiate procedures that used to be regarded totally as the purview of a PICU and which are now increasingly within the therapeutic armamentarium of competent physicians in other areas such as emergency rooms and smaller hospitals, and thereby to improve the outcome for critically ill and injured children.

Traditionally, books on pediatric critical/intensive care have been written from the standpoint of care within the regional PICU setting. This book is intended for all those who must provide intensive care in the much broader context of real-world clinical practice, where there are few, if any, more challenging and alarming situations than being called upon to care for a critically ill or injured child. To help expedite appropriate care in these situations, this text describes:

- the initial approaches necessary to support systems in failure
- the key points to consider in providing initial intensive care
- the major management errors and secondary insults to avoid
- the process and priorities for timely, safe, interhospital transport
- the first steps that can be made towards a definitive diagnosis
- the likely course of the child's subsequent care in the PICU

✓ KEY POINTS

➤ Basic intensive care is provided in many settings, and the extent of care provided is dependent on the level of expertise and facilities available in the particular setting

➤ Anticipation of problems and optimal management prior to transfer to the PICU is:
(a) possible
(b) a prerequisite for optimal outcome

➤ When care beyond basic intensive care is required, the outcome for critically ill children is better if they are cared for in tertiary pediatric intensive care units rather than in district hospitals or adult ICUs

➤ The PICU and its senior staff act as an advice and consultation resource for medical or paramedical personnel caring for any critically ill child in the region

➤ Friendly, accessible staff and an effective transfer service are vital elements of an effective PICU

➤ Provision of pediatric intensive care requires tact and strategic organizational skills in addition to the obvious medical/surgical skills, and effective multidisciplinary collaboration (medicine, surgery, subspecialty, nursing, and paramedical staff)

➤ Intensive care is a mixture of meticulous and unrelenting attention to detail and ongoing reevaluation of priorities for intervention, investigation and care

➤ The PICU offers the environment, staff, and state-of-the-art technology necessary to monitor a child's progress, to support life in the presence of organ failure, and to provide continuity of care in an atmosphere in which the needs of the whole child and family are understood

➤ Parents require information and communication that is comprehensive and honest and to have their child's care provided in an environment that is oriented to their individual family's needs, particularly regarding involvement in decision-making, visiting, their level of involvement in care, and customs surrounding death

FURTHER READING

1. Levin DL, Morriss FC, editors. Essentials of pediatric intensive care, 2nd ed. New York: Churchill Livingstone; 1997
   – (*Comprehensive, user-friendly text which addresses care in the PICU and conceptual, procedural, and logistic considerations related to critical care*)

2. Pearson G, Shann F, Barry P, Vyas J, Thomas D, Powell C, Field D. Should paediatric intensive care be centralized? Trent versus Victoria. Lancet 1997; 349: 1213–1217

3. Pollack MM, Alexander SR, Clark N, Ruttimann UE, Tesselaar HM, Bachulis AC. Improved outcome from tertiary center pediatric intensive care: a statewide comparison of tertiary and non-tertiary facilities. Crit Care Med 1991; 19: 150–159
   – (*Evidence that pediatric intensive care provided in specialized regionalized centers results in improved outcome for critically ill and injured children*)

4. Hourihan F, Bishop G, Hillman KM, Daffurn K, Lee A. The Medical Emergency Team: a new strategy to identify and intervene in high-risk patients. Clin Intensive Care 1995; 6: 269–272
   – (*This paper describes the concept of a team for the rapid identification, assessment and management of seriously ill patients with abnormal physiological variables, indicating that assessment prior to cardiorespiratory arrest results in better outcome*)

1.2 Special needs of the critically ill child

Quen Q. Mok

Children need to be treated differently from adults, in separate areas, where appropriately sized equipment is available, and by people who understand their special physical and psychological requirements. It is particularly important to recognize the early signs of failure of respiratory, cardiovascular or nervous system function in order to prevent progression to respiratory and cardiac arrest whenever possible.

The spectrum of illnesses from which children suffer is different from that of the adult population, as is a child's response to illness and injury. Congenital abnormalities, chromosomal and genetic syndromes, illnesses related to birth injury and inborn errors of metabolism are common causes of illness in childhood. Trauma due to nonaccidental injury (physical or sexual abuse), and factitious illnesses (Munchausen syndrome by proxy) perpetrated by a caregiver should also be considered in the differential diagnosis of an acutely ill child. Even a condition such as asthma, which is relatively common in both adults and children, presents different diagnostic and management problems in the child.

ANATOMY AND PHYSIOLOGY

Weighing a critically ill child may be impractical, and in these circumstances formulae, charts or calibrated tapes (e.g. Broselow tape) or extrapolation from a recent accurate weight should be used. If the age is known, the formulae in Table 1.2.1 can be used for rapid assessment of the patient and to

---

TABLE 1.2.1 **Useful formulae, based on age of child in years**

- Weight of child in kg = 2 (age + 4)
- Size of endotracheal tube in mm = (age/4) + 4
- Length of endotracheal tube in cm = (age/2) + 12 for an oral tube
- Length for oratracheal tube = internal diameter (mm) × 3 (add 3 cm per nasal length)

---

choose the equipment needed during resuscitation. A child's weight changes rapidly during growth spurts, particularly during the first year of life and during puberty, thus the formula for weight is most accurate between 1 year and 10 years of age.

A child's body surface area varies as body proportions change with age. Young children with a high ratio of body surface area to weight are more prone to heat loss which can easily go unrecognized, especially when attention is focused on procedures, and close monitoring of core temperature is required. Thermoregulation is virtually nonexistent with the immature homeostatic reflexes and thin skin of young infants, who therefore behave like 'poikilotherms' with their temperature quickly approximating that of the environment. The resulting hypothermia has a number of metabolic consequences, and leads to an increase in metabolic rate and oxygen demand which may adversely affect the outcome of the child. The larger surface area of the head and trunk in younger children must also be considered when calculating fluid replacement in burns, or when computing certain drug dosages. Small children have limited fluid reserves and rapidly develop adverse effects from reduced intake or increased loss. A history of intake decreasing to less than 50% of the child's normal fluid volume for 24 hours is always important.

RESPIRATORY SYSTEM

The anatomy of the airway and the surrounding structures changes with age. With a prominent occiput and short neck, there is a tendency for the neck to be flexed in the supine child. This flexion distorts the airway, and placing a small roll under the shoulders will extend the neck slightly, which facilitates endotracheal intubation. The relatively large tongue and small mandible can make intubation more difficult, and adenotonsillar hypertrophy in children 3–8 years old may cause difficulty with the passage of nasal tubes. The floppy horseshoe-shaped epiglottis and a high anterior larynx may cause problems with visualization of the airway for intubation. A straight rather than a curved laryngoscope blade is preferable for optimal visualization of the larynx in neonates and infants. The narrowest part of the airway in the child is the cricoid ring, unlike adults in whom the larynx is the narrowest part of the airway. The clinical implication of the narrow cricoid region is simply that endotracheal tubes which will pass easily through the larynx may wedge tightly at the cricoid, leading to mucosal edema or necrosis and development of scarring and subglottic obstruction. It is usual to attempt to prevent such complications by using uncuffed endotracheal tubes in children under 8 years old, and by ensuring that an audible gas leak is present when the breathing system is pressurized to 25 cm H$_2$O, which indicates an adequate 'space' around the tube.

Infants under 6 months old are obligate nose breathers, making upper airway obstruction and respiratory compromise common in this age group. The trachea is short, and as the carinal angles are symmetrical, foreign bodies readily enter either mainstem bronchus, as opposed to preferentially entering the more vertical right mainstem bronchus as occurs in older children and adults. Also, as small children spend so much time supine, the upper lobes are just as frequently affected as the lower lobes in aspiration episodes. The relatively small cross-sectional area of the lower airways also means that a minor reduction in the radius of the airway produces a marked increase in resistance to air flow (Poiseuille's law), and hence respiratory difficulty. This is exemplified in the presentation of small infants with bronchiolitis caused by respiratory syncytial virus. Small airway edema is poorly tolerated in the first months of life, unlike the relatively minor symptoms experienced by older children whose larger airways are subject to much less severe impairment from the same degree of edema. Small children thus present earlier with respiratory distress and more frequently require ventilatory support.

The lungs are relatively immature at birth and the alveoli continue to grow and develop in the first few years of life. Resting respiratory rate is higher in children because of their relatively high metabolic rate and oxygen consumption, and grad-

ually reduces with age to the adult level (Table 1.2.2). As the lungs are relatively noncompliant after birth compared with the chest wall, respiratory distress presents with sternal retraction and intercostal and subcostal recession, in addition to tachypnea. Grunting frequently occurs as a sign of severe respiratory distress in infants; this is produced by exhalation against a partially closed glottis which generates a positive end-expiratory pressure that prevents alveolar or conducting airway collapse. Signs of accessory muscle use and increased work of breathing include flaring of the nostrils. Fatigue can mask the signs of respiratory distress, and when a reduction in symptoms occurs due to exhaustion this is an ominous sign which indicates imminent respiratory failure and the need for intervention and support.

The diaphragm is the dominant inspiratory muscle in infants. The 'bucket handle' intercostal muscle–rib system is mechanically inefficient because the ribs lie in a horizontal plane. In addition, the chest wall is made up of both cartilaginous ribs and poorly muscularized interspaces which are drawn inwards during forced inspiration, which adds to the mechanical inefficiency of the infant respiratory pump mechanism. The diaphragm tends to fatigue quickly because there are fewer type I muscle fibers, especially in the preterm infant. The very limited reserves of the thoracic pump owing to these mechanisms, combined with noncompliant immature lungs, make the neonate and young infant extremely prone to develop respiratory failure if any additional adverse event occurs.

Ventilation is preferentially distributed to the uppermost lung in the lateral decubitus position in children. Thus with unilateral parenchymal

TABLE I.2.2 Changes in normal parameters with age			
Age (years)	Respiratory rate (breaths/min)	Heart rate (beats/min)	Systolic blood pressure (mmHg)
<1	30–40	110–160	70–90
2–5	20–30	95–140	80–100
6–12	15–20	80–120	90–110
>12	12–16	60–100	100–120

lung disease, or unilateral diaphragmatic impairment, nursing the child with the unaffected side uppermost improves gas exchange. This postural redistribution of ventilation changes late in the second decade of life to the adult pattern of preferential ventilation of the dependent lung. Perfusion however follows the adult pattern, with better perfusion to the inferior segments of the lung.

Another factor influencing tissue oxygenation in neonates is the type of circulating hemoglobin. At birth fetal hemoglobin (HbF) accounts for 70% of the circulating hemoglobin. The oxygen dissociation curve of HbF is shifted to the left, resulting in higher oxygen Hb saturations for the same Po_2 for HbF. This would produce a lower Pao_2 for the same level of oxygen saturation with (adult) hemoglobin. The HbF level gradually declines to negligible amounts by the age of 6 months. Irritability or agitation are often signs of hypoxemia.

CARDIOVASCULAR SYSTEM

In the first weeks after birth the pulmonary vasculature retains a relatively muscular intima, and pulmonary hypertension may persist or be induced in certain situations. Hypoxia and acidosis potently stimulate pulmonary vasoconstriction. Pulmonary hypertensive crises are seen in children where congenital heart disease is associated with increased pulmonary blood flow. Pulmonary hypertension, in the form of persistent pulmonary hypertension of the newborn (PPHN), is central to the pathophysiology of many types of neonatal respiratory failure. After birth the right ventricle remains muscular until pulmonary pressure falls, and the left ventricle subsequently becomes the dominant ventricle (from about 6 months of age). This is reflected in the changes in axis and progression of QRS complexes in the electrocardiogram, which may be misinterpreted if one is unaware of the normal variations in the different stages of childhood.

The infant has a higher cardiac output indexed to body weight than at any other stage in life: 300 ml/min·kg as opposed to 70–80 ml/min·kg in the adult. The neonate and infant cardiac ventricles are relatively noncompliant; stroke volume increases little as ventricular filling pressure increases, for

instance with colloid administration. Since stroke volume is fixed, cardiac output is largely dependent on heart rate in these children, and bradycardia is poorly tolerated. Blood pressure increases with age (Table 1.2.2 and BP percentiles p. 605) owing to a rising systemic vascular resistance. To ensure accurate noninvasive recording of blood pressure, care should be taken to use a cuff appropriate to the child's size (use a cuff that covers more than half but less than two-thirds of the length of the upper arm or thigh used for measurement).

Circulating blood volume in the child is highest per kilogram of body weight at birth (80–90 ml/kg), dropping to 70–80 ml/kg by 3–6 months, and to an adult value of approximately 70 ml/kg beyond 1 year of age. In neonates, absolute volumes involved are small, and what may appear to be insignificant blood loss may in fact be critical to the child. Hypotension occurs late in children, with blood pressure maintained initially even with losses of 15–25% of circulating blood volume. Other signs of circulatory insufficiency such as cold extremities, delayed capillary refill, pallor, weak pulses, and changes in mental status may be more useful for early detection of circulatory failure.

Cardiac arrest in childhood is rarely due to primary heart disease, and is more frequently secondary to respiratory insufficiency with hypoxia. This combination of hypoxia and acidosis often means that there is damage of other more sensitive organs (e.g. brain, liver and kidneys) before myocardial damage is severe enough to cause cardiac arrest. Thus although cardiac output can be restored more easily than in adults with primary myocardial dysfunction, the chance of intact neurological survival is poor following a cardiorespiratory arrest in children. It is thus important to recognize the early signs of cardiorespiratory insufficiency so that appropriate steps can be taken to anticipate and prevent the chain of events leading to respiratory and cardiac arrest.

CENTRAL NERVOUS SYSTEM

Although the brain constitutes a large part of the body at birth, it is still relatively immature. In the first few years of life the cerebral cortex continues to develop, and myelination proceeds rapidly, with the progressive loss of primitive reflexes and attainment of developmental milestones at various ages. Severe illness commonly causes temporary developmental regression, but during crucial growth and developmental stages of the brain it can compromise or halt development, causing a variety of neurological problems. Seriously ill children tend to be obtunded and hypotonic, lying with their limbs in a 'floppy', frog-like position. Persistence of primitive reflexes or abnormal posturing (e.g. decerebrate or decorticate posturing) indicate severe brain dysfunction.

Owing to limited myelination and developmental immaturity, investigations of cortical function should be correlated with the age of the child. Electroencephalography and tests of brain-stem function must be interpreted with care in children, and by experts conversant with the variations with age. In addition, interpretation of structural imaging of the brain and spinal cord requires an understanding of normal growth and anatomical development.

The relative immaturity of the central nervous system does not decrease responses to pain. It is now well established that even premature neonates show adverse behavioral and physiological responses if analgesia is inadequate during or after painful procedures (Ch. 5.2).

RENAL TRACT

Fetal lobulations that may remain in the first year can give the impression of scarring on imaging to the untutored eye. Many investigations that rely on renal function (e.g. isotope scans) cannot be performed reliably until after the first few months of life.

The kidney tubules have a poor concentrating ability in the first 6 months of life, consequently infants are unable to respond to dehydration or hypovolemia by decreasing urine production. (Oliguria is considered to be present when urine output is less than 2 ml/kg per hour in infants or less than 1 ml/kg per hour in children). If urine output is less than 1 ml/kg per hour in children of any age, full evaluation should be undertaken. It should, however, be noted that in stable, low-risk term infants urine output may be minimal or even absent for the first 24 hours of life.

Immature kidney function also means that drugs that are normally excreted through renal metabolism will accumulate and remain pharmacologically active for longer periods in the body, even when used in correct dosages for weight (Ch. 5.1).

HEPATOBILIARY SYSTEM

Immaturity of liver metabolism results in physiological jaundice in the newborn period, and pathological hyperbilirubinemia from deranged liver function occurs earlier in children during multisystem illness. Drugs that are normally metabolized by the liver also accumulate more readily in children during the first few months of life, when liver function remains immature.

IMMUNE SYSTEM AND INFECTION

The newborn infant is immunologically incompetent, and is therefore prone to serious infections. At birth humoral immunity is provided by maternal antibodies that have crossed the placenta in the last trimester of pregnancy, and these progressively decline to low levels during the first 6 months after birth. The infant's own antibody production is slow to mature, particularly the production of immunoglobulin A (IgA) which is the secretory antibody in the respiratory and gastrointestinal tracts. Respiratory and enteral infections are therefore frequent occurrences in the first year of life. Also, IgG_2 production does not reach adult levels until the second year of life, which explains the predisposition of infants and toddlers to infections with encapsulated organisms (e.g. coliforms and *Haemophilus*).

Symptoms of infection are nonspecific in children. Lethargy, poor appetite and irritability are frequently the only presenting features. Signs of serious infection are just as nonspecific and unhelpful in localizing the source, with respiratory distress and pallor common to any severe infection. Neck stiffness is frequently absent in young children with meningitis, and fever is not always present, particularly with a fulminating infection. Laboratory tests do not always show a neutrophilia, as the bone marrow is immature and unable to respond to an infective stress in the same way as an adult. The likely result is suppression of the bone marrow, with neutropenia, anemia and thrombocytopenia the more common responses to serious infection in children. A localized infection can rapidly lead to septicemia and it is therefore important to screen any acutely ill child for infection and to start treatment with broad-spectrum antibiotics without waiting for microbiological proof of infection.

Congenital viral or parasitic infections result from maternal infections during pregnancy, but may not present until a few months of age (usually with failure to thrive). Maternal infection may only become apparent after an infection is diagnosed in the child. Because testing for infection in a child can reveal the status of the mother, counseling and consent of the parents is necessary prior to testing for the human immunodeficiency virus (HIV), to explain the implications on the family of a positive test in the child.

THE CHILD AND FAMILY

Children are entirely dependent on their adult carers to provide for all their physical and emotional needs. Children are often unable to communicate their concerns effectively, especially when very young or acutely ill. This and the nonspecific nature of their illnesses make recognition of the problems of a child dependent on the observation and experience of the carer; this is particularly crucial in the critically ill child. Communication is difficult for many reasons (e.g. lack of language development or fear of strangers), and therefore nonverbal cues play a major role in the examination and management of the acutely ill child. Explanation of procedures and treatment in appropriate language and terminology is mandatory. Play therapy and providing an alternative focus (e.g. reading stories with parents, familiar music, or blowing bubbles to control breathing) provide an element of near-normality for the child. Such measures contribute to the child's feelings of choice and control, and can help the child's understanding of what is happening, and contribute positively to recovery.

The child is an individual but also a part of the family unit, and parents provide a special contribution to their child's care that cannot be duplicated by staff members. Most parents will express feelings of frustration and helplessness at the loss of their usual caretaker and protector roles (Ch. 5.5), especially when staff take charge (insensitively) in the hospital setting. Excluding parents only increases anxiety in both the child and the parents. Staff must be sensitive to these feelings, involve parents in their child's care, and not underestimate them (Ch. 5.6).

The emotional and social burdens of a child's life-threatening illness on the family are undeniable. A child's admission to hospital, especially with a critical illness, causes stress and major disruption to the entire family unit. People under stress are often unable to function at their normal level, and parents may appear difficult, irrational or demanding. Professionals must recognize that retention of information is limited in a stressful situation, hence the need for explanation and repetition. A good balance is required between technological scientific support for the child and the psychological emotional support for the family. The impact on the whole family, including siblings, and their need for emotional and spiritual support needs to be recognized and dealt with compassionately. Most parents are unprepared for the uncertainty and isolation that accompany the devastating news of sudden and unexpected illness. Disbelief about the critical nature of an illness makes the tragedy of sudden loss and the reality of death even more difficult to accept. Parents need to feel that everything possible has been done for their child—hence the need sometimes to continue support even where it is futile, to give parents time to come to terms with reality. Involvement of other compassionate agencies (pastors, counselors, parental self-help groups) often helps parents deal with their grief, denial and fear. The quality and timing of professional help is relevant. Having a psychologist or social worker on the staff to deal with urgent stressors may help defuse the situation (Chs 3.10, 5.5). In the event of death, the family should be given the opportunity to return for bereavement follow-up, to discuss questions or concerns regarding the events surrounding their child's death. Their support and care do not end with the death of their child (Ch. 5.8).

✔ KEY POINTS

➤ Understanding the normal anatomical and physiological variations with age will lead to early recognition of the abnormal; physiological parameters may, however, be altered by anxiety and fear

➤ Symptoms and signs of acute severe illness in children are often nonspecific

➤ The clinical condition can change rapidly, and therapy needs to be immediate

➤ Early intervention may produce a better outcome

➤ Therapy in children must be related to their age and weight

➤ Supportive management of the family is as important as medical management of the child

✗ COMMON ERRORS

➤ Treating the child as a small adult

➤ Failure to use appropriate-sized equipment

➤ Misinterpreting normal developmental variations as abnormal

➤ Failure to recognize the signs of potential respiratory, circulatory and neurological failure, leading to delay in instituting therapy

➤ Forgetting that the family needs as much support as the child to come to terms with acute illness

FURTHER READING

1. Aynsley-Green A. Pain and stress in infancy and childhood. Where now? Paed Anaesth 1996; 6: 167–172

2. Hey EN, Katz G. The optimum thermal environment for naked babies. Arch Dis Child 1970; 45: 328–334

3. Openshaw P, Edwards S, Helms P. Changes in rib cage geometry during childhood. Thorax 1984; 39: 624–627

4. Heaf DP, Helms P, Gordon I, Turner HM. Postural effects on gas exchange in infants. N Engl J Med 1983; 308: 1505–1508

5. Mackway-Jones K, Molyneux E, Phillips B, Wieteska S. Advanced pediatric life support. The practical approach. London: BMJ Publishing; 1993

6. Baum JD, Dominica F, Woodward RN. Listen. My child has a lot of living to do. Caring for children with life threatening conditions. Oxford University Press; 1990

7. Hazinski MF. Nursing care of the critically ill child, 2nd ed. St Louis: Mosby YearBook; 1992

8. Kuttner L. A child in pain. How to help, what to do. Hartley & Marks; 1996

1.3   Epidemiology of severe illness in childhood

Elizabeth Segedin

A wide range of conditions can cause children to become critically ill: from common childhood illnesses such as croup, bronchiolitis or gastroenteritis, to congenital malformations or inborn errors of metabolism or acquired conditions such as trauma, seizures or septic shock.

Most critically ill children remain so for only a short time (1–4 days) during an acute acquired illness or following major surgery. Between 80% and 97% of patients survive admission to the pediatric intensive care unit (PICU). The health status of 75% of these is equal to or better than their preadmission state and healthy survivors can expect a full productive life (Ch. 5.11).

FACTORS AFFECTING PICU ADMISSION

AGE

About 1.2% of children in developed countries will become sufficiently ill to require ICU admission. Up to 10% of these children are less than 1 month old, more than 50% are less than 2 years old and two-thirds are less than 5 years old. This age pattern reflects:

- early presentation of inherited or congenital disease
- anatomical and physiological immaturity including a poor immune response to infections, both viral and bacterial, and lack of prior exposure to pathogens
- size disadvantage (e.g. airway size in croup or bronchiolitis)

Disease patterns vary with age:

- *infancy*: apnea, bronchiolitis or complications of congenital malformations, many of which rarely present after infancy
- *later childhood*: accidental poisoning, asthma, severe upper airway obstruction
- *adolescence*: trauma, asthma, diabetic ketoacidosis or scoliosis repair

Some diseases have a different severity and mode of presentation at different ages. Whooping cough in older children or adults, for example, in the absence of encephalopathy, is often mild enough to be treated at home, but in the infant can lead to life-threatening apnea and bradycardia, pneumonia and respiratory failure requiring skilled emergency care and prolonged hospital admission. Respiratory syncytial virus (RSV) infection in the preterm infant is frequently associated with bronchiolitis or apnea, but causes only upper respiratory symptoms in children and adults. Head injuries in the school-aged child are usually due to road traffic injuries or falls, whereas in patients under 2 years of age, significant head trauma is often caused by a nonaccidental injury. Isolated head injuries are common in infants and preschool children, while in older children they are more often associated with injuries to the limbs or trunk. Infants and toddlers are vulnerable to nonaccidental injury because of their small size and fragility, and because their behavioral immaturity can provoke disproportionately violent responses in some adults.

SOCIOECONOMIC FACTORS

Factors such as family income, standard of housing and parental education strongly influence the risk of a child's becoming critically ill (Table 1.3.1). The risk of pedestrian injury or penetrating trauma (stab

TABLE 1.3.1 **The effects of socioeconomic disadvantage: mortality rate in the most disadvantaged 20% of Australian children compared with the least disadvantaged 20%**

	Boys	Girls
Respiratory disorders	× 2.5	× 3.7
Drowning	× 3	Same
Congenital heart disease	Same	× 2
Complications of prematurity	Same	× 2
Automobile accidents	× 1.53	× 1.95
Hypoxia and birth asphyxia	× 1.9	× 1.9
Sudden infant death syndrome	× 1.2	× 1.69
All causes	× 1.5	× 1.67

or gunshot) is greater in children whose families are poor or underprivileged. Bronchiolitis is more common in children from poor housing areas, and rheumatic carditis and meningococcemia are more common in children living in crowded conditions.

Low income

Low income significantly impedes access to primary health care in countries where health care for small children is not readily available, or where a system of free primary care is poorly developed. This can lead to low immunization rates for preventable diseases, late presentation of diseases such as gastroenteritis and meningococcal sepsis, and inadequate early treatment of minor complaints, such as infected skin lesions, which can lead to invasive staphylococcal infection or post-streptococcal diseases such as rheumatic fever or glomerulonephritis. In poor communities, congenital illnesses including heart disease and inborn metabolic errors are often diagnosed too late, to prevent severe and perhaps irreversible deterioration.

Unrestrained passengers are much more likely to die or be seriously injured in road crashes than those restrained by seat belts. Preventive measures cannot be implemented where families cannot meet the costs of installing seat belts or effective car restraints for babies, purchasing cycle helmets or fencing properties.

Housing

High-density housing with vehicle access to several dwellings predisposes to off-road pedestrian injuries, especially in toddlers.

Social problems

Social disorganization of the family in stress leads to poor supervision of children, noncompliance with medical therapy and poor attendance at antenatal care.

Diet and drug use

Parental behavior can also affect the health of infants and children. Poor maternal diet increases the risk of central nervous system abnormalities in the fetus. Overconsumption of alcohol in pregnancy can lead to fetal alcohol syndrome and the use in pregnancy of cocaine, nicotine and other drugs may cause fetal malformations, growth retardation and drug withdrawal in the newborn. Parental smoking increases the incidence of respiratory disease in infants.

RACE

Some critical childhood illnesses are more common in specific racial groups. Sickle cell disease (Ch. 3.6) for instance, is rare in children who are not of African or Mediterranean descent. Cystic fibrosis is almost entirely confined to children of European origin. Some inborn errors of metabolism are more common in particular racial groups: for example the storage diseases in Scandinavians, Puerto Ricans and Ashkenazi Jews.

Cultural and socioeconomic factors may be hard to separate from racial influences in many communities (for example, diarrheal disease, pneumonia and rheumatic heart disease in indigenous populations in the New World). Racial and climatic factors may combine to increase the prevalence of asthma in Vietnamese emigrés.

VARIATION IN DISEASE PATTERN WITH TIME

Table 1.3.2 shows the numbers of children with common medical disorders requiring intensive care in a population of 1.5 million children. It shows that the incidence of severe disease has increased over the 14-year period in some illnesses

TABLE 1.3.2 **Change with time in all PICU admissions for critical illness due to medical conditions in a population of 1.5 million children**

	1982	1985	1988	1991	1994	1996
Asthma	20	34	43	98	103	78
Bronchiolitis	16	14	21	19	15	30
Croup	79	63	124	89	60	40
Drug ingestion	24	31	33	41	36	32
Epiglottitis	52	47	46	58	6	4
Status epilepticus	30	29	41	45	53	39
Near-drowning	12	8	13	16	13	6
Meningitis	16	19	18	26	11	23

Figures are from the PICU, Royal Children's Hospital, Melbourne

(asthma and bronchiolitis); has decreased in others owing to improved prevention or early treatment measures (e.g. croup and epiglottitis); but has remained fairly constant in many conditions (e.g. near-drowning, poisoning and meningitis).

SEASON AND WEATHER

Figure 1.3.1 shows the breakdown by month of children requiring pediatric intensive care. There is a higher incidence of severe respiratory illness in autumn and early winter (i.e. March to June in the southern hemisphere) which substantially increases presentation with critical illness during those months. During periods of smog and atmospheric temperature inversion, and as the pollen density increases in spring, severe attacks of asthma occur more frequently.

CONGENITAL ANOMALIES

Most congenital malformations that require treatment do so during infancy, often during the first few days of life. Malformations of the gastrointestinal tract such as tracheoesophageal fistula or gastroschisis may require a lengthy stay in intensive care, depending on the presence of associated congenital anomalies or complications such as respiratory failure. Airway anomalies may require surgery and prolonged intensive care management. Laryngomalacia or tracheobronchomalacia may require respiratory support with continuous positive airway pressure (CPAP) for several months. Those who survive intensive care often have little or no disability in the long term.

Congenital abnormalities tend to group together, often in recognized combinations, the most common of which is the VATER association (vertebral, anorectal, tracheoesophageal, renal and radial anomalies). Other known associations include midline defects such as omphalocele with cardiac disease, and renal anomalies with anorectal defects. Awareness of such combinations allows multisystem investigation and support in children presenting with critical illness. Before definitive treatment of any malformation is undertaken, such children should be screened for cardiac and renal abnormalities. In some instances it may be appropriate not to offer definitive therapy to children with multiple severe abnormalities, particularly when permanent bowel and bladder incontinence, chronic renal failure or severe intellectual disability combine to make independent living very unlikely (Ch. 5.7). Immediate care in emergencies usually employs all measures of care. However, be aware that written care plans limiting treatment may exist and that urgent telephone

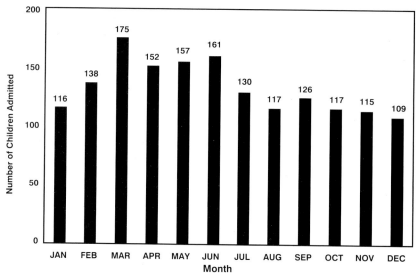

Figure 1.3.1 Seasonal admission rates to an Australian PICU showing higher rates in autumn and early winter (March to June)

discussion with regular caregivers and referral centers should be initiated whenever doubt arises.

HEREDITARY AND CHROMOSOMAL ABNORMALITIES

Age of presentation

Many inherited conditions present in the first year of life. Defects in intermediary metabolism usually become apparent in infancy, although the atypical, late-presenting forms of some disorders such as ornithine transcarbamylase deficiency may not be recognized until later in childhood. Late recognition and treatment can severely impair the child's neurodevelopmental outcome. In some of these conditions, such as the urea cycle disorders, severe exacerbations recur throughout childhood, sometimes associated with intercurrent febrile illnesses.

Children with chromosomal abnormalities usually present within the first year of life, mostly because of their associated malformations. These children often have multiple abnormalities involving several organ systems and limited intellectual capacity.

Clustering of anomalies

Clustering of anomalies in individual children greatly increases their risk of critical illness, and these children form a disproportionately large part of the population referred for PICU care. Because their best (pre-illness) quality of life and level of intellectual function are often limited, their best outcome after an ICU stay is also reduced (Ch. 5.11).

ANTENATAL TESTING

Antenatal testing for inherited conditions (including fetal ultrasonography, amniocentesis and chromosomal testing) now gives families at risk and their caregivers warning that an infant will be abnormal at birth. This allows for critical care interventions to be planned and explained in advance, and also permits the option of termination of pregnancy for some conditions (including Duchenne's muscular dystrophy or cystic fibrosis). Overall, antenatal testing may reduce the incidence of severe inherited and congenital disorders.

Fetal echocardiography is now widely available, and via the option of termination may reduce the incidence of severe anomalies such as hypoplastic left heart syndrome. Antenatal diagnosis of other malformations such as diaphragmatic hernia has not influenced the incidence of this condition in liveborn babies, as many families elect to give their affected babies a chance at extrauterine life.

HEART DISEASE

AGE OF PRESENTATION

Children with congenital heart disease often become severely ill in the neonatal period with cyanotic lesions (e.g. transposition of the great arteries, TGA) or circulatory obstruction (e.g. aortic stenosis). Infants whose circulation depends on the patency of the ductus arteriosus (e.g. hypoplastic aortic arch or pulmonary atresia) will become severely ill with shock or cyanosis when the ductus closes in the first few days of life. Infants with congestive cardiac lesions with left-to-right shunts usually present after the first few weeks when falling pulmonary vascular resistance allows the development of cardiac failure (Ch. 3.2).

CARDIOMYOPATHY

Congenital cardiomyopathy may present at birth or on antenatal ultrasound examination as hydrops fetalis, while acquired cardiomyopathy may be associated with a viral illness or may follow anthracycline chemotherapy for solid tumors in childhood or adolescence.

RHEUMATIC FEVER

Rheumatic fever is the biggest cause of acquired cardiac disease in childhood worldwide but is extremely uncommon in most Western communities. It is more prevalent in less developed countries or in underprivileged communities with poor access to primary health care.

ASSOCIATED ILLNESS

Congenital and acquired disorders of other body systems such as renal tract abnormalities, tracheobronchomalacia and stroke are very often associated with congenital heart disease and its treatment.

RESPIRATORY DISEASE

Between one-quarter and one-third of all children requiring admission to a PICU in a developed country (Table 1.3.3) have disease of the upper or lower respiratory tract. Most cases are due to viral infections causing croup, bronchiolitis, pneumonia or precipitating acute asthma. Bacterial infections such as pneumonia, whooping cough, epiglottitis or retropharyngeal abscess

TABLE 1.3.3 **Admissions to a general pediatric intensive care unit in 1996**	
Disorder	**Percentage of total admission (n = 1300)**
Respiratory	
Asthma	6
Bronchiolitis	2.5
Croup	3
Pneumonia	1
Upper airway obstruction	2
ARDS	2.5
Other respiratory disorders	7
All	24
Trauma	
Burns	0.5
Near-drowning	0.5
Poisoning	2.5
Other trauma	7.5
All	11
Cardiovascular	
Post cardiac surgery	35
Other cardiac disorders	2
All	37
Neurological	
Status epilepticus	4
Meningitis or encephalitis	3
Other neurological disorders	2
All	9
Miscellaneous	
Septic shock	2
Diabetic ketoacidosis	1
Diaphragmatic hernia	1
Post cardiac arrest	2
Other	13
All	19

ARDS, *acute respiratory distress syndrome.*

are less common but carry significant morbidity. Most severe respiratory illness occurs in the first 3 years of life. Bronchiolitis and pertussis in the first 6 months and pneumonia in the first 2 years are responsible for much of the mortality and morbidity.

CONTRIBUTORY FACTORS

Small babies are most vulnerable to acute respiratory disease because of:

- their flexible rib cage and horizontal rib position which reduces respiratory muscle efficiency
- high resistance to airflow in small obstructed airways
- airway closure during tidal expiration (Ch. 3.1)
- immunological naïvety (lack of prior exposure to most pathogens)
- immature immune system (e.g. low levels of immunoglobulins, complement and phagocyte function and poor immune response to encapsulated organisms) which impairs the defence against bacterial and viral pathogens

Acute respiratory infections account for half of all illnesses in children under 5 years old and a third of all illnesses in those aged 5–12 years.

CONGENITAL ANOMALIES

Congenital anomalies of the upper airway and lung usually present in early infancy with upper airway obstruction, failure to thrive or wheezing. They may be primary developmental anomalies (e.g. laryngomalacia, laryngeal cysts or webs) or secondary to neonatal intubation (subglottic stenosis) or external airway compression from a vascular ring.

CROUP

Croup (laryngotracheobronchitis) is an acute syndrome of hoarse voice, barking cough and inspiratory stridor which occurs throughout childhood but mostly in children younger than 5 years. It is most common in children aged 6 months to 2 years, when most cases are due to a viral infection. Later in childhood, recurrent croup is more common, usually with a history of asthma, eczema or hay fever in the child or a first-degree relative. Recurrences of croup may not be associated with a viral infection. Croup is more common in boys than girls (ratio 1.5:1), is more common in autumn and early winter, and shows peaks in incidence every 2 years. Although there is geographical variation in the incidence and severity of croup, in Australia about 25% of children with croup require hospital admission (because of stridor at rest) and 0.5–3% are admitted to intensive care. The proportion requiring PICU admission and tracheal intubation has fallen by about 70% since the introduction of steroid treatment in the late 1980s for all children admitted for croup (Ch. 3.1).

EPIGLOTTITIS

Epiglottitis (acute bacterial supraglottitis) is a serious and occasionally fatal cause of acute upper airway obstruction. Before the introduction of *Haemophilus influenzae* type b (Hib) vaccine, epiglottitis was responsible for 5–20% of hospital admissions for upper airway obstruction. Most cases occur in children 6 months to 6 years of age, with a peak incidence at 2–3 years. In younger children most cases are caused by Hib, but in older children and adults the rare cases are more commonly due to other organisms such as *Staphylococcus aureus* and pneumococci. The introduction of Hib vaccine has dramatically reduced the incidence of epiglottitis. The few cases now seen in Western countries are due to vaccine failure or nonvaccination because of underlying disease or by parental choice. Although all children with epiglottitis are bacteremic, metastatic infection (e.g. meningitis or septic arthritis) is rare.

BRONCHIOLITIS

Bronchiolitis is a common viral respiratory illness in the first year of life: 80% of infants hospitalized for bronchiolitis are less than 6 months old. Admission to a PICU is required for 7–10% of infants admitted to hospital with bronchiolitis, but less than 3% require mechanical ventilation (Ch.

3.1). Bronchiolitis is more common if the following factors are present:

- crowded living conditions
- siblings at school or crèche
- parents smoke
- never breastfed
- atopy

Respiratory failure in bronchiolitis is more severe in:

- younger infants
- ex-premature infants
- boys
- congenital heart disease (especially in complex lesions)
- underlying lung disease (e.g. bronchopulmonary dysplasia or cystic fibrosis)
- neuromuscular disorders (e.g. spinal muscular atrophy)
- immunosuppressed children

Most morbidity and almost all mortality occurs in these conditions. Bronchiolitis is more severe in young infants because exudate or mucosal edema causes more resistance to air flow in small bronchi. Apnea is especially common in younger infants and the premature. Seventy per cent of cases are due to RSV in annual epidemics over later autumn to early spring, while the remainder are due to other respiratory viruses including parainfluenza virus 1, 2 or 3, influenza A, rhinovirus or adenovirus.

PNEUMONIA

Most cases of pneumonia in children in Western countries are caused by viruses.

Viral pneumonia

Respiratory syncytial virus can cause severe pneumonia in infants (most commonly under 6 months old), usually in late winter and early spring. While adenovirus may also cause classical bronchiolitis without seasonal variation, certain types (3, 7, 21) may cause a severe, sometimes fatal, necrotizing pneumonia or bronchiolitis obliterans. Parainfluenza virus type 3 causes bronchiolitis and occasionally pneumonia, especially in spring in older infants and toddlers. Influenza A causes severe pneumonia during winter, especially in children with underlying lung disease, but is a far less common cause of pneumonia than RSV or parainfluenza, even during influenza epidemics. The other respiratory viruses (including rhinovirus, influenza B, parainfluenza 1 and 2 and the enteroviruses and herpes simplex) cause pneumonia which can be severe, but do so much less frequently.

Bacterial pneumonia

Community-acquired bacterial pneumonia occurs less frequently than the viral disease but causes severe systemic illness, often with septicemia.

Newborn

Causes in the newborn include:

- group B streptococci (associated with septic shock)
- Gram-negative bacilli from the birth canal or nosocomial transmission
- *Chlamydia trachomatis*: afebrile respiratory failure at age 4–12 weeks

Older children

Mycoplasma pneumoniae is the most common cause of pneumonia. Staphylococcal pneumonia may be a primary infection, but risk factors include:

- age less than 3 months
- viral pneumonia, especially influenza or measles viruses
- immune deficiency
- antibiotics
- hematogenous spread from a staphylococcal lesion elsewhere (e.g. osteomyelitis)

Nosocomial pneumonia

Nosocomial pneumonia occurs in immunocompromised children (e.g. due to congenital or acquired immune deficiency, starvation, severe trauma including burns, tumor chemotherapy or immunosuppressive drugs), and in hospitalized severely ill children. Those with impaired conscious state, neuromuscular or cardiorespiratory failure or requiring tracheal intubation are particularly at risk. The usual organisms include Gram-negative bacilli (e.g. *Klebsiella* and *Pseudomonas*) and indolent organisms such as *Acinetobacter* and upper respiratory commensals such as *Moraxella catarrhalis*.

Nosocomial pneumonia is usually acquired from the hands of carers owing to inadequate handwashing practices, and antibiotic-resistant organisms are usually transmitted between patients in this way, especially when staff are looking after more than one patient. Hospital equipment such as ventilators, humidifiers, nebulizers and sinks frequently harbor organisms such as *Pseudomonas* or *Serratia* spp. which are then transferred to the child's lungs.

WHOOPING COUGH

Whooping cough in infants is more prevalent in communities with a low immunization rate and may require prolonged hospital admission for apnea, severe cyanosis and bradycardia during coughing spells.

NEUROLOGICAL DISEASE

EPILEPSY

Epilepsy is defined as the occurrence of at least two nonfebrile seizures. In the USA, 4% of white middle-class children and 8% of poor children have had a seizure by age 20 years. Eighty-six per 100 000 infants have a fit in the first year of life. The incidence declines to 40–50 per 100 000 per year until age 60 years, then increases sharply. Epilepsy and status epilepticus are more common in children with:

- structural brain abnormalities such as absent corpus callosum
- hydrocephalus
- brain injury including trauma, infection and hypoxic–ischemic injury
- inborn errors of metabolism
- cerebral palsy

About 2–5% of children have at least one febrile seizure between ages 6 months and 6 years, the peak incidence being between 18 months and 2 years. In 25–50% of these children seizures recur: more commonly if the first seizure occurs before age 12 months and when the fit occurs at a lower temperature or in a child with a family history of seizures.

Episodes of status epilepticus in a child with a seizure, or accompanying an acute brain condition, often result in the need for admission to a PICU following initial emergency care, because of ventilatory inadequacy during the postictal phase or because of respiratory depression by anticonvulsants. Some children need respiratory support (Chs 2.1, 6.4) because of aspiration pneumonia after vomiting during a seizure. Others require aggressive treatment and monitoring for control of status epilepticus (Ch. 2.5). Of such cases, 25% are precipitated by a febrile seizure.

CENTRAL NERVOUS SYSTEM INFECTIONS

Acute CNS infections such as meningitis or encephalitis may require intensive care if associated with:

- status epilepticus (Ch. 2.5)
- hypoventilation (Ch. 2.1)
- shock due to bacterial or viral septicemia (Ch. 2.3)
- evidence of raised intracranial pressure (Ch. 2.4) or severely depressed conscious state
- severe metabolic derangement: hyponatremia (Ch. 2.10) or hypoglycemia

Although immunization against Hib has greatly reduced the incidence of bacterial meningitis, pneumococci and meningococci (Chs 3.3, 3.8) cause life-threatening meningitis.

Placental transfer of antibodies confers immunity to both organisms in the first months of life, but between 6 months and 2 years of age the production of antibodies to encapsulated organisms is poor, causing susceptibility to both bacteria. At any moment, the pharynx of 25–50% of children is colonized with pneumococci (of the same serotypes that cause invasive disease) and most children are colonized at some time each year. Black children in the USA are up to five times as susceptible as white children to pneumococcal

meningitis, partly because of the prevalence of sickle cell disease (Ch. 3.6) in the African-American population.

The epidemiology of meningococcal disease is discussed below. Meningitis and brain abscess (due to pneumococci, *Haemophilus* or anaerobic streptococci) may follow paranasal sinusitis, otitis media, meningomyelocele or head trauma with fracture through the paranasal sinuses, and may sometimes be recurrent. In the newborn, organisms acquired in the birth canal (e.g. group B streptococci and *Listeria*) and Gram-negative bacilli (sometimes acquired in hospital from the hands of carers or via indwelling tubes or catheters) are responsible for most cases of meningitis.

CONGENITAL DEFECTS

Congenital abnormalities of the brain are responsible for many cases of critical neurological illness in children, including cerebral hemorrhage or heart failure due to cerebral arteriovenous malformations (AVMs) and status epilepticus due to structural brain anomalies.

HYPOXIC–ISCHEMIC INJURY

Hypoxic–ischemic injury following cardiac arrest occurs throughout infancy and childhood (Ch. 2.2), while that following near-drowning is more common in toddlers and teenagers (Ch. 4.9).

CEREBROVASCULAR DISEASE

Unlike adults, children rarely suffer primary cerebral hemorrhage (other than bleeding into a tumor or AVM) and cerebral thrombosis is rare except in some inherited conditions—e.g. sickle cell disease (Ch. 3.6), neurofibromatosis or deficiencies of antithrombin III or proteins C or S—or following trauma to the neck vessels. Embolic strokes are seen in children with congenital heart disease in the following circumstances:

- older children and teenagers with uncorrected right-to-left shunts
- intravenous injection of air or clot in children with right-to-left shunts
- following cardiac surgery
- bacterial endocarditis (also accompanies rheumatic heart disease)

INFECTION

Infections—viral, bacterial or protozoal—are responsible for 10% of childhood deaths in developed countries and more than 60% worldwide. Community-acquired or hospital-acquired infections cause or contribute to many cases of critical illness in children.

SEPTICEMIA

In previously healthy children, septicemia (e.g. with coagulase-positive staphylococci, *Streptococcus pneumoniae* or *Neisseria meningitidis*) may occur de novo. Septicemia with Gram-negative bacilli, *Staphylococcus aureus*, yeasts or fungi may complicate other severe illnesses and their treatment, especially if treatment involves surgery, broad-spectrum antibiotics or invasive catheterization of the trachea, bladder or central veins. Children with impaired immunity for any reason (such as malnutrition; severe illness including nephrotic syndrome; glucocorticoid; immunosuppressive or cytotoxic drug therapy; or congenital immune deficiency) are at risk of developing septicemia and other infections due to opportunistic organisms (e.g. cytomegalovirus or *Pneumocystis carinii* pneumonia, fungal brain abscess, or septicemia caused by *Pseudomonas*, *Serratia* or mixed Gram-negative organisms).

NEISSERIA MENINGITIDIS INFECTION

The incidence of meningococcal disease has increased significantly in several parts of the Western world including Great Britain, parts of the USA, Europe and New Zealand since 1991. The baseline incidence in most Western countries is 1–2 cases per 100 000, but during epidemics the incidence increases 7–10-fold for 5–15 years. The incidence in infants from high-risk populations may be as high as 120 per 100 000. Three-quarters of cases occur in winter and early spring, with 60–90% of patients being children. Half of newborns carry bactericidal titres of placentally transferred antibody, but antibody levels decline to a minimum between 6 months and 24 months of age, when 50% of childhood cases occur, then slowly increase to adult levels by age 12 years.

Neonatal infection is uncommon. Outbreaks of strains A and C may be controlled by vaccination, but no vaccine is available for the B strain which is responsible for many of the current outbreaks.

About 50% of children with meningococcal disease have meningitis and 25% have septic shock. The latter is more common in:

- girls
- outbreaks involving specific serotypes, e.g. ET-15
- prior infection with influenza A or B virus

TOXIC SHOCK SYNDROME

Severe staphylococcal or streptococcal toxic shock syndrome (TSS) may follow bacterial contamination of a burn, skin wound (surgical or accidental), or mucosal ulcer. A few cases of staphylococcal TSS are due to tampon use in adolescent girls.

NEOPLASTIC DISEASE

Oncology patients usually become critically ill because of:

- respiratory failure (due to pneumonia involving opportunistic organisms such as cytomegalovirus, *Pneumocystis carinii* or fungi; pleural effusion or large airways compression by tumor)
- septic shock
- renal failure (due to sepsis, chemotherapy or nephrotoxic antibiotics)
- cardiac failure (anthracycline cardiomyopathy)

HIV

At least half a million children worldwide are infected with human immunodeficiency virus (HIV), most of whom will become critically ill but will never receive comprehensive care as they live in remote rural areas in developing countries. The great majority (86%) of children with HIV are perinatally infected. Most of the remainder are infected by contaminated blood products. Even among adolescents, transfer by sexual contact or intravenous drug use is less common than congenital or blood product transfer. As the prognosis for HIV-infected children who require intensive care admission for respiratory failure improved greatly in the 1990s (Ch. 3.7), more such children will survive, possibly to have multiple episodes of critical illness.

ENVIRONMENTAL RISKS

Trauma, burns, envenomation, drowning and poisoning represent failure of environmental safety mechanisms for children and account for 10–15% of PICU admissions (Table 1.3.3). Mobility, inexperience, adventurousness and degree of supervision determine who is at risk. Boys are more at risk than girls from most types of trauma, including burns, poisoning, drowning, falls, automobile/pedestrian and cycle injuries.

AGE

After the age of 1 year, inexperience and increasing mobility render toddlers at risk of drowning, falls, poisoning, burns and scalds.

SOCIAL CLASS AND EDUCATION

Supervision and training may contribute to the vulnerability of children of families from social classes IV and V, and those whose mothers have low educational attainments. These children are more at risk of falls, burns, poisoning, motor vehicle accidents and penetrating injury (stab or gunshot).

SEASON

Physical injuries (including falls and automobile-related trauma) are more common in summer than in winter, especially in Europe and North America.

TIME OF DAY

All forms of childhood injury, including poisoning, are more common between 3 p.m. and 7 p.m., after children have emerged from school and parents' attention is diverted to meal preparation, bathing siblings, etc. Another, smaller, peak occurs before school, between 7 a.m. and 9 a.m.

SOCIAL DEVELOPMENT

Bravado and broadening horizons increase the risk of bicycle-related and automobile driver injuries, penetrating trauma and drowning in older children and teenagers, especially boys. Critical illness due to experimental or habitual drug abuse and deliberate self-harm also increases in this group (Ch. 3.10).

RACE AND GEOGRAPHY

There is considerable geographic and racial variability in injury pattern: stab and gunshot wounds account for 1.5% of child trauma admissions and 10% of child trauma deaths in the USA and are more common among African-American and Hispanic boys, but are uncommon in most other countries. Drowning is far more common in warm climates than in cold.

POSTOPERATIVE ILLNESS

After some forms of major elective and semielective surgery, it is anticipated that many children will be severely ill, with failure or instability of one or more organ system. For example, cardiac failure, respiratory and renal failure, coagulopathy and gastrointestinal stasis are common after open heart surgery. The epidemiology of the severe postoperative illness of these children is therefore that of the underlying condition, its complications and the health status of the child at the time of surgery (e.g. preoperative malnutrition or failure of one or more organ systems increases the duration of recovery from surgery and the risk of severe postoperative complications). The timing of surgery and the nature and difficulty of the surgery also contribute to the child's postoperative state.

CARDIAC SURGERY

Children who are severely though briefly unstable after cardiac surgery represent a considerable proportion of critically ill children in many Western countries (Table 1.3.3). The incidence of congenital heart disease is 7 per 1000 live births, of which the most common lesions are ventricular septal defect (VSD, 32%), patent ductus arteriosus

(12%), pulmonary stenosis (8%), atrial septal defect (ASD, 6%), aortic coarctation (6%), tetralogy of Fallot (6%), aortic stenosis (5%) and transposition of the great arteries (5%). There is little difference between countries and racial groups and over time in one country in the overall incidence of congenital heart disease and in the incidence of the individual lesions.

As more and more preterm infants survive neonatal intensive care, the incidence of patent ductus arteriosus (PDA) is increasing, although the mortality and morbidity of surgery for this condition is very low. The incidence of some congenital heart lesions (especially the more severe disorders such as hypoplastic left heart syndrome) in the liveborn population has been reduced in some Western countries by antenatal ultrasound diagnosis and elective termination of pregnancy.

ASSOCIATED CONDITIONS

Congenital heart lesions are more common in children with chromosomal disorders including trisomies (e.g. atrioventricular septal defect in Down syndrome), and chromosomal deletions and translocations; in first-degree relatives of people with congenital heart lesions and in some constellations of congenital abnormalities such as the CHARGE association (Fallot's tetralogy) and Williams' syndrome (supravalvar aortic stenosis). Some maternal illnesses are associated with particular congenital heart lesions, for example diabetes mellitus (VSD, TGA), rubella (PDA, peripheral pulmonary stenosis) and systemic lupus erythematosus (heart block). Mortality and postoperative morbidity are higher for complex lesions, especially for combinations of lesions, and are higher for those lesions that require repair in infancy than in those that can safely be repaired later in life.

AGE AT SURGERY

The repair of some congenital and acquired disorders of childhood is undertaken at particular stages of development, e.g. craniofacial procedures for cranial synostosis are performed in infancy, while repair of idiopathic scoliosis is performed in early adolescence. Conditions such as gastroschisis, omphalocele, bowel atresias, esophageal atresia and tracheoesophageal fistula require repair early in the newborn period. The need for prolonged respiratory and gastrointestinal support is anticipated in many of these infants.

GASTROINTESTINAL SURGERY

Gastrointestinal emergencies such as volvulus and necrotizing enterocolitis (NEC) may present in the newborn period with shock and abdominal distention and may need prolonged respiratory and nutritional support after surgery. Necrotizing enterocolitis is more common in preterm infants, in twins, after birth asphyxia or fetal distress, in children with respiratory distress or sepsis, and in those whose umbilical vessels have been cannulated.

✔ **KEY POINTS**

➤ In developed countries 1.2% of children need PICU care; 10% are less than 1 month old and 50% are less than 2 years old

➤ Socioeconomic disadvantage increases the risk of most kinds of severe childhood illness

➤ Antenatal screening fails to diagnose many structural congenital abnormalities

➤ Clustering of congenital anomalies in a child increases the risk of critical illness and reduces the best outcome after the PICU stay

➤ Severe respiratory illness accounts for 25–35% of PICU admissions in autumn and early winter

➤ Study of the epidemiology of critical illness guides the rational provision of services and may help reduce childhood mortality and morbidity

FURTHER READING

1. Pless IB, editor. The epidemiology of childhood disorders. Oxford University Press; 1994
 – (*Thorough reviews of epidemiology of major groups of childhood illnesses including respiratory infections, trauma and structural birth defects. Section on methodology and terminology*)

2. Forfar JO. Demography, vital statistics and the pattern of disease in childhood. In: Campbell AGM, McIntosh N, editors. Forfar and Arneil's Textbook of paediatrics, 4th ed. Edinburgh: Churchill Livingstone; 1992
 – (*Overview of pediatric epidemiology from a UK and global perspective*)

3. Canosa CA, Willoughby A, Yaffe SJ, editors. HIV infection in children. Acta Paediatr (Suppl.) 1994; 400
–   (*Several articles on the epidemiology of the HIV pandemic, including its infective complications*)

4. Division of Injury Control, Center for Environmental Health and Injury Control, Centers for Disease Control. Childhood injuries in the United States. Am J Dis Child 1990; 144: 627–646
–   (*This issue of the journal contains several detailed epidemiological reviews of aspects of child trauma in the US*)

1.4 Prevention of critical illness and injury

Simon Young

Injuries are the leading cause of death in pre-school and school-aged children, adolescents and young adults. A significant proportion are both predictable and preventable. Physicians must be advocates of appropriate child care, safe practices, improvement of unsafe items and appropriate legislation. Many prevention strategies are known to be effective in reducing injury, mortality and morbidity. A preventive strategy is most likely to be effective if it:

- is carefully planned
- incorporates data collection and analysis
- identifies issues and trends in the target population
- provides information and a developed preventive plan
- includes monitoring of the effectiveness of the strategy
- provides for modification, and feedback to the organizations and individuals involved

DEVELOPING PREVENTION STRATEGIES

DEFINITIONS

Primary prevention is any measure intended to reduce the incidence of a disease. Examples include bicycle helmet laws, vaccination programs and measures to ensure a safe, continuous water supply. Some primary prevention benefits the community as well as the individual. For example, herd immunity produced by widespread diphtheria vaccination of susceptible children reduces the risk of diphtheria infection, even in unvaccinated children.

Secondary prevention is screening for diseases: for example antenatal ultrasound examination, routine testing for hypothyroidism and phenylketonuria in the newborn period, and examination in well-baby clinics.

Tertiary prevention includes measures to prevent deterioration in established disease: for example,

regular air flow monitoring in asthmatic children and early surgery for many congenital heart lesions.

DATA COLLECTION AND ANALYSIS

Accurate and reliable data, collected in a standard form from a series of related incidents, are used to identify trends. An open format, suitable for collecting broad data, is used when the aim is general surveillance (e.g. to gain information about the contents of home drug cupboards for a future education campaign). If the goal is more specific (for example, to prevent a particular type of sporting injury), then the format should be much more directive, eliciting responses to specific questions.

Whom to study

If the aim is to prevent the complications of diabetes in teenagers, then the study sample should be representative of all teenage and pre-teenage diabetic patients, including representative proportions of geographical, racial, sex and socioeconomic subgroups. On the other hand, if the intention is to prevent illness due to solvent abuse in a particular racial subgroup, then children of that race should be studied, including urban and rural children, both sexes and all socioeconomic groups.

The study method selected must be capable of providing the information required. For example, a telephone survey will give only information about children whose families are affluent enough to own a telephone, and who speak the language of the surveyors. If the response is voluntary, then the results will reflect those of a motivated, literate and often middle-class population who frequently have a personal interest in the survey outcome, but not those of other socioeconomic and linguistic groups.

Data selection

Data should be collected as soon as possible after the event to which they refer. Compliance with injury surveillance data collection is variable and enthusiasm for data collection often wanes with time.

A data set that is simple, clinically relevant but not repetitive will enhance compliance. The injury surveillance section of the Victorian Emergency Minimum Data Set (Table 1.4.1) is an example of a computerized database on all illnesses and injuries sustained by children presenting to emergency departments in the state of Victoria, Australia.

Valuable information on the circumstances and occurrence of preventable illness and injury can sometimes only be obtained outside the pediatric emergency environment (e.g. when the event is not serious enough for emergency services to be involved). Monitoring during anesthesia illustrates the importance of detecting minor events which although harmless in themselves can lead to harm over time. At the other end of the spectrum, the death of a child outside hospital will often be investigated by police and/or the coroner.

Epidemiological information may come from pediatric or general hospital emergency or outpatient departments or intensive care units, or from other health services such as maternal and child health nurses, local medical practitioners, sports medicine clinics, smaller public hospitals and private clinics. Poison information centers, infectious diseases laboratories, the coroner, police and government health departments all collect and collate information pertaining to children. Other sources, such as local medical practitioners, are likely to collect information but store it in individual case notes where it is less accessible.

Illness prevention requires data from many sources. For example, to identify the best way to prevent accidental childhood poisoning requires the following information:

- the age distribution of children in the population (census data)
- how frequently the medication is prescribed or sold over the counter (Department of Health)
- how many children are reported to take the medication accidentally (poisons information center, hospital emergency department, family physicians)
- how many are advised not to seek further medical care (poisons information center, medical sources)
- how many present to an emergency department (emergency department)
- how many are treated and discharged from the emergency department (emergency department)
- how many are admitted to an intensive care unit (unit records)
- what medical interventions are given (ambulance, emergency department, ICU)
- how many die following ingestion of the drug (emergency department, ICU, coroners' records)

IDENTIFICATION OF TRENDS IN INJURY AND ILLNESS

Trends in the incidence of injury or illness in the community may be recognized by an astute clinician, but increases in the incidence of injury or illness perceived by one individual may not be statistically significant, and some trends (especially those involving infrequent events) may easily be missed. Pooling data from several clinicians within a single hospital, or from various hospitals within a city, a state or a nation, will improve the identification of statistical trends. Many countries already have linked databases for trauma, cancer and infectious diseases.

Regular surveillance of the collated data and subsequent statistical analysis by investigators who understand childhood illness, statistical principles and the cultural background of the

TABLE 1.4.1 **State of Victoria emergency minimum data set**	
Name	Sex
Date of birth	Address
Arrival transport mode	Arrival (date and time)
Triage (date and time)	Seen by treating
Departure destination	doctor (date and time)
Investigations	Departure (date and time)
Primary emergency	Procedures
department diagnosis	Body region
(ICD9 code for	Human intent
noninjuries)	Nature of main injury
Type of place where	Injury cause
injury occurred	Activity when injured
Description of injury event	

community provide a picture of the incidence of serious injury and illness in the target population. Although much of the information obtained will reflect the incidence of known problems such as motor vehicle trauma, unexpected findings will occasionally appear: for example, a spate of serious injuries in young children falling from shopping trolleys, which may require preventive action. In practice, many important preventive programs are born when a clinician, alerted by recent clinical involvement in a case, interrogates the database looking for similar cases and discusses the findings with other clinicians. In the light of the trend data and of published information on the subject, steps are taken to prevent the problem. For example, in 1971 in Melbourne, emergency department and intensive care staff noticed a huge increase in the number of children presenting with tricyclic antidepressant (TCA) overdose. Several children were critically ill and two died. A survey found that most were less than 3 years of age, so a study of the accessibility of tablets in various types of containers (including 'palm-and-turn' bottles, clear wrap and foil wrap) was undertaken, using preschool children in a suburban crèche. Foil-wrapped tablets proved to be significantly less accessible to younger children than those in other containers and after representations were made to the Minister for Health, pharmaceutical companies were encouraged by the government to package TCAs in foil. Most complied and over the next 2 years, hospital admissions for child TCA overdose fell by 60% despite a 50% increase in TCA prescriptions in the state.

The data should also be available to respond to interest in the subject from the public, the media or from politicians. Warding off a misguided 'preventive' strategy may be just as important as starting an effective one.

PROVISION OF INFORMATION

Media reports usually produce an immediate but short-lived response, especially when the topic is newsworthy (e.g. snakebites in summer, or an outbreak of gastroenteritis) and can be conveyed briefly with a simple message to parents. This publicity may be used as the start of a much larger campaign. Media publicity about the drowning of a 2-year-old child in a backyard pool may stimulate parents to examine their pool security arrangements. The excellent immediate effects of this publicity are likely to be short-lived as the memory of the emotional event subsides. To achieve an effective and sustained reduction in early childhood drowning requires a strategy with many facets including raising parental awareness during infant 'well baby' center visits and possibly also by a highly visible advertising campaign. Legislation on mandatory fencing of backyard swimming pools, enforcement of that legislation, and cardiopulmonary resuscitation training are also necessary.

Information provided by the injury surveillance system may be presented to a local Child Injury Prevention Task Force which selects appropriate courses for community action.

Pamphlets, posters and video presentations in the waiting areas of hospital outpatient clinics can be used to provide information to families and stimulate thought on issues of illness and injury prevention. The same publicity material can also be displayed in local doctors' waiting rooms, in maternal and child health clinics and in schools to reach a wider audience.

Selection of the most appropriate organization to receive and act on the data depends on the organization's resources (financial and personnel), access to the target audience and political influence. For example, yachting and fishing clubs may assist in promoting the wearing of lifejackets by children. Appropriate groups may include parent organizations, schools, safety action groups, service clubs, motoring organizations, sporting clubs, local doctors, pediatricians, local councils, police and government.

Coordination between groups involved in preventive strategies is crucial. Using current safety campaigns and publicity vehicles saves time and effort as well as avoiding the risk of confusing the public with conflicting messages or tiring them with repetition. The form (written, oral, video or computer-based presentations) and content of information must be appropriate to the target audience. The message should be simple and straightforward with minimal use of medical terminology. Publicizing actual clinical events is an effective way of drawing media attention to a problem, but if the child is identified, the possible effects of the consequent publicity on the child must be carefully considered and consent obtained from the legal guardian and (usually) from the child.

MOBILIZING RESOURCES

Individuals in positions of influence who are willing and able to assist in this process should be identified, as strong leadership at clinical and community level will contribute to the success of a preventive campaign.

Any large strategy must be properly funded, usually by hospitals, service groups, businesses or government. Association with a safety campaign may help a business market its product (e.g. children's play equipment or kitchen furniture). Other businesses may be well known locally for their altruism in supporting 'good causes'. Local government departments that offer child care facilities or immunizations may be able to assist a preventive campaign. Funds donors should be acknowledged, but prevention not advertising must remain the primary goal.

Primary prevention often requires changes to legislation or regulations, for example those governing compulsory child car restraints, bicycle helmets and home swimming-pool fencing.

EVALUATION

Random sampling by questionnaires or telephone polls can determine whether the preventive program is being understood or implemented by the target audience. A sustained reduction in the incidence of the illness or injury is the 'gold standard' by which the success of a strategy is assessed. Unfortunately, the lack of a true control population and the presence of many confounding variables may impede adequate statistical analysis of the effect of the strategy. For example, an apparent decrease in child passenger deaths after the introduction of seat-belt regulations may actually be due to safer car construction, safer roads or a reduction in the number of child car journeys. If the evaluation suggests that a preventive campaign has not been effective, all stages of the process, from the epidemiological evaluation and analysis to the preventive measures adopted, should be reassessed to determine the reasons for the failure.

The results of the evaluation, whatever its findings, should be fed back to all health workers who have contributed, to health authorities, both local and national, and if possible, to the public. These steps will reinforce the effects of a successful campaign and will increase public awareness of the problem even if the campaign is ineffective.

✔ KEY POINTS

➤ Choose the right sample group and method of study for the information being sought
➤ Collect data as soon as possible after the event
➤ Media publicity campaigns are effective but the effect is often short-lived
➤ Evaluate the effectiveness of the preventive strategy and use the information obtained to improve it

PREVENTION OF SPECIFIC ILLNESSES

TRAUMA

General preventive measures

Advice about child safety can be given to parents by the family doctor, at well-baby clinics and by the child's school (Table 1.4.2). There are opportunities for education of the child in television advertisements, in schools and in sporting clubs.

Falls

Falls in infants are usually due to unattended infants falling off a table, a bed or down stairs. Discussions and pamphlets can be given at antenatal classes and at well-baby clinics, warning parents against leaving infants unattended, advocating the use of stair guards, window guards and cot sides, and advising against baby walkers. Parents should be reminded that the child will learn to roll and to climb.

In older children, publicity at school about safe behavior, risk-taking and resisting peer pressure may help to reduce the danger from falls.

TABLE 1.4.2 **Child safety education**	
Parent education	**Child education**
Antenatal classes	**School**
Automobile restraints	Electrical safety
Safe baby furniture	Safety with poisons
Never leave baby unattended	Strangers
Safety in the sun	Road safety
Bath safety	Bicycle safety
Home hot water temperature 49°C (120°F)	Drugs, tobacco and alcohol
Infant welfare clinic	Sport safety
Dealing with anger	Water safety
Rolling	Risk-taking behavior
Hot liquids	Substance abuse
Electrical safety: cords and outlets	Driving safety
Keep small objects out of reach	CPR training
Childproof medicine cupboards	Sexually transmitted diseases
Stair gates and window guards	
Swimming-pool fencing	
Safety with animals	
CPR advice	

CPR, cardiopulmonary resuscitation.

Supervision of play equipment and talks about its safe use can reduce the risk of injuries. National design standards for child furniture (if monitored and enforced) also reduce these risks.

Road trauma

Pedestrian

At well-baby clinics, parents can be taught (by discussion or pamphlet) about unsupervised play in driveways and near roads; about teaching road safety drills to toddlers, and the role of example-setting. Classroom discussion about pedestrian and cyclist safety, and about safe behavior when catching or alighting from school buses, can help schoolchildren think about the issues. These discussions may involve teachers, parents, police or other traffic experts.

Automobile passenger

Pamphlets and discussion groups on infant safety capsules, seats and restraints should be part of antenatal classes and should be available at infant welfare clinics. Legislation making seat-belts compulsory for front and rear seat passengers has contributed to a dramatic reduction in death and severe injury to automobile passengers. Infant safety seats are a comparable advance, although airbag technology remains imperfect as far as children are concerned. They should be placed in the rear seats in vehicles with airbags. Strict laws, reinforced by heavy penalties, governing speeding and intoxication with alcohol or other drugs while driving have also reduced the risk to passengers. Improved design of automobiles and roads in recent years has made a modest contribution to passenger safety, and monitoring the role of defective vehicles or roads in automobile passenger injuries may indicate where further preventive measures can be applied. Television campaigns aimed at drivers and their families can reduce mortality and morbidity by increasing awareness of the role of alcohol, speed, tiredness, aggression and vehicle disrepair in passenger injuries.

Penetrating trauma

Penetrating wounds may be accidental (e.g. from machinery) or from assault, homicide or attempted suicide (knife and gunshot). The appropriate means of prevention depends on the causation in each society, and effective prevention requires accurate local epidemiological information (Ch. 1.3). When most penetrating trauma is due to machinery in the home and on farms or is due to the presence of children in dangerous workplaces, the most effective methods may be intensive publicity campaigns aimed at parents and children. Enforceable regulations (with regular inspection) governing the safety of machinery and access of children to machinery may also help.

Prevention of suicide is discussed in Ch. 3.10. When adolescents at risk are identified, limiting access to guns and therapeutic drugs (the most common and preventable means of suicide) may reduce the risk of completed suicide. Strict laws regulating access of the general population to firearms and regulating the type of weapons that can be kept in the home not only reduces the incidence of injury due to these weapons, but also discourages any prevailing perception that firearm use is acceptable. The role of violent films and videos in the prevalence of violence among adolescents is uncertain, and the effectiveness of censorship as a preventive measure is even more so.

Although most trauma deaths occur at the scene and are unavoidable, some deaths and morbidity can be prevented by:

- centralization of specialist trauma services within a region
- a rapidly responding, well-trained paramedic ambulance service
- education of the public in basic cardiopulmonary resuscitation (CPR)
- education of doctors and other health workers in advanced trauma life support and advanced pediatric life support by attending the appropriate courses

POISONING

The main groups at risk are toddlers (accidental ingestion, Ch. 4.5) and adolescents (suicide and parasuicide, Ch. 3.10). The most useful measures in prevention of poisoning are minimization of exposure and detection of adolescents at risk.

Education

Education of the parents of infants (Table 1.4.2) and young children should include:

- information on which household substances are poisonous
- advice on appropriate storage of pharmaceuticals, cleaning agents, insecticides, hydrocarbons and other poisons
- recognition of poisonous plants and fungi
- appropriate first aid

Publicity

Publicity on these topics should be available in schools, public libraries, physicians' waiting rooms, hospital outpatient departments and other public places.

Media advertising and news releases about poisoning incidents and preventive measures may be helpful.

Legislation

Laws and regulations govern:

- childproof packaging of drugs
- coloring and unpleasant flavoring of poisonous liquids
- limits on prescribable quantities of pharmaceuticals

BURNS

Prevention of childhood burns and scalds includes general measures (primary and tertiary prevention) and those that apply specifically to children. Instructing parents to turn down the thermostat on the hot water supply to 49°C (120°F) so that water at the tap cannot cause scalds is simple and particularly effective.

General

General preventive measures include:

- publicity about risks such as flammable building materials and furnishings; safety of house wiring and electrical appliances
- publicity about flammable clothing, especially sleepwear
- building regulations: smoke alarms, sprinklers and fire exits
- national standards on electrical wiring, smoke alarms and flammability of building materials and clothing
- effective firefighting and fire investigation services
- public education by the media, on home fire extinguishers, escape from a burning building and first aid

Child-specific

Parental education (e.g. in well-baby clinics, physicians' waiting rooms and in schools) should warn them about hazards in the home: matches; flammable clothing and furnishings; scalds in infants and toddlers from hot beverages; pots on stoves; hot baths; risks of bar radiators.

Child education at school should focus on fire risks, including matches and use of fire accelerants.

Publicity in the media may include:

- the dangers of children playing with matches and with flammable liquids
- scalds from hot liquids
- planning for escape from a fire in the house

DROWNING

The appropriate preventive methods depend on the most common circumstances of drowning in a community. For example, in the USA, New Zealand and Australia, many child drownings involve domestic swimming pools, so the measures most likely to be effective include mandatory installation of high fences with childproof gates around private pools and public education campaigns about pool fencing, and supervision of children swimming. In other societies, publicity about the risks of infants and children near baths, buckets of water, lakes, rivers and the sea may be more appropriate, with emphasis on the need for supervision. Encouragement of education of teenagers and adults in basic life support is important, as bystander CPR saves many lives among the near-drowned.

Education of teenagers about the risks of swimming alone, of diving, of unseen underwater hazards and of alcohol should be given at school and in the media. Signs at dangerous swimming spots and the presence of an effective, trained lifeguard service at popular swimming places save the lives of children as well as adults.

✔ KEY POINTS

➤ Parental education on supervision and sources of risk is vital to the prevention of burns, poisoning and drowning in children

➤ Antenatal classes, well-baby clinics and schools offer opportunities for education of parents and children on injury prevention

➤ Driver education, speed cameras, compulsory use of seat-belts and bicycle helmets, drink-driving laws and random breath testing greatly reduce deaths and severe injuries among automobile drivers and passengers, cyclists and pedestrians

INFECTIOUS DISEASE

The basis of prevention of all infectious disease is an effective government epidemiological service which undertakes general surveillance, data collection and analysis, investigates specific outbreaks, and gives advice to the government on preventive measures. Compulsory case notification, quarantine, testing of at-risk groups (e.g. Mantoux testing of recent immigrants from areas of endemic tuberculosis) and treatment of contacts are part of the preventive function of a government health department.

Community-acquired severe infection in children

General preventive measures include the provision of a safe, continuous water supply and safe sewage disposal for all communities within a country. A government-supported system of urban and rural health care and well-baby clinics can help educate parents on personal and domestic hygiene, as well as delivering and monitoring a vaccination program. Clinic workers can also deliver education messages to schools, in cooperation with teachers. Distance and local customs such as the subordinate role of women in some societies may hamper primary prevention and surveillance and screening for infection, and may mean that children from poor rural communities present late in the course of an infective illness, greatly increasing their risk of dying or suffering severe morbidity. Education (especially of women), improved transport and increased numbers of itinerant government health workers can help to alleviate this problem.

Promotion of breastfeeding reduces the prevalence of severe gastrointestinal and respiratory illness in infants. Breast milk is sterile, cheap and inhibits the replication of viruses including influenza and mumps. Immunoglobulin A in breast milk reduces the enteric absorption of ingested pathogens.

Immunization has greatly reduced the prevalence of several severe childhood illnesses, including poliomyelitis, pertussis and measles. During the 1990s, intensive care admissions for acute epiglottitis and meningitis due to *Haemophilus influenzae* type b (Hib), previously common, have almost ceased in countries that have introduced widespread Hib vaccination. Where immunization programs have broken down (e.g. in countries involved in civil war), the prevalence of severe diseases such as measles has dramatically increased. Table 1.4.3 shows a suitable immunization program.

TABLE 1.4.3 **Immunization schedule**	
Age	**Vaccine**
2 months	DPT, Hib, Hep B, oral polio
4 months	DPT, Hib, Hep B, polio
6 months	DPT, Hib, polio
12 months	Hep B, MMR
18 months	DPT, Hib
4 years	DPT, polio
10 years	MMR
15 years	DPT, polio

DPT, *diphtheria, pertussis, tetanus; Hep B, hepatitis B; Hib, Haemophilus influenzae type b; MMR, measles, mumps, rubella.*

Immunization should be postponed in the presence of acute febrile illness (other than minor respiratory infection) or developing neurological illness, to avoid diagnostic confusion. Severe reactions to previous doses of a vaccine are a contraindication to further doses. Live vaccines such as oral polio vaccine should be avoided in immunocompromised children. When immunization rates fall (because of fear of vaccine-related complications or lack of confidence in the vaccine), the benefits of herd immunity for the unimmunized decline (e.g. pertussis in the newborn). In these circumstances, media publicity campaigns involving case reporting are effective preventive measures.

Children in countries, regions or communities where tuberculosis is prevalent should be screened regularly (at 12 months, 4 years and 15 years), as should children at risk in other communities (Table 1.4.4).

TABLE 1.4.4 **Children at risk of tuberculous infection**
• Child or parents from a country where TB is prevalent
• Contact of a patient with active TB
• Institutionalized child
• Immunodeficient child
• HIV-positive child
• Reduced immunity
– steroid therapy
– cancer chemotherapy
– malnutrition
– diabetes mellitus
– lymphoma
– chronic renal failure

TB, *tuberculosis.*

Severe hospital-acquired infection

Approximately 5% of hospitalized patients develop a hospital-acquired infection, and 4% of these infections cause or contribute to death. Critically ill children are 10–20% more likely—and neonatal intensive care patients are 4–5 times more likely—to acquire a nosocomial infection than general hospital patients.

Primary prevention

Primary prevention measures include:

- handwashing by all staff (especially medical) and visitors; active campaigns, visible surveillance and publicity are known to be effective
- infection control programs:
  - surveillance of outbreaks and their cause
  - education of staff and visitors
  - review of antibiotic use and resistance
  - supervised infection control procedures
- minimize antibiotic use:
  - firm hospital guidelines
  - early consultation with infectious diseases staff
  - avoid broad-spectrum antibiotics and third-generation cephalosporins whenever possible
  - Avoid antibiotic prophylaxis
- take several cultures before starting antibiotics
- use the antibiotic to which the organism is sensitive
- only treat clinically important infection
- never treat colonization (e.g. asymptomatic *Pseudomonas* in a tracheal aspirate)
- remove endotracheal and nasogastric tubes and central venous and urinary catheters as soon as possible
- use a clean, no-touch technique in breaking intravenous, arterial and central venous lines
- use a sterile technique in inserting urinary and indwelling vascular catheters
- care with operative technique
- remove dead tissue

- ban staff with active infections from patient care, especially in operating rooms and intensive care units

Secondary prevention

Secondary prevention (screening of patients and staff) is of doubtful efficacy, even in the presence of an active outbreak. Isolation and treatment of carriers have not been shown to be effective in the prevention of nosocomial infection. Surveillance of hospital buildings and equipment may indicate a source of organisms (e.g. *Serratia*, *Pseudomonas* or *Acinetobacter* in washbasins, water traps or ventilators). This may suggest a change in procedures or equipment to correct the problem.

Tertiary problem

The most effective means of tertiary prevention is frequent clinical observation of hospitalized children for signs of infection. The total white cell count and the ratio of immature to total neutrophil numbers (especially if this ratio is increasing) are useful indicators of sepsis in a sick child.

Unproven or ineffective preventive measures

The following measures have not been proved to be effective:

- antibiotic prophylaxis (more than a single dose before surgery)
- elective change of central venous catheters
- selective decontamination of the digestive tract
- antibiotic or antiseptic-impregnated central venous or urinary catheters
- in-line i.v. filters
- skin decontamination
- occlusive dressings or antibiotic cream to i.v. or central venous puncture sites

✓ KEY POINTS

➤ Promotion of breastfeeding reduces the prevalence of severe gastrointestinal and respiratory illness in infants
➤ Falling immunization rates deny the benefits of herd immunity to unimmunized infants

➤ Handwashing, minimization of antibiotic use, and care with aseptic technique during all invasive procedures are central to the prevention of nosocomial infection
➤ The ratio of immature to total neutrophil numbers (especially if this ratio is increasing) is a useful indicator of sepsis in a sick child

HEREDITARY AND CONGENITAL DISORDERS

Primary prevention

The likelihood of developmental abnormalities of the fetus may be reduced by:

- rubella immunization of preadolescent girls
- education in schools, clinics and the media to reduce smoking, alcohol consumption and drug use in pregnancy
- education of physicians and the public on the teratogenic properties of therapeutic drugs and benefits of folic acid supplements

When a hereditary disorder is detected in a child, or when there is a high risk of chromosomal or hereditary disorder (e.g. advanced maternal age, consanguineous parents, teratogenic exposure), parents should be offered genetic counseling before subsequent pregnancies, and if necessary, diagnostic tests such as amniocentesis or chorionic villous sampling. Fetal ultrasound examination is routinely performed at 18 weeks' gestation in Western countries, and repeated if necessary. It detects major structural abnormalities, especially of the renal and musculoskeletal systems, but many serious structural abnormalities remain undetected, and even when they are detected, termination of pregnancy is not always performed, especially in societies where termination of pregnancy is unacceptable. Antenatal diagnosis of a major structural abnormality may allow transfer of a baby in utero to a specialist center, or may lead to delivery by cesarean section or to intrauterine or early postnatal intervention (e.g. intrauterine drainage in a child with massive hydronephrosis due to urethral valves), reducing the severity of subsequent illness.

Routine neonatal screening for phenylketonuria (Guthrie test) and other inborn metabolic errors including hypothyroidism allows treatment to begin early and prevents later critical illness. Screening of siblings and other near relatives of children with inborn errors of metabolism and other disorders may also lead to early intervention.

Maintaining extensive records of affected children and their families improves the detection and survival of children with life-threatening congenital and hereditary disorders.

✓ **KEY POINTS**

➤ Antenatal ultrasonography has a low sensitivity for serious structural lesions
➤ Antenatal screening is only useful if early intervention is feasible or if elective abortion is acceptable

CONGENITAL HEART DISEASE

Primary prevention

There are few means available for primary prevention:

- rubella immunization prevents a few cases of congenital heart disease associated with congenital rubella
- education of adolescent girls may prevent some cases of fetal alcohol syndrome

Secondary prevention

Antenatal ultrasound examination reveals some major structural lesions but is dependent on operator expertise and has a low sensitivity: many lesions remain undiscovered until birth. Routine well-baby examination reveals some lesions (not all lesions have obvious clinical signs at birth); repeated examination at well-baby clinics is therefore the best form of secondary prevention.

Tertiary prevention

Regular follow-up of known heart lesions is important so that the optimal time for surgery can be chosen. Early surgery (in the first months of life) prevents irreversible deterioration and critical illness in some lesions (e.g. pulmonary hypertension in truncus arteriosus) and allows the optimal operation and the best long-term outcome to be available.

ASTHMA

There is no good evidence that environmental manipulation can completely prevent asthma. Parental education to prevent passive smoking may reduce the frequency of wheezing attacks. Secondary prevention can detect a trend to deterioration and permit early intervention:

- regular clinical follow-up
- use of peak flowmeters: recorded two or three times daily to establish each child's best baseline flow—a 20% reduction or more below baseline is significant
- history and skin testing for household allergens may allow some acute attacks to be prevented:
  - avoid feathers, some pollens and animal danders
  - minimize house dust (to reduce mite exposure)
  - immunotherapy is of doubtful effectiveness

Effective interval therapy is the most useful means of preventing severe acute attacks. Ongoing, regular education should be organized by the government health department or by the regional pediatric hospital to help asthmatic children, their families and school staff to avoid triggering factors, recognize acute wheezing attacks and plan what to do in the event of an acute attack (e.g. effective administration of bronchodilator drugs and access to a doctor or to hospital). Information leaflets should be available in schools, hospitals and physicians' offices. Adoption (by child asthma specialists), acceptance and wide distribution of asthma treatment protocols improve the standard of asthma management, and may reduce the frequency of acute attacks and prevent some sudden asthma deaths. The following measures are also helpful:

- keeping injectable bronchodilators in the home for emergency use together with clear, individualized protocols for acute attacks in severely asthmatic children

- the wearing of 'alert' bracelets to indicate that the child has severe asthma
- priority listing of severely asthmatic children by the local paramedic ambulance service

KEY POINT

➤ Regular clinical follow-up is the foundation of tertiary prevention in asthma

LOWER RESPIRATORY TRACT INFECTION

The most effective means of reducing the prevalence of severe lower respiratory tract infection would be an attack on poverty, malnutrition and overcrowding, but these are not usually within the control of health services. Campaigns to reduce indoor pollution (e.g. by regulations governing standards of building ventilation and of indoor heating) and to discourage smoking by family members may reduce the incidence of severe pneumonia in infants and children.

Immunization (see above) dramatically reduces the childhood mortality from pertussis and from pneumonia due to measles. Vaccination against tuberculosis with BCG should be offered to Mantoux-negative children at risk of developing this disease (Table 1.4.4).

Although immunologically competent children can mount an adequate immune response to the pneumococcus, pneumococcal vaccination should be offered before splenectomy (elective, semielective or emergency) and to any child with nephrotic syndrome, sickle cell disease (Ch. 3.6) or any form of immune compromise, including steroid or immunosuppressive drug therapy.

Children with immune compromise who have been in close contact with varicella are susceptible to catastrophic varicella pneumonia and should be given varicella-zoster immune globulin prophylactically.

UPPER AIRWAY OBSTRUCTION

Foreign body inhalation

Primary prevention (through antenatal classes, well-baby clinics and pamphlets) consists of:

- parental education about the dangers of small objects (food items for infants, and toys, pins, buttons and coins for toddlers)
- parental education in basic life support, including methods of clearing the airway
- education of ambulance and emergency department personnel in basic and advanced life support
- a rapidly responding emergency ambulance service (Ch. 1.5)

Croup

Tertiary prevention consists of the administration of steroids, which dramatically reduces the severity of croup, shortens hospital stay and reduces the need for tracheal intubation.

Epiglottitis

Epiglottitis and other severe childhood illnesses due to Hib have almost disappeared in countries that have introduced Hib vaccination.

INBORN ERRORS OF METABOLISM

Primary prevention

Genetic counseling of parents at risk of having children affected by a severe hereditary metabolic disorder may lead to a decision to abandon childbearing, or to selective termination of pregnancy based on the results of amniocentesis or chorionic villous sampling.

Secondary prevention

Universal screening (e.g. the Guthrie test) is only worth while for conditions whose incidence is high and where effective treatment is available. For other conditions, the most effective screening measures are a high level of suspicion of metabolic disease in any child with an unexplained illness, and selective screening of those children and others at risk (e.g. related to a known sufferer).

Tertiary prevention

Tertiary prevention depends on:

- education of the parents and the older child or adolescent about:
  - diet
  - prompt response to any intercurrent illness
  - signs of deterioration
  - early consultation with the pediatric hospital
- early referral to a specialist center
- advice, literature and support groups being readily accessible to the family
- fast-track hospital admission in the event of acute illness

FURTHER READING

1. Mortimer EA. Preventive pediatrics and epidemiology. In: Behrman EA, editor. Nelson Textbook of pediatrics, 14th ed. Philadelphia: WB Saunders; 1992
   - (*Overview of preventive approaches commonly used in pediatrics, especially immunization*)

2. Rivara FP. Injury prevention. In: Reisdorff EJ, Roberts MR, Wiegenstein JG, editors. Pediatric emergency medicine. Philadelphia: WB Saunders; 1993
   - (*US approach to the prevention of blunt and penetrating trauma, burns, drowning and poisoning*)

3. American Journal of Diseases of Children 1990; 144: June issue
   - (*This whole issue is devoted to the epidemiology and prevention of child trauma*)

4. Wall MA, Moe EL. Prevention of lung disease. In: Loughlin GM, Eigen H, editors. Respiratory disease in children: diagnosis and management. Baltimore: Williams & Wilkins; 1994
   - (*Good review of methods available for preventing asthma and respiratory infections*)

1.5 Interfacility transport

Andrew J. Macnab, Shirley M. Alexander, Duncan J. Macrae and Gordon Green

Advances in technology and the delivery of medical care for critically ill neonates and children have resulted in reduced morbidity and mortality, and have necessitated the development of regionalized, designated intensive care units. Regionalization and rationalization of specialized services have resulted in the need to transfer a growing number of patients from the institution where they first received care to a specialized unit. Increasingly, this interfacility transfer of patients is managed by transport teams because of recognition that injured infants and children can be extremely vulnerable during interhospital transfer.

Transport programs vary considerably, depending upon local geography, logistics and population. However, the priorities for transport teams in different locations are often similar and standards of care have now been established to enable the majority of these patients to be transported without harm from the inherent risks of the transport process itself. These programs are expensive, but prove cost-effective if long-term morbidity and duplication of specialist services are reduced. For some centers, transportation of critically ill patients over large distances is now an everyday occurrence. More often the distances between the referring and the receiving facilities are relatively short, and the practical difficulties stem from traffic congestion and the lack of availability of transport teams.

PRINCIPLES OF SAFE TRANSPORT

The principles of safe and appropriate transport can be summarized under the following headings.

WHO SHOULD BE TRANSPORTED?

Seriously ill or injured children are transported between hospitals because of their need for specialized facilities or treatment. The request for transfer is usually made when a referring physician perceives that further management of a child is—or soon will be—beyond the capabilities and resources of the local institution.

RESUSCITATION

Efficient and ongoing resuscitation is essential to successful transport outcome. Transport teams can contribute effectively to the extended resuscitation and stabilization of critically ill children. When necessary, the resuscitation effort should be guided by the transport director from the time of referral, and continued by the team upon arrival.

COMMUNICATION

Prompt, early, detailed and ongoing communication between the referring and receiving hospital is vital and must be documented. A written procedure should be established (and in place) in every institution likely to use the transport team's services. It is helpful for the referring hospital to be told the estimated time of arrival for the team, of any unexpected delays in the outward journey and of safe arrival at the receiving hospital. The transport director's experience should ensure that no key issues regarding care or transfer are overlooked by personnel at referring institutions who may rarely manage cases of such complexity. The transport director must communicate with the team to confirm that stabilization is as complete as possible prior to transfer, and have the ability to communicate during the transport to provide advice concerning the ongoing management of the patient if necessary.

STABILIZATION

Morbidity is lowest following transfer where maximum stabilization has occurred prior to the journey. In some patients only a relative degree of stabilization is feasible, but the maximum possible should be achieved before the child is transported. All appropriate services and specialists available at the referring hospital should be utilized, in addition to relevant advice from staff at the receiving institution.

It is common for the stabilization process to take an hour for patients requiring ventilation and longer for complex cases. Leaving the referring hospital means leaving the support of other staff and all investigative and laboratory facilities, hence the need for optimal stabilization prior to departure. Teams should not yield to inappropriate pressure from referring hospital staff to leave prematurely. Any areas of dispute should be discussed with the physician directing the transport who must be prepared to intervene to ensure appropriate action by the team on behalf of the patient.

Outreach education is an important means of educating the staff at referring hospitals. The stabilization process is not an indirect criticism of their care, but an essential part of safe and comprehensive transport. Education also promotes earlier recognition and referral of children requiring transfer and greater understanding of the benefits of two-way transport using trained teams. It has been observed that the more cases a hospital refers, the better their initial management becomes.

Specific treatment measures for stabilization and preparation for transport are included under individual conditions in the text. The priorities are shown in Table 1.5.1.

OPTIMAL TRANSPORT

Following stabilization, vital signs must be followed using monitoring equipment. Immediately prior to transport all patients should be checked to ensure the adequacy and security of lines and tubes and to evaluate physiological stability. It is particularly important to confirm that the patient is being appropriately ventilated (following initiation of assisted ventilation or transfer to the trans-

port team's ventilator). Many teams consider telephone discussion with the transport director obligatory at this point. A care plan must be made to cover the duration of the transport (Table 1.5.2).

ORGANIZING TRANSPORT IN AN EMERGENCY

If a protocol exists at your institution, follow it! If not, follow Table 1.5.3 and the outline below and initiate a protocol for subsequent transports.

Call early to obtain advice from the most suitable facility. If you delegate this call, give your delegate the questions you need answered regarding patient care management and transport logistics. Speak to the most senior physician possible at the receiving institution. Ask for a call back from this individual if your initial contact is with a member of junior staff. Obtain advice regarding further resuscitation, additional investigations, the stabilization process, starting definitive treatment, and plans and options available for treatment following transfer.

Speak with the child's relatives. Consider giving them the opportunity to visit their child briefly while treatment is in progress. Do not promise that a relative can travel with the child, but reassure the family that this issue will be discussed with them by the transport team. (There are benefits to a relative accompanying the child, but space

---

TABLE 1.5.1 Priorities for stabilization

1. Airway patency and adequate oxygen delivery (ventilation)
2. Intravenous access and support of the circulation
3. Control of bleeding
4. Stabilization of fractures or wounds
5. Provide sufficient, secure vascular access
6. Start diagnostic studies and definitive care

TABLE 1.5.2 Key elements of transport care plan

1. Respiratory support
2. Intravenous fluid requirements
3. Medications
4. Monitoring intervals for vital signs and neurological status
5. Specific interventions for potential complications (e.g. further respiratory compromise, hypotension, seizures, cardiac failure, arrhythmia, or high fever)
6. Consideration should also be given to special needs due to impending transfer over a long distance or at high altitude, and confirmation made that adequate supplies of oxygen, drugs, and fluid are carried to allow for rerouting or delays
7. Review of care plan with transport coordinator/physician at the receiving hospital

---

TABLE 1.5.3 **Sequence for emergency transport**
1. Call the receiving institution early
2. Obtain advice for ongoing resuscitation and stabilization
3. Speak with relatives
4. Prepare documents for transfer
5. Repeat blood tests and relevant investigations prior to arrival of team
6. Collaborate with team to optimize pretransport care (stabilization)
7. Review transport protocol after the journey as a quality assurance measure

is often limited in transport vehicles—hence the ultimate decision has to be made by the team.)

During pretransport care, have copies prepared of the history, laboratory data, radiographs, consent forms, and the patient's family and family physician information, and include specimens, e.g. blood for crossmatch, cerebrospinal fluid, blood cultures or placenta. Repeat relevant blood tests, radiography or other investigations prior to the arrival of the team. When the team arrives, collaborate with them to optimize care and complete the process of stabilization. Look for opportunities to learn from the exchange to benefit future patients requiring transfer. Anticipate that in preparation for transfer there will be checks made on or replacement of tubes, lines or treatments already initiated. This process is necessary because of the unforgiving nature of the transport environment and the extreme difficulty of replacing lost access in transit.

Following transport, review all aspects of case management with the aim of improving your hospital's future management of transport emergencies. Consider contacting the transport director and requesting continuing medical education in the area of transport.

EMERGENCY TRANSPORT IN THE ABSENCE OF A DEDICATED TEAM

If there is no dedicated transport team available to perform a two-way transfer from your institution, the following procedure is recommended.

Call the most suitable local facility for advice on pretransport patient management and confirm the ability of that institution to accept your patient. Stabilize the patient as fully as possible using the treatment suggestions made by the receiving institution. Pay particular attention to assessment of the airway and oxygen delivery, bearing in mind that it is likely that respiratory function will deteriorate during the journey, i.e. have a low threshold for electively intubating and assisting ventilation, particularly where ventilation is impaired through obtunded consciousness, central depression or cerebral hypoxia. Ensure that the tube is correctly placed and optimally secured. Also confirm that the method of assisted ventilation to be used in transit achieves appropriate gas exchange (if you are hand-bagging, check that the rate and pressure used is not adversely affecting PaO_2 or $PaCO_2$).

Make sure resuscitation of the circulation is optimal (restoration of normal blood pressure), that vascular access has been achieved with i.v. lines of sufficient size and number to guarantee sustained access, and that the lines are optimally secured.

Make a treatment plan that anticipates possible major problems (high fever, seizures, respiratory failure, hypotension, hypoglycemia) and prepare the necessary range of medications, with spare supplies to allow for error or delay. Provide warmth, pain relief and consider antiemetic medication. Have a low threshold for passing a nasogastric tube and urinary catheter in complex patients. Monitor the patient's oxygen saturation and heart rate as a minimum. Follow respiratory rate by auscultation if electronic monitoring is not available.

Avoid undue haste or inappropriate delay. Ensure the receiving hospital knows of your patient's status prior to departure, and review your care plan for transport with their receiving physician.

MODE OF TRANSPORT

Initially, trauma management concepts dictated rapid transfer and a 'scoop and run' philosophy. It is now recognized that the time taken to stabilize the patient in the referring hospital prior to transport dramatically decreases the incidence of secondary complications in transit. Also, neonatal survival improves if the fetus is transported in utero while the mother is in labour rather than the neonate transported after birth.

'One-way' transport with personnel from the referring hospital accompanying the child in transit was common. It is now known that there are major disadvantages associated with this practice, particularly with regard to the lack of familiarity of the transporting personnel with the transport environment, the likelihood of the equipment available proving inadequate and the high incidence of secondary complications which can occur during the journey. Moreover, small hospitals can rarely afford to part with staff necessary to escort the patient, even temporarily. Even less acceptable is to commit patients to the care of ambulance personnel unless they have specialized interhospital transport training. Generally these individuals lack the expertise required to monitor the patient's clinical status comprehensively or provide ongoing treatment for complex conditions and support vital functions appropriately. 'Two-way' transport can eliminate many of these difficulties, as a team from a receiving hospital travels to the referring hospital, to stabilize and then transfer the patient back. There are comprehensive guidelines for the organization and training of such teams. They have specialized equipment available designed for the transport environment, are directed by physicians and have experience with patient care during transport which ensures a high standard of care. There is no substitute for experience with large numbers of patients to optimize outcome.

One problem inherent in two-way transports is the time factor. The team must be able to respond promptly and achieve a safe, rapid transit to a referring hospital. The time taken for teams to be dispatched and reach the patient is often an issue for the referring hospital. However, the benefits of two-way transport generally outweigh the drawbacks, particularly if good communication is established early and advice provided regarding resuscitation and patient management in the interim.

TEAM COMPOSITION

The personnel on a transport team are its most important resource. Institutions use individuals from diverse backgrounds. The personnel involved and the skills available are dictated by the characteristics of the institution coordinating the team, and the geography and population of the area it serves. Some teams use specially trained ambulance personnel because these individuals are required to manage the ambulance and load the equipment and are therefore available to assist with the stabilization process at the referring institution. Other teams rely predominantly upon nursing personnel with additional training in transport medicine. In North America a team often includes a respiratory technician for the management of ventilated patients.

A physician may be part of the transport team. Studies attempting to assess the need for a physician on a specific transfer indicate that the subjective judgment of a transport director is at least as good as any scoring system. The level of training of physicians who participate in transports is variable, although the majority of programs use senior house officers/residents or fellows. Whatever the composition of a given team, success in transporting a patient safely generally relates most closely to the team's level of experience in dealing with the complex logistics of the transport process.

TRANSPORT DIRECTION

The physician directing the transport process at the receiving hospital is a crucial element for effective transport. This individual's role is to make correct decisions regarding the need for transport, provide advice for continuing resuscitation and care, and achieve prompt dispatch of an appropriate team. Commonly, the transport director is a member of the intensive care team on call. This individual has a major role in the standards of care provided during interfacility transport. The responsibilities of the transport director can be divided into those involving patient care (Table 1.5.4) and those involving team management (Table 1.5.5).

The value of expert direction of transport teams is increasingly recognized and such individuals are now a defined part of most national guidelines for air and ground transport of pediatric patients. These individuals not only improve the quality of care but are cost-efficient. In a well-established system, consultation with the referring hospital upon receipt of a transport request helps rationalize the

---

> **TABLE 1.5.4 Patient care responsibilities of a transport director**
>
> - Receiving requests for transport
> - Taking and documenting the medical facts
> - Providing immediate advice on resuscitation, investigation and care to the referring physician
> - Deciding whether transport is appropriate
> - Mobilizing a team of individuals with the necessary skills and provided with appropriate equipment and medication
> - Choosing a desirable mode of transportation
> - Advising the team while at the referral center and in transit
> - Organizing hospital admission

need for transport. In certain instances advice and assistance from the transport director may make it unnecessary for the patient to be transferred from the referring institution. Ideally, referring hospitals can access the transport director via a dedicated telephone line so that only one call is required to refer a patient. Where junior staff answer such calls initially, they should provide answers to the basic questions asked, obtain the name and location of the referring physician and relevant telephone numbers, then immediately contact the on-call physician acting as transport coordinator so that this individual can take over responsibility for the transport.

The vehicles used for transport vary. Ambulances and aircraft are generally not owned by the transferring institution and carriers such as the local ambulance services, air charter companies and the police or military are used. The needs of each community will vary and the important issue is that a defined structure is in place for appropriate vehicles to be made available promptly when transport is required. Air or road transport vehicles must be designed to accommodate the patient and personnel and all necessary equipment safely. The majority of transports involve road ambu-

lances, but helicopters have a defined place for rapid transfer, particularly from the scene of a motor vehicle injury or between institutions separated by traffic density or unusual geography. A variety of small, fixed-wing aircraft are suitable for longer transfers. Major factors affecting vehicle selection are summarized in Table 1.5.6. Local factors will influence the vehicles available in a given location. The equipment carried will be mandated by the training and role of individual teams, and should be selected and prepared in advance.

THE TRANSPORT ENVIRONMENT

The transport environment is 'user unfriendly', with restricted space and patient access, and isolation from familiar support services and equipment. In addition, lighting is often suboptimal and there is background noise and vibration. Restricted access and conditions within the transport vehicle may make it difficult or impossible to perform procedures such as intubation, intravenous insertion, or even a meaningful physical examination of the patient. Background noise makes auscultation of the chest and heart imprecise, and even relatively gross signs such as unequal air entry or arrhythmia are difficult to assess. Lighting within different vehicles varies but is often poor, and physical indicators of changes in oxygenation such as pallor or cyanosis must be substantial to be visible and recognized reliably.

Ensuring the warmth and security of the patient is part of basic transport care. Vibration, turbulence and noise can occur in the air and on the ground and contribute to motion sickness, which can cause discomfort, vomiting, aspiration or elevation of intracranial pressure; in addition, vibration can affect equipment settings, and interfere

---

> **TABLE 1.5.5 Team management responsibilities of the transport director**
>
> - Selecting, training, testing and skill maintenance of personnel
> - Equipment evaluation
> - Protocol development
> - Outreach education for units using the team
> - Quality assurance and research activities

> **TABLE 1.5.6 Factors affecting selection of transport mode**
>
> - The location and condition of the patient
> - Traffic volume
> - Distance between referring and receiving hospitals
> - Complexity of care required during transport
> - Potential cost

with or produce artefact on monitors. Cold stress is a particular concern in neonates and small children; frequent or continuous temperature monitoring is essential in these patients.

Both expected and unexpected movement occurs during transport, threatening all medical equipment and monitoring devices. All tracheal tubes, chest tubes, intravenous lines, arterial lines and urinary catheters must be secured carefully to avoid displacement during loading and unloading of the patient and during acceleration, deceleration or turbulence. Equipment must be loaded and anchored where it is visible or readily accessible, or placed in storage if not required.

The transport of patients by air raises potential problems in addition to those related to ground transport. The basic principles of aviation physiology must be appreciated before transporting any child by air. These include the risk of hypoxia due to the fall in oxygen tension and Pao_2 with increasing altitude, and dysbarism where gas expansion occurs with decreases in atmospheric pressure. Dysbarism causes particular problems in regard to pneumothorax, pneumomediastinum and air in the bowel wall or cranium. Knowledge of these issues and aircraft pressurization characteristics is part of the mandate of the transport director, and an expectation of transport team personnel. The transport team must be aware of the special attention that their equipment requires at altitude, e.g. all tracheal tube cuffs and Foley catheter balloons must be filled with 0.9% saline to avoid pressure problems due to expansion at altitude. Inflatable splints should not be used and intravenous flow rates will vary unless they are controlled by infusion pumps. Potentially fatal hemolysis of crossmatched blood can occur during transport. All blood components require correct packaging and care. Follow the directions of the issuing laboratory conscientiously and refer any questions to them. Guidelines for packaging blood components for transport are summarized below.

PACKAGING PROCEDURES FOR SAFE TRANSPORT OF BLOOD COMPONENTS

All blood components (packed red cells, frozen plasma and platelets) should be packaged and shipped according to the following general procedures (developed by the Canadian Red Cross Blood Service) or comparable guidelines from your regional blood center. Care must be taken with all blood products to avoid damage to the containers or leakage. Whole blood, especially fresh whole blood, is rarely available. Packed red blood cells with a hematocrit of 0.55 are most often supplied.

- All blood components should be transported enclosed within a plastic liner (plastic bag) inside an insulated Styrofoam shipping box. The lid should be attached securely.
- When shipping only a few units per box, packing material such as newspaper should be used to fill the dead space and prevent the items from moving during transport. This will also help stabilize the internal temperature of the cooler.
- The blood components should be placed inside the plastic bag liner inside the box and the top of the plastic liner should be twisted or tucked to close it. Then, depending on the nature of the products, cardboard should be inserted as insulation, with a cooling pack on top (for packed red blood cells or thawed plasma) or a dead space filler should be inserted (for platelets). The lid of the Styrofoam box should be secured. If a Red Cross shipping box is used, the outer cardboard container should be closed and the belt should be secured (these belts should not be tied in knots or cut to open the container).
- All documentation in relation to the blood products should be placed on top of the Styrofoam lid inside the cardboard container. These documents should not be placed inside the plastic liner or inside the Styrofoam box in case of spillage. Packaging procedures for each blood product must ensure appropriate storage temperatures to maintain the viability of each specific product. Packaging instructions with the product should be found and checked with the blood bank issuing the material.

Packed red cells

Up to 10 units of packed red cells can be placed upright in a Red Cross storage box. A piece of insulating cardboard must be placed on top of the plastic bag containing the red cell units to separate them from the cooling pack. The cooling pack is placed on top of the cardboard and must not be under the red cells or come into direct contact with the red cell units (to avoid hemolysis). A large enough piece of cardboard should be used to completely separate the cooling pack from the blood unit. Dry ice must not be used. General packaging instructions should be checked with the issuing laboratory.

Plasma (previously frozen, thawed for transfusion)

Plasma intended for use during transport will be supplied thawed in a Red Cross storage box. Packaging procedures can be the same as for packed red cells (see above). After thawing, and before infusion, plasma should be kept cool ($1–10°C$) ($33.8–50.0°F$) in transit. Hemolysis will not occur because of excessive cooling, but plasma should not be infused until it has thawed completely.

Platelet concentrate

Platelet concentrate is shipped at room temperature i.e. about $20°C$ ($68°F$). Measures must be taken to ensure that excessive cooling or warming does not occur in transit. The specific nature of each team's transport environment must be considered for each shipment. Transport in the type of container used for other blood products is generally adequate, but platelet concentrate must be stored separately (i.e. not carried in the same container as packed red cells). Additional advice can be obtained from the issuing laboratory.

Platelet packs are placed flat in the base of the shipping box within the plastic liner. Dead space can be filled with newspaper.

(*Note* – the above guidelines are reproduced from Macnab AJ, Pattman B, Wadsworth LD. Potentially fatal hemolysis of cross-matched blood during interfacility transport: standards of practice for safe transport of safe blood products. Air Med J 1996; 15(2): 69–72.

Specific packaging instructions and/or the issuing laboratory should be checked.

TRANSPORT MONITORING

Because conditions in the transport environment make clinical judgement potentially unreliable, monitoring equipment specifically designed for transport is essential. Transport equipment, now widely available, is sophisticated, compact, reliable and capable of battery operation. Most of the difficulties with earlier equipment (vibration sensitivity, loss of signal during radio transmission, electromagnetic interference with aircraft avionics, large size and weight, high power consumption and limited monitoring capabilities) have been overcome.

The new monitors significantly increase the ability of escorts to detect impending problems during transport. The monitoring of heart and respiratory rate, temperature and oxygen saturation has become standard practice. In addition, central venous or arterial pressure monitoring and end-tidal carbon dioxide monitoring are now commonplace. Portable analyzers are now available that allow blood gas analysis and basic hematology and chemistry investigations to be done in transit or to speed stabilization and decrease transport time.

TRANSPORT POPULATION

Although the range of medical and surgical conditions that a transport team may encounter is extensive, respiratory and neurological problems predominate in pediatrics. Amongst neonates, prematurity, respiratory distress, 'presumed sepsis' and congenital abnormalities are the major diagnoses. Children needing transplant procedures require meticulous pretransport planning as many have multiple special needs or are critically ill. Transport of a child presumed to be brain-dead may be necessary on largely compassionate grounds, for metabolic autopsy, or if the child is a potential organ donor. Optimal physiological stability in transit (Ch. 5.9) increases the chances of successful transplantation.

Whatever the diagnosis or age, the risks for the transported child include those from the underlying disease, the treatment instituted and the transfer itself. Transported patients are particularly vulnerable to deterioration resulting from their underlying illness, respiratory failure and secondary insults that may occur during transport. These must be actively anticipated by the team prior to the journey and measures taken to prevent—or at least moderate—these potential consequences of transport. This process is aided by making a transport care plan for each patient and using a predeparture checklist (Table 1.5.7). This anticipation and 'preventive' approach to transport care can considerably reduce the incidence of secondary insults resulting from avoidable deterioration or complications in transit. The standards of care for provision, organization and performance of interfacility transport that have been adopted in most countries can minimize these risks. Quality assurance measures such as physiological stability during the call, postcall review by the transport coordinator and appropriate feedback for the transport team and referring hospital staff also contribute to this process (continuing education). The electronic exchange of data or images (telemedicine) is beginning to rationalize decisions regarding transport. The misreading of cervical spine radiographs in referring hospitals is a frequent cause of unnecessary patient transfer.

RESEARCH AND QUALITY ASSURANCE

The transport environment is not an easy one to research; neither patients nor the referring institution can realistically become a control group, and patient populations and level of treatment vary greatly between centers. Despite these obstacles the standard and scope of research are improving. Comparisons and audits are increasingly commonplace in intensive care using a variety of scoring methods. Data collection using such objective score criteria (e.g. the Paediatric Index of Mortality score, PIM) and continuous quality improvement review should be a part of every transport program to ensure that appropriate standards of care are maintained and improve over time.

TABLE 1.5.7 **Predeparture checklist**	
• Airway, ventilation	Need intubation?
	ETT position correct and secure?
	Blood gas satisfactory?
	ETT patent — suction handy?
	Ventilator settings checked?
	Oxygen supply adequate?
	Bag and mask handy?
• Circulation	Fully resuscitated?
	Volume handy for journey if required?
	Blood pressure monitored?
	Secure venous/arterial access?
	Inotropes infusing?
• Drugs, fluid	All potentially necessary drugs handy?
	All infusions functioning and secure?
	Enough drugs and fluids for journey?
	Biochemical abnormalities corrected?
• Monitors	Functioning and alarms set?
	Secured?
• Miscellaneous	Nasogastric tube in place, on free drainage?
	Urinary catheter in place?
	Chest drain connected to Heimlich valve?
• Information, communication	Referral letter and investigation results?
	Parents fully informed?
	Any consent needed for procedure at receiving hospital?
	Receiving hospital staff aware of patient and transport details?
	Transport providers ready?

ETT, endotracheal tube.

Although the principles of transport management appear simple, they are effective and can virtually eliminate transport-related mortality and morbidity. Moreover, they now constitute the accepted standard of care medicolegally in many jurisdictions. Transport by specialized teams is an integral part of regionalized health care delivery. A well-equipped, properly trained and appropriately directed team can provide a level of care closely comparable to that provided in most intensive care units.

✔ **KEY POINTS**

➤ The potential need for interhospital transport of any critically ill child should be discussed promptly with a regional specialist PICU

➤ Interhospital transfer of critically ill children should be undertaken by specialist pediatric emergency transport teams

➤ Transport teams should operate according to clear administrative and clinical protocols

➤ Patients should not be transferred without prior resuscitation and preparation

➤ Clear communication is essential throughout the transport process

➤ Air transport presents additional unique problems and should be undertaken only by specially trained personnel

✗ **COMMON ERRORS**

➤ Communication delayed or not initiated; only occurs between junior staff; or dialog not maintained as patient changes

➤ Inadequate resuscitation

➤ Incomplete stabilization (particularly of airway, breathing and circulation)

➤ Failure to anticipate respiratory failure or other potential deterioration in transit

➤ Lack of awareness of complications possible from ascent to altitude

➤ Failure to notify referring hospital staff of the safe arrival of the child/team at the receiving institution

➤ Not using a trained transport team when available

FURTHER READING

1. Day SE. Intra-transport stabilization and management of the pediatric patient. Pediatr Clin North Am 1993; 40(2): 263–274
   – (*A review of pretransport stabilization of children*)

2. Macnab AJ. Optimal escort for inter-hospital transport of pediatric emergencies. J Trauma 1991; 31: 205–209
   – (*The reduction in morbidity achieved by avoidance of secondary insults during transport*)

3. McCloskey KA, Orr RA. Pediatric transport issues in emergency medicine. Emerg Med Clin North Am 1991; 9: 475–489

4. Macrae DJ. Paediatric intensive care transport. Arch Dis Child 1994; 71: 175–178

5. Henning R. Pediatric transport. In: Morton NS, Pollack MM, Wallace PGH, editors. Stabilization and transport of the critically ill. New York: Churchill Livingstone; 1997

6. American Academy of Pediatrics. Task force on interhospital transports: guidelines for air and ground transport of neonatal and pediatric patients, Elk Grove: AAP; 1993

7. Society for Critical Care Medicine Joint Task Force. Guidelines for the safe transfer of critically ill patients. Crit Care Med 1993; 21: 931–937

8. Macnab AJ. Paediatric interfacility transport: organization and principles. Paed Anaesth 1994; 4: 351–357
   – (*Six papers on the principles, organization and standards of care for pediatric transport*)

9. Whitfield JM, Buser NNP. Transport stabilization times for neonatal and pediatric patients prior to interfacility transfer. Ped Emerg Care 1993; 9: 69–71
   – (*Documentation of mean times for stabilization at the referring hospital*)

10. Macnab AJ, Richards J, Green G. Family oriented care practices during paediatric interfacility transport. Patient Education and Counselling 1999; 36: 3247–3257
    (*Evaluation of communication practices preferred by families*)

11. Shann F, Pearson G, Slater A, Wilkinson K. Paediatric index of mortality (PIM): a mortality prediction model for children in intensive care. Intens Care Med 1997; 23: 201–207
    – (*The PIM score*)

12. McCloskey K, Orr R, editors. Pediatric transport medicine. St. Louis: Mosby; 1995
    – (*A comprehensive text covering all areas of pediatric transport*)

13. Devellis P, Thomas SH, Wedel SK, Stein JP and Vinci RJ. Prehospital fentanyl analgesia in air-transported pediatric trauma patients. Ped Emerg Care 1998; 14(5): 321–323
    (*No adverse effects in 211 uses of fentanyl over 5.5 years on retrospective review of 131 patients, mean age 6.2 years mean GCS 9*)

Organ system failure

2

2.1 Respiratory failure

Robert Henning

Respiratory failure is the inability of the respiratory system to maintain adequate oxygen and carbon dioxide homeostasis. In a child with respiratory failure, the respiratory system is unable to transfer the volumes of oxygen and carbon dioxide needed by the body's metabolism, or can only do so at the expense of a decreased partial pressure of oxygen or an increased partial pressure of carbon dioxide in arterial blood.

Although one can arbitrarily select values of arterial P_{O_2} and arterial P_{CO_2} beyond which respiratory failure is said to be present—for example, Pa_{O_2} 6.5 kPa (<50 mmHg) and Pa_{CO_2} >6.5 kPa (50 mmHg), breathing >50% oxygen at sea level these values can only be a guide in practice. For example, a Pa_{O_2} of 4 kPa (30 mmHg) may represent severe respiratory failure in a previously normal child but may be usual in an infant with cyanotic congenital heart disease, in whom the cause of the low Pa_{O_2} is unrelated to respiratory disease. The arterial P_{O_2} depends on the F_{IO_2} which often cannot safely be reduced merely to establish the diagnosis of 'respiratory failure'.

Management and prognosis in most cases of respiratory failure are guided by a combination of factors including the underlying disease, the child's clinical state and its rate of change and response to treatment, rather than a label of respiratory failure. For example, one would commence mechanical ventilation at a much lesser degree of hypoxemia or hypercarbia in a preterm baby or a child with shock or a severe head injury, than in a fit adolescent with asthma.

CAUSES OF HYPOXEMIA

The causes of hypoxemia in a child breathing air at sea level may be classified as ventilatory or non-ventilatory.

VENTILATORY

When the alveolar ventilation is inadequate; the Pa_{CO_2} increases and the Pa_{O_2} falls. The most common causes are diseases of the large and small airways or of the lung parenchyma; disorders of the central nervous system, the neuromuscular pathways or of the chest wall contribute fewer cases. In children with disease of the lung parenchyma or small airways with ventilation–perfusion inequality or intrapulmonary right-to-left shunting, the child can maintain a normal or even low Pa_{CO_2} by overventilating the alveoli that remain ventilated and perfused. When too few of these are left, or when respiratory muscle fatigue or central nervous depression (e.g. due to sedative drugs) supervenes, the Pa_{CO_2} will rise. This occurs for example, in a child with severe acute asthma.

NON-VENTILATORY

In non-ventilatory hypoxemia, the Pa_{CO_2} is low or normal provided that the respiratory system can increase the ventilation of the remaining perfused alveoli sufficiently to maintain CO_2 homeostasis. Its causes are:

- right-to-left shunt which may be intrapulmonary or extrapulmonary
- diffusion block
- ventilation–perfusion inequality

These causes may coexist. For example, a child with heart failure and pulmonary edema may have ventilation–perfusion inequality in some partly ventilated alveoli; shunt due to perfusion of alveoli which are filled with edema fluid and unventilated; diffusion block caused by thickening of alveolar septa; and hypoventilation because of respiratory muscle fatigue. Breathing air with a low P_{O_2} (e.g. due to low barometric pressure in an aircraft during interhospital transport) causes hypoxemia and exacerbates that due to other causes.

It is important to determine if the cause of respiratory failure in a given child is mainly ventilatory (requiring treatment to improve the alveolar ventilation such as bronchodilator therapy in asthma, nebulized epinephrine (adrenaline) or tracheal intubation in croup, or mechanical ventilation in neuromuscular disease) or mainly an oxygenation defect (requiring oxygen therapy by mask or nasal catheter, administration of continuous positive airway pressure (CPAP) by mask, nasopharyngeal tube or endotracheal tube), or mechanical ventilation with positive end-expiratory pressure (PEEP).

Abnormalities at several sites in the respiratory pathway often contribute to the respiratory failure (for example, in an asthmatic child, small airways disease, a pneumothorax and respiratory muscle

fatigue may combine to cause respiratory failure). Correcting one of those abnormalities (e.g. drainage of the pneumothorax) may be enough to relieve the respiratory failure.

APPROACH TO A CHILD WITH SUSPECTED RESPIRATORY FAILURE

During the initial assessment of any seriously ill child, the airway, breathing and circulation are assessed, and resuscitation measures commenced simultaneously (Ch. 2.2).

DIAGNOSIS OF RESPIRATORY FAILURE

INADEQUATE GAS EXCHANGE

A hypoxic child may be restless, confused or unconscious. Central cyanosis implies the presence of at least 30–50 g/L of unsaturated hemoglobin, although anemia, skin vasoconstriction and artificial lighting may prevent detection of cyanosis even when the saturation is low. Hypercarbia causes drowsiness, stupor or coma, warm sweaty skin, tachycardia and bounding pulses.

Although the diagnosis of respiratory failure is usually made on clinical grounds, arterial blood gas analysis is used to confirm the diagnosis and assess the severity of the problem. A raised arterial P_{CO_2} means hypoventilation or, in the presence of lung disease, inability of the respiratory system to increase alveolar ventilation sufficiently to maintain a normal Pa_{CO_2}. In the presence of hypoxemia, the magnitude of the oxygenation defect can be estimated by the alveolar-arterial oxygen difference (Aa_{DO_2}) (see box).

$$Aa_{DO_2} = P_{A_{O_2}} - Pa_{O_2})\ kPa$$
$$P_{A_{O_2}} = (P_{I_{O_2}} - Pa_{CO_2}/R)\ kPa$$

Pa_{O_2} and Pa_{CO_2} (which is approximately equal to $P_{A_{CO_2}}$) are obtained from blood gas analysis
$P_{I_{O_2}} = F_{I_{O_2}} \times$ (barometric pressure − 47) in mmHg = $F_{I_{O_2}} \times$ (barometric pressure − 6.3) in kPa
R is the respiratory quotient (approximately 0.8 in children on a normal diet)

The Aa_{DO_2} is high 6–7 kPa (45–55 mmHg) in the newborn, but decreases to normal adult values of

1–2 kPa (7–15 mmHg) after a few weeks. In a hypoxemic infant, measuring the Pao_2 while the child breathes 100% oxygen may distinguish between ventilation-perfusion mismatch (due to lung disease) and right-to-left shunt (usually due to cyanotic congenital heart disease). Administration of 100% oxygen greatly increases the Pao_2 in V/Q mismatch but not if right-to-left shunt is a major cause of the hypoxemia.

Gas exchange in a child with suspected respiratory failure should be monitored continuously by noninvasive means such as pulse oximetry or transcutaneous Po_2 or Pco_2 measurement (Ch. 6.6). In a child with lung disease, the relationship between the end-tidal Pco_2 and the arterial Pco_2 is too unsteady and unpredictable for end-tidal Pco_2 monitoring to be a useful indicator of $Paco_2$, while the accuracy of transcutaneous Po_2 and Pco_2 measurement is reduced when the skin perfusion is poor. Insertion of an arterial cannula for repeated blood gas analysis is justified if the child's respiratory failure is severe and is not responding rapidly to treatment, or if the child's blood pressure is sufficiently unstable to require invasive monitoring.

INCREASED RESPIRATORY EFFORT

A child whose respiratory drive is increased may feel dyspneic and appear distressed; tachypnea, an expiratory grunt and flaring of the alae nasi appear. Table 2.1.1 shows the normal respiratory rate at different ages. A steadily rising respiratory rate, especially if associated with an increasing tachycardia, is an ominous sign of imminent respiratory failure. When the lungs are noncompliant or the airway resistance is high, a more negative intrapleural pressure is needed to inflate the lungs during inspiration: this causes intercostal, subcostal and sternal retraction and a tracheal tug. The use of the accessory muscles of respiration such as the sternomastoids implies severely increased respiratory effort.

CAUSES OF RESPIRATORY FAILURE

The causes of respiratory failure in children are summarized in Table 2.1.2.

The presence of stridor implies an abnormality of the extrathoracic airway (Table 2.1.3), while wheezing heard at the lips or on auscultation of the chest indicates a problem in the intrathoracic airways. In an unconscious child, respiratory failure associated with stridor may sometimes be relieved by adjusting the position of the child's neck or jaw (implying that poor muscle control of the pharynx or tongue is the main problem) or by gentle pharyngeal suction (if pooling of saliva due to an inadequate swallowing reflex is obstructing the airway). Investigation of respiratory failure due to upper airway obstruction may require a lateral neck X-ray (if the presence of a foreign body or retropharyngeal abscess are suspected, and in the few children in whom the diagnosis of acute epiglottitis cannot be established clinically and who have minimal airway obstruction).

Awake fiberoptic pharyngoscopy or laryngoscopy under local anesthesia may be useful to establish the cause of obstruction if a supraglottic foreign body or anatomical lesion is suspected, although these procedures are clearly inappropriate and dangerous if one suspects the presence of acute epiglottitis or retropharyngeal abscess. When the lesion appears clinically to be below the glottis, laryngeal examination under anesthesia and rigid or fiberoptic bronchoscopy or esophagoscopy may be needed. Functional studies such as flow volume loops are rarely useful in the diagnosis and acute management of severe upper airway obstruction in children.

Once the nature of the upper airway obstruction causing respiratory failure has been established, management involves securing the airway: if possible by conservative means such as administration of nebulized epinephrine (adrenaline) in croup, or adjustment of the jaw position in an unconscious child, but if necessary by tracheal intubation (Ch. 6.2). Rarely, emergency or semi-elective tracheostomy may be required (e.g. in a child with severe obstruction due to laryngeal trauma, or a subglottic hemangioma). In most cases requiring tracheal intubation, passage of a nasotracheal or orotracheal tube by an

TABLE 2.1.1 **Changes in the normal respiratory rate with age**							
	Age (years)						
	Newborn	1	2	5	10	15	Adult
Breaths per minute	36	25	25	22	19	18	15

experienced intubator is safer than emergency tracheostomy. After intubation or tracheostomy, the child's safety depends on close observation, secure fixation of the tube, adequate humidification of inspired gas and on adequate tracheal suction (Ch. 6.2). Details of the indications for and duration of intubation in individual conditions are given in Ch. 3.1.

Wheezing at the lips associated with widespread crackles on chest auscultation in an infant suggests the diagnosis of viral bronchiolitis. Although an attack of bronchodilator-responsive wheezing in a known asthmatic patient is not usually a problem in diagnosis, other diagnoses than asthma should be considered in a first attack of wheezing, especially when there is little response

---

TABLE 2.1.2 Causes of respiratory failure in childhood

Diseases of the central nervous system
- **Drugs**
  Sedatives, narcotics, general anesthetic agents
  Poisoning
- **Metabolic disorders**
  Hypoxia, hypercapnia
  Hyper/hypoglycemia
  Hyponatremia
  Hypocalcemia
  Hyperammonemia
- **Infections**
  Meningitis
  Encephalitis
  Bulbar poliomyelitis
- **Postinfectious**
  Guillain-Barré syndrome
- **Brain-stem abnormalities**
  (e.g. Arnold–Chiari malformation)
- **Bone disorders affecting the brain-stem**
  Osteogenesis imperfecta
  Achondroplasia
- **Other**
  Seizures
  Raised intracranial pressure of any cause
  Brain-stem trauma
  Central alveolar hypoventilation

Neuromuscular diseases
- **Drugs**
  Muscle relaxants
  Anticholinesterases
  Glucocorticoids
- **Trauma**
  Spinal cord
  Phrenic nerve
  Diaphragm
- **Metabolic**
  Starvation
  Uremia
  Hypermagnesemia
  Acute intermittent porphyria
  Hypophosphatemia

- **Infection**
  Tetanus
  Botulism
  Diphtheria
- **Other**
  Myasthenia gravis
  Spinal muscular atrophy
  Other muscular dystrophies
  Envenomations (tick, tetrodotoxin, snake)
  Respiratory muscle fatigue

Disorders of pulmonary bellows function
- **Chest wall**
  Kyphoscoliosis
  Asphyxiating thoracic dystrophy
  Chest wall burns or edema
- **Pleura**
  Hemothorax
  Pneumothorax
  Pleural effusion

Airway disorders
- **Upper airways obstruction**
  Nose
  Pharynx
  Larynx
  Trachea
  Bronchi
- **Small airways disease**
  Asthma
  Viral bronchiolitis
  Bronchiolitis obliterans
  Burn inhalation injury

Disorders of the lung parenchyma (e.g. pneumonia, pulmonary edema, pulmonary fibrosis, pulmonary alveolar proteinosis)

Congenital malformations of the lung (e.g. pulmonary hypoplasia, congenital lobar emphysema, lung sequestrations)

Pulmonary vascular disorders (e.g. primary pulmonary hypertension, pulmonary arteriovenous malformations and pulmonary embolism)

TABLE 2.1.3 Differential diagnosis of upper airway obstruction

	Croup	Epiglottitis	Foreign body	Tracheitis	Retropharyngeal abscess
Stridor:					
pitch	High	Low	High	High	Low
timing	Insp	Exp	Variable	Insp + Exp	Insp
Fever	Moderate	High	Nil	High	High
Toxic	−	++	−	++	++
History of choking	−	−	+	−	−
Cough	++	−	+	++	−
Dysphonia	−	+	±	−	+
Tender trachea	−	+	±	++	±
Trismus	−	−	−	−	+

Exp, expiratory; Insp, inspiratory.

to bronchodilators (Table 2.1.4). Unless the cause of wheezing is obvious from the child's history and physical examination, an anteroposterior (AP) and lateral chest X-ray should be obtained, which may show a radio-opaque foreign body, narrowing or deviation of the tracheal air column (e.g. due to a mediastinal cyst) or patchy alveolar infiltrates (e.g. in recurrent aspiration). Other investigations which may be needed to elucidate the cause of wheezing are discussed in Chapter 3.1.

In a child with severe respiratory failure and wheezing, if no further diagnostic information is immediately available, it is reasonable to give a trial of a nebulized β_2-sympathomimetic drug (Ch. 3.1) and assess the effect on the child's clinical signs and gas exchange. Unless the bronchodilator reverses the narrowing of the small airways, it may reduce the hemoglobin saturation even further by inhibiting hypoxic pulmonary vasoconstriction in the presence of alveolar disease. Uncommonly, children with wheezing and respiratory failure continue to deteriorate despite treatment and require ventilatory support (see below).

Reduced air entry or inspiratory crackles on auscultation, dullness on percussion or poor chest wall movement may indicate disease of the lung parenchyma or pleura. In children with impaired consciousness or reduced muscle power, the presence or absence of significant lung or chest wall disease and the rate of progression of the child's respiratory failure may show whether the unconsciousness is causing the respiratory failure or vice versa.

The priorities of management in children with neuromuscular, chest wall or parenchymal lung disease are:

1. Maintain the child's life by supporting gas exchange if necessary during examination and investigation.
2. Establish (by history, examination and blood gas analysis) whether the main problem is hypoventilation, or an oxygenation defect (see above).
3. Adopt the appropriate means of respiratory support (see below).
4. Investigate and treat any treatable causes of respiratory failure (e.g. perform a urine drug screen and give naloxone for opiate intoxication, or perform cultures of tracheal aspirate, blood or lung biopsy specimen and give antibiotics for bacterial pneumonia).

SUPPORT OF ALVEOLAR VENTILATION

When the cause of hypoventilation is upper airway obstruction, treatment is aimed at securing an adequate airway by adjusting the jaw position in an unconscious child, giving nebulized epinephrine (adrenaline) for croup or postextubation stridor, by removing a foreign body and, if necessary, by inserting an endotracheal tube (Ch. 6.2). Artificial ventilation is not necessary unless disease of the lung parenchyma or small airways is also present (e.g. postintubation pulmonary edema in severe croup, or extensive bronchomalacia). In some cases of disease of the small airways or alveoli (e.g. viral bronchiolitis, mild to moderately severe ARDS, or *Pneumocystis carinii* pneumonia), a trial of noninvasive support using CPAP by nasal mask, full face mask or nasopharyngeal

TABLE 2.1.4 **Causes of wheezing in childhood**	
	Age group involved
Acute	
Asthma	Infant or child
Viral bronchiolitis	Infant
Foreign body	Infant or child
Mycoplasma pneumoniae infection	Child
Anaphylaxis	Child
Recurrent or chronic	
Asthma	Infant or child
Cystic fibrosis	Infant or child
Recurrent aspiration pneumonitis	Infant or child
Tracheobronchomalacia	Infant or child
Tracheal stenosis	Infant or child
Vascular ring	Infant or child
Bronchiolitis obliterans	Infant or child
Mediastinal tumors, cysts or tuberculous lymphadenopathy	Infant or child

cannula may allow endotracheal intubation and its complications (Ch. 6.2) to be avoided.

SUPPORT OF OXYGENATION

A child with hypoxemia due to hypoventilation requires support of alveolar ventilation (Ch. 6.4), but when the hypoxemia is not due solely to hypoventilation, added oxygen should be given by mask (4–8 L/min), nasal catheter, nasal prongs or head box.

Nasal catheters should be inserted into the nostril for a distance 1 cm less than the distance from the nares to the tragus. An oxygen flow of 150 ml/kg min through a catheter in this position gives an FIO_2 of 0.4–0.6. Nasal prongs and catheters inserted a shorter distance are not capable of delivering as high an FIO_2, although they are less likely to suffer the problems of catheter blockage with mucus and gastric distention which are sometimes seen with nasopharyngeal catheters.

In small infants, oxygen-enriched air may be more conveniently given by headbox. The larger the head box, the higher the gas flow needed to prevent rebreathing of CO_2 within the box: in general, flows not less than 12 L/min are required. The concentration of oxygen in the gas entering a head box should be controlled by an air–oxygen blender or, in the absence of a supply of compressed air from pipes or cylinders, by using an oxygen-driven, air-entraining Venturi device.

Controlling the oxygen concentration in the head box by varying the flow rate of oxygen causes rebreathing and hence hypercarbia at low oxygen flow rates.

The concentration of oxygen in the head box should be monitored continuously or at least hourly, using an oxygen meter, usually of the fuel cell type. The gas should be humidified, as gas from cylinders or from the hospital oxygen supply is much drier than room air and its inhalation leads to heat loss, airway obstruction and atelectasis due to mucus crusting in airways.

Adequate oxygen therapy is sometimes mistakenly withheld from children with acute exacerbations of conditions such as asthma for fear of suppressing the hypoxic respiratory drive and causing severe respiratory acidosis. This is only likely to occur in children with severe exercise limitation due to chronic respiratory failure in conditions such as muscular dystrophy and terminal cystic fibrosis. It virtually never occurs in childhood asthma. In conditions in which the risk is significant, the safest course is to give 30–35% oxygen and monitor the blood gases (including the $PaCO_2$) carefully. Transcutaneous PCO_2 monitoring is often useful.

If oxygen therapy alone fails to restore adequate levels of PaO_2, CPAP may be needed. This may be delivered by a normal ventilator circuit and a nasopharyngeal tube (a conventional endotracheal tube positioned in the nasopharynx as described above) or by nasal mask. Pressures of 5–15 cmH$_2$O (0.5–1.5 kPa) may be applied in this way and this method has been used successfully in the management of acute bronchiolitis and pertussis in infants, and in pulmonary edema, ARDS and viral and *Pneumocystis carinii* pneumonia in older children.

Should nasopharyngeal CPAP fail to improve the child's oxygenation, or if hypoventilation is present as well as an oxygenation defect, mechanical ventilation with PEEP 5–15 cmH$_2$O (0.5–1.5 kPa) may be needed. This requires tracheal intubation (Ch. 6.2). Appropriate modes of mechanical ventilation are described in Chapter 6.4. As discussed above, controlled mechanical hypoventilation is now regarded as the most appropriate technique of mechanical ventilation in children with impaired oxygen transfer within the lung.

If adequate gas exchange cannot be sustained by conventional mechanical ventilation using airway pressures and F_{IO_2} which are low enough to minimize the risk of chronic iatrogenic lung injury, then a trial of high-frequency oscillatory ventilation is justified. This method is most likely to be useful in parenchymal lung disease which is unevenly distributed throughout the lung (e.g. lobar pneumonia) or in the presence of major air leak (e.g. bronchopleural fistula). It has never been shown to be useful in the ventilation of patients in status asthmaticus.

When all methods of conventional ventilation have failed to support adequate gas exchange, some form of extracorporeal life support may be needed (Ch. 6.7). This is usually venovenous ECLS unless the heart and circulation cannot maintain an adequate cardiac output and blood pressure to supply the metabolic needs of the tissues (e.g. when septic shock and respiratory failure coexist), in which case venoarterial ECLS is required. The use of ECLS is justifiable only if:

- the child's lung disease is potentially reversible
- the child is most unlikely to survive without ECLS
- the child has a reasonable prospect of enjoying an acceptable quality of life after recovery from the lung disease

OTHER METHODS OF IMPROVING GAS EXCHANGE

BRONCHODILATORS

By reducing the resistance of narrowed bronchioles, bronchodilatory drugs (Ch. 3.1) increase the total alveolar ventilation (reducing $Paco_2$), decrease the intrapulmonary right-to-left shunt and improve ventilation–perfusion matching (thereby reducing $AaDo_2$ and increasing arterial Po_2). Beta-2-sympathomimetic drugs such as salbutamol (albuterol) also reduce hypoxic pulmonary vasoconstriction, which tends to increase the $AaDo_2$. If these drugs are given to a child with lung disease such as pneumonia, the hemoglobin saturation falls further unless bronchodilator-responsive bronchoconstriction is a major cause of the hypoxemia. Intravenous preparations are more likely to have this effect than inhaled preparations.

CORTICOSTEROIDS

Corticosteroids are known to improve gas exchange (in combination with β_2-sympathomimetic drugs) in asthma and to relieve airway obstruction in viral croup. They have been shown to improve gas exchange in AIDS-associated *Pneumocystis carinii* pneumonia and to shorten time on a ventilator in infants with bronchopulmonary dysplasia. They are commonly used with reported success in postextubation upper airway obstruction, in bronchiolitis obliterans organizing pneumonia (e.g. after adenovirus infection) and in interstitial pneumonitis (e.g. drug-associated).

DIURETICS

Diuretics reduce lung water in cardiogenic and noncardiogenic pulmonary edema, improving gas diffusion and ventilation–perfusion matching in the lung. Excessive diuresis sufficient to cause hypovolemia, however, may impair gas exchange by reducing the cardiac output (see below). A trial of diuretic therapy is commonly used to accelerate weaning from ventilation in infants with bronchopulmonary dysplasia.

EXOGENOUS SURFACTANT

Exogenous surfactant, as prophylaxis or as rescue therapy, reduces the risk of mortality and morbidity in newborns with hyaline membrane disease. Numerous anecdotal reports have been published of the successful use of surfactant in newborns with congenital diaphragmatic hernia or meconium aspiration syndrome and in older children with ARDS or viral pneumonia, but the results of controlled trials are not yet available.

NITRIC OXIDE

Nitric oxide inhalation (1–10 parts per million) reduces pulmonary vascular resistance in infants and adults with labile (but not with fixed) pulmonary hypertension. Nitric oxide inhalation also increases blood flow to ventilated alveoli and thereby improves ventilation–perfusion matching in ARDS and probably also in other lung diseases such as pneumonia. Nitric oxide therapy requires care and experience in administration, scavenging and monitoring to avoid toxicity to the lung (from NO_2) and to staff.

INCREASING CARDIAC OUTPUT

Measures to increase the cardiac output (e.g. plasma volume expansion and inotropic drug infusion) may improve gas exchange, especially in the ventilated patient, by improving the perfusion of underperfused alveoli.

PRONE POSITIONING

Prone positioning may improve gas exchange in children who need mechanical ventilation for severe lung disease, by improving the ventilation of well-perfused alveoli in dorsal areas of the lung.

✔ KEY POINTS

➤ It is important to determine whether the main problem is impaired ventilation (high $PaCO_2$) or whether it is oxygenation defect (normal or low $PaCO_2$)

➤ If oxygenation improves markedly on giving 100% oxygen, the hypoxemia is due to lung disease rather than to cyanotic congenital heart disease

➤ In respiratory failure due to large airway obstruction, mechanical ventilation is not necessary unless there is also parenchymal lung disease

➤ A child in a head box needs at least 12 L/min of gas flow to prevent rebreathing and CO_2 retention

➤ Giving 'too much' oxygen virtually never suppresses respiratory drive in childhood asthma

➤ To monitor the progress of gas exchange, either calculate $AaDO_2$ or measure the SaO_2 after breathing air for 2 minutes.

➤ If oxygen by mask or head box fails to improve oxygenation, reassess the diagnosis and consider using CPAP via mask or endotracheal tube, or IPPV plus PEEP

✘ COMMON ERRORS

➤ Failure to anticipate incipient respiratory failure and to intervene to support respiration

➤ Reliance on pulse oximeter readings during oxygen therapy to monitor changes in alveolar ventilation (e.g. in asthma or upper airway obstruction)

FURTHER READING

1. McWilliams B. Respiratory disorders. In: McCloskey KAL, Orr RA, editors. Pediatric transport medicine. St Louis: Mosby; 1995
   – (*Describes a useful approach to the acute management of a child with respiratory failure*)

2. Truog WE. Pulmonary gas exchange. In: Chernick V, Mellins RB, editors. Basic mechanisms of pediatric respiratory disease: cellular and integrative. Philadelphia: BC Decker; 1991
   – (*Reviews the pathophysiology of respiratory failure in childhood*)

3. Sivan Y, Newth CJL. Acute upper airway obstruction. In: Loughlin GM, Eigen H, editors. Respiratory disease in children. Diagnosis and management. Baltimore: Williams & Wilkins; 1994
   – (*Good review of the problem and its management*)

4. Feihl F, Perret C. Permissive hypercapnia: how permissive should we be? Am J Respir Crit Care Med 1994; 150: 1722–1737
   – (*Review of the safety of permissive hypercapnia*)

5. Shann F, Gatchalian S, Hutchinson R. Nasopharyngeal oxygen in children. Lancet 1988; ii: 1238–1240
   – (*An assessment of FIO_2 at various oxygen flow rates and body sizes*)

6. Ring JC, Stidham JL. Novel therapies for acute respiratory failure. Pediatr Clin North Am 1994; 41(6): 1325–1363
   – (*Overview of various forms of respiratory support and their place in childhood respiratory failure*)

7. Martin LD, Bratton SL, Walker LK. Principles and practice of respiratory support and mechanical ventilation. In: Rogers MC, editor. Textbook of pediatric intensive care, 3rd ed. Baltimore: Williams & Wilkins: 1996
   – (*Thorough review of mechanical ventilation in children and its physiology, indications and side-effects*)

2.2 Cardiopulmonary resuscitation

Duncan J. Macrae

Primary cardiac arrest is extremely rare in children, in whom cardiac arrest typically follows a prodromal period of profound respiratory or circulatory and respiratory failure. It follows therefore that cardiac arrest in children can often be averted through prompt recognition and treatment of prodromal events. In contrast, adult cardiac arrest usually has a primary cardiac cause and is a sudden event, which cannot usually be anticipated. Thus when cardiac arrest does occur, in contrast to the adult with sudden onset of ventricular fibrillation, profound hypoxemia, acidosis or neurological and other end-organ damage may already be present. This is thought to account for the very poor outcome reported for cardiac arrest in childhood.

Guidelines for pediatric life support have been published by many national organizations. In 1992 an international liaison group was established to examine differing national guidelines and the scientific evidence supporting recommendations. Fortunately for the editors of this 'multinational' book, 1997 saw the publication, by the International Liaison Committee on Resuscitation (ILCOR) to which European, North and South American and Australasian representatives contribute, of a series of advisory statements from which it is hoped all national guidance will flow and soon lead to international pediatric CPR guidelines. The Resuscitation Council of the United Kingdom (RCUK) has decided to adopt the ILCOR advisory statements and to pilot these on behalf of the European Resuscitation Council. The CPR algorithms described in this chapter are those published by the RCUK based on the ILCOR statements. These represent the most recently revised and internationally agreed protocols on pediatric CPR.

PEDIATRIC BASIC LIFE SUPPORT

DEFINITIONS

The practicalities of resuscitation must take into account the age of the child. Two age categories are recognized by ILCOR: infants, defined as a child less than 1 year of age; and children, aged between 1–8 years. The upper age limit has been proposed as the age up to which a child receives adequate chest compression from a one-handed technique. Older children and teenagers should be resuscitated using adult algorithms and techniques. Variability in size and maturity of children leave a rescuer no choice but to judge the effectiveness of the resuscitation technique chosen and modify it accordingly. In the following discussion, 'child' includes 'infant' except where clearly indicated.

ASSESSMENT

Before initiating basic or advanced life support it is important to assess the patient's level of consciousness and response. Responsiveness indicates that oxygen delivery to the brain is intact, whereas unresponsiveness requires urgent assessment. If a child responds to voice or gentle shaking, check the child's condition, send for assistance and reassess continually. If the child does not respond, send for help and start resuscitation immediately through application of the basic life support algorithm (Fig. 2.2.1). Assessment should take no longer than 10 seconds. Help should be summoned immediately if more than one rescuer is present. A lone rescuer should perform resuscitation for about a minute before going for help, and should if possible take the child along while doing so.

Suspected neck injury

If neck injury is suspected:

- do not shake the child
- do not use the head tilt airway maneuver; use the alternative jaw thrust method

AIRWAY AND BREATHING

Is the child breathing? Look for chest and abdominal movement and confirm by feeling or

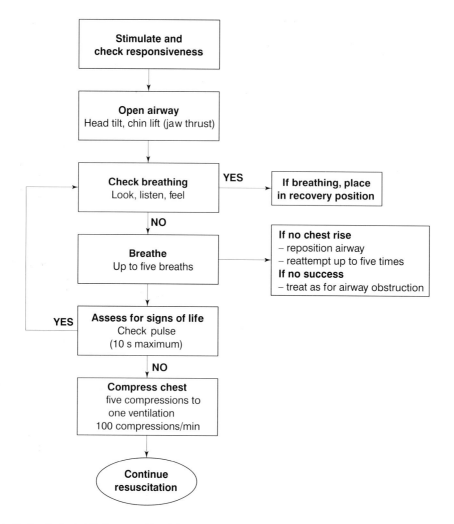

Figure 2.2.1 Pediatric Basic Life Support Algorithm

listening that air is moving in and out of the mouth or nose effectively. Remember that vigorous respiratory effort can be seen in children with severe or complete airway obstruction. If in doubt about airway patency, perform airway opening maneuvers.

The relatively large tongue of the child is a frequent cause of airway obstruction. Airway patency should be ensured by the head tilt–chin lift maneuver (see Fig. 6.3.1), that is, gently tilting the head back by placing a hand on the child's forehead while at the same time lifting the point of the chin with a fingertip to open the airway. The jaw thrust maneuver is an alternative and is the only maneuver recommended if neck injury is suspected.

BREATHING

Assess adequacy of breathing: *look* for chest movement; *feel* at the mouth and nose for air movement; *listen* over the airway for breath sounds. Spend up to 10 seconds assessing breathing before declaring it absent. If a child is not breathing effectively open the airway (see above) and start expired air ventilation, or bag-and-mask ventilation where trained personnel have access to such equipment. Five slow breaths, lasting 1–1.5 seconds are administered initially. Obtain chest movement equivalent to a deep breath. This should ensure firstly that the airway is open and that the tidal volume delivered is not excessive, which could result in gastric distention. If the chest does not rise when attempting ventilation, repeat airway clearing maneuvers, and if chest movement still cannot be obtained, treat as foreign body airway obstruction (Fig. 2.2.2).

CIRCULATION

After clearing the airway and delivering effective rescue breaths, check for signs of life. If breathing is reestablished, place the child in the recovery position and continue to observe. If the child remains unresponsive and apneic, feel for a pulse at either the carotid (child) or brachial (infant) site. Only if the pulse can be felt with absolute certainty or there is clear evidence of recovery of consciousness or clearly effective breathing, should progression to the next stage of resuscitation, chest compression, be averted. *If there are no signs of effective circulation or the rescuer is unsure, it is recommended that chest compressions be added to rescue breathing.* The technique is described in Table 2.2.1).

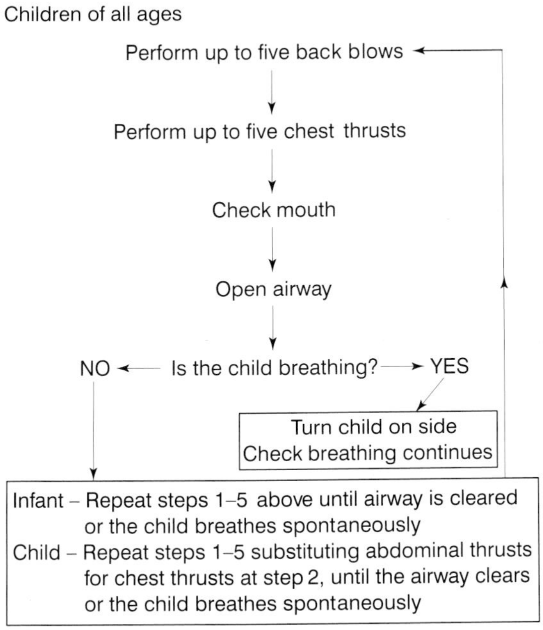

Children of all ages

Figure 2.2.2 Foreign body obstruction sequence

Foreign body obstruction of the airway

There are a number of different algorithms for dealing with foreign body obstruction of the airway, each with its own advocates. Algorithms similar to that shown in Figure 2.2.2 are widely accepted.

- if breathing spontaneously, the child's own efforts to clear the obstruction should be encouraged; intervention is only necessary if these efforts are clearly ineffective and breathing is becoming compromised
- do not attempt to remove the obstruction blindly, as the object may be further impacted by such attempts
- if effective breathing is absent or ineffective, follow steps listed in Figure 2.2.1.

PEDIATRIC ADVANCED LIFE SUPPORT

Even in skilled hands, basic life support measures are essential at the beginning of all resuscitation sequences. Basic life support however, may progress to pediatric advanced life support (PALS) if appropriately skilled personnel and necessary drugs and equipment are available.

The RCUK algorithm for PALS, based on the ILCOR guidelines, assumes that asystole is the primary arrhythmia, since ventricular fibrillation has been detected in fewer than 10% of cases assessed early in their evolution. The algorithm in the Figure 2.2.3 stresses the importance of airway and oxygenation maneuvers in children.

MONITORING DURING CPR

An electrocardiogram (ECG) monitor or ECG monitoring defibrillator should be attached early in the PALS resuscitation sequence to diagnose heart rhythm. The application of defibrillation shocks and pharmacological treatment of rhythm disturbances must be guided by monitored ECG.

The effectiveness of CPR may be judged clinically by palpation of peripheral pulses or more objectively during in hospital CPR by measurement of end-tidal carbon dioxide (*good*: high) or invasively monitored arterial pressure waveform (*good*: high

TABLE 2.2.1 **Technique of chest compression**		
Infant < 1 year	**Child 1–8 years**	**Child > 8 years or adult**
Position Locate sternum and place two fingertips one finger's breadth below nipple line	Place heel of hand over lower half of sternum Lift fingers off ribs Press down vertically with arms straight to 1/3 depth of chest	Place one hand over the other, over the lower half of the sternum Keep fingers away from ribs Press down vertically with arms straight to 1/3 depth of chest
Compression rate 100 per minute *Breath : compression ratio* 1 : 5	100 per minute 1 : 5	100 per minute 2 : 15

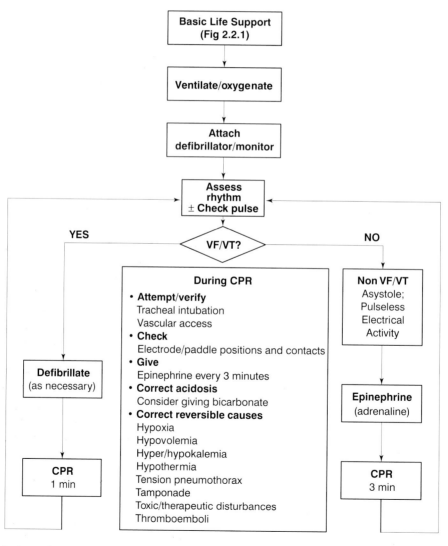

Figure 2.2.3 Pediatric Advanced Life Support Algorithm

mean pressure and substantial area-under-curve).

It is good practice to obtain a sample of blood for blood gas, electrolyte and glucose analysis as early as possible during CPR. Hyperglycemia, hypoglycemia, preexisting acidosis and major electrolyte disturbances should be treated.

ASYSTOLE AND PULSELESS ELECTRICAL ACTIVITY

Asystole and pulseless electrical activity (PEA) are by far the most common rhythms in childhood cardiac arrest.

> **ASYSTOLE or PEA: ADMINISTER EPINEPHRINE (ADRENALINE)**

Give epinephrine (adrenaline):

- preferred route *intravenous* or *intraosseous*
  - initial dose 10 μg/kg (0.1 ml/kg of 1:10 000 solution)
  - second and subsequent doses 100 μg/kg (1 ml/kg 1:10 000 or 0.1 ml/kg 1:1000 solution)
- OR where venous access has not been established, give 100 μg /kg via tracheal tube
- epinephrine (adrenaline) doses should be followed by 3 minutes of CPR followed by repeat epinephrine dosing; a higher dose of epinephrine (100 μg/kg) is recommended for second and subsequent i.v. or intravenous doses.

VENTRICULAR FIBRILLATION AND VENTRICULAR TACHYCARDIA

> **VF or VT: DEFIBRILLATE**

Ventricular fibrillation (VF) and ventricular tachycardia (VT)—although uncommon in pediatric cardiac arrest—are treated, as in adults, by DC cardioversion:

- defibrillate the heart with up to 3 shocks:
  - first shock 2 J/kg
  - second shock 2 J/kg
  - third shock and subsequent 4 J/kg

- paddle placement:
  - paddle A on chest wall below right clavicle
  - paddle B on chest wall – anterior axially line

In small infants where adequate physical separation between defibrillator paddles cannot be achieved on the front of the chest, apply the paddles to the front and back of the chest.

SUMMARY OF PALS

- Perform BLS algorithm
- Attempt to establish definitive airway with tracheal intubation and continuously verify tube position and patency
- Ventilate with 100% oxygen
- Establish reliable vascular access: direct venous access or intraosseous access
- Give epinephrine (adrenaline) every 3 minutes
- Consider giving bicarbonate to correct documented severe metabolic acidosis
- Correct reversible causes

OPEN CHEST CARDIAC COMPRESSION

There is clear evidence that open chest 'direct' cardiac massage is superior to closed chest techniques. Open chest cardiac massage is the technique of choice in a patient with a recent median sternotomy incision who has sustained an in hospital cardiac arrest, as skilled cardiac surgical assistance is immediately available. Open chest cardiac massage should not be attempted without skilled surgical assistance.

Coronary perfusion may be further optimized during the initial stages of open chest resuscitation by raising proximal aortic pressure by partial clamping of the ascending aorta and systemic – pulmonary artery shunts where present.

TRACHEAL DRUG ADMINISTRATION

Use of the tracheal route to administer lipid-soluble drugs such as atropine, lidocaine (lignocaine), naloxone and epinephrine (adrenaline) before vascular access is obtained has been recommended in

CPR guidelines. Impaired absorption and unpredictable pharmacodynamics have led newer CPR guidelines to stress the importance of achieving venous or intraosseous access. If the tracheal route of drug administration is used, it is recommended that at least 2–3 times the intravenous dose of drug is used and that this is given diluted in 3–10 ml 0.9% sodium chloride via a tracheal catheter.

ATROPINE

Bradycardia in children is usually due to severe myocardial hypoxia or hypoperfusion which is overcome by restoration of myocardial oxygenation and cardiac output. Unlike isoproterenol (isoprenaline), atropine has little potential to do harm if used to 'treat' bradycardia other than delaying more appropriate definitive treatments. Atropine (0.02 mg/kg, minimum dose 0.1 mg/kg) may be used to antagonize excessive vagal activity during tracheal intubation.

ADRENERGIC AGONISTS

Epinephrine (adrenaline)

Epinephrine is well established as the essential drug in successful resuscitation from cardiac arrest. Once thought to act by improving the contractile state of the heart through its β-adrenergic activity, it is now known that the essential action of epinephrine during CPR is to induce peripheral vasoconstriction, an alpha effect. Although other pure α-adrenergic agonists such as norepinephrine and phenylephrine have been suggested as alternatives to epinephrine in CPR, none has been shown to be consistently superior to epinephrine.

Isoproterenol (isoprenaline)

Isoproterenol is a synthetic catecholamine, which possesses both β_1- and β_2-agonist properties. It is used occasionally during specialized cardiac intensive care to promote atrioventricular conduction in children with heart block or to increase sinus rate of the denervated heart following cardiac transplantation. However, isoproterenol has no place in routine CPR owing to its adverse influence on myocardial oxygen balance. The drug causes *vasodilatation* through its β_2-agonist effect at a time when *vasoconstriction* is required to promote vital organ perfusion and it also has the potential to induce a damaging increase in myocardial oxygen demand through its β_1-agonist effect.

CALCIUM

It is now recommended that administration of calcium (which was once administered as frequently as epinephrine during CPR) be restricted to specific situations where relative hypocalcemia exists. This caution has been exercised because of concerns that calcium may worsen postischemia reperfusion injury and hasten intracellular toxic events. Indications for calcium administration include:

- documented hypocalcemia
- calcium channel blocker overdose
- hyperkalemia
- hypermagnesemia

ACIDOSIS

Metabolic acidosis develops during CPR due to anerobic metabolism forced on tissues by absent or suboptimal oxygen delivery. Added to this, many children will have already developed acidosis as a result of prearrest problems. Myocardial contractility is impaired in the presence of severe acidosis.

The most commonly used alkalinizing agent, sodium bicarbonate, generates carbon dioxide which can produce a transient intracellular acidosis during the buffering process. This may be clinically significant when ventilation and perfusion and thus carbon dioxide elimination are impaired during CPR. Excessive administration of alkalinizing agents induces a state of metabolic alkalosis which will cause a left shift in the oxyhemoglobin dissociation curve, further limiting tissue oxygen delivery. Sodium bicarbonate solutions deliver sodium in equal molar quantities to bicarbonate with the potential to induce hypernatremia. There is no evidence to support the routine use of bicarbonate in the early stages of pediatric resuscitation. It may occasionally be used transiently to increase pH to render epinephrine (adrenaline) more effective, especially where substantial prearrest base deficits exist.

FLUID ADMINISTRATION

Expanding circulating volume complements the effects of epinephrine (adrenaline) in maintaining central circulation volume and pressure. Documented preexisting deficits must be replaced as early as possible during resuscitation with colloid or glucose-free crystalloid solutions. A bolus of 10–20 ml/kg should be considered in any child not responding to epinephrine alone even if prearrest euvolemia is certain.

GLUCOSE

Blood glucose level should be determined as soon as possible during resuscitation. Severe hypoglycemia (blood glucose <2.5 mmol/L) may occasionally be seen in a child sustaining cardiac arrest and must be treated by careful delivery of glucose solutions. Hyperglycemia worsens neurological outcome. Glucose-containing solutions should be avoided during CPR except in the treatment of documented hypoglycemia.

STABILIZATION AFTER RESUSCITATION

Resuscitation does not end with the return of spontaneous circulation as efforts must then be directed towards supporting and improving cardiac output, and optimizing tissue reperfusion, as myocardial function continues to deteriorate for a few hours after arrest. It is usual for the post-arrest myocardium to require inotropic support as the effect of resuscitative epinephrine (adrenaline) recedes. Ventilation of the lungs should be continued until cardiorespiratory stability is achieved, avoiding both hypercapnia (risk of raising intracranial pressure) and hypocapnia (risk of excessive restriction of cerebral blood flow). Cerebral resuscitative strategies such as thiopental (thiopentone), lidoflazine (a calcium channel blocker), steroids and mannitol have at times been recommended, although none has been shown consistently to be effective in controlled trials and such treatments should be avoided. Metabolic normality should be obtained through gradual correction of metabolic acidosis and other documented biochemical abnormalities.

OUTCOME OF PEDIATRIC RESUSCITATION

The outcome of children requiring CPR remains poor. In a series of out-of-hospital cardiac or respiratory arrest cases presenting to the emergency room of a children's hospital, 10 of 21 children were alive 12 months after presenting apneic but with a pulse, of whom six were neurologically normal or near-normal. The same survey documented outcome of 80 children presenting with cardiac arrest, of whom six survived to discharge from hospital, three with moderate deficits and three in persistent vegetative state. There were no survivors of those requiring more than 20 minutes of CPR in the emergency room. Other series of both in-hospital and out-of-hospital cardiac arrest document similarly poor outcomes with relatively few unimpaired survivors. Factors associated with better outcomes include respiratory arrest without cardiac arrest and short duration of CPR. Early institution of open chest cardiac massage certainly improves organ perfusion and may improve patient outcome from in-hospital cardiac arrests.

 KEY POINTS

➤ Airway patency must be continually reassessed during basic life support
➤ Infants and children who undergo cardiac arrest have a very poor prognosis
➤ Respiratory arrest alone is associated with better outcome
➤ By far the most effective treatment of cardiac or respiratory arrest is prevention: recognition and urgent treatment of prodromal states are essential.

FURTHER READING

1. Paediatric advanced life support: an advisory statement by the Pediatric Life Support Working Group of the International Liaison Committee on Resuscitation. Resuscitation 1997; 34: 115–127
2. Schindler MB, Bohn D, Cox P et al. Outcome of out-of-hospital cardiac or respiratory arrest in children. N Engl J Med 1996; 335: 1473–1479
3. Sheikh A, Brogan T. Outcome and cost of open- and closed-chest cardiopulmonary resuscitation in pediatric cardiac arrests. Pediatrics 1994; 93: 392–398
4. Zideman DA. Pediatric and neonatal life support. Br J Anaesth 1997; 188–197

2.3 Shock

Michael D. Seear

The full spectrum of shock is difficult to sum up in a simple definition. It is a syndrome of events fundamentally caused by failure of adequate peripheral perfusion, leading in advanced or untreated cases to diffuse organ damage and ultimate death. Put more simply, it is a state of respiratory failure at a cellular level.

Peripheral delivery of oxygenated blood depends on a functioning cardiorespiratory system plus adequate vascular tone and intravascular volume. Classification and investigation tend towards the primary inciting injury, such as heart failure, dehydration, anaphylaxis or sepsis. More recent work has concentrated on the final common pathway of organ damage, which appears to result from an interaction between damaged endothelium and activated leukocytes.

Although the management of traumatic shock has improved greatly, we are still far from understanding advanced septic shock and its continuum of multiple organ system failure. Inevitably, advances in the management of shock have brought their own problems. Acute (adult) respiratory distress syndrome and multiple organ failure have only been described relatively recently because patients need to survive the initial shock-inducing episode before these complications can develop.

INITIAL INJURY

Many descriptive terms have been used to define and classify the causes of shock. However, there is no single pure cause of shock.

Adequate cellular perfusion requires a normal cardiac output with good vascular tone. Recognizing that there will always be overlap between different stimuli, some use may be gained from the classification system in Table 2.3.1.

The first step in managing shock is to treat any identifiable underlying cause. Consequently, diagnosis and classification of the inciting agent is of some value. However, once the state of shock is

---

TABLE 2.3.1 Classification of shock

1. Abnormalities of preload—hypovolemic shock

In children the most common cause is dehydration following gastroenteritis, although burns, gastrointestinal and traumatic hemorrhage, heat stroke, diabetic ketoacidosis, third space losses, reduced intake and adrenal insufficiency are other causes

2. Abnormalities of contractility—cardiogenic shock

Common causes in children include prolonged cardiopulmonary bypass, hypoxic–ischemic damage, myocarditis, tamponade, drug overdose and sepsis. Depression of cardiac function due to a variety of circulating substances is a common end result of shock from any cause

3. Abnormalities of afterload—obstructive shock

In children, pulmonary emboli are rare. The most common obstructive lesions are congenital and include coarctation of the aorta, aortic or pulmonary stenosis, and occasionally post-traumatic aortic injury

4. Abnormalities of vascular tone— distributive shock

The most common causes in children are anaphylaxis, septicemia, and drug overdose or toxicity; rarely the cause is neurogenic (e.g. spinal injury). Overwhelming sepsis can be due to:
- Neonate:
  - group B streptococcus
  - *Escherichia coli* or other Gram-negative bacteria
  - *Listeria monocytogenes*
  - *Staphylococcus*
  - *Candida*
  - herpes simplex virus
- Infant or older child:
  - *Haemophilus*
  - *Streptococcus*
  - *Neisseria meningitidis*
  - *Enterobacteriaceae*
  - *Staphylococcus*
- Immunocompromised (e.g. bone marrow transplant) patient:
  - *Streptococcus*
  - *Staphylococcus*
  - *Gram-negative bacteria*
  - *Candida* or *Aspergillus*
  - herpesvirus

established, a self-perpetuating inflammatory cascade is established that is largely independent of the original cause. Recognizing the potential for shock to develop and prompt intervention to prevent or minimize its effect is therefore a key element of comprehensive care in critical illness or injury.

Shock can be considered simply as inadequate cardiac output to meet tissue demands. More accurately, it describes inadequacy of oxygen delivery to the tissues.

> Oxygen delivery (DaO_2)
> = cardiac output (CO) × oxygen carrying capacity (CaO_2)
> = CO × (Hb × SaO_2 × 1.34 + 0.003 × PaO_2)

Metabolic acidosis results from lactic acid formation. Compensated shock refers to a condition where blood flow to the tissues is redistributed to the vital organs and oxygen consumption is maintained by an increased extraction of oxygen. Venous blood has a lower oxygen saturation. Mixed venous oxygen saturation can be a useful monitor of cardiac function in some situations.

> Extraction ratio = $(CaO_2 - C\bar{v}O_2)/CaO_2$
> = $(SaO_2 - S\bar{v}O_2)/SaO_2$
> (ignoring the small amount of plasma dissolved oxygen)

Blood pressure may be normal. Pulse pressure narrows next. Hypotension is a LATE sign of shock. Hypovolemic shock from loss of volume results in reduction in venous return because of a decrease in mean systemic filling pressure. Compensation occurs by altering the ratio of pre- and postcapillary resistance to allow movement of fluid from the interstitial space to the intravascular space, increased oxygen extraction, reduced venous compliance, or a reduction in resistance to venous return. A response to volume is diagnostic.

Cardiac failure of any cause results in a decrease in the cardiac function curve and a shift to the right, for any given filling pressure. No matter what the degree of ventricular dysfunction in cardiogenic shock, cardiac output may still be improved with a judicious volume challenge.

Septic shock is a form of distributive shock which results from mediator-induced circulatory and cellular metabolic abnormalities. The hemodynamic consequences are complex. Cardiac function, intravascular volume and vascular tone may simultaneously be affected. Cardiac output may be increased or decreased. Peripheral resistance and afterload may be either increased or decreased. Capillary permeability abnormalities or bleeding diatheses and blood loss associated with sepsis contribute to the loss of intravascular volume.

The consequences of prolonged or untreated shock are often irreversible and reperfusion injury may result which is largely untreatable. Myocardial depressant factors are released and contribute to the inadequacy of oxygen delivery. Coagulation and fibrinolysis become activated in an uncontrolled fashion resulting in bleeding diatheses. Vital organ function becomes deranged. Multiple endocrine abnormalities arise. Multisystem organ failure (Ch. 2.12) can occur after any of the shock states described above, and carries a very high mortality.

Shock ultimately compromises cerebral blood flow (CBF) – early where cerebral autoregulation is impaired. Inadequate CBF results in cerebral metabolic requirements for oxygen ($CMRo_2$) being unmet. Hypotension is synergistic in this regard with anemia and hypoxemia, and with states that increase $CMRo_2$ (fever, seizures).

FINAL COMMON PATHWAY

Although there are many vasoactive substances circulating in the body, including both vasoconstrictors (catecholamines, angiotensin) and vasodilators (histamine, serotonin, prostacyclin), vasomotor tone is mainly controlled by autonomic innervation and local interaction between endothelial cells and the surrounding smooth muscle. Muscle tone is locally controlled by substances produced in the endothelial cells. Relaxation is produced by nitric oxide (previously known as endothelial-derived relaxing factor) and constriction by endothelin-1. During states of poor perfusion, the local build-up of carbon dioxide, lactate and hydrogen ions probably overrides other controls and causes local vasodilation.

The endothelium acts as a semipermeable barrier between blood and the organs. It can itself be looked on as an organ. Only relatively recently has it been realized that the endothelium has a central role in the metabolism and production of a large range of substances. Apart from regulation of the circulation and various synthetic functions, the endothelial layer plays a central role in coagulation and also has an important immunological function.

The term 'endotheliopathy' has been coined to describe the self-perpetuating secondary injury that follows some states of shock and ultimately progresses to multiple organ failure. If endothelial cells are injured by ischemia or circulating inflammatory cytokines such as tumor necrosis factor, they express endothelial leukocyte adhesion molecules (ELAMs). Large, composite molecules called integrins (composed of CD18 and CD11 subunits) on activated monocytes and neutrophils bind to the endothelial receptors. Leukocytes subsequently move through the vascular barrier, releasing cytokines, prostanoids, supraoxides and other mediators of tissue damage that further perpetuate the inflammatory cycle. Numerous studies using neutrophil depletion or monoclonal antibodies against adhesion receptors have shown improved survival in sepsis or reperfusion injury models. Subsequent therapies will undoubtedly be directed towards controlling the leukocyte endothelium interaction with specific antagonists to various levels of the inflammatory cascade.

CLINICAL PICTURE AND DIAGNOSIS

Early and aggressive intervention is the best guarantee of a successful outcome in the management of shock. Consequently, there must be a high index of suspicion for the development of shock in appropriate clinical settings. There are no tests or measurements that define the existence of shock; it is entirely a clinical diagnosis. Clinical signs of shock are shown in Table 2.3.2.

Advanced states of shock are easily recognized. Poor peripheral perfusion leads to a reduced conscious level; cold, clammy peripheries; weak, rapid pulse; poor urine output; and low blood pressure. Unfortunately, by the time these fea-

tures have developed, the chance of successful outcome is small.

The earliest sign of poor perfusion is decreased capillary refill and cool peripheries. These signs are not quantifiable and can only be learned by experience. Hence the need to recognize that a wide range of situations can be complicated by shock (Table 2.3.3). Anxiety regarding possible overtreatment is unfounded in virtually all cases; if the clinical setting suggests the possibility of shock, then it is best to treat or investigate without waiting for the child to develop clear overt signs (Table 2.3.4).

TABLE 2.3.2 **Clinical signs of shock**

System	Signs
Cardiovascular	Tachycardia, weak or impalpable pulses, cold and/or mottled extremities, sluggish or absent capillary refil (> 2 s), pallor, hypotension (late sign indicating severe shock)
Respiratory	Tachypnea, peripheral or central cyanosis, irregular respiration or apnea, compromised airway patency
Central nervous system	Disturbed level of consciousness, agitated initially followed by lethargy, weakness or coma
Renal	Oliguria

TABLE 2.3.3 **Conditions associated with shock**

Condition	Signs
Hypovolemia	Dehydration, poor skin turgor, sunken eyeballs, dry mucosae, distended tense abdomen, signs of multiple trauma
Sepsis	May be wide pulse pressure initially, flushed appearance, fever, hypothermia
Cardiogenic shock	Absent femoral pulses, hepatomegaly, cardiomegaly, gallop rhythm, chest crepitations

TABLE 2.3.4 Laboratory features of shock	
Investigation	**Results**
Complete blood count with differential and platelet count	WBC may be increased, normal or decreased in sepsis, often with a left shift of immature leukocytes. After hemorrhage Hb can be normal or ↓ and reticulocytes normal or ↑ Thrombocytopenia, anemia occur with sepsis or over time
Coagulation screen:	PT, PTT increased in sepsis Fibrinogen may be low in sepsis or shock of any cause D-dimers elevated typically in sepsis
Electrolytes and renal function	Exclude hypoglycemia, hyperglycemia is a common feature of the stress response Differentiate prerenal and renal causes of oliguria
Arterial blood gases	Acidosis secondary to inadequate tissue perfusion (pH < 7.35) Cultures and urinary bacterial antigens
Metabolic screen serum ammonia (neonates and infants) CXR	Urinary amino acids and organic acids if suspicion of congenital metabolic disease Cardiomegaly suggests a cardiac cause

TREATMENT

As yet, there is no specific treatment that will reverse or inhibit the inflammatory cascade once it has started. The best treatment of shock is prevention based on early, aggressive resuscitation combined with treatment of the underlying cause. An algorithm for treatment is shown in Figure 2.3.1.

GENERAL PRINCIPLES

Priority 1

The first priority is attention to the adequacy of the airway and breathing. Avoiding hypoxia is essential (Pao_2 > 10.7 kPa, 80 mmHg). Administer oxygen. Physiological compensation includes increased respiratory drive. Progressive hypoxemia and acidosis secondary to deterioration of cerebral perfusion compromise this drive. Respiratory effort falls, conscious level deteriorates, airway patency is jeopardized and apnea will precipitate cardiac arrest. An unconscious and moribund patient requires intubation and assisted ventilation with 100% oxygen initially. Place the patient in a supine position and elevate the legs.

Blood samples should be taken at the time of insertion of the peripheral venous or central line, but should not interfere with the resuscitation.

Priority 2

Priority 2 is rapid restoration of perfusion to the critical vascular beds and hence oxygen delivery. This is aimed at preventing the activation of the secondary and as yet largely untreatable mediator cascades.

Priority 3

Treatment of the underlying cause occurs simultaneously.

Ongoing support is essential. This involves close and careful monitoring, measuring responses to any therapeutic interventions. Fine tuning the metabolic condition of the patient—correction of acid–base abnormalities (consider giving $NaHCO_3$ if pH < 7.2), correcting electrolyte abnormalities, avoiding hypoglycemia—is an essential component of ongoing care. Much of the intensive care of these patients involves multiple organ support until the homeostatic mechanisms normalize and the patient recovers.

Insertion of an indwelling urinary catheter is required after the resuscitation has begun.

CARDIOVASCULAR SUPPORT

The principles are to normalize cardiac output and perfusion pressure rapidly. Blood pressure and pulse rate should be normalized for age.

Preload

Large-bore intravenous access is a prerequisite for rapid infusion of fluids during volume resuscitation to achieve rapid restoration of circulating blood volume and hence venous return. Isotonic

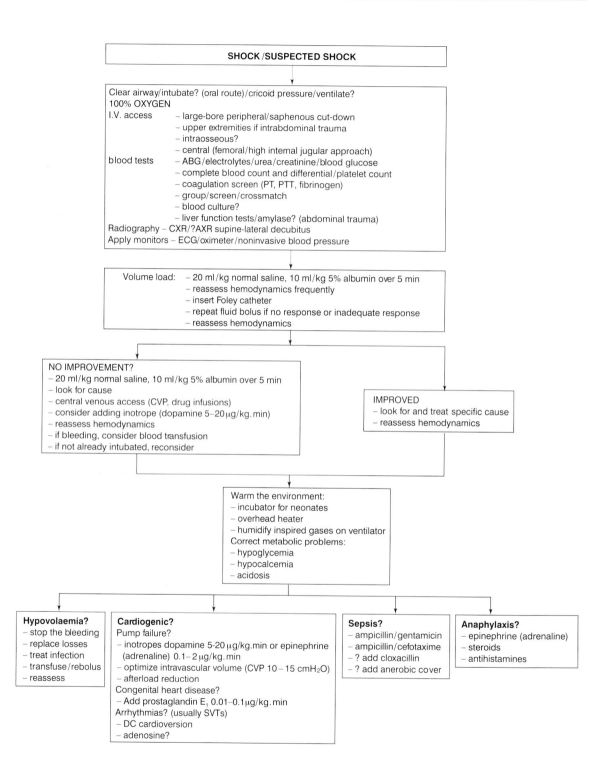

Figure 2.3.1 Treatment of shock

fluids (0.9% saline, Ringer-lactate solution, or 5% albumin) should be infused rapidly over 5–10 minutes (dose 20 ml/kg 0.9% saline, or 10 ml/kg 5% albumin). Repeat the fluid challenge immediately if the clinical effect is assessed to be inadequate (no improvement in heart rate, blood pressure, peripheral perfusion, or conscious level).

Monitor the adequacy of a volume challenge by assessing the post-challenge central venous pressure if a central line has been placed (aim for 10–12 cmH$_2$O), peripheral pulse volume, improvement in base deficit on blood gas, production of urine (0.5–1.0 ml/kg·h), and reduction in liver size. Signs of fluid overload include rales in the lungs, gallop rhythm, hepatomegaly.

Contractility

In cardiogenic shock and often in septic shock, the addition of an inotrope is often required after restoring normovolemia, to optimize cardiac output and perfusion pressures. The inotrope of choice in children is dopamine (up to 10–15μg/kg·min). If this is ineffective reassess volume status and try epinephrine (adrenaline) in a dose of 0.1–2μg/kg·min. Amrinone is a useful inotropic agent in the postoperative cardiac surgical patient because of its inotropic action and effect as a peripheral vasodilator. The dose ranges from 5–10 μg/kg·min after an intravenous load of 1–2 mg/kg, given over 30–60 minutes. Inotropes can be used alone or in combination. A neonate has immature norepinephrine (noradrenaline) stores and sympathetic supply, and hence may have an inadequate response to dopamine.

Neonates may respond to a calcium infusion. Follow with ionized calcium levels. *Note* – care is necessary with a calcium bolus as it may precipitate hypertension, bradycardia and cardiac standstill if an excessive dose is inadvertently administered. Place the child on a cardiac monitor, start the i.v., infusion and give calcium gluconate 10% (dose 2 ml/kg i.v. over 30 min).

Avoid hypoglycemia. Check the glucometer levels frequently. If hypoglycemia develops, correct immediately with a bolus of 1–2 ml 25% dextrose solution, followed by a dextrose infusion of 5–8 mg/kg·min, using either 5% or 10% dextrose solution.

Optimize afterload

Neonates and infants are particularly sensitive to increased afterload. Children with a primary cardiac disorder will respond to peripheral vasodilators such as nitroprusside. Inhaled nitric oxide acts specifically as a pulmonary vasodilator and hence can unload the right ventricle in states associated with acute pulmonary hypertension.

Children in septic shock and vasodilated will respond well to a titrated infusion of norepinephrine (noradrenaline) in the same dose range as epinephrine (adrenaline). Children with extensive burns not only have large volume losses but also develop a systemic inflammatory response which responds well to norepinephrine.

Rate and rhythm

Oxygen should minimize the risk of bradycardia. Specific arrhythmias are initially treated by correcting the metabolic disorders commonly precipitating them (hypoxemia, systemic acidosis, electrolytes).

RESPIRATORY SUPPORT

Shock results in hypoxemia because of an inadequate perfusion pressure in the lungs, with a resultant increase in dead space ventilation and increased ventilation–perfusion mismatching. Some children may have alveolar infiltrates of cardiac or noncardiac origin which contribute to the hypoxemia.

The patient with severe respiratory dysfunction will benefit from intubation and assisted mechanical ventilation by optimizing the delivery of 100% oxygen and reducing the work of breathing.

The patient with severe cardiac dysfunction will also benefit from intubation and assisted mechanical ventilation. Great care must be taken to avoid agents that will depress contractility further, as well as avoiding hypoxemia during the intubation procedure. The benefits derived from ventilation are as follows:

- ensuring delivery of adequate oxygen to the patient (who may be disoriented and continually remove the oxygen mask)
- reducing the work of breathing (substantial in a critically ill shocked patient from any cause)

- redirecting blood flow to vital organs away from the respiratory muscles
- improving afterload of the left ventricle by reducing the transmural pressure

Care must be taken to ensure that preload is optimized so a reduction in venous return does not complicate the institution of positive pressure ventilation.

SUPPORTIVE MEASURES

Supportive measures include:

- clotting factor replacement for symptomatic coagulopathy (fresh frozen plasma)
- fluid/electrolytes adjustment
- antibiotics if suspicion of septicemia and longer-term intensive care
- surgery to control hemorrhage or stabilize long-bone fractures
- gastric stress ulcer prophylaxis using either H_2-antagonists or sucralfate (both equally effective)
- metabolic support
- dialysis for renal failure
- nutrition (preferably enteral)
- general support for liver failure
- surveillance for secondary complications and nosocomial infections

CONTROVERSIES IN CARE

There has been debate concerning the ultimate physiological goals of resuscitation. Some would argue that resuscitating a patient to normal levels of hemodynamic function is insufficient to counteract the progressive nature of the peripheral endothelial damage. However, the so-called 'supernormal' or 'supraphysiologic' approach has been criticized on a number of grounds. The fact that resuscitated patients with above-normal hemodynamic parameters tend to do better may simply mean that these patients are able to achieve these levels and consequently represent a good risk group.

Measurement of mixed venous oxygen or arterial lactate can give some indication of the patient's state, but there is no absolute measure that adequate resuscitation has occurred. At pres-

ent, there is little support for the practice of trying to drive a patient's hemodynamic variables well above what might be considered a normal range. Generous use of fluid resuscitation, inotropes and vasodilators should be continued until the primary physician feels that adequate perfusion is present. Subsequent management depends upon obsessive attention to the maintenance of cardiorespiratory and metabolic variables.

Use of large doses of steroids is not of benefit in septic shock where patients probably have a blunted pituitary and adrenal response. They may benefit from stress replacement of hydrocortisone. The adrenal response can be assessed by the ACTH stimulation test.

It is likely that the future will bring us treatments that will allow manipulation of the inflammatory cascade. Therapies ranging from passive immunization against Gram-negative antigens, to monoclonal antibodies to tumor necrosis factor or adhesion molecules have all been tested at an animal level. Large studies in humans have failed to show any benefit from the use of monoclonal antibodies directed against tumor necrosis factor or interleukin-1. Clearly, there is a long way to go before shock and multiple organ failure are adequately understood. Until this day arrives, the basis of treatment of shock is early resuscitation, treatment of the inciting cause and careful continuous support.

MONITORING

The subject of monitoring is controversial. The spectrum runs from those who believe invasive lines should never be used, to those who frequently put in pulmonary artery catheters. This topic is discussed in Chapter 6.5.

Although there is no consensus on all parameters that should be measured, some variables should be monitored continuously in any patients receiving treatment for shock. The most sensitive signs of progress are obtained by repeated, careful clinical examination by an experienced caregiver. Many of these variables such as respiratory pattern, type of pulse, peripheral perfusion and color are subjective, but changes in heart rate, blood pressure and conscious level are more objective and, with experience, a good assessment of the child's general status can be obtained. Careful clinical examination should always be the foundation for management decisions.

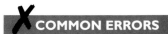

KEY POINTS

➤ Shock should be anticipated and preventive measures instituted

➤ The hallmarks of established shock are hypotension and evidence of poor perfusion; these signs are the final results of a complex systemic response to a wide range of insults

➤ Shock results in reduced CBF and inadequate oxygen delivery to meet CMR_{O_2}

➤ Early and aggressive treatment of the inciting cause combined with good supportive care of the circulation are the best therapeutic options

➤ Despite optimal therapy, some cases will still progress to multiple organ system failure and death

✘ COMMON ERRORS

➤ Failure to anticipate shock

➤ Failure to optimize airway patency and respiratory support

➤ Failure to vigorously restore normovolemia/blood pressure via fluid challenge

➤ Assuming the absence of hypotension excludes a diagnosis of shock

➤ Mistaking the flushed appearance of septic shock as evidence of adequate perfusion

➤ Giving inotropes without adequate provision of preload

FURTHER READING

1. Tobias J. Shock in children: the first 60 minutes. Pediatr Ann 1996; 25: 330–338
    – (*This article provides a practical approach to the management of common shock states in children*)

2. Seear M, Wensley D, Macnab A. Oxygen consumption—oxygen delivery relationship in children. J Pediatr 1993; 123: 208–214
    – (*V_{O_2} and D_{O_2} relationship over a range of metabolic demand—normal children during exercise and children after cardiac surgery*)

3. Abello P. Shock and multiple organ failure. Adv Exp Med Biol 1994; 366: 253–268

4. Mouchawar A. A pathophysiological approach to the patient in shock. Int Anaes Clin 1993; 31: 1–20
    – (*Two detailed reviews of the underlying pathophysiology of shock*)

2.4 Coma

Robert C. Tasker

The normal conscious state is characterized by sleep-wake cycles and by the ability to arouse and respond to the environment. The term 'coma' or 'encephalopathy' implies a disorder of consciousness: it may be applied to a state or continuum of worsening consciousness from being fully alert and responsive to deep coma. Terms such as 'stupor' and 'semi-coma' are best avoided because they are imprecise. Arousal is impaired in encephalopathy and absent in deep coma.

In the normal state, consciousness is maintained by the integrity of certain areas in the cerebral cortex, thalamus and brain stem, particularly the portion of the reticular formation located in the upper pons and midbrain. Awareness or cognition, another feature of the normal conscious state, depends on the integrity of the cerebral hemispheres. Usually levels of arousal and awareness are closely associated, but they may be dissociated as in the persistent vegetative state when arousal is preserved but awareness or cognition is lost.

CAUSES

A number of disorders may lead to encephalopathy and the primary disease may arise from within or outside the CNS (Table 2.4.1). Some have found it helpful to classify the various conditions under those associated with structural cerebral abnormalities and those with a predominantly metabolic dysfunction. This distinction is somewhat arbitrary, however, and frequently a structural cause of disturbed consciousness may be associated with metabolic dysfunction, e.g. inappropriate antidiuretic hormone secretion may complicate herpes simplex encephalitis. Conversely, a metabolic cause of disordered consciousness such as diabetic ketoacidosis may be associated with the anatomical abnormalities of cerebral edema. Specific investigation should be directed by the differential diagnosis based on the history and examination.

TABLE 2.4.1 **Causes of coma**
1. **Trauma**   Accidental   Non-accidental
2. **Hypoxic–ischaemic injury**   Cardiorespiratory arrest   Near-miss sudden infant death syndrome   Near-drowning   Smoke inhalation   Shock syndromes
3. **Intracranial infection**   Meningitis   Encephalitis   Postinfectious
4. **Mass lesion**   Hematoma   Abscess   Tumor
5. **Fluid, electrolyte and acid–base disorders**   Hypernatremia   Hyponatremia   Water intoxication   Acidosis   Alkalosis
6. **Acute ventricular obstruction**
7. **Seizure disorders**
8. **Complications of malignancy**
9. **Systemic infection**   Sepsis syndrome   Septic encephalopathy
10. **Poisoning**
11. **Vascular**   Arteriovenous malformation   Hypertensive encephalopathy   Embolism   Migraine   Venous thrombosis   Arteritis   Homocysteinuria
12. **Endocrine dysfunction**   Hypoglycemia   Diabetes mellitus   Diabetes insipidus
13. **Respiratory failure**
14. **Renal failure**
15. **Hepatic failure**
16. **Reye's syndrome**
17. **Inherited metabolic disorder**   Lactic acidosis   Urea cycle disorder   Aminoacidopathies
18. **Hypothermia, hyperthermia**
19. **Iatrogenic**   Overcorrection of acidosis   Overhydration   Drug overdosage

CLINICAL EVALUATION

Evaluation of the encephalopathic patient in general, with assessment of all organ systems is essential, if secondary or complicating factors such as impending respiratory failure or incipient myocardial dysfunction are to be identified, limited or avoided. Concerning the specific central nervous system features of an encephalopathy on examination, most causes produce a relatively stereotyped array of symptoms and signs. These should be evaluated in a methodical and meticulous manner. In the infant and child, interpretation must take into account the stage of development and expected normal responses. In general, however, the neurological findings will fall into one of the following categories:

1. Generalized depression of hemisphere function — in these patients consciousness is depressed, motor tone becomes diminished, pupils are small but reactive, and reflex eye movements are disinhibited. Asterixis (postural unattentiveness of outstretched limbs), is one of the hallmarks of such metabolic encephalopathy and may relate to intermittent depression of motor function.

2. Heightened excitability of neural tissue occurs and results from a direct lowering of the threshold for neuronal excitability or from selective depression of inhibitory influences on neuronal function. Cheyne–Stokes respiration may result from bilateral hemispheric inhibition, and certain types of seizures from neuronal excitability.

3. Selective vulnerability or focal involvement of a specific brain region to a systemic metabolic insult may be due to regional differences in tissue metabolic requirements for oxygen, glucose, or amino acids or, alternatively, regional differences in neurotransmitters and receptors. It is not uncommon for focal findings to remain unexplained, e.g. those occurring during hypoglycemia, hyperglycemia, uremia, and hypercalcemia, or possibly to be representative of an anamnestic response to a previous neurological injury.

4. Central syndrome — progressive rostrocaudal deterioration with features and signs indicative of raised intracranial pressure and brain tissue shifts may occur with any cause of cerebral edema or space-occupying lesion (Figure 2.4.1).

SCORING SYSTEMS

In patients needing frequent neurological review to monitor for significant change or evaluate the need for specific cerebral protective therapy, there are obvious advantages to using a screening assessment that can be carried out quickly and reliably by different bedside attendants. A number of such clinical neurological scoring systems have been applied to infants and young children in coma. All of these have similarities with the description of progressive rostrocaudal neurological deterioration or 'central syndrome'.

The best-known assessment for coma is the Glasgow coma scale (GCS) (Table 2.4.2) which is a modification of the 'central syndrome' that assigns scores for clinical findings that develop (in the course of deterioration) following head injury. Although many advocate the use of a pediatric scale to facilitate rapid screening review and assessment, in practice multiobserver interpretation of 'vocal sounds', 'cries' and arousal behavior is very difficult and for the most part probably inadequate and not reproducible between different observers. An alternative scoring assessment, which can also be used effectively in intubated patients, relies predominantly on brain-stem reflexes (Table 2.4.3).

CLINICAL STRATEGY

General supportive care of the unconscious patient, management of raised intracranial pressure (Ch. 2.6), and control of status epilepticus and seizures (Ch. 2.5) are the main intensive care problems encountered in the comatose patient. A general management outline follows and specific management issues for prehospital, emergency and ward care for common encephalopathies such as head injury, postresuscitation disease and poisoning are discussed in Chapters 2.6, 3.2, and 4.5.

Stage	Level of consciousness	Respiration	Pupil size and reactivity	Oculocephalic and oculovestibular responses	Posture and tone
Diencephalic (early – late) ↓	agitation drowsiness stupor ↓	deep sighs or yawns Cheyne-Stokes or periodic breaths ↓	small 1-3 mm with brisk reaction to light ↓	conjugate at rest and respond quickly ↓	normal ↓ generalized muscular hypertonus
Midbrain– upper pons ↓	coma ↓	central hyperventilation ↓	midposition 3-5 mm with sluggish reaction to light ↓	dysconjugate ↓	decorticate posture and increased tone bilateral decerebate rigidity
Lower pons– upper medulla ↓	deep coma ↓	irregular breathing interrupted by deep sighs or gasps ↓	midposition and fixed ↓	absent ↓	flaccid: – retained bilateral extensor plantars – occasional flexor responses in the lower limbs
Medullary (terminal)	deep coma	terminal apnea	may be unequal	absent	flaccid

Figure 2.4.1 Stages in progressive deterioration or central syndrome (reading across the chart gives the clinical features for each stage)

MANAGEMENT OUTLINE

ABCs

Protect the airway. Stabilize the cervical spine

URGENT ACTION

Consider:

- immediate therapy:
  - hypoglycemia (dextrose 25% 1–2 ml/kg i.v.)
  - opiates (naloxone 0.1 mg/kg i.v.)
  - benzodiazepines (flumazenil 0.2 mg i.v. slowly, consider repeat)
  - increased ICP (mannitol, intubate and hyperventilate for brief periods until CT scan)
  - signs of infection (antibiotics, lumbar puncture if stable, but generally this should be deferred if patient comatose or abnormal neurologically; blood cultures)
- immediate CT:
  - trauma?
  - focal CNS signs?
  - signs increased ICP?
  - signs mass lesion?
  - hemorrhage?

HISTORY

Duration, onset, evolution, past history, trauma, medication, drugs, toxins.

INVESTIGATIONS

Glucose, calcium, blood gases, blood count, electrolytes, BUN, creatinine, osmolality, toxicology screen.

Consider also ammonia, AST, ALT, coagulation studies, metabolic screen, EEG, ECG.

PHYSICAL SIGNS

Conscious level

Assess Conscious level:

- lethargic (drowsy)
- obtunded
- stuporose (barely rousable)
- comatose
- vegetative (brain-stem signs only)

Vital signs

- temperature:
  - ↑ infection
  - ↓ exposure
- heart rate:
  - ↑ trauma (shock), cardiac failure metabolic (DKA)
  - ↓ (with ↑ BP) raised ICP, drug ingestion
- BP:
  - ↑ hypertensive encephalopathy
  - ↓ shock, adrenal crisis

Other diagnostic clues

- colour:
  - cyanosis: hypoxia, cardiac disease (? emboli in CHD)
  - cherry red: smoke, carbon monoxide exposure
  - jaundice: hepatic failure, drugs
  - pigmentation: hypoadrenalinism
  - bruises: trauma, NAI, drug effects
  - petechiae: bleeding disorder, drug effects
- Eyes:
  - retinal hemorrhages: NAI
  - raccoon eyes: NAI, skull fracture
  - periorbital edema: infection, sinus thrombosis
  - pupil anomaly: see Table 2.4.4

TABLE 2.4.2 The Glasgow coma scale

- **Eye opening**

Spontaneously	4
To speech/verbal command	3
To pain	2
None[a]	1

- **Verbal response**

Oriented (appropriate conversation/reaction, for age to stimuli or surroundings)	5
Confused (disoriented, uncooperative, uses words/cries and consolable, aware of surroundings)	4
Inappropriate words, vocal sounds or crying; awareness and responses inconsistent	3
Incomprehensible sounds, cries, unaware and unresponsive to surroundings	2
None	1

- **Best motor response**

To verbal command: obeys (spontaneous)	6
To painful stimulus[b]	
localizes stimulus (vocalizing)	5
withdraws (flexion)	4
abnormal flexion (decorticate)	3
extensor response (decerebrate)	2
none	1

- **Total score**
  eyes (1–4) + verbal (1–5) + motor (1–6)
  Range 3–15

From Teasdale G, Jennett B. Assessment of coma in impaired consciousness. A practical scale. Lancet 1974; i: 81
Simpson D, Riley P. Pediatric coma scale. Lancet 1982; ii: 450.
[a]Award full score to children under 2 years old for crying response after stimulation (CPS. Management of children with head trauma. Can Med Assoc J 1990; 142(9): 949).
[b]Stimuli for motor response: nail bed pressure (upper limb) or supraorbital pressure (localizing response—hand movement to the chin)

TABLE 2.4.3 Clinical assessment of cortical and brain-stem function

Best response	Score
Cortical function (scores 0–6)	
• Purposeful, spontaneous movement	6
• Purposeful movement to command	5
• Localizing pain	4
• Nonpurposeful movement, withdrawal response	3
• Decorticate posturing	2
• Decerebrate posturing	1
• Flaccidity	0
Brain-stem function (scores 0–3)	
Pupillary light reflex, corneal reflex, oculovestibular and oculocephalic response:	
• All normal	3
• Some absent or diminished	2
• All absent, but breathing	1
• All absent and apneic (normal carbon dioxide)	0
Total score:	
Cortical (0–6) + brain stem (0–3)	**0–9**

From Morray JP, Tyler DC, Jones TK et al. Coma scale for use in brain injured children. Crit Care Med 1984; 12(12): 1018–1020.

TABLE 2.4.4 Pupil examination

Appearance	Reaction	Term	Causes
Small			
Bilateral	Reactive	Miosis	Narcotics, barbiturates, organophosphates, pilocarpine
			Encephalitis, abscess
			Tumor, bleed
Unilateral	± reactive		Normal in neonate
			Sympathetic lesion (ipsilateral)
Bilateral	Fixed		Lesion in pons
Bilateral	Light response negative, accommodation response positive	Argyll-Robertson pupil	Encephalitis, tumor
Bilateral	Light response positive, accommodation negative	Reverse Argyll-Robertson pupil	Meningitis, tumor
Large			
Bilateral	Reactive	Mydriasis	Postictal
	Light reflex slow, accommodation normal	Adie's pupil	Normal
Bilateral	Fixed		Cycloplegia
			Anorexia
			Toxic (drugs, metabolic)
			Tumour, injection
			Mania
Unilateral	Fixed		Uncal herniation
			Third cranial nerve/midbrain
Midsize			
Bilateral	Reactive		Normal
Bilateral	Fixed		Midbrain lesion, glass eye
Rapid alternate dilation/constriction		Hippus	Midbrain lesion
			Drug or alcohol excess
			Trauma to optic nerve
			Homocystinuria
'Multiple' pupil		Polycoria	Trauma, surgery, congenital
Unequal sizes		Anisocoria	Normal variant, iritis, eye medication, cerebral herniation, cervical sympathetic lesions, glaucoma, glass eye
Asymmetric			Trauma
Asymmetric on deviation (abducted side larger than adducted)		Tournay's sign	Normal
Absent iris		Aniridia	Wilms' tumor

- ears and nose:
  - hemotympanum: basal skull fracture
  - CSF leak
- neck:
  - stiffness: meningitis, meningism secondary to bleeding
  - pain: trauma
- head:
  - scars or mass: surgery, ventriculoperitoneal shunt
- breath:
  - alcohol (ethanol/methanol)
  - diabetic coma (acetone)
  - organophosphates (garlic)
  - cyanide (almonds)

Abnormal movements

See Table 2.4.5.

Motor examination

- Response to noxious stimuli (sternal pressure, pinched finger or toe):
- purposeful: absent with coma (Note—reflex withdrawl persists)
- asymmetric: present with confusion, stupor, delerium. Focial lesion likely
- decorticate (arms and wrists flex, legs and feet extend): cortex problem (above thalamus) (see Fig. 3.3.3)
- decerebrate (arms, legs, feet in tonic extension): brain-stem problem – high (below thalamus) (see Fig. 3.3.3)
- hypotonic/flaccid: brain-stem problem
- hypertonic: corticospinal trauma

TABLE 2.4.5 **Characteristics of abnormal movements**			
Term	**Description**	**Site**	**Timing**
Athetosis	Writhing movements: axial rotation with hyperextension (hypoxic–ischemic birth injury)	Distal extremities	Irregular but often continuous, particularly with excitement
Chorea	Rapid, involuntary, nonrhythmic jerking	Proximal and distal elements of the limbs are involved, face and trunk may also be affected	Rapid, spontaneous and often brief (e.g. up to a few seconds)
Dystonia	Irregular movements caused by simultaneous contraction of opposing muscle groups	The extremities, head and trunk can be affected	Depends on the speed of contraction and is often twisting in nature with slower pattern of relaxation
Myoclonus	Irregular, very rapid, repetitive, involuntary contraction of muscle groups	Various (can involve a single muscle)	Brief (up to 5 s)
Tick	Irregular, rapid, stereotyped movements that often rotate away from the midline	Frequently involving areas in the distribution of the cranial nerves (face, neck, shoulder)	Irregular, frequently less than 1 s in duration with repetition for several minutes and increased frequency with excitement.
Tremor	Rhythmic, regular movement, usually with equal range, speed and power of movement in each direction	Frequently in the hand or foot, can involve a whole limb	Brief (approximately 1 s)

LOCATION OF LESION

The location of the lesion may be identified from the following signs:

- supratentorial:
  - abnormal pupils
  - asymmetric motor signs
  - focal cerebral dysfunction
- subtentorial:
  - doll's eye reflexes
  - cold caloric stimulus abnormal
  - cranial nerve palsies
  - abnormal respiration
  - history of sudden onset
- metabolic:
  - pupils normal or dilated ± fixed
  - symmetric motor signs
  - seizures, tremor, myoclonus, acidosis
  - history of gradual onset (confusion/stupor)
- psychiatric:
  - pupils normal (or large)
  - reflexes symmetrical
  - eye closure inappropriate
  - increased or variable respiration

GENERAL CARE

The first priority in the management of comatose patients is preservation of vital function, i.e. airway protection, maintenance of ventilation, assurance of oxygenation, and support of the circulation (to maintain cerebral perfusion and oxygen delivery). The patient should be positioned to avoid aspiration, suffocation, or physical injury. If neck injury is suspected, the neck must be immobilized and great care taken during intubation maneuvers. Adequate aeration should be ensured, and an airway may be placed if it can be done easily. The forced insertion of an airway or the use of tongue blades or metal objects may cause severe oral injury and should be avoided. In the presence of poor air exchange, the child should be intubated and mechanically ventilated. It is wrong to await the development of florid systemic complications such as cyanosis, severe acidosis, or hemodynamic instability before proceeding to intubation.

To accomplish intubation, neuromuscular blockade is often necessary. Moreover, because all such patients should be assumed to have a 'full stomach' and be at significant risk of aspiration, a rapid sequence technique (Ch. 6.2) with cricoid pressure is mandatory. After intubation is accomplished, the child should be placed in 100% oxygen to avoid the development of hypoxia. Subsequent oxygen therapy should be guided by arterial blood gas analysis and other appropriate oxygen monitoring.

General clinical surveillance should include regular observations of motor, sensory, and pupillary function; blood pressure, pulse, oximetry and temperature, and electrocardiographic state. In severely affected patients, more complete and invasive monitoring should be undertaken, e.g. capnography and central venous pressure monitoring. It is also important to review which investigations will facilitate supportive therapy (Table 2.4.4).

Nursing care is also vitally important. Tracheobronchial secretions may be excessive and bronchial or endotracheal tube obstruction is a significant hazard. Scrupulous attention should therefore be given to airway care. In addition, early tube feeding for nutrition, regular turning to avoid pressure sores, and protective eye care should be instituted.

TABLE 2.4.6 Investigations that will facilitate supportive therapy
Arterial blood gas
Urea, electrolytes and creatinine
Blood glucose
Osmolality of plasma and urine
Urine testing for ketones, sugar, and pH
Full blood count
Coagulation screen
Infection screen
Blood levels of anticonvulsants
Virology
Chest X-ray
Electrocardiogram
Electroencephalography
Brain-stem auditory, visual and somatosensory evoked potentials
Cerebral imaging

✓ KEY POINTS

➤ Stabilize the patient:
- by ensuring adequate cardiorespiratory function and oxygenation
- by correcting and preventing metabolic imbalance of hydration, electrolytes, glucose, and lactate

➤ Treat the treatable:
- by preventing or correcting any systemic complications
- by controlling raised intracranial pressure (Ch. 2.6)
- by stopping seizures promptly (Ch. 2.5)
- by evaluating and treating specific causes

FURTHER READING

1. Teasdale G, Jennett B. Assessment of coma and impaired consciousness. A practical scale. Lancet 1974; ii: 81–84
2. Reilly PL, Simpson DA, Sprod R, Thomas L. Assessing the conscious level in infants and young children: a paediatric version of the Glasgow coma scale. Child Nerv Syst 1988; 4: 30–33
3. Eyre JA. (ed). Coma; Clinical paediatrics, international practice and research. Baillière Tindall, London, 1994; 2: 1

2.5 Seizures

Robert C. Tasker

Infants and children can have both convulsive and nonconvulsive forms of prolonged seizures. This chapter addresses only convulsive episodes of status epilepticus, which is strictly defined as two or more seizures occurring consecutively without an intervening period of full recovery of consciousness, or as recurrent epileptic seizures lasting for more than 30 minutes. Unfortunately, such a precise definition of status epilepticus—although useful for epidemiological analysis and evaluation of therapeutic interventions—conceals a sometimes frenetic approach to acute care and the urgency experienced by clinicians when confronted with a convulsing child, irrespective of how long the episode has lasted. It therefore seems more appropriate to take a pragmatic view and consider 'status epilepticus' as the severe end of a continuum encountered during the progressive evolution of an unrelenting seizure, which heralds a potentially life-threatening sequence of complications in central, metabolic and systemic physiology (Table 2.5.1).

CLINICAL PERSPECTIVE

Both the clinical context and natural history of acute seizures and status epilepticus are important considerations when evaluating choice of anticonvulsant therapy. In many parts of the world the most common cause of status epilepticus in childhood is an acute febrile illness in an otherwise healthy child although a wide variation exists in the actual proportion of such patients, who may comprise one-quarter to one-half of any index population.

MANAGEMENT

CLINICAL STRATEGY

The majority of acute seizures in children stop spontaneously. In out-of-hospital seizures, the period of transit is usually long enough for most episodes to have resolved or responded to initial interventions. The inference is that a child who is still convulsing on arrival in the emergency

---

TABLE 2.5.1 **Central, metabolic and systemic physiological changes and derangements during prolonged seizures**

Parameter	Duration of seizure		
	< 30 min (phase I)	> 30 min (phase II)	Hours (refractory)
Blood pressure	Increased	Decreased	Hypotention
Arterial oxygen	Decreased	Decreased	Hypoxemia
Arterial carbon dioxide	Increased	Variable	Hypercapnia
Lung fluid	Increased	Increased	Pulmonary edema
Autonomic activity	Increased	Increased	Arrhythmias
Temperature	Increased by 1°C	Increased by 2°C	Fever — hyperpyrexia
Serum pH	Decreased	Variable	Acidosis
Lactate	Increased	Increased	Lactic acidosis
Glucose	Increased	Normal or raised	Hypoglycemia
Serum potassium	Increased or normal	Increased	Hyperkalemia
Serum creatine phosphokinase	Normal	Increased	Renal failure
Cerebral blood flow	Increased 900%	Increased 200%	Cerebral edema
Cerebral oxygen consumption	Increased 300%	Increased 300%	Cerebral ischemia
Cerebral energy state	Compensated	Failing	Deficit — ischemia

department will continue to do so unless actively treated. How rapidly such treatment should be given then becomes the most important issue. Status epilepticus in the 1990s has a relatively low morbidity and mortality directly attributable to the seizure itself, and an overexuberant approach using anticonvulsants has been criticized as exposing patients to the iatrogenic risks of respiratory depression and hypotension unnecessarily. An important question to ask is, 'does the morbidity of the immediate treatment of seizures in the sick child to prevent status now exceed the morbidity of the status epilepticus itself?' In the absence of any clear clinical data to answer this question fully, the onus on those involved with acute seizure treatment is to ensure that it is administered safely, and in a standardized fashion which is understood by all the personnel involved.

EMERGENCY SUPPORTIVE THERAPY

Anyone who is actively convulsing should receive basic supportive therapy immediately.

Airway and oxygenation

Hypoxemia can be both a cause and a consequence of a seizure. When the episode is severe enough, complicating hypotension and bradycardia may also arise. To begin with, the head and neck should be positioned to keep the airway open, and if necessary the airway should be suctioned to ensure patency. If feasible, an oral airway can be inserted, although this should only be undertaken if there is no likelihood of trauma to the mouth and teeth; oxygen should be administered by nasal cannula or mask and bag-valve-mask ventilation. If the need for respiratory assistance persists after the patient has been supported by bag-valve-mask ventilation, endotracheal intubation should be considered. However, administering an anticonvulsant is a priority because managing the airway and assisting respiration are much easier after the convulsion has stopped. If persistent convulsive activity causes hypoventilation necessitating intubation, seizure activity can be temporarily stopped with a high dose of a short-acting barbiturate or midazolam (Fig. 2.5.1) and a neuromuscular blocking agent.

Glucose

Hypoglycemia is a rare cause of prolonged seizures in children. Nevertheless, all patients should have a prompt measurement of blood glucose (a profound disruption of autoregulation of cerebral blood flow can develop). If hypoglycemia (blood glucose concentration below 3 mmol/L) is documented or if it is impossible to obtain the measurement, intravenous glucose should be administered as 10% glucose, 5 ml/kg.

Blood pressure

Hypotension can potentiate or exacerbate any derangement in cerebral physiology and function. Systolic blood pressure should be maintained at normal levels. If there is no evidence of shock, minimal isotonic fluids should be given initially at a rate of 2–3 ml/kg·h.

EMERGENCY INVESTIGATIONS

In the convulsing patient initial supportive, therapeutic and diagnostic measures need to be conducted simultaneously. When status epilepticus is present measurement of blood gases, pH, blood glucose, renal and liver function, calcium and magnesium levels, hematological parameters (including platelet count), and anticonvulsant levels should be carried out. In addition blood and urine should be kept for toxicological or metabolic screening later, if this is subsequently deemed necessary. Further investigation will depend on the presenting clinical circumstances, whether or not there is a history of epilepsy, and age of presentation. When the episode of status is unexplained, focal, or coexistent with an acute illness, cranial computed tomographic scanning is warranted. Examination of the cerebrospinal fluid should only be carried out when there is no risk to the patient. Lumbar puncture can induce apnea, hypotension and respiratory arrest in addition to potentially causing direct CNS damage where there is significant elevation of intracranial pressure. The absence of papilledema does not exclude possible elevation of ICP.

ANTICONVULSANT THERAPY

The goal of anticonvulsant therapy is the rapid termination of clinical and electrical seizure activity

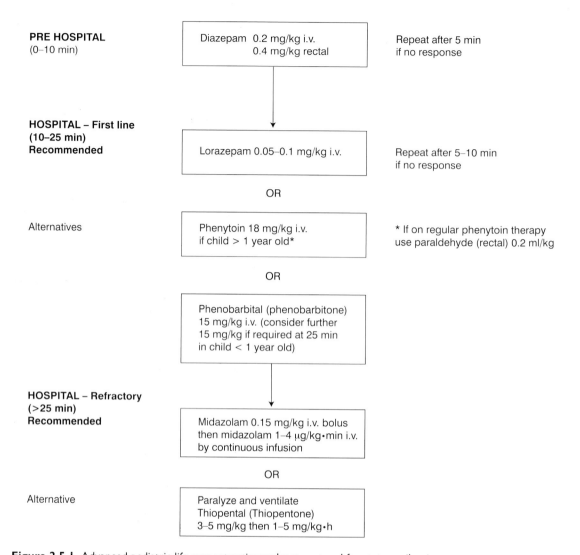

Figure 2.5.1 Advanced pediatric life support anticonvulsant protocol for status epilepticus

by the prompt administration of appropriate drugs in adequate doses, with attention to the possibility of complicating apnea, hypoventilation, hypotension and other metabolic abnormalities.

Prolonged seizures and anticonvulsant responsiveness

The concept of an acute seizure and status epilepticus being on a continuum is useful in regards to administering anticonvulsant therapy. For example, using diazepam in controlled experimental studies of prolonged seizures has established that the longer the duration of a seizure episode prior to treatment (ranging from 7 minutes to 130 minutes) the more difficult it is to control and the more likely it is that diazepam will convert an overt motor episode into another subtle or electroencephalographic form of seizure activity. Since similar findings have been reported in humans, the need for rapid, definitive treatment of acute seizures, irrespective of whether 30 minutes has elapsed, is clearly underscored.

Anticonvulsant protocol

There is no evidence that any one particular anticonvulsant protocol is the best for treating acute seizures. However, a clear path or treatment plan is necessary and recommended for effective and consistent management. One such approach is that recommended by the Advanced Life Support Group (Fig. 2.5.1). While endorsing wholly this specific approach, not least because it is taught widely and has been adopted as an international standard of care, we should also consider the emerging strategies using only benzodiazepine agents (Fig. 2.5.2), which may in the future simplify considerably the emergency treatment of acute seizures.

Prehospital therapy

The efficacy of intravenous diazepam for the treatment of status epilepticus is well recognized, with termination of episodes in some 80% of cases. However, safety is a significant concern, with apnea and respiratory depression as common complications. Therefore, except in known cases of recurrent prolonged seizures, drug treatment has traditionally been reserved for administration after arriving in hospital. However, if diazepam is not only effective therapy but also better when administered earlier, then why not give it before the patient reaches hospital—providing this can be done safely?

One reported approach has been to use in the prehospital setting 15 minutes of seizure activity as a threshold for administering intravenous diazepam (0.2 mg/kg) or rectal diazepam (0.5 mg/kg) by paramedical staff. As a safety issue, respiratory depression from rectal diazepam (0.2–0.5 mg/kg) is rare among children (a review of 13 papers on rectal diazepam by Siegler in 1990 identified only three cases of reversible respiratory depression in 843 cases). Some patients, however, may be at greater risk of respiratory depression, e.g. those with major comorbidities and those on regular anticonvulsants or with chronic CNS abnormalities. In these patients a lower rectal dose of 0.25 mg/kg is advised.

Taken together, research supports the use of a single prehospital dose of rectal diazepam, although attendants should be aware of the possibility of respiratory depression and be able to support breathing if necessary.

First-line hospital therapy

A child who is still convulsing on arrival in hospital can be assumed to have had a seizure lasting at least 10 minutes and therefore will require

Multi-agent (standard) 1 Protocol

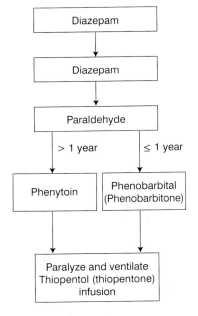

Benzodiazepine –1 only Protocol

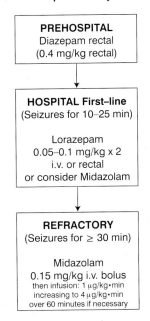

Figure 2.5.2 Seizure Control: comparison of (standard) 'multi-agent' and 'benzodiazepine-only' protocols

emergency treatment. Some children may have already received rectal diazepam. In this phase of management, the issues are whether diazepam is the treatment of choice, and if it is, whether it should be used more than once. Dealing with the latter issue first, although the precise serum diazepam concentration required for a therapeutic effect is not known, levels of 150–336 ng/ml are associated with arrest of seizure activity. These are achieved with a single dose of rectal diazepam, which questions the notion that further doses would be of benefit in those whose seizure has not come under control—unless administration of the first dose has been unreliable or a second episode has occurred. Few studies in children have looked specifically at the effectiveness of serial doses of diazepam when the first dose has failed to control the seizure.

Choices from phenobarbital (phenobarbitone), phenytoin and lorazepam as candidate alternative drugs for status epilepticus have been debated. Lorazepam, a hydroxylated benzodiazepine, is an effective anticonvulsant with a response latency comparable with that of diazepam, and it has the advantage of a longer duration of anticonvulsant effect than diazepam. Although there are few studies comparing lorazepam with established standards, it has been recommended as one of the first-line agents for status epilepticus for the above reasons. There is also the suggestion that it causes less respiratory depression than diazepam.

Despite the favourable aspects of lorazepam, there are still indications for the other agents. Lorazepam appears to be less effective in patients chronically treated with other benzodiazepine anticonvulsants and in those who will need the drug more than once. In both of these instances phenobarbital (phenobarbitone) appears to be superior, although there is little comparative clinical evidence. Phenytoin has a role when there is concern about impaired cerebral function and the need for clinical assessment of neurology.

Refractory seizures

Refractory status epilepticus has been defined as a seizure that is unresponsive to an adequate dose of a first-line parenteral anticonvulsant, or a seizure that is unresponsive to at least two doses of diazepam intravenously or rectally in succession followed by phenytoin, phenobarbital (phenobarbitone) or both, 20 mg/kg given over 30 minutes as an infusion, or failure to respond to the latter alone or in combination; or, a seizure that continues for 60–90 minutes after the initiation of therapy. This lack of consistency in definition is important when one considers the treatment and its consequences. Traditionally, for the most severe cases of status epilepticus induction of general anesthesia has been recommended using a short-acting barbiturate such as thiopental (thiopentone) 3–5 mg/kg as a bolus followed by infusion of up to 5 mg/kg·h along with supportive endotracheal intubation and mechanical ventilation. An alternative, effective approach has been to use, if necessary, repeated bolus doses of intravenous phenobarbital (10 mg/kg) every 30 minutes, without reference to a predetermined maximum level or dose, after one dose of intravenous diazepam has failed to control a seizure. A number of questions arise: for example, at what point is induction of anesthesia overexuberant? Is it really necessary to wait 60–90 minutes before deciding that standard anticonvulsants are ineffective? When is it inevitable that standard anticonvulsants are unlikely to work—after the second dose of diazepam, after the second drug, or after the third drug? Some of these issues have been addressed already. The main disadvantage of thiopental relates to its high lipid solubility and slow metabolism, which results in a prolonged period of intensive care support being necessary before a child is completely awake and cooperative once treatment has been stopped. Similarly, prolonged intensive care will be necessary when using very high doses of phenobarbital.

An approach recently delineated in children has been to use midazolam, an imidazobenzodiazepine. This drug has a relatively short elimination half-life of 1.5–3.5 hours, and preclinical and clinical analysis indicates that it shares anxiolytic, muscle relaxant, hypnotic and anticonvulsant actions with other benzodiazepines. Intravenous midazolam given as a bolus of 0.15 mg/kg followed by continuous infusion of 1 μg/kg·min (with increasing increments of 1 μg/kg·min every 15 minutes until seizure control) can be used, and after stopping the infusion the average time to full consciousness is in the range 2–9 hours.

NEUROLOGICAL INTENSIVE CARE

A number of medical complications may arise in patients being treated for status epilepticus (Table 2.5.2). General coma care is the same as that described for head injuries (Ch. 2.6).

CONTROVERSIES IN CARE

Devising a protocol for the management of status epilepticus with the optimal selection of anti-convulsant drugs is fraught with problems. Inevitably, factors other than pharmacology will influence the specific approach adopted. What is right for a practice seeing predominantly head injury as the cause of status epilepticus may not be appropriate for those seeing central nervous system infection as their leading etiology. The clinical context, cost and logistics of delivering effective treatment and care are important. Diagnostic studies and the type and timing of investigation are also a concern.

Perhaps not surprisingly, there is a paucity of clinical data comparing drug regimens for status epilepticus which means that there is still much to learn about this emergency. There is scope for a number of important clinical studies concentrating on the prehospital, first-line and refractory phase of drug treatment. Is prehospital administration of rectal lorazepam by paramedical staff of benefit? Can midazolam be used as monotherapy—using the intranasal or rectal route in the prehospital setting, and parenterally thereafter? Can we predict better those patients who will eventually prove to be refractory to treatment? Research is needed to answer these and other questions.

✔ KEY POINTS

➤ Prompt, effective basic life support is essential
➤ In the emergency room it should be assumed that any seizure will continue unabated unless actively treated
➤ Adhere to a standard protocol

TABLE 2.5.2 Medical complications of status epilepticus

- **Interictal coma**

- **Cumulative anoxia**
  cerebral and systemic

- **Cardiovascular complications**
  tachycardia, bradycardia
  cardiac arrest
  hypertension
  cardiac failure, hypotension, cardiogenic shock

- **Respiratory system failure**
  apnea
  Cheyne–Stokes breathing
  tachypnea
  neurogenic pulmonary edema
  aspiration, pneumonia
  pulmonary embolism
  respiratory acidosis
  cyanosis

- **Renal failure**
  oliguria, uremia
  acute tubular necrosis
  rhabdomyolysis
  lower nephron necrosis

- **Autonomic system disturbance**
  hyperpyrexia
  excessive sweating, vomiting
  hypersecretion (salivary, tracheobronchial)
  airway obstruction

- **Metabolic and biochemical abnormalities**
  acidosis (metabolic, lactate)
  anoxemia
  hypernatremia, hyponatremia
  hyperkalemia
  hypoglycemia
  hepatic failure
  dehydration
  acute pancreatitis

- **Infections**
  pulmonary
  bladder
  skin

- **Other**
  altered autoregulation and CBF
  increased cerebral metabolic rate for oxygen ($CMRo_2$)
  disseminated intravascular coagulation
  multiple organ system dysfunction
  fractures, thrombophlebitis

FURTHER READING

1. Meldrum BS, Horton RW. Physiology of status epilepticus in primates. Arch Neurol 1973; 28: 1–9
2. Meldrum BS, Brierley JB. Prolonged epileptic seizures in primates. Arch Neurol 1973; 28: 10–17
3. Meldrum BS, Vigouroux RA, Brierley JB. Systemic factors and epileptic brain damage. Prolonged seizures in paralyzed, artificially ventilated baboons. Arch Neurol 1973; 29: 82–87
4. Lothman E. The biochemical basis and pathophysiology of status epilepticus. Neurology 1990; S2: 13–23
5. Maytal J, Shinnar S, Moshe SL, Alvarez LA. Low morbidity and mortality of status epilepticus in children. Pediatrics 1989; 83: 323–331
6. Siegler RS. The administration of rectal diazepam for acute management of seizures. J Emerg Med 1990; 8: 155–159
7. Crawford TO, Mitchell WG, Fishman LS, Snodgrass SR. Very-high-dose phenobarbital for refractory status epilepticus in children. Neurology 1988; 38: 1035–1040
8. Tasker RC, Boyd SG, Harden A, Matthew DJ. EEG monitoring of prolonged thiopentone administration for intractable seizures and status epilepticus in infants and young children. Neuropediatrics 1989; 20: 147–153
9. Rivera R, Segnini M, Baltodano A, Perez V. Midazolam in the treatment of status epilepticus in children. Crit Care Med 1993; 21: 991–994
10. Lal Koul R, Raj Aithala G, Chacko A, Joshi R, Seif Elbualy M. Continuous midazolam infusion as treatment of status epilepticus. Arch Dis Child 1997; 76: 445–448

2.6 Trauma: cranial, spinal and multiple

Peter W. Skippen

Blunt trauma remains the leading cause of death in children over 1 year old. In the USA, nonaccidental injuries (NAI) are the most common cause of trauma death in children under 4 years of age; the other most common cause of injuries is trauma involving motor vehicles with the child as an occupant, pedestrian or bicyclist. Falls and recreational injuries are also common. Only a small proportion of traumatized children (10–15%) require a rapid systematic approach to initial management that will affect their outcome. This chapter describes that approach.

INITIAL RETRIEVAL

The prehospital care of these children involves initiation of medical therapy before and during transport to the location of definitive care. Communicating the status of the patient's condition to the receiving hospital allows appropriate triage upon arrival. A variety of trauma scores have been developed to assist with communication.

Particular attention is directed to:

- the cervical spine and skeletal injuries with careful extrication and appropriate immobilization techniques
- clearing the airway with basic airway maneuvers
- supporting inadequate ventilation
- control of any obvious external bleeding sites
- expeditious transport to the nearest medical facility
- stabilization and transport to the nearest facility offering specialized pediatric treatment (e.g. medivac evacuation process)

Prolonged resuscitation attempts delay definitive patient care. Most authorities advocate evacuation of the patient from the accident site to the nearest medical facility with minimal delay. However, in the severely injured child with altered level of consciousness and poorly palpable pulses, if the emergency medical transport team can rapidly access the circulation this is beneficial (intraosseous needle or intravenous cannula access).

PRIMARY SURVEY

The basic components of the primary survey strategy were formulated by the American College of Surgeons during the development of the Advanced Trauma Life Support (ATLS) course in the 1970s, and have become a standard of care throughout the world. The survey emphasizes immediate assessment of the airway and cardiorespiratory function, basic airway support maneuvers and vascular access during the initial few moments of arrival in the emergency room for any child with multiple injuries. History is performed after stabilization. The individual components of the primary survey are performed concurrently.

Immediately upon arrival, life-threatening conditions are identified and managed:

- attempt to arouse the child if unconscious, to assess the level of consciousness
- feel for the pulse rate and its quality; observe the child's color
- observe for signs of upper airway obstruction or respiratory distress
- control obvious external hemorrhage
- apply essential monitors (BP cuff, ECG monitor, pulse oximeter, temperature probe)
- establish baseline vital signs and record them

AIRWAY

The first minute should provide relief of upper obstruction airway and augmentation of gas exchange. Oxygen should be applied to any child sustaining significant trauma (while maintaining cervical spine precautions). In-line cervical stabilization rather than in-line traction is used. The preferred *methods for clearing the airway include chin lift and jaw thrust.* Head tilt should be avoided because of the potential for cervical spine trauma. Oropharyngeal debris should be cleared under direct vision. Oral airways can induce gagging and vomiting and nasal airways may induce a significant nosebleed.

Once the airway is cleared, other immediate respiratory life-threatening injuries are searched for and managed accordingly:

- open pneumothorax
- tension pneumothorax
- flail chest

BREATHING

The smaller the child, the more its reliance on diaphragmatic function and the greater risk of respiratory muscle fatigue. Air swallowing is common, which increases the risk of gastric dilatation and aspiration. The decision to intubate a child with multiple trauma should take into consideration:

- whether the airway is normal or abnormal
- the clinical condition of the patient

The most common indications to intubate in the trauma setting include:

- coma (children with a Glasgow coma scale score below 8)
- shock states
- failure to oxygenate or ventilate/chest wall dysfunction
- fatigue
- prophylactic:
  - suspected airway burn
  - for transport
  - airway protection

> The Glasgow coma scale is set out in Table 2.6.1

It is essential to assess the neurologic status of the patient quickly prior to intubation. Considerations while preparing to intubate include:

- children desaturate quickly
- a full stomach increases the risk of aspiration

- gastric dilatation is likely with improper clearance of airway secretions and bag-and-mask support

Is there:

- associated hypovolemia?
- possible intracranial injury?
- an abnormal airway?
- other injury that precludes a routine oral intubation?

All children require sedation or anesthesia for intubation unless they have sustained severe injury and present with a GCS score of 3 or 4. Children desaturate quickly upon induction of apnea, especially if there is partial upper airway obstruction or associated chest injury. Pre-oxygenation and continuous monitoring of pulse oximetry and blood pressure during and immediately following induction of anesthesia and intubation are important. Giving anesthetic drugs and starting intermittent positive pressure ventilation can result in hypotension and hypoventilation in the hypovolemic child. Depending on the clinical situation, having resuscitation drugs such as a prepackaged syringe of 1 in 10 000 epinephrine (adrenaline) readily available to support hemodynamics may be useful. Anesthetic drugs and muscle relaxants (Chs 6.2, 7.1) should be used cautiously if there is a risk of losing a clear airway and being unable to support ventilation. Options for sedation and anesthesia include:

1. *Ketamine* in a dose of 1–1.5 mg/kg will usually have minimal effect on the blood pressure but its use in a patient with a closed head injury is controversial.
2. *Thiopental* (*Thiopentone*) can precipitously lower cardiac output and blood pressure but a small dose (1–2 mg/kg) may be judiciously used so long as volume resuscitation is in progress. In a normovolemic patient, a full anesthetizing dose of thiopental (3.5 mg/kg) should be used together with a bolus of isotonic crystalloid to help support the blood pressure.
3. *Fentanyl* in a dose of 5–10 μg/kg can also be used but may indirectly lower blood pressure. This dose may result in some muscle rigidity.

4. *Midazolam* in a dose of 0.1 mg/kg can be used as an adjunct but is also associated with hypotension in a hypovolemic patient.

5. *Lidocaine* (*lignocaine*) is a safe adjunct in a dose of 1–1.5 mg/kg i.v., particularly in a child with an associated head injury.

Even small doses of these agents can cause hypotension in the hypovolemic child.

The muscle relaxant of choice for the acute trauma patient remains succinylcholine (suxamethonium). It has the most rapid onset and shortest duration of action. Dosage is 2–3 mg/kg for infants and 1.5–2 mg/kg for the older child. The only absolute contraindications to the use of succinylcholine in the emergency setting are:

- the child with a known upper airway obstruction where any muscle relaxation is contraindicated
- a patient presenting with a known muscular dystrophy (unlikely)
- a known history of malignant hyperpyrexia

Proper airway management should always take precedence over the relative contraindications (e.g. raised ICP) to the use of succinylcholine (suxamethonium). When indicated, it is safe to use in the face of spinal cord injury, burns and crush injuries during acute resuscitation.

There is no role for the use of a small dose of a nondepolarizing muscle relaxant prior to the administration of succinylcholine to prevent fasciculations. It serves no useful purpose in children and delays intubation, and occasionally can cause undue muscle weakness. In a patient with a known contraindication to the use of succinylcholine, rocuronium has the fastest onset of the currently available nondepolarizing muscle relaxants. The intubating dose is 1 mg/kg. Expect a long duration of action with this dose.

In children with a normal upper airway, oral intubation using a rapid sequence induction (RSI) technique (to prevent regurgitation of gastric contents) is safest and involves:

- preoxygenation using an anesthetic mask and reservoir bag with 100% oxygen
- intravenous access and fast-running i.v. solution

- suction device and appropriately sized Yaunker suction catheter at the right hand of the intubating physician
- an appropriately sized oral endotracheal tube according to age (selecting the size of the ETT is based on the simple formula of age/4 + 4, or approximates the patient's nares or little finger). Use an uncuffed ETT in children under 8 years of age unless there has been major thoracic trauma
- a lubricated stylet
- sedatives and muscle relaxants prepared prior to intubation and administered rapidly into a free running intravenous line
- application of cricoid pressure while drugs are administered (by a suitably instructed assistant), maintained until the endotracheal tube has been successfully placed and/or the cuff of the tube inflated

In trauma cases, use appropriate modification of RSI technique with drug administration into a fast-flowing intravenous line:

- atropine 10–20 μg/kg
- lidocaine (lignocaine) 1–1.5 mg/kg, 30–60 seconds prior to inducing anesthesia
- anesthetic agent
  ketamine 1–2 mg/kg in the absence of neurotrauma
- or thiopental (thiopentone) 1–2 mg/kg in the presence of hypovolemia
- or thiopental (thiopentone) 3–5 mg/kg in the absence of hypovolemia
- or fentanyl 5–10 μg/kg can be used as the anesthetic agent in the presence of hypovolemia or neurotrauma
- succinylcholine (suxamethonium) 1.5–2 mg/kg

Directly visualize the endotracheal tube pass through the cords. Pass the endotracheal tube only as far as the black line on the ETT. After visualizing the ETT pass through the cords, hold the tube firmly between the fingers and rest them at the corner of the child's mouth. Make a mental note of where the tube is, at the lips or the teeth at the corner of the mouth, so as the tube does not slip in or out while it is being secured. Confirm the position of the ETT with an end-tidal CO_2 monitor and chest

X-ray. Auscultation is notoriously unreliable in children. The decision to change from an oral to a nasal endotracheal tube depends on the ease of intubation, the indications for intubation, the stability of the child, and the clinical experience of the intubating physician.

Following successful intubation, gentle support of ventilation is commenced using either a Jackson-Rees circuit or a self-inflating bag. Assess the lung compliance. Check the adequacy of chest expansion and that both sides of the chest move equally.

- *Decreased lung compliance* in a recently intubated trauma patient suggests:
  - secretions or blood in the airway, an obstructed ETT or a foreign body in the airway (e.g. a broken tooth)
  - ETT down too far (on the carina or right mainstem bronchus)
  - pneumothorax
  - air space disease (contusion, aspiration)
- *Hypoxemia* that develops following intubation suggests:
  - esophageal intubation
  - dislodged ETT
  - obstructed ETT
  - air space disease
  - tension pneumothorax
  - relevance of checking expired/end-tidal CO_2 value
- *Hypotension* following induction of anesthesia and intubation suggests:
  - hypovolemia
  - tension pneumothorax
  - tension hemothorax
  - cardiac tamponade

An urgent chest X-ray is required for either persisting hypoxemia or hypotension following intubation. A needle thoracentesis may be warranted while awaiting the chest X-ray to exclude a tension pneumothorax or hemothorax. Use a catheter over the needle device (e.g. an angiocatheter or disposable intravenous cannula) with a syringe attached. Continuously aspirate while inserting the needle between the ribs. The safest site is between the mid and anterior axillary line on the interspace between ribs five and six. A significant tension pneumothorax will be drained equally well by this

approach as by the anterior approach. An intercostal catheter of appropriate size for the age of the patient should be inserted once the pneumothorax or hemothorax is confirmed with a chest X-ray.

Once the patient has been stabilized, aim for an expired tidal volume of 10–12 ml/kg and a respiratory rate appropriate for age (e.g. Table 2.1.1). Ideally, ventilation should be monitored with capnography aiming for an end-tidal CO_2 reading of approximately 35 mmHg in most patients. The ventilatory strategy for neurotrauma patients is considered under the section dealing with head injuries. Blood should be drawn if facilities allow for blood–gas analysis to confirm adequacy of ventilation and oxygenation. Maintain anesthesia while the patient is intubated, using morphine (intermittent boluses of 0.1–0.2 mg/kg followed by an infusion of 20–40 µg/kg·min), fentanyl (1–2 µg/kg bolus followed by an infusion of 1–2 µg/kg·h), or a midazolam infusion of 1–2 µg/kg·min.

An *abnormal airway* requires expert management (e.g. by anesthesia). It may require a surgical approach (by ENT). In a patient with a complicated airway, avoid the use of sedatives, muscle relaxants or attempts at passing the endotracheal tube blindly. In a patient with a suspected difficult airway, but where oral intubation is to be attempted, the neck should be prepared for immediate percutaneous cricothyrotomy should intubation fail. In the event of a failed intubation, an appropriate management protocol should be followed (Table 6.2.5.)

A sump–type orogastric tube is inserted to decompress the stomach and aspirate gastric contents. Adult sump tubes are inappropriate as their side holes extend too far proximally into the esophagus and will not adequately drain the child's stomach.

CIRCULATION

Early recognition and aggressive treatment of shock in children with multiple trauma reduces mortality and long-term morbidity rates. The evaluation by an experienced surgeon is essential in any hypotensive child who has sustained multiple trauma. *Hypovolemia is the most common cause of shock in children.* Common causes of hypovolemia include intraabdominal and retroperitoneal bleeding and lower limb long-bone fractures. Large scalp lacerations in infants can cause hypovolemia. Hypotension should never be attributed to head injury alone until more common causes are sought.

> An algorithmic approach to managing shock is presented in Chapter 2.3, Figure 2.3.1.

Immediately life-threatening causes of shock include:

- tension pneumothorax
- massive hemothorax
- cardiac tamponade

The cardiac output of an infant is rate-dependent. The autonomic control of the cardiovascular reflexes in children is vagal dominant. Bradycardia is an ominous finding in infants and children. The most common cause of bradycardia in children is hypoxemia but it is also caused by severe hypotension.

Children can maintain a normal blood pressure despite a loss of up to 25% of their intravascular blood volume primarily by tachycardia and increased peripheral vascular resistance. Pain, fear and psychological stress can produce a similar response and make clinical evaluation of these children difficult. Other useful clinical signs include pulse quality, capillary refill, skin mottling, peripheral and central temperatures, and measurement of urine output with a Foley catheter. Blood loss exceeding 25% of estimated blood volume results in poor peripheral pulses, hypotension and an altered level of consciousness. Blood loss exceeding 45% of estimated blood volume results in impalpable pulses, bradycardia on the ECG monitor and unconsciousness.

A vigilant clinician remains the best monitor of a child's response to resuscitation. Frequent reassessment of clinical signs can be supplemented with noninvasive blood pressure measurement, ECG monitoring, oximetry, and occasionally central venous pressure readings.

Management of hemorrhagic shock

The priorities of managing hemorrhagic shock are:

- control of any active external hemorrhage (avoid tourniquets and MAST suits)
- intravenous access (at least two sites in a hypotensive patient)
- aggressive volume resuscitation (to restore normotension)
- oxygenation
- adequate circulating hemoglobin
- optimizing cardiac output (avoiding bradycardia)

Establishing intravenous access can be difficult in hypovolemic and chubby infants. The peripheral veins on the back of hands, forearms, antecubital fossa and feet are best tried first. Valuable resuscitation time should not be wasted with repeat peripheral punctures if two or three attempts are unsuccessful. Unless the clinician is familiar with the technique, time wasted attempting a peripheral cut-down is also unwarranted. Alternative approaches to secure venous access include:

1. *Intraosseous needle*: fastest and easiest, preferably inserted into the proximal upper third of the medial surface of the tibia. Bilateral intraosseous needles can be inserted within a couple of minutes after appropriate sterile preparation and local anesthetic infiltration using 1% lidocaine (lignocaine) of the skin of the periosteum. Rapid volume infusion can be enhanced by using either a pressure bag or a syringe and three-way stopcock attached to the infusion circuit.
2. *Femoral venous access* may be attempted (using Seldinger's technique Ch. 6.1), but is difficult in a hypotensive child and ill-advised with active intraabdominal bleeding.
3. *Internal and external jugular veins*: this approach has the disadvantages that it can be difficult to gain access to the head of the bed and care is required with potential cervical spine injuries.
4. *Subclavian venous access* is often the preferred site in PICUs in children who are intubated or are in shock. As with all medical procedures, complications of this approach are related to the experience of the operator. With appropriate attention to

detail and skill, this technique is associated with a very low complication rate in all age groups. If the child already has a chest drain, insert the subclavian catheter on the side with the intercostal catheter. Otherwise, use a left-sided approach. Sterility in the emergency setting is difficult. Lines should be changed to a sterile site following stabilization.

Resuscitation fluid

The choice of resuscitation fluid is less important than ensuring that an adequate volume of fluid is used to restore hemodynamic status to normal. Volume requirements and drug dosages are often given based on an estimate of the child's weight in the emergency room. This is notoriously inaccurate. The estimated weight should be used only as a guide and the child resuscitated to stable hemodynamic parameters for age as indicated by a slowing of the heart rate, improving pulse pressure and pulse volume, improving blood pressure to at least 80 mmHg, decrease in skin mottling and an increasing warmth of the peripheries, increasing urine output and improved level of consciousness.

Isotonic crystalloid solutions are cheapest, readily available and the preferred initial choice. Saline (0.9%) or Ringer-lactate solution are most commonly chosen. The requirements for isotonic crystalloid solutions can be much greater than the 3:1 rule of thumb typically quoted. Loss of capillary integrity and significant third space losses from the tissue trauma can increase requirements considerably. Isotonic crystalloid solutions remain in the intravascular compartment for a maximum of only 30 minutes. A persisting tachycardia is an indication for further resuscitation.

Suitable colloids include 5% albumin and various commercially formulated plasma substitutes. Initial volumes administered in a hypotensive child would typically be 20 ml/kg of isotonic crystalloid or colloid, repeated as necessary.

Red blood cells should be administered early to any child presenting with 35–40% estimated blood loss. Colloid and reconstituted packed cells can be used to replace blood loss in a volume of 1:1. If administering red blood cells, group-specific blood is preferred and can be released from the blood bank within 10 minutes of receipt of the blood sample. This includes the patient's blood group and an immediate spin crossmatch of the recipient's serum with donor cells.

Hypertonic saline and other hypertonic solutions currently under investigation are not indicated as routine therapy as they have not proved to be superior to the more commonly available solutions. Dextrose solutions should *not* be used for resuscitation or in children who have sustained a severe closed head injury.

Resuscitation problems

There is debate regarding the possible adverse effects of full-volume resuscitation in the trauma patient. The concern is that this will disrupt hemostatic plugs as well as dilute coagulation factors. It has been suggested that the initial aim should be to resuscitate to the point of low normal blood pressure followed by immediate surgical intervention should that be indicated. At present, most authorities recommend early and aggressive resuscitation with surgical involvement as indicated.

The most common cause of a coagulopathy in a multiply-injured child is hemodilution as a consequence of the volume resuscitation. Delays in resuscitation and persisting tissue ischemia activate clotting and fibrinolytic systems and set the scene for the development of disseminated intravascular coagulation.

The principles of preventing or treating a coagulopathy are:

- control the source of bleeding
- ensure adequate oxygenation
- restore or maintain normothermia
- correct metabolic acidosis with aggressive volume resuscitation
- monitor laboratory parameters (International Normalized Ratio (INR), PTT, fibrinogen, fibrin degradation products)
- restore deficient factors or platelets

A common pitfall in resuscitating children with skeletal trauma is to underestimate the amount of blood lost from fractures of the long bones and pelvis. These children are often normotensive on initial presentation. Unless further loss is anticipated and volume replacement initiated, these children will decompensate during transport to a tertiary care center. It is essential these children receive a bolus of crystalloid of at least 20 ml/kg and further boluses as necessary dependent on clinical reassessment. As much as 10–20% of the child's blood volume can be lost into the surrounding soft tissues with these fractures.

Always consider hidden, coexisting intraabdominal, intrathoracic or skeletal injuries if there is persisting unexplained tachycardia or hypotension.

Try to control heat loss:

- use warm intravenous fluids
- use overhead warmers
- minimize exposure once the examination is completed

DISABILITY AND DIAGNOSIS

A brief neurologic examination should be performed during the primary examination. A Glasgow coma scale score is most commonly used (Table 2.6.1). The motor component is most predictive of the patient's long-term neurologic outcome. Look for asymmetry of motor movements. Examine pupils for size, symmetry and reaction to light. The examination should be repeated at intervals to assess progress and the effect of treatment. Pitfalls in the interpretation of the GCS score include drug ingestion, postictal state, inadequate volume resuscitation and hypoxemia.

SECONDARY SURVEY

The secondary assessment is often delayed until life-threatening injuries have been managed, an orogastric tube is in place and a Foley catheter inserted to monitor urine output. It must be emphasized that the patient's vital signs should be continually checked during the secondary assessment.

All injuries are determined, documented and management initiated. A complete head-to-toe examination, including both front and back, is performed. Examination of the back in a patient with a suspected cervical spine injury is best performed with one person maintaining the head and neck in the axial line of the thoracolumbar spine while two other people perform a log roll. Injuries should be managed in descending order of urgency.

TABLE 2.6.1 **The Glasgow coma scale**	
● **Eye opening**	
Spontaneously	4
To speech/verbal command	3
To pain	2
None[a]	1
● **Verbal response**	
Oriented (appropriate conversation/reaction, for age to stimuli or surroundings)	5
Confused (disoriented, uncooperative, uses words/cries and consolable, aware of surroundings)	4
Inappropriate words, vocal sounds or crying; awareness and responses inconsistent	3
Incomprehensible sounds, cries, unaware and unresponsive to surroundings	2
None	1
● **Best motor response**	
To verbal command: obeys (spontaneous)	6
To painful stimulus[b]	
localizes stimulus (vocalizing)	5
withdraws (flexion)	4
abnormal flexion (decorticate)	3
extensor response (decerebrate)	2
none	1
● **Total score** eyes (1–4) + verbal (1–5) + motor (1–6)	
Range 3–15	

From Teasdale G, Jennett B. Assessment of coma in impaired consciousness. A practical scale. Lancet 1974; i: 81
Simpson D, Riley P. Pediatric coma scale. Lancet 1982; ii: 450.
[a]Award full score to children under 2 years old for crying response after stimulation (CPS. Management of children with head trauma. Can Med Assoc J 1990; 142(9): 949).
[b]Stimuli for motor response: nail bed pressure (upper limb) or supraorbital pressure (localizing response—hand movement to the chin)

In the event that NAI is suspected, careful documentation of all external injuries and fundoscopic examination are required. Consider photographic documentation of the injuries later. Contact the police and the appropriate agencies.

EXTREMITIES

The extremities are examined for abrasions, contusions, hematoma, obvious bony deformity and neurovascular function. A compartment syndrome must be suspected and diagnosed early. Measurement of compartmental pressures is not always reliable. The decision to perform a fasciotomy most often is dependent on clinical examination of peripheral pulses, pallor, parasthesia and paralysis if the patient is conscious. Prophylactic antibiotics (e.g. cefazolin, cloxacillin, gentamicin) may be necessary for compound orthopedic injuries. Tetanus toxoid and immunoglobulin should be given if the immunization history is uncertain.

HISTORY

A detailed history of the onset of the injury or illness is essential. Knowledge of the forces of the injury associated with the trauma is important in determining the extent of possible injuries and further investigations such as an aortogram. If the history does not adequately explain the severity of the injuries (especially intracranial hemorrhage in infants), consider NAI and investigate appropriately. The past medical history is important, as are any ongoing systemic illnesses. A medication and allergy history should also be obtained. Much of the background history can be obtained from family members or eyewitnesses by a nurse during the clinical examination and resuscitation. A complete and detailed history is obtained following stabilization of the patient.

INVESTIGATIONS

Relevant investigations can be divided into laboratory and radiologic, urgent and nonurgent. Urgent laboratory tests include:

- blood group and screen, crossmatch
- hemoglobin, platelets
- blood glucose, electrolytes
- urea and creatinine
- AST, ALT
- INR, PTT
- urinalysis

Urgent radiologic investigations include:

- AP and lateral cervical spine
- AP chest X-ray

Other investigations are performed as required depending on clinical suspicion and clinical findings. Consider a skeletal survey if NAI is suspected.

In the critically ill, multiply-injured child, the primary and secondary survey and investigations should have been accomplished within an hour of arrival in the emergency room.

HEAD TRAUMA

The leading cause of death in children following multiple trauma is CNS injury. Significant head trauma occurs in over 50% of children who have sustained a blunt injury. Head trauma is frequently associated with the faciomaxillary, chest, and intraabdominal injury. Most NAI is associated with some form of head trauma. Outcome is worse in the very young (< 3 years) compared with the older child. Outcome is better in children than in adults with a similar severity of GCS score. Children with severe, closed head injury and multiple other injuries have a higher mortality rate than children with an isolated head injury. The classification of pediatric head injury is given in Table 2.6.2.

TABLE 2.6.2 Classification of pediatric head injury by severity

Mild
Asymptomatic
Mild headache
Three or fewer episodes of vomiting
Glasgow coma scale score of 15
Loss of consciousness for less than 5 minutes

Moderate
Loss of consciousness for 5 minutes or more
Progressive lethargy
Progressive headache
Vomiting protracted (more than three times) or associated with other symptoms
Post-traumatic amnesia
Post-traumatic seizure
Multiple trauma
Serious facial injury
Signs of basal skull fracture
Possible penetrating injury or depressed skull fracture
Suspected child abuse
Glasgow coma scale score of 11–14

Severe
Glasgow coma scale score of 10 or less or a decrease of two points or more not clearly caused by seizures, drugs, decreased cerebral perfusion or metabolic factors
Focal neurologic signs
Penetrating skull injury
Palpable depressed skull fracture
Compound skull fracture

Modified from Canadian Pediatric Society. Management of children with head trauma. Can Med Assoc J 1990; 142(9): 949.

PHYSIOLOGY

Cerebral blood flow varies somewhat with age but reaches adult levels by early childhood (3–4 years of age). Intracranial pressure (ICP) is low in infancy (< 5 mmHg) but increases with age to a normal adult pressure of 10 mmHg by late childhood. The primary determinants of cerebral blood flow and cerebral oxygenation are:

1. *Autoregulation*: the autoregulation curve describes the ability of the brain to maintain constant blood flow over a wide range of cerebral perfusion pressure (mean arterial pressure – ICP). Normal CPP varies according to the age of the child. The autoregulation curve is shifted to the right by head trauma. It has been demonstrated in adults that a higher than normal CPP is required to maintain an adequate cerebral blood flow following neurotrauma. This is likely to be the case for children also. Maintaining an adequate CPP and cerebral blood flow minimizes the risk of ICP plateau wave development.
2. *Partial pressure of arterial CO_2*: there is a 3% change in cerebral blood flow for each 1 mmHg (0.13 kPa) change in Pa_{CO_2}. This response is retained in all but the most severely traumatized brain. Hypercarbia abolishes cerebral autoregulation. The combination of partial airway obstruction and hypotension is devastating in patients with neurotrauma. Hypocarbia can also result in a severe reduction in cerebral blood flow.

Cerebral ischemia is common after severe head trauma in both adults and children. Post-traumatic cerebral hyperemia is far less common in pediatric neurotrauma than once thought. The combination of these intrinsic low flow states and hypotension predisposes to a more severe injury. Post-traumatic ischemic injuries are common at post mortem in these patients. Inappropriate hyperventilation probably does more harm than good.

An individual's cerebral blood flow is unpredictable following head trauma and may change during the course of recovery from the injury. The metabolic requirements of a comatose brain are less than those of a normal brain and relative hyperemia is common (i.e. oxygen delivery adequate to meet metabolic requirements). However, elevation of temperature and seizures dramatically increase the brain's requirement for O_2 (CMR_{O_2}). Co-existing acidosis or hypoglycemia can disrupt autoregulation. Importantly these factors act syngergistically, i.e. levels of acidosis, fever, hypoxia and hypertension which alone pose no threat can together significantly compromise CBF. All patients except the most severely injured (GCS score of 3) will respond to acute changes of CO_2. There is no consistent relationship between cerebral blood flow and raised intracranial pressure (ICP) or between cerebral blood flow and GCS score. A normal global cerebral blood flow does not exclude significant regional abnormalities of CBF.

Elevated ICP is common after closed head injuries. Most likely factors include:

- increased intracranial blood volume
- cerebral vasodilation
- cerebral edema
- intracranial mass lesions
- obstructed CSF drainage

Increased ICP is significant for two reasons:

1. It impairs CPP and contributes to ischemic damage.
2. The regional effects of pressure increases within the cranium result in secondary brain injury and/or transtentorial herniation.

BRAIN INJURY

Head injury can be divided into a primary and a secondary injury. The primary injury occurs at the time of the trauma. Any coincident events such as asphyxia from airway obstruction can be included in this injury. Following the primary injury, a cascade of events is initiated including free radical production and release of neuroexcitatory transmitters such as glutamine. These agents are believed to cause neuronal death. Secondary brain injury significantly contributes to morbidity and mortality following head trauma. Common causes include:

- hypotension (any episode doubles mortality associated with head trauma)
- hypoxemia

- raised ICP
- hyperpyrexia
- hyponatremia, hyposmolality
- seizures

The most common types of intracranial injury following head trauma in children include:

- diffuse axonal injury
- contusion
- intracranial hematomas
- raised ICP and cerebral edema
- direct vascular injury (carotid, vertebral)— consider when CNS deficit is not explained by CT findings
- cerebral vasospasm

PRIMARY SURVEY

The initial management of the child presenting with acute neurotrauma involves:

- relieving upper airway obstruction
- securing the airway with an oral ETT under general anesthesia with a rapid sequence induction technique as previously outlined if:
  – GCS less than 8
  – the child is combative and disoriented with multiple other injuries
  – transport of the patient to CT scan or tertiary referral center is required.
- supporting ventilation with 100% oxygen
- restoration and maintenance of an adequate circulating blood volume and CPP. There is no place for restricting fluids *during resuscitation* in a patient with neurotrauma. Normovolemia should be maintained at all times using isotonic crystalloids of colloid to avoid possible hyponatremia. Dextrose-free solutions should be used.

Routine monitoring of a head-injured patient includes ECG, oximetry, non-invasive BP and ET_{CO_2} measurement. The ideal range of CO_2 values in a patient without localizing signs of raised ICP is 35–40 mmHg ET_{CO_2}, confirmed by arterial blood gas analysis. Unmonitored hyperventilation may result in regional cerebral ischemia and a secondary injury. A GCS score should be assessed

prior to induction of anesthesia and intubation if time allows. Never forget the possibility of a cervical spine injury with associated head or faciomaxillary injury. Clinical signs of elevated ICP such as a sluggish and dilating pupil, a fixed and dilated pupil, or Cushing's triad should prompt:

- brief periods of hyperventilation guided by capnography and arterial blood gas analysis: aim for Pa_{CO_2} 3.3–4.0 kPa (25–30 mmHg) initially.
- 20% mannitol 0.25–0.5 g/kg administered over 20 minutes (multiple doses of mannitol can induce hypovolemia and severe electrolyte disturbances, especially hypernatremia).
- urgent head CT scan to exclude a space-occupying lesion which may require neurosurgical intervention

SECONDARY SURVEY

An outline of the intensive care required by neurotrauma patients is shown below. Meticulous attention to detail, maintenance of CPP and avoidance of excessive hyperventilation are essential. The full neurologic examination is performed at this time. Remember that NAI is a major cause of neurotrauma in young children. These patients need to be examined and investigated accordingly. Fundoscopic examination with careful documentation of the findings is essential.

COMPLICATIONS

Complications that should be anticipated during intensive care following resuscitation include:

1. Worsening cerebral edema for 72–96 hours may occur with elevated ICP.
2. Cerebral vasospasm occurs in up to 40% of adults sustaining head trauma with associated subarachnoid hemorrhage and similar frequency is likely in children. Prophylactic nimodipine therapy may be warranted in children with subarachnoid blood seen on the initial CT scan. Ensure normal intravascular volume prior to its use as hypotension is possible. Consider monitoring these children with sequential

transcranial Doppler imaging. Hypervolemic and hypertensive therapy should be considered if vasospasm is confirmed with angiography.

3. Salt-losing states and water retention can occur in these children and result in profound hyponatremia unless special care is taken with fluid and electrolyte management.

4. Neurogenic pulmonary edema can result in significant hypoxemia. The cause is likely to be multifactorial. Management is supportive with increased inspired oxygen concentrations and the judicious application of positive end-expiratory pressure (PEEP) to recruit alveoli.

5. Combined closed head injury and thoracic injury presents the most complicated management problem. Management of the lung injury may require high levels of PEEP to ensure adequate systemic and cerebral oxygenation. Current strategies tolerate mild to moderate hypercarbia to reduce ventilator-induced lung injury. Under these conditions intracranial pressure may be difficult to control. These patients should be monitored with external ventricular drains for monitoring of ICP and drainage of CSF. The development of ARDS is not uncommon in these patients.

6. hypertension is not uncommon in the absence of clinical and radiographic evidence of raised ICP. Ensuring that the child is sedated and pain-free (local anesthesia for procedures) is all that is required in most cases. Maintenance of euvolemia should be the priority at all times. Ensure bladder distention is avoided (Foley catheter) as well as disturbance from loud noise and unnecessary movement.

Most ICUs manage patients without muscle relaxants. If paralysis is induced for active control of temperature or for severe elevations of ICP, phenytoin seizure prophylaxis should be instituted (dose 15–20 mg/kg initially i.v. over 20 min), especially if the child has already had a seizure or if there is cerebral contusion or intracranial hematoma. Nutritional support is instituted early via a nasogastric or naso-

jejunal tube within the first 24 hours of the injury. There is no place for steroid or barbiturate coma in the management of these children. Mild hypothermia (32–33°C) appears to have merit in young adults with severe injury or unstable ICP, and warrants consideration in the management of children with this degree of injury during the initial 24 hours.

PROTOCOL FOR MANAGING CHILDREN WITH HEAD INJURY AND A GCS SCORE BELOW 8

MANAGEMENT WITHOUT ICP MONITOR

Basic principles:

- head position neutral
- head of bed elevated 30°
- normovolemia—maintain Hb >100 g/L (i.e. usual cardiovascular principles) by following pulse rate, blood pressure, urine output, tissue perfusion and CVP (if the patient has a central line)
- normothermia (35.5–37°C)
  - cooling blanket beneath all patients, turn on if the patient's temperature rises
  - consider hypothermia (32–33°C): set blanket at 32.5° C for 24 hours in severe injury/unstable ICP.
  - *Note*—rewarming should then be passive (< 1°C per hour) and monitor for potential hyperkalemia
- normocarbia—$PaCO_2$ 4.7–5.3 kPa (35–40 mmHg)
- no paralysis—i.e. routinely unparalyzed (unless the cooling blanket/hypothermia is used or patient is rewarming—then paralyze)
- anticonvulsants (phenytoin)—routinely for cerebral contusions or intracranial blood, and for all paralyzed patients
- routine blood investigations:
  - initial 48 hours, electrolytes and blood gases every 6 hours
  - frequency to be reviewed thereafter
- arterial line for routine indications

AGGRESSIVELY TREAT HYPOTENSION
(any episode of hypotension doubles the mortality after a severe closed head injury)

- fluids at 80% maintenance initially:
  - the usual maintenance fluid for patients with severe acute head injuries should be 0.9% saline. (Ringer-lactate solution and 0.45% saline are hypotonic)
  - avoid dextrose-containing solutions unless hypoglycemia is demonstrated or the child is less than 6 months old (and then only with close monitoring of blood glucose levels)—MAINTAIN NORMOVOLEMIA AT ALL TIMES
- intravenous $MgSO_4$, 0.15 mmol/kg (40 mg/kg), every 6 hours for 48 hours. Measure serum magnesium levels daily – continue Mg therapy as long as serum Mg is below 2 mmol/L
- nutrition—commence no later then 24 hours, preferably by the enteral route. If gastric paresis persists beyond 48 hours, a jejunal feeding tube should be placed (*remember to restrict free water*)
- steroids—*never,* for the uncomplicated head injury
- repeat head CT scan routinely after 24–48 hours, or for any unexpected or unexplained deterioration in clinical status

ADDITIONAL MANAGEMENT WITH ICP MONITORING

The ultimate decision about monitoring should be made by the neurosurgeon. An external ventricular drain (EVD) is the preferable method:

- no prophylactic antibiotics
- position EVD at 20 cm above the tragus (15 mm Hg on the ICP monitor)
- maintain ICP monitor below 20 cm H_2O or 15 mmHg
- jugular venous bulb catheter—infuse regular heparinized 0.9% saline at 2 ml/h; *NO DRUGS TO BE INFUSED OR INJECTED VIA THIS LINE*
- monitor cerebral extraction ratio: $CEo_2 = (Sao_2 - Sjo_2)100/Sao_2$

ACUTE NEUROLOGIC DETERIORATION

Management without ICP monitor

In a child who shows signs of neurological deteriation such as acute pupillary dilatation:

- hyperventilate with 100% oxygen
- call ICU pediatrician or neurosurgeon
- give mannitol 20%, 1 g/kg over 20 minutes
- arrange urgent CT scan of head, simultaneously with all of the above

Management with measured elevation of ICP

Acute neurologic deterioration is evidenced by persistent elevation of the ICP above 15 mmHg for more than 5 minutes, or alteration in pupillary reponses. *Note*—ICP is normally elevated in healthy patients by such maneuvers as coughing and turning, and is usually coincident with an elevation in blood pressure. This is *normal.*

An elevated ICP becomes abnormal when it:

- remains elevated and becomes a plateau rather than a spike
- becomes elevated without a coincident rise in arterial blood pressure
- remains elevated for less than 5 minutes, but is associated with a falling arterial BP while the ICP stays high
- exhibits frequent and recurrent unstimulated spikes in pressure

i.e. it is associated with a fall in cerebral perfusion pressure CPP

Interventions

- Open the EVD—allow to drain for 5 minutes.
- If the CSF is not draining, or if opening the drain does not result in lowering of the ICP, administer mannitol 0.25–1 g/kg for ICP over 15 mmHg. Mannitol may be used repeatedly if clinical effect persists—MAINTAIN NORMOVOLEMIA, and follow electrolytes closely (Na 140–150 mmol/L). Discontinue mannitol if hypernatremia develops.

- It may be prudent in some patients to leave the drain open 'continuously' (for example, if a sustained effect on lowering ICP is not produced by mannitol, and the drain requires opening more frequently than twice hourly). If this clinical decision is made, it is important to turn the three-way stopcock every 30 minutes to read the actual ICP. If the drain is not working (i.e. not draining CSF fluid), contact the neurosurgeon and ask to reassess function of the drain.

Do not record the ICP reading from the monitor when the drain is open.

However, if when the drain is closed the pressure rises to above 35 mmHg and appears to be continuing to rise, the drain should be reopened before a 'stable' ICP recording is reached and the ICP recorded as '> 35 mmHg' for that measurement.

- hypocarbia – to a minimum of 30 mmHg, unless using jugular venous oxygen extractions to monitor the therapy.

Other than for brief periods of hypocarbia, the effect should be monitored (preferably with the guidance of a xenon CT scan) using the jugular venous catheter. Acceptable CEO_2 values in a pediatric patient lie below 30%. A low extraction ratio (less than 20%) if associated with a high ICP indicates that cerebral blood flow is excessive and may be contributing to the high ICP. If the CEO_2 is low and the ICP is high, gentle lowering of the $Paco_2$ is appropriate. Hyperventilation can also be used as a rescue maneuver if there is sudden acute CNS deterioration such as a dilated pupil.

- should problems with intracranial hypertension occur when the patient is not already cooled, moderate hypothermia (32–33°C) may be instituted
- hypertensive therapy—optimizing cerebral perfusion pressure. Hypertensive therapy must be discussed with the neurosurgeon and the PICU physician. If the ICP remains problematic and unresponsive to all of the above maneuvers, consideration should be given to increasing the systemic blood pressure. A central venous catheter should be inserted. The intravascular volume should be 'full', i.e. give boluses of fluid to increase the CVP to 8–10 mmHg. Add dopamine 5–10 µg/kg·min. If this does not bring the CPP above the age-dependent CPP level (Table 2.6.3), consider the introduction of either phenylephrine or norepinephrine (noradrenaline) via a central venous catheter to increase the systemic BP in an effort to improve the CPP and hence cerebral blood flow to the injured brain.

- barbiturate therapy if all else fails

REMEMBER: these are lower limits of CPP autoregulation. Head-injured patients have the CPP autoregulation curve shifted to the right, which means that these patients will not tolerate a low CPP, and may require a higher than normal pressure for their age to maintain adequate cerebral blood flow (e.g. a 5-year-old with a normal lower limit of CPP of 50 mmHg may not have normal flow as judged by either a xenon CBF study or cerebral extractions unless the CPP is raised to 60–70 mmHg).

MANAGEMENT OF JUGULAR VENOUS CATHETERS

- infuse heparinized saline at 2 ml/h
- lateral cervical spine X-ray of base of brain and vertebrae to assure correct position
- measure cerebral oxygen extractions for acute changes in therapy (e.g. hyperventilation), otherwise every 8–12 hours

TABLE 2.6.3 **Age ranges for normal mean blood pressure (BP), intracranial pressure (ICP) and cerebral perfusion pressure (CPP).**

AGE (years)	BP (mmHg)	ICP (mmHg)	CPP (mmHg)
0.5	70	2	50
1	76	5	50
2	76	10	50
5	70	10	50
12	74	12	60
15	95	15	60

MANAGEMENT OF CEREBRAL OXYGEN EXTRACTION

Normal CEo_2 in children is 20–30%

1. If CEo_2 exceeds 30%, this implies either excessive oxygen consumption by the brain, or inadequate oxygen delivery or inadequate blood flow to the brain. Hence interventions are required to either reduce oxygen consumption or increase blood flow.
2. If CEo_2 is below 20%, this implies that there is either a low oxygen consumption by the brain (very low extractions occur with the most severe injuries and brain death), or excessive cerebral blood flow.
3. If there is an associated increased ICP, then interventions may be undertaken to reduce the excessive flow in an attempt to reduce the ICP, but *not* at the expense of maintaining an adequate CPP (e.g. consider lowering the $Paco_2$ in an effort to reduce CBF) any intervention undertaken to manipulate blood flow should be monitored with CEo_2 to ensure that the blood flow remains acceptable. If the CPP and ICP are reasonably controlled, and the CEo_2 is below 30%, there is no need to intervene.

SPINAL CORD INJURIES

ANATOMY AND PHYSIOLOGY

There are significant differences in the anatomy and biomechanics of the pediatric vertebral column which affect the type of injury sustained. These include:

- relatively large, heavy head
- weak cervical supporting musculature
- lax interspinal ligaments and joint capsules
- intervertebral facet joints oriented horizontally (pseudosubluxation as defined by a 3 mm or greater vertebral displacement of C-2 upon C-3 occurs in more than 50% of normal children)
- mostly cartilaginous vertebrae causing disc spaces to appear wide
- vertebral bodies maintain a wedge shape and appear more narrow anteriorly until

about 7 years of age, after which they become more square, to resemble those of the adult vertebral column
- the vertebral column is similar to adults by 10 years of age

Blood supply to the spinal cord is unique for its segmental distribution. The anterior spinal artery supplies the anterior two-thirds of the spinal cord and originates from the vertebral arteries. It is fed by a number of cervical, lumbar and sacral radicular vessels. The largest of these vessels originates from the mid-lower thoracic region. Potential watershed areas exist between the cervical, thoracic, lumbar and pelvic regions and also between the anterior and posterior cord. The posterior third of the spinal cord is supplied by the two posterior spinal arteries, also originating from the vertebral arteries. Blood drains from the cord to the valveless venous plexus surrounding the cord.

The control of spinal cord blood flow is similar to that of the cerebral circulation. It is primarily dependent on an adequate spinal cord perfusion pressure, such that a decrease in systemic mean arterial pressure or increased venous pressure (e.g. raised intraabdominal pressure) will impair spinal cord blood flow. There is also a linear response to changes in CO_2 as in the cerebral circulation. There are obvious implications for resuscitation and management of spinal cord injuries.

SPINAL TRAUMA

Vertebral column and spinal cord injuries are uncommon in children. High cervical spine injuries (C-1 to C-3) are more common in infants, whereas lower cervical spine injuries are more common in the older child. Thoracolumbar injuries are also more common in the older child. Younger children are prone to purely ligamentous injuries. The SCIWORA syndrome (spinal cord injury without radiologic abnormality) refers to these purely ligamentous injuries in children and is thought to result from the hypermobile pediatric vertebral column. Most children suffering from SCIWORA syndrome have complete cord lesions and a poor prognosis. Teenagers more often sustain injuries of the vertebral body and/or the posterior elements. The absence of pain in a conscious patient does not exclude a significant cervical spine injury.

The most common causes of cervical spine injuries in children less than 8 years old are motor vehicle injuries, falls, birth trauma and child abuse. Athletic injuries (diving, skiing or snowboarding) become more prominent in adolescent years. Injuries sustained during motor vehicle crashes and NAI are often associated with closed head injuries.

The use of lap belt restraints in motor vehicles has created the syndrome of Chance fractures. These are lumbar spine hyperflexion injuries secondary to inappropriately applied lap seat-belts which ride above the pelvis of small people. They are often associated with major intraabdominal hollow viscera injury (contusion, perforation, avulsion).

Conditions such as Down syndrome, achondroplasia and juvenile rheumatoid arthritis predispose children to cervical spine and cord injury following minor trauma.

PRIMARY SURVEY

Management at the scene of the injury involves immobilization techniques that splint both head and torso to a rigid board with bilateral sandbags at the head. These techniques are superior to collars in reducing movement of the vertebral column. Soft collar 'immobilization' should not be used.

The primary survey of a child presenting with suspected spinal cord injury is identical to that already described. In an unconscious child arriving in the emergency room with a rigid collar, safe access to the head and neck can be achieved by removing the collar while maintaining the head and neck in a neutral position with in-line manual cervical stabilization. This will also be required for intubation. Ventilatory assistance with bag-and-mask ventilation may be required for high cord lesions involving the phrenic nerve (C-2 to C-4) or for associated hypoxemia and hyperventilation from other causes.

If the child requires intubation, direct laryngoscopy under anesthesia is not associated with aggravation of the cord injury so long as the head and neck are maintained in a neutral position. Small amounts of spinal movement occur with all basic and advanced airway maneuvers, including application of cricoid pressure. Rapid sequence induction is the preferred approach. Cervical spine injury by itself is not an indication for blind nasotracheal intubation or cricothyrotomy.

Restoration of intravascular volume and correction of hypotension is urgent. Neurogenic shock can occur with high cord lesions and manifests as hypotension unresponsive to aggressive volume resuscitation. There will usually be a bradycardia and warm, vasodilated peripheries. It is imperative to exclude other causes of hypotension: in particular, intraabdominal injuries are notoriously difficult to detect. Once spinal shock is confirmed, care is required to avoid overaggressive resuscitation. Pulmonary edema in this setting is not uncommon and is multifactorial in etiology:

- neurogenic
- fluid overload
- aspiration

These children may require inotropic support to maintain an acceptable systemic blood pressure and spinal cord perfusion pressure.

A full neurologic examination is reserved for the secondary survey. The back is carefully examined for evidence of bruising and obvious deformities while palpating the intervertebral spaces from head to sacrum. The functional integrity of the cord is assessed, including motor and sensory function, and bulbocavernosus reflex and anal tone. The sensory components of the examination are difficult to assess in small children, and in unconscious and intubated patients.

RADIOLOGIC EXAMINATION

The plain cervical spine X-ray remains the best method to diagnose cervical spine injuries but may require supplementation with CT scan and three dimensional reconstruction, or an MRI examination. Essential plain X-ray views include:

- lateral cervical X-ray to include the cervicothoracic junction (an assistant may be needed to apply gentle traction to the arms, to pull the shoulders down and out of the way); a swimmer's view may be required to delineate the cervicothoracic junction
- AP view
- open mouth or odontoid views are difficult to obtain in intubated patients and children

Bony ossification centers in the cervical vertebrae (especially the atlas, axis and odontoid) makes interpretation of the pediatric cervical spine X-ray difficult. Seventy per cent of these children can have a straight appearance of the spine in a neutral position as opposed to the normal lordotic curvature. Soft tissue swelling anterior to the cord is common in normal children, especially if they are crying. *The safest approach, if in doubt, is to maintain cervical spine precautions until the radiographs have been examined by an experienced radiologist or neurosurgeon.* Flexion/extension views under neurosurgical supervision may be warranted.

The SCIWORA syndrome presents with normal plane X-ray views and CT scan. However, MRI demonstrates cord swelling or intramedullary hematomas.

SPECIFIC THERAPY

The principles of management of children with acute spinal cord injury include meticulous attention to supporting the circulation to achieve adequate spinal cord perfusion pressure and oxygenation. In addition, high-dose methylprednisolone is currently recommended for acute care. It is administered intravenously, with a bolus of 30 mg/kg commenced within 8 hours following the injury, and maintained with a continuous infusion of 5.4 mg/kg over 23 hours. The studies demonstrating improved outcome did not include children, but most pediatric neurosurgeons recommend this therapy.

CHEST TRAUMA

Blunt chest trauma is common in children. Motor vehicle trauma or falls account for most cases. Mortality is high. Most deaths occur after the child reaches the hospital. Associated injuries are common, particularly closed head injuries. Penetrating chest injuries are uncommon. The child's compliant chest results in few rib fractures but pulmonary contusion is common. The mobile mediastinum predisposes children to tension pneumothoraces but makes major vascular and airway injuries unlikely. Diaphragmatic injuries must still be considered.

PRIMARY SURVEY

Identification and treatment of the following life-threatening injuries is a priority during the primary survey:

- airway obstruction
- open pneumothorax
- tension pneumothorax
- massive hemothorax
- flail chest
- tamponade

Diagnosis of these conditions depends on clinical examination, chest X-ray, and possibly an ECG or echocardiogram.

Pneumothorax

Treatment of an open or tension pneumothorax requires:

- closure of the chest wall defect with a sterile closure dressing
- insertion of an intercostal catheter connected to an underwater sealed drain, best inserted between the mid and anterior axillary lines and in either the 5th or 6th interspace.
- suction pressure of -20 cmH$_2$O.

Intercostal catheters are difficult to manage if the child is transported by air. A Heimlich valve device can be used during land or air transport but can be problematic with a significant hemothorax.

Flail chest

Flail chest is uncommon but presents clinically with paradoxical movement of the chest wall with inspiration and expiration. The major problem is not the chest wall defect so much as pain interfering with adequate chest excursion, as well as the underlying pulmonary contusion associated with the chest wall defect. Management of a significant flail chest may require:

- epidural analgesia
- intubation and mechanical ventilatory support

Cardiac tamponade

Cardiac tamponade is uncommon and difficult to diagnose (distended neck veins may be difficult to visualize in the small, chubby child or the hypovolemic child). It should be suspected in the child with persisting hypotension despite adequate intravascular volume replacement and a chest X-ray excluding a tension pneumothorax. A transthoracic echocardiogram can confirm the diagnosis if time permits. Management includes:

- restoring intravascular volume
- inotropic support
- needle pericardiocentesis using a catheter over needle device (14 or 16 gauge) attached to a syringe and inserted under the xiphoid at an angle of 30°, aiming for the left shoulder; the needle is advanced while continuously aspiration is maintained on the syringe. Echocardiographic or ECG guidance is preferable
- a subxiphoid pericardial window remains the definitive therapy once the diagnosis is confirmed

Myocardial depressants should be avoided in suspected cardiac tamponade. Ketamine may be used for sedation or anesthesia.

SECONDARY SURVEY

Potentially life-threatening injuries are identified during the secondary survey and may include:

- pulmonary contusions, lacerations, hematoma
- tracheobronchial tear
- myocardial contusion
- diaphragmatic rupture
- partial aortic arch disruption
- esophageal perforation

Contusion is suspected with hemoptysis or suctioning of blood from an endotracheal tube. Chest X-ray changes occur early and resolve over 2–6 days. Similar chest X-ray appearances can occur with aspiration or ARDS. Management ranges from supplemental oxygen to full ventilatory support.

Pulmonary *hematomas* generally resolve spontaneously but can become secondarily infected. Antibiotic coverage may be warranted to minimize the risk of a lung abscess. Most parenchymal *lacerations* will heal spontaneously with supportive care and an intercostal catheter to drain the air leak.

Direct laryngeal trauma presents with hoarseness, hemoptysis, surgical emphysema and possibly upper airway obstruction. Intubation of these patients requires expert assistance for a possible cricothyrotomy or surgical tracheostomy. Fiberoptic bronchoscopy and ENT consultation for upper airway endoscopy may be indicated prior to intubation.

A *tracheobronchial tear* is suggested by a large persisting air leak with surgical and mediastinal emphysema. Diagnosis is clinical and confirmed with flexible fiberoptic bronchoscopy. These patients can present major ventilatory problems. Options for managing ventilation include:

- isolation of the lung with a double-lumen endotracheal tube (these are too large to be used in most children)
- high-frequency jet ventilation or oscillation
- extracorporeal life support

Surgical repair via a lateral thoracotomy may be required in these cases.

Myocardial contusion is rare but should be considered if tamponade has been previously diagnosed for persisting hypotension despite seemingly adequate intravascular volume resuscitation. Diagnosis is clinical and supported by a 12-lead ECG (right bundle branch block, ST segment changes, arrhythmias) and echocardiography. Therapy is supportive.

A *diaphragmatic rupture* should be suspected following a major compressive injury to the lower chest and upper abdomen or pelvis. There seems to be an increased frequency in children with lap belt injuries. Left-sided ruptures are more common. Diagnosis should be suspected in the presence of an elevated or obscure left hemidiaphragm, a left hemothorax or a nasogastric tube in the left chest. It may be an incidental finding at laparotomy. Definitive therapy requires a laparotomy and surgical repair.

Partial aortic ruptures should be suspected when there is a history of major impact with sudden deceleration. It most commonly occurs at the origin of the left subclavian artery, near the attachment of the ligamentous arteriosum. A chest X-ray may demonstrate:

- a wide mediastinum with obliteration of the aortic knob
- pleural cap
- deviation of the trachea to the right
- depression of the left mainstem bronchus
- deviation of an orogastric tube to the right
- fractured first and second ribs and/or fractured scapula

The definitive diagnosis of partial aortic disruption and other major vascular intrathoracic injury is made with aortography. Transesophageal echocardiography is useful if the facility is available but will probably miss the other major vascular injuries. Definitive therapy requires surgical repair.

Emergency room thoracotomy is unwarranted. However, urgent thorocotomy in the operating room may be indicated for partial aortic and major vascular injury, massive air leak from a tracheobronchial tear, a massive hemothorax or management of cardiac tamponade.

ABDOMINAL INJURIES

Blunt abdominal injuries are common in children. A surgeon must be involved in the care of these patients. The most common causes include pedestrians struck by motor vehicles, and falls. Bicycle handlebar injuries are not uncommon. The most common lethal injuries are splenic or liver lacerations. The hollow viscera may be torn or avulsed at their sites of attachment by deceleration injuries.

Assessment of the abdomen takes into consideration the fact that the diaphragm can rise as high as the fourth intercostal space during expiration. The upper abdominal cavity is covered by the bony thorax and can be injured by penetrating trauma to the ribcage. It contains the liver, spleen, stomach and transverse colon. The lower abdominal cavity includes the remainder of the intraabdominal organs.

Clinical suspicion and frequent reexamination complemented by appropriate radiologic examination are necessary to make the diagnosis of an intraabdominal injury. Increasing abdominal tenderness, absent bowel sounds and abdominal distention in association with clinical signs of shock suggest a major intraabdominal injury. Clinical signs of peritonitis from a perforated viscus will be delayed. An examination of the perineum and rectum completes the abdominal examination.

Initial assessment of a suspected intraabdominal injury is focused on possible intraabdominal hemorrhage. Priorities include resuscitation and insertion of a nasogastric tube and Foley catheter in the absence of urethral injury. Investigation of the child with suspected intraabdominal injury includes:

- laboratory: Hb, platelets, group and screen, crossmatch, PT, PTT, ALT, AST, amylase, urinalysis
- radiology: the abdominal CT scan with contrast enhancement accurately diagnoses injury to all the solid organs including the retroperitoneum and pelvis:
  - the presence of free fluid suggests intraabdominal hemorrhage
  - the presence of free air indicates a torn hollow viscus
  - this scan is an essential part of the examination of the unconscious child with multiple trauma
- peritoneal lavage is rarely indicated in the assessment of intra-abdominal injuries in a child as it gives no indication of the source of the bleeding and can compromise CT examination

DEFINITIVE CARE

Most major pediatric intraabdominal trauma is now managed nonoperatively. Over 90% of major splenic injuries and 80% of hepatic injuries are successfully managed with a nonoperative approach. This should only be undertaken in a tertiary pediatric center under the supervision of a surgeon. The decision not to operate is surgical. Persisting volume resuscitation (transfusion requirement in excess of 40 ml/kg), falling hemoglobin level and rising pulse rate suggest continuing bleeding and the need for surgical intervention. Nonoperative management involves:

- intravascular resuscitation with crystalloid and blood products as necessary
- observation in an ICU for 24–48 hours
- frequent monitoring of hemoglobin and amylase with regular monitoring of vital signs

- observation on the ward for a further 5 days following discharge from the ICU
- CT or ultrasound follow-up prior to discharge from the hospital
- strict avoidance of any contact sports or physical activity for 6 weeks following discharge from hospital, with a follow-up ultrasound scan

✗ COMMON ERRORS

CNS

➤ Failure to anticipate hypotension during sedation, anesthesia and intubation will aggravate the primary cerebral insult: avoid by preloading with intravascular volume (isotonic crystalloid or colloid) and careful titration of the sedative drugs

➤ Using elective hyperventilation in the head injured child during the first 24 hours of care (maintain $PaCO_2$ at low end of normal range 4.7–5.3 kPa/35–40mmHg). Hyperventilation has an important place in therapy but only for elevated ICP clearly evident on clinical or neuroradiological grounds

➤ Excluding a spinal cord injury in a comatose trauma patient on the basis of your opinion that the cervical spine radiograph is normal. Maintain cervical spine precautions during the acute period of stabilization until the child is reviewed by neurosurgical staff. Consider a cervical CT or MRI scan

➤ Not assessing the airway for obvious anatomical features that will make intubation difficult. Failed intubation in a paralyzed patient can compound neurologic injury

➤ Performing a lumbar puncture in a child with depressed level of consciousness

CARDIOVASCULAR

➤ Using drugs indiscriminately to assist intubation in a hypotensive patient: the result can be lethal. Select your agents cautiously, and titrate to effect. Small doses should be used

➤ Treating the 'numbers' rather than clinical response. An absolute number can be misleading during monitoring. The number (e.g. CVP) is less important than the trend or patient's response to

a therapeutic challenge (e.g. fluid bolus).

➤ Not recognizing that hypotension requires immediate reaction and action; delays in resuscitation can be lethal

RESPIRATORY

➤ Allowing hypercarbia in patients with acute CNS insults or pulmonary hypertension

➤ The use of sedation and muscle relaxants by inexperienced physicians when intubating

➤ Forgetting the risks associated with attempting awake intubation of a struggling patient with CNS injury

➤ Attempting to normalize the blood gases by overaggressive ventilation in a previously hypercarbic patient. This will potentially result in acute electrolyte changes and lung injury. Avoiding hypoxia should be the priority, *not* normalizing the blood gases

TRAUMA

➤ Not maintaining cervical spine precautions in children with multiple injuries while stabilizing the airway. Treating a suspected cervical spine injury is NOT the time to practice nasal intubation. An oral approach using a laryngoscope with manual in-line cervical spine stabilization remains the technique of choice

➤ Repeated attempts at gaining intravenous access in a 'shocky child', rather than using the intraosseous route

➤ Aiming for more than 1 ml/kg urine output. Children require 0.5–1 ml/kg·h; any more indicates overaggressive fluid resuscitation

FURTHER READING

1. Skippen P, Seear M, Poskitt K et al. Effect of hyperventilation on regional cerebral blood flow in head-injured children. Crit Care Med 1997; 25(8): 1402–1409

2. Editorial. Hyperventilation in traumatic brain injury: friend or foe? Crit Care Med 1997; 25(8): 1275–1278

  – *(Two papers addressing the effect of hyperventilation in management)*

3. Kirkpatrick PJ. On guidelines for the management of the severe head injury (editorial). J Neurol, Neurosurg Psych 1997; 62: 109–111

4. Chestnut RM. Avoidance of hypotension. The 'conditio sine qua non' of successful severe head injury management. J Trauma 1996; 42: (5 Suppl): 54–59

5. Rosner M, Rosner S, Johnson A. Cerebral perfusion pressure: management protocol and clinical results. J Neurosurg 1995; 83: 949–962

–   *(Three papers discussing key aspects of management after traumatic head injury)*

6. APLS: The pediatric emergency medicine course, 2nd ed. Elkgrove/Dallas: American Academy of Pediatrics/American Academy of Emergency Physicians. 1993

–   *(Manual of APLS course which teaches excellent trauma and resuscitation skills; good summaries of practical elements of trauma management and key references, outstanding section on cervical spine injury and radiology findings)*

7. Rogers MC (ed). Textbook of pediatric intensive care. 3rd ed. Williams and Wilkins: 1996

8. Schindler MB, Bohn D, Cox P et al. Outcome of out-of-hospital cardiac or respiratory arrest to children. N Engl J Med 1996; 335: 1473–1479

–   *(Two additional sources of key material)*

9. Bullock R, Chesnut R, Clifton G. Guidelines for the management of severe head injury. American Association of Neurological Surgeons, Brain Trauma Foundation, July 1995. J Neurotrauma 1996; 13(11): 639–734

–   *(Standards, guidelines and options for adult management, but with evidentary tables, scientific foundation and key areas for future investigation plus extensive references)*

10. Rumana CS, Gopinath SP, Uzura M, Valadka AB, Robertson CS. Brain temperature exceeds systemic temperature in head injured patients. Crit Care Med 1998; 26(3): 562–567

–   *(A study supporting the importance of temperature control in severely injured patients)*

11. Cruz J. The first decade of continuous monitoring of jugular bulb oxyhemoglobin saturation: Management strategies and clinical outcome. Crit Care Med 1998; 26(2): 344–351

2.7   Sepsis and fever

Mark J. Peters, Simon Dobson, Vas Novelli, Jennifer Balfour and Andrew Macnab

The morbidity and mortality rates of sepsis remain high despite widespread advances in treatment, in large part because we are able to provide care to more severely ill patients with advanced disease states. Critical illness secondary to infection can be caused by a variety of microorganisms, including Gram-positive, Gram-negative, rickettsial, viral and fungal agents. Importantly, the epidemiology and etiology vary significantly around the world and within different parts of the same country, and even within a single institution. Depending on the population of the children cared for you must know the important pathogens prevalent within your area to provide comprehensive care.

Treatment of the critically ill child with sepsis must address the immediate support of failing systems prior to using specific therapy against the presumed causative agent of the illness. Consequently, attention to the airway, adequacy of respiratory effort and gas exchange, and effectiveness of cardiac output and overall circulation are the elements necessary to preserve life. Comprehensive care then addresses the most likely cause and adds to the treatment regimen other therapeutic entities including the antibiotics most likely to be effective against the probable infecting microorganisms.

DEFINITIONS

Hayden has adapted the American College of Chest Physicians and Society of Critical Care Medicine consensus conference terminology for childhood illness:

- **bacteremia**—presence of viable bacteria in the blood
- **infection**—a microbial process characterized by an inflammatory response to the presence of microorganisms (bacteria, viruses, parasites) or the invasion of normally sterile host tissue by those organisms
- **systemic inflammatory response syndrome** (SIRS)—a system's response to a range of severe clinical insults (e.g. infection, trauma, burns). The syndrome is present where there are two or more of the following:
  - temperature is > 38°C or < 36°C
  - heart rate per minute > 2 SD above the normal for age
  - respiratory rate per minute more than 2 SD above the normal for age
  - leukocyte count > 12 × 10⁹/L (12 000/mm³), < 4 × 10⁹/L (4000/mm³) or > 10% band cells
- **sepsis**—systemic response to infection (SIRS plus infection)
- **severe sepsis**—sepsis with associated organ dysfunction, hypotension or hypo-perfusion; perfusion abnormalities can include (but are not limited to) lactic acidosis, oliguria or acute deterioration in mental status
- **septic shock**—sepsis where hypotension occurs, in spite of adequate fluid resuscitation, plus perfusion anomalies as in severe sepsis (Ch. 2.3). Children can have disordered perfusion even in the absence of measurable hypotension or while receiving inotrope or pressor support
- **hypotension**—a systolic blood pressure of more than 2 standard deviations below the mean (the European Society of Intensive Care Medicine suggests mean arterial pressure should be used for this definition, as MAP represents the organ perfusion pressure). Circulatory failure is defined as:
  - MAP < 40 mmHg at age 3–6 months
  - MAP < 45 mmHg at age 6–12 months
  - MAP < 50 mmHg at age 1–4 years
  - MAP < 55 mmHg at age 4–10 years
  - MAP < 60 mmHg at age 10–14 years
  - MAP < 65 mmHg at age 14–18 years
  MAP is either measured directly or calculated via the formula MAP = (systolic arterial pressure) + (2 × diastolic arterial pressure) ÷ 3.

- **multiple organ dysfunction syndrome** (MODS)—the occurrence of altered organ function in an acutely ill child so severe that homeostasis cannot be maintained without intervention.

PHYSIOLOGY

A systemic inflammatory response occurs when foreign substances in the blood or tissue are recognized by the host. This response to neutralize microorganisms and their products aids microbial clearance, but, negative effects on the host, especially tissue damage, can result. Proinflammatory and antiinflammatory cytokines activated in the vascular compartment through the presence of microbial material are particularly damaging. A SIRS can follow bacteremia or release of toxic products at the site of infection.

In Gram-negative sepsis the cytokine tumor necrosis factor alpha can be induced by circulating endotoxin and interleukin 1 then released. These two agents underlie many of the physiological sequelae of the septic state, e.g. alteration of the temperature set point producing either fever or hypothermia, changes in vascular resistance and vessel permeability, altered cardiac function, effects on bone marrow, including increased white blood cell production, plus metabolic effects mediated through direct action on enzymes and indirect alteration of substrate levels.

With escalating severity of the response, multiple end-organ cytokine effects are caused by mediators such as nitric oxide, prostaglandins, platelet activating factor and lipooxygenase derivatives. Such mediators ultimately disturb the coagulation and fibrinolytic systems and produce disseminated intravascular coagulopathy.

PRESENTATION

Serious infections may develop suddenly, follow a recognized prodrome or appear clinically minor before major symptoms develop. The possible clinical manifestations of early and advanced disease are numerous but largely age-specific. The septic infant, for example, is often lethargic, feeds poorly,

has temperature instability, respiratory difficulty and a tendency to hypoglycemia. In contrast, an older child may show signs of elevated temperature perhaps be inconsolable by a parent, or have headache, nausea or rigors, become confused or present with seizure or coma. It is important to recognize the multiple potential causes for each sign and symptom e.g. increased respiratory effort may be secondary to hypoxemia, hypercarbia, central nervous system inflammation, disruption of normal acid–base balance or primary lung pathology.

COMMON CLINICAL MANIFESTATIONS

Systemic

Systemic manifestations include fever (often > 38.5°C), regardless of age this temperature warrants investigation. In neonates fever may be absent. If present, a level of 38°C is an indication for septic investigation. In children under 3 years high fever (> 39.5°C) should raise concern of occult bacteremia. In infants temperature instability is present when core temperature fluctuates above 37°C or below 36°C over 4 h.

The overall appearance is important. Does the child appear unwell? If so are they sick (distressed or agitated), or critically ill (lethargic, unresponsive)? In infants how is their interest in and ability to feed? The unwell but apparently stable child requires frequent careful reassessment to detect any change in status suggesting disease progression, which can be rapid particularly in the very young.

Neurologic

The presence of neurologic signs may indicate serious infection. These signs include marked alteration in the sensorium, e.g. irritability, lethargy, lack of interest in surroundings, failure to respond appropriately to stimuli, weak cry, hypotonia or hypertonia, abnormal movements or frank seizures.

Cardiovascular

Cardiovascular signs of serious infection are elevation of heart rate (bradycardia may be seen in neonates), inadequate peripheral perfusion, prolonged capillary refill (> 2 s), cold extremities, decreased urine output (< 1 ml/kg·h). The presence of shock, either warm (hypotension and peripheral vasodilation) or cold (hypotension and peripheral vasoconstriction) or signs of impending circulatory failure are central to the presentation of critical infectious illness.

Respiratory

Elevated respiratory rate or effort of breathing (neonates also tend to become apneic) causing varying degrees of respiratory distress, poor color, and possibly frank cyanosis.

Gastrointestinal

Gastrointestinal signs include poor feeding, a tendency to vomit or have diarrhea (frank anorexia may occur), abdominal distention with or without pain, organomegaly (particularly of the liver), and possibly ileus.

Skin

The skin may be pale and mottled or ashen, and a rash may be evident, certain exanthems are associated with specific disease states (see Table 2.7.2). Look carefully for petechiae, purpura or signs of bleeding in the mucous membranes (indicative of possible disseminated intravascular coagulopathy).

Other

Every organ system can malfunction related to specific aspects of sepsis, e.g. metabolic effects including hypoglycemia, hypocalcemia, or consequences of hepatic or renal failure.

PRIMARY CLINICAL ASSESSMENT

Assess the vital signs (heart rate, respiratory rate, blood pressure, temperature). A febrile child with significant bradycardia probably has impending circulatory failure. Tachycardia, particularly in a small child, probably represents compensatory increase in heart rate to maintain cardiac output. Elevation of respiratory rate may indicate a local pulmonary infectious focus, pulmonary edema, or respiratory compensation or lactic acidosis secondary to compromised perfusion. Assessment of the adequacy of circulation should include measurement of blood pressure but must also include the broad indicators of perfusion (pallor, skin temperature, pulse quality) and mental status (agitation, lack of awareness of surroundings and inappropriate response to stimulus, or marked depression of conscious level).

Airway protection and provision of supplemental oxygen are essential in critically ill children with presumed sepsis. Vascular access should be obtained promptly and a fluid bolus of 10–20 ml/kg of 0.9% saline should be considered if perfusion appears borderline or inadequate. An improvement in heart rate and perfusion following such a bolus confirms functional hypovolemia. Fluid boluses must often be repeated many times in severe sepsis.

SUBSEQUENT CARE

DETAILED PHYSICAL EXAMINATION

Physical examination should include:

- repeat vital signs (make sure blood pressure is not omitted); consider documenting Glasgow Coma Scale
- head: check fundi (papilledema or signs of infective endocarditis), always examine ears for otitis media as infective focus. Exclude significant cellulitis, sinusitis, nasal foreign body, peritonsillar or dental abscess, pharyngitis
- neck: neck stiffness should always be looked for (and its presence or absence documented). When meningitis is suspected, assess the safety of a diagnostic lumbar puncture: the infant must have a patent airway, adequate respiratory effort and no obvious degree of circulatory compromise (the positioning required for lumbar puncture is restrictive and can precipitate acute deterioration). In any child, localizing neurological signs, suspicion of a space-occupying lesion or likelihood of raised intracranial pressure require CT scan

prior to lumbar puncture. Cervical lymphadenopathy is common in infants but large glands or multiple gland enlargement are likely to be significant. The jugulodigastric gland at the angle of the jaw drains the middle ear and tonsillar bed. Posterior cervical glands are commonly enlarged with scalp infections or infections involving the posterior nasal space, and also with rubella.

- lungs: local signs may be evident;
- cardiac: new murmurs should raise suspicions of endocarditis
- abdomen: look for localized tenderness, masses or signs of ileus. Have a low threshold for doing a rectal examination when no infectious focus is found elsewhere (check for tenderness, masses, or the presence of blood). In infants, if the taking of a rectal temperature stimulates explosive passage of loose stool, gastroenteritis is likely. Pelvic examination may be indicated for pelvic inflammatory or sexually transmitted disease in teenagers.
- musculoskeletal system: tenderness, joint swelling, effusions, masses and erythema may indicate an infective focus. Exquisite tenderness over bones suggests osteomyelitis.
- skin: look for cellulitis, abscess, purpura, petechiae, evidence of emboli, the presence of rashes which may be diagnostic (see Table 2.7.2), and carefully examine any sites where skin integrity is broken (e.g. children with indwelling lines, IV sites or implanted devices such as shunts).

MEASURES TO CONTAIN INFECTION

Any recent source of infection must be reassessed, physical sites inspected and likely extensions of the process looked for. Laboratory studies are always necessary where there is known bacteremia, or pneumonia or meningitis is suspected. A venous blood culture is obligatory unless it delays initiation of urgent resuscitation. This is still the optimal method of detecting occult bacteremia.

INVESTIGATION

1. White blood cell count—Leucocytosis (though not specific) suggests infection particularly when $> 15 \times 10^9$/L (1500/mm^3) with left shift; leukocytopenia may accompany severe sepsis. In neonates a white blood cell response may not be mounted owing to a lack of an appropriate immune response in the newborn. White cell counts below 5×10^9/L (5000/mm^3) or above 30×10^9/L (30 000/mm^3) are suggestive of infection, particularly with an elevated band cell count (See Ch. 7.3 normal values hematology).

   Neutropenia is defined as an absolute neutrophil count (ANC) below 1.0×10^9/L (1000/mm^3). The lower the count the greater the risk of serious infection (causes include aggressive cancer chemotherapy and immuno-suppression following organ transplantation).

2. Platelet count—with thrombo-cytopenia $< 100 \times 10^9$/L (100 000 mm^3) consider coagulation studies fibrinogen and fibrin split products (re disseminated intravascular coagulopathy).

3. Cultures and Gram staining of blood, CSF, urine and swabs or fluid from other potentially infected sites. Be prepared to repeat cultures performed earlier (particularly with suspected meningeal infection), where suggestive symptoms occurred but cultures were negative. A key diagnosis can be missed if the opportunity for repeat cultures is not taken.

4. Urinalysis – looking for red cells, white cells, bacteria and nitrites, Hb or casts.

5. Sedimentation rate (ESR)—abnormal > 15 mm/h during day 1 of life, > 30 mm/h subsequently. Measurement errors occur with excess alcohol application prior to capillary samples, clots, DIC and Coombs' test positive hemolytic disease.

6. Chest radiograph—usually relevant, especially in younger children with suspected sepsis but where no focus of infection is evident. Other radiology based on history and physical signs.

7. Countercurrent immunoelectrophoresis, latex agglutination test and enzyme-linked immunoabsorbent assay should be considered to identify bacterial antigens in urine, blood or other fluids (e.g. group B streptococci, *E. coli* K1, Hib, pneumococcus, meningococcus).

8. Laboratory—arterial blood gas, urea, electrolytes, glucose, liver function tests.

9. Buffy coat Gram's stain (blood sample) has 50% predictive value for bacterial sepsis.

10. Specific studies as indicated by physical examination or history.

MONITORING

1. Close observation for signs of impending respiratory compromise.

2. Close observation for signs of deteriorating perfusion or evidence of impending shock.

3. Pulse oximetry and ECG monitoring of cardiac rate and rhythm.

4. Regular vital signs, with close attention to trends and response to (a) basic life support and (b) treatment interventions.

5. Repeat laboratory studies where abnormal values are obtained (4 hourly-blood gases/chemistry, 12 hourly-hematology, daily-LFTs).

6. Other monitoring as indicated by the presence of shock, respiratory failure or ongoing therapy for system support, e.g. arterial and/or central venous pressure.

ANTIBIOTIC ADMINISTRATION

Children with signs of serious sepsis with or without shock require prompt treatment with broad-spectrum antibiotics. Logical initial regimens are shown in Table 2.7.1.

Children who have sepsis and evidence of immunocompromise (e.g. neutropenia, see Ch. 3.8), are receiving cancer chemotherapy, are HIV-positive, or are known to be asplenic, also require urgent antibiotic treatment.

The younger the child and the more toxic the presentation, the sooner appropriate antibiotics should be given. In the neonate antibiotics should be started promptly in anticipation of possible positive cultures, and a diagnosis of sepsis should be considered in any sick infant. The following are risk factors but any or all can be absent: prematurity, rupture of the maternal membranes (> 24 h), intrapartum maternal fever (> 38°C), heavy maternal colonization with group B streptococcus, perinatal asphyxia, meconium aspiration or other significant perinatal problems.

The choice of antibiotic(s) is determined by:

- The most likely infecting organisms in a child of that age (Table 2.7.1)
- The results of culture and sensitivity tests
- Known drug allergies

Children do not require antibiotics until a diagnosis of the cause of their infection is made if they (a) are not toxic; (b) are immune competent; and (c) have no specific source for their fever and have no specific signs or elements of history of concern. The decision not to treat is easier in older patients, but a lower threshold for antibiotic treatment should be applied to infants, particularly in the first year of life. This group also requires particularly careful follow-up arrangements.

MANAGEMENT

The overall goals for care of the critically ill child with sepsis are comparable to those with other types of critical illness:

1. Comprehensive initial stabilization in the hospital to which the child presents.

2. Collaboration with all appropriate specialists in the local institution and the nearest intensive care unit in order to complete the stabilization process, to begin the diagnostic process.

3. Establish the optimum location for subsequent treatment.

4. Early and safe transfer to a higher level of care if this is necessary.

5. Provision of definitive care, additional diagnostic studies, appropriate monitoring, provision of additional treatment measures sufficient to achieve resolution of the underlying cause for the illness or improvement to a point where continuing care can be provided back at the referring institution.

TABLE 2.7.1 Antibiotic choice for specific clinical situations

Indication	Comments	Antibiotic
Probable sepsis		
Infants 0–1 month	Onset < 7 days (peak about 15 h) usually maternal origin: group B streptococcus, E. coli, Listeria	Ampicillin and gentamicin (cephalosporins have poor Listeria cover so do not use alone) (Ampicillin plus cefotaxime is an alternative
	Onset > 7 days hospital origin Staphylococcus aureus, S. epidermidis, group B streptococcus, Listeria, E. coli and other Gram-negative bacteria	
Infants 1–3 months	Roughly 5% of infants with high fever (> 38°C) and high WBC are bacteremic. Neisseria meningitidis, Streptococcus pneumoniae (Haemophilus influenzae type b now rare where Hib immunization programs in place), group B streptococcus, Gram-negative organisms	Ampicillin and cefotaxime or Ampicillin and ceftriaxone
Children 3 months–5 years	Use the underlying disease as a guide (e.g. osteomyelitis or pneumonia); if nothing obvious clinically, always check the urine. Neisseria meningitidis; Streptococcus pneumoniae; Haemophilus influenzae type b; Staphylococcus aureus (see note a); Streptococcus pyogenes (group A) (see note b)	Cefotaxime or ceftriaxone (a) If sepsis with S. aureus (or toxic shock syndrome) is likely, then an antistaphylococcal agent such as flucloxacillin should be added. IVIG should also be considered for TSS (b) If necrotizing fasciitis is a likely cause of shock then penicillin and clindamycin should be used. Consider IVIG also
Children > 5 years	Neisseria meningitidis; Streptococcus pneumoniae; Staphylococcus aureus (see note a); Streptococcus pyogenes (group A) (see note b)	(a) If sepsis with S. aureus (or toxic shock syndrome) is likely, then an antistaphylococcal agent such as flucloxacillin should be added. IVIG should also be considered for TSS (b) If necrotizing fasciitis is a likely cause of shock then penicillin and clindamycin should be used. Consider IVIG also
Immunocompromised or asplenic child	Staphylococcus aureus, S. epidermidis, pneumococcus, Gram-negatives including Pseudomonas	Ampicillin (or piperacillin in high-risk patients) plus cloxacillin plus tobramycin For a patient with penicillin allergy, give vancomycin plus ceftazidime
Pneumonia		
Newborn	Congenital: TORCH infections and Listeria < 7 days: group B streptococcus, E. coli, Listeria, Gram-negatives	Ampicillin and gentamicin
	> 7 days: respiratory viruses, Chlamydia, Staphylococcus aureus, Pneumocystis, group B streptococcus, E. coli, Listeria	Add cloxacillin for S. aureus cover in older babies
Child (mild illness)	Usually viral in children < 5 years (RSV, parvovirus flu, adenovirus flu, etc.); other pathogens include Streptococcus pneumoniae, Staphlococcus aureus, group A streptococcus, Mycoplasma, Haemophilus influenzae	Amoxicillin or erythromycin, cefixime or cefaclor or TMP-SMX (cotrimoxazole) as alternatives
Child (severe illness)	Rarely tuberculosis, Legionnaires' disease, Chlamydia; Streptococcus pneumoniae, Staphylococcus aureus, group A streptococcus, Mycoplasma, H. influenzae	Cefuroxime IV Erythromycin for atypical pneumonias
Cystic fibrosis	Pseudomonas and Staphylococcus aureus; H. influenzae in young child	Cloxacillin and cefotaxime for young child Tobramycin and ticarcillin for older child

Indication	Comments	Antibiotic
Immunocompromised child	Any organism, but particularly *Pneumocystis*, CMV, Gram-negatives, *Staphylococcus aureus* or fungi	Cloxacillin and gentamicin plus TMP-SMX (co-trimoxazole) IV (oral TMP-SMX reserved for mild disease, or when pneumonitis resolving) BAL or lung biopsy often necessary for diagnosis
Lung abscess	Anaerobic oral flora, occasionally *Staphylococcus aureus* and *Klebsiella*	Clindamycin, cloxacillin or cefuroxime
CNS infection Infants < 3 months	Group B streptococcus, *E. coli Listeria*, other Gram-negatives	Ampicillin and gentamicin (neonates) Ampicillin and cefotaxime (infants 1–3 months)
Child 3 months–18 years	*H. influenzae, N. meningitidis, Streptococcus pneumoniae*, rarely streptococcus and Gram-negatives; if *Staphylococcus aureus*, consider SBE as an underlying cause	Cefotaxime or ceftriaxome (adjust antibiotic regimen when organism is known)
Brain abscess	Mixed oral organisms (aerobic and anaerobic) *Staphylococcus aureus*, *Streptococcus pneumoniae*	Vancomycin, cefotaxime and metronidazole (not clindamycin since no CSF penetration) until organism is known
Bowel infections Peritonitis	Gram-negatives, anaerobes	Gentamicin and clindamycin
Necrotizing enterocolitis	*Staphylococcus epidermis*, Gram-negatives, anaerobes	Vancomycin and cefotaxime
Bone and joint infections Neonates	Group B streptococcus, *Staphylococcus aureus*, Gram-negatives	Cloxacillin and cefotaxime
Infants	*Haemophilus influenzae*, group A streptococcus or staphylococcus	Cefuroxime or cefotaxime or cloxacillin
Children (> 4 years)	*Staphylococcus aureus*, group A streptococcus and pneumococci	Cloxacillin Alternative is β-lactamase or clindamycin
Miscellaneous Cellulitis	Group A streptococcus, *Staphylococcus aureus*, *H. influenzae* in young children	Cefuroxime or ceftriaxone
Otitis media	Pneumococcus, *H. influenzae*, group A streptococcus, *Moraxella catarrhalis*, *Staphylococcus epidermis*	Amoxicillin or erythromycin plus sulfa, or TMP-SMX (co-trimoxazole) or cefaclor or cefixime or oral cefuroxime
Pharyngitis	Usually viral; group A streptococcus, rarely *Candida, Corynebacterium diphtheriae*	Penicillin or erythromycin
Sinusitis	*Haemophilus influenzae*, pneumococcus and anaerobes	See otitis media
Urinary tract infections	*E. coli* then other Gram-negatives *Proteus*, Pseudomonas, *Klebsiella*, *Streptococcus faecalis* and *Staphylococcus aureus*; *Staphylococcus epidermis* if catheterized	Amoxicillin or TMP-SMX (co-trimoxazole) or sulfasoxazole
Encephalitis	Herpes simplex	Acyclovir 30 mg/kg per day (8 hourly for 10–14 days)
Toxic shock syndrome		Nafcillin or oxacillin
Necrotizing fasciitis	*Streptococcus pyogenes* (group A)	Penicillin and clindamycin (consider IVIG)

TMP-SMX, trimethoprim and sulfamethoxazole. Modified from Forbes J. and Dobson S. Infections Diseases. In: The Pocket Pediatrician. Seear M. (ed) Cambridge University Press, 1996.

INITIAL STABILIZATION

Attend to airway, breathing and circulation. Additional care is required with intubation if there is a coagulopathy, particularly to avoid bleeding from the posterior nasopharynx with nasotracheal intubation. Vascular access must be sufficient to guarantee the ability to infuse the necessary volume and commence inotropes when required.

Provide supportive and specific therapies for each system in failure or in imminent risk of failure.

Consider early assisted ventilation. Anticipate the need for higher than normal levels of end-expiratory pressure (pulmonary edema is common in septicemia and ARDS may develop). Sedation and/or paralysis lowers the risk of bleeding from endotracheal tube, trauma aids ventilation, and reduces oxygen consumption.

Optimal oxygen delivery is paramount, particularly through aggressive support of the circulation (adequate preload and myocardial contractility, vascular tone and renal blood flow).

Initial fluid resuscitation can require more than 40 ml/kg during the first hour. Definitive data as to the optimal type of fluid does not exist. Ringer-lactate solution and 0.9% saline are both suitable; packed red cells are required where there is significant anemia or active bleeding to optimize oxygen-carrying capacity; coagulation anomalies necessitate fresh frozen plasma and/or platelets (Ch. 2.8). Albumin is currently less in favour but individual patients may require its use.

Frequent reassessment of the cardiovascular system is essential (including urine output—aim for approximately 1 ml/kg·h).

Inotropes

If there is no improvement in blood pressure or signs of perfusion following the administration of two fluid boluses, each of 20 ml/kg (Chapter 2.3), inotropic drugs should be infused. Dopamine is usually the first choice starting with a dose of 10 µg/kg·min and increasing the dose if necessary. Norepinephrine (noradrenaline) is a vasopressor as well as an inotrope and is used for hypotension resistant to fluid boluses plus high dose dopamine.

Epinephrine sometimes improves blood pressure and perfusion in children who have failed to respond to other inotropes.

Dobutamine is not useful in sepsis unless impaired myocardial contractility is the main cause of a child's hypotension and circulatory failure.

The inotope dose is titrated against blood pressure, heart rate and indications of organ perfusion (Ch. 2.3). The drug and dose are chosen to avoid excessive tachycardia and abrupt changes in blood pressure or vascular resistance. The haemodynamic effects of sepsis make inotrope adjustment difficult. *Changes* in haemodynamic variables following inotrope adjustments are the best indicators of effect. In the hyperdynamic state that results from the infectious process the heart rate and cardiac output usually increase and the blood pressure and systemic vascular resistance decrease. Worsening sepsis is accompanied by deteriorating ventricular function and cardiac output. Consequently, beneficial effects of inotrope therapy usually produce a reduction in heart rate stabilization of BP, and an improvement in perfusion and urine output.

Give appropriate antibiotics (Table 2.7.1) in correct dosage and optimal combination for the presumed diagnosis and age of the patient.

Consider the risk of adverse drug effects and incompatibilities (e.g. competition for the cytochrome P-450 system—particular care is necessary when macrolide agents are required).

Obtain all relevant assistance available locally (anesthesia, pediatrics, surgery) and from the regional PICU.

TRANSPORT CARE

There is a need for ever-present suspicion of the possibility of sepsis, either causing or complicating serious illness. Similarly, rapid deterioration or progression should be anticipated in those with early or seemingly mild infection. Another key to providing optimal care is awareness that certain patients (the very young, those with particularly serious infections, e.g. meningococcemia, and the immunocompromised) are particularly vulnerable to rapid deterioration.

All children critically ill with sepsis are vulnerable to the physiological stresses of transport, particularly on longer journeys or where more than one vehicle (or aircraft) must be used. These children generally require as much or more care of their circulation as of their airway and ventilation. Pulmonary edema should be anticipated and clinical signs of increased moist sounds in the chest, worsening saturation and/or perfusion should prompt increased ventilation pressures. The security of the endotracheal tube and vascular access must be ensured (Ch. 1.5). Discuss and confirm optimal fluid resuscitation rates to establish a transport treatment plan. Plentiful supplies of intravenous fluid should be carried and it is prudent to have inotropes mixed ready for infusion prior to departure if not already running.

Ensure that the transport treatment plan specifies when the next antibiotic doses are required so that the regimen can be continued without dose delay in order to optimize blood levels.

Monitor SpO_2, perfusion, blood pressure, heart rate, respiratory rate and temperature and maintain a flow sheet to identify trends in these values. Many children will have a urinary catheter in place in which case hourly measures of urine output are useful to guide adjustments to therapy. Blood products may be infusing or need to be carried in case of difficulties with coagulopathy or anemia. The correct storage and identification of blood products are essential (Ch. 1.5). Point of care testing is of particular benefit in this group of children if available to the transport team (to follow acid-base status, hemoglobin, glucose and electrolytes).

SEPTIC SHOCK AND MULTIORGAN DYSFUNCTION SYNDROME

The immediate care of a child with suspected sepsis and actual or impending shock must follow the principles of 'A, B, C' (airway, breathing and circulation) followed by specific therapy for the probable causative organism.

Recognition

The initial symptoms preceding a collapse are extremely variable, especially in infants. Hence the need for careful reassessment(s). Any child with an unexplained change in conscious level (irritability or lethargy), poor feeding, vomiting, pallor, or a new rash must be assessed with the possibility of systemic infection in mind. Early recognition, starting supportive treatment, and initiation of antibiotic(s) may prevent or alleviate the severe clinical consequences described below.

Initial assessment

On first contact, assessment must be made of the patient's conscious level, ability to maintain an adequate airway and respiratory function. When these have been noted, and if necessary treated, a thorough assessment of the state of the circulation must be undertaken.

The heart rate, blood pressure and capillary refill time (normal < 2 s) should be assessed and secure intravenous access obtained. A prolonged capillary refill time (> 5 s) should be immediately treated with 20 ml/kg of intravenous fluids (e.g. 0.9% saline); usually this can be safely repeated while management is continuing if the desired clinical effect does not occur.

Investigations

Include in the initial resuscitation collection of blood for culture, full blood count, blood glucose, electrolytes, coagulation screen, and acute-phase reactants such as C reactive protein. In the critically ill septic child further investigations which will localize a focus or define the extent of infection such as a lumbar puncture or chest X-ray can wait until stabilization is achieved.

Antibiotics

The administration of empiric antibiotic therapy to cover the likely pathogens (Table 2.7.1) is essential. Patients with nosocomial infections and/or central lines often require added Gram-negative coverage (e.g. an aminoglycoside) and/or the addition of vancomycin.

Subsequent management

Further resuscitation must be guided by regular assessment of vital signs. Persistent tachycardia and hypotension with a prolonged capillary refill time after 40 ml/kg of fluid resuscitation indicates a child with significant cardiovascular compromise.

Consider semielective intubation and ventilation in such a child to secure the airway, maximize respiratory function and to control pulmonary edema (which is likely present and possibly increasing). The decision about who intubates must be made by a senior physician and will reflect local expertise and staffing. When laboratory results are available they can add to (but not replace) the clinical estimate of disease severity, e.g. low WBC and/or platelet count, low blood glucose level.

Ideal subsequent management will involve the siting of central venous access and the titration of fluid administration to maintain right heart filling pressures (usually 8–12 cmH$_2$O). In the presence of persistent hypotension despite adequate filling inotropic agent choice varies between institutions but a reasonable starting regimen would be dopamine at 5–15 μg/kg·min, followed by epinephrine (adrenaline) 0.1–0.5 μg/kg·min (or more) if there is no response.

It is important to emphasize that optimal resuscitation of a child presenting with sepsis and shock cannot be undertaken single-handedly. On recognition that a child requires the above approach, senior help, including anesthetic or intensive care assessment if available, is essential. Early referral to a regional pediatric intensive care unit for management advice and/or transport should be considered.

✗ COMMON ERRORS

➤ Failure to establish intravascular access in a severely shocked child:
- attempt peripheral IV access (for a maximum of 1.5 min)
- if unsuccessful, intraosseus needle placement into anterior tibia allows high fluid infusion rates and drug administration
➤ Inadequate fluid resuscitation:
- 20 ml/kg fluid boluses initially, repeated as required; may need total of >100 ml/kg
- high requirement for fluid indicates severe disease; consider ventilation and titration of fluid administration to CVP
➤ Intubation and ventilation not initiated until cardiorespiratory arrest. Consider semielective intubation and ventilation in presence of:
- decreased conscious level

- severe cardiovascular compromise, e.g. hypotension, high fluid requirement
- significant respiratory dysfunction, e.g. increasing requirement for supplemental oxygen
- presence of markers of severe disease (see below)
➤ False security after initial response to resuscitation. Disease severity indicators must be assessed. Severe disease likely if:
- low WBC count
- low platelet count
- high requirement for fluid resuscitation
- short history (< 6 h)
- rapidly spreading rash
- no meningitis
  (the last two indicators suggest meningococcal disease)
The presence of meningitis is associated with a 50% mortality.

FEVER IN THE CRITICALLY ILL CHILD

PATHOPHYSIOLOGY

Fever is an elevation of temperature above the normal daily variation that occurs when various infectious and noninfectious processes interact with the host immune system. The thermoregulatory center, located in the anterior hypothalamus, controls body temperature by balancing heat loss from the periphery with heat production from tissues. Usually the thermoregulatory center is set to maintain a body temperature of 37°C. This set point is readjusted when phagocytic host inflammatory cells release endogenous pyrogens (cytokines), which act on the thermoregulatory center through the mediation of prostaglandins. Cytokine release is stimulated by a variety of agents (e.g. bacteria, endotoxin, antigen/antibody complexes) and induces core temperature to rise through increased heat production (shivering), increased heat conservation (peripheral vasoconstriction) and decreased sweating.

MANAGEMENT

There is much debate as to whether fever may be beneficial to host survival during some infectious episodes. However, it is clear that feverish states lead to increased metabolic demands on the critically ill child who may have compromised cardiopulmonary or neurologic status, which may result in serious consequences, e.g. raised intracranial pressure, pulmonary vasoconstriction. It is also well known that a rapid increase in temperature in young children may induce febrile convulsions and that temperatures in excess of 42°C may lead to irreversible brain damage. Aggressive treatment of fever is therefore appropriate in some critically ill children. Inhibitors of cyclooxygenase act as potent antipyretics. Acetaminophen (paracetamol), aspirin and NSAIDS are all useful antipyretic agents, although aspirin because of its association with Reye's syndrome is rarely used.

Other measures to control temperature can be used in addition to standard antipyretic drugs. Always remove most clothing, and provide extra fluids.

Corticosteroids have an antipyretic effect; as well as blocking cyclooxygenase, they block production of endogenous mediators. Phenothiazines act as antipyretics by blocking vasocontriction, and therefore are contraindicated in children with cardiac disease. Dantrolene blocks heat production by inhibiting muscle contractions. External cooling via a hypothermia blanket and/or tepid water sponging can be used. Cooling blankets tend to induce shivering—so if cooling is essential, assisted ventilation and neuromuscular blocking agents are generally used as well.

FEVER IN CHILDREN UNDER 3 YEARS OLD

Common final diagnoses in this age group are:

- otitis media 37%
- nonspecific illness 25%
- pneumonia 15%
- recognizable viral illness 13% (exanthem, croup, gastroenteritis, aseptic meningitis)
- recognizable bacterial illness 10% (cellulitis, meningitis, bacteremia, urinary tract infections)

Several serious bacterial illnesses have their highest occurrence in this age group; bacteremia is most frequent in children with higher temperatures. The bacteria most often isolated from blood of children without a source for their fever, are *Streptococcus pneumoniae*, *Haemophilus influenzae*, *Neisseria meningitidis*, *Staphylococcus aureus*, *Streptococcus pyogenes* and *Salmonella* spp. Since the immunization of infants with *H. influenzae* type B vaccine, the proportion of children with invasive disease caused by this pathogen has diminished significantly.

High fever ($> 39.5°C$) warrants immediate hands on evaluation in this age group. The likelihood of serious disease increases with fever above 40°C, petechiae, a toxic-looking child, age less than 3 months, and abnormal test results, e.g. white blood count above $15 \times 10^9/L$ ($15\,000/mm^3$) or below $5 \times 10^9/L$ ($5\,000/mm^3$), platelets count below $100 \times 10^9/L$ ($100\,000/mm^3$).

History

The history should include:

- child's state of wellbeing (irritability, alertness, appetite)
- characteristics of fever (duration, severity)
- associated symptoms, e.g. abnormal movements, jerking, stiffening suggesting seizures. *Note*—It is rare for bacterial meningitis to present with a febrile seizure as the *sole* finding)
- past history (immunizations, previous illness or fever, medications)
- social history (infectious source, e.g. daycare, school friends, recent travel)
- family history (any ill family members or visitors)

Examination

Careful examination is required:

- record temperature
- vital signs—pulse, respiratory rate (likely to be increased) and general status (malaise, discomfort, irritability or decreased responsiveness likely)
- respiratory (impending failure, laboured, unequal air entry, adventitious sounds)
- cardiovascular (circulation status, cardiac failure, presence of murmurs)
- rash (describe and locate)
- lymphadenopathy (local or generalized)
- ENT (important to see eardrums)

- abdomen (rectal examination if indicated)
- musculoskeletal (swelling, joint movements, focal tenderness)
- CNS (meningism frequently not present, fontanelles, sensorium)

Investigations

Investigations are indicated if clinical risk factors are present, no specific cause of fever is evident, or the degree of illness is inappropriate for proposed diagnosis:

- initial investigations:
  - CBC (WBC total ↑ or ↓ for age, elevated absolute band and/or absolute neutrophil counts, thrombocytopenia)
  - urinalysis
- subsequent investigations:
  - lumbar puncture (unless decreased level of consciousness or focal signs)
  - blood cultures (if leukocytosis or abnormally low WBC present)
  - urine culture if urinalysis abnormal
  - CSF examination if lumbar puncture done
  - throat swab (usually insensitive)
  - viral (stool, urine, CSF, nasopharyngeal washing)
- antigen analysis: urine and CSF may be helpful, especially if prior treatment given
- chest X-ray: particularly important for children < 3 months old, with respiratory symptoms, fever > 40°C or WBC > 15 × 10⁹/L (15 000/mm³)

Management

Fever with a focus of infection

Confirm and treat the underlying cause.

Fever without a focus of infection

There is no completely reliable indicator of sepsis other than positive blood cultures, consequently have a low threshold for starting therapy. The antibiotics used depend on the physician's subjective impression, and the child's age, most likely diagnosis and condition, and are not readily expressed in a protocol. All febrile infants, and toxic children should ideally be in hospital for 24 h (pending results of cultures). Children >3 months with a temperature above 39°C need a WBC, and if this exceeds 15 × 10⁹/L (15 000/mm³) a blood culture. Children discharged following emergency assessment should be re-examined within 24 h.

FEVER OF UNKNOWN ORIGIN

Fever of unknown origin is defined as the presence of a documented fever of above 38.5°C in a child for more than 7 days, who has been investigated for the more common causes of fever.

Etiology

About one-third of cases prove due to unusual disorders, one-third to atypical presentations of common conditions, and one-third remain undiagnosed. Principal causes of FUO in children are infections, collagen vascular diseases and malignancy. The younger the child, the more likely there is to be an infective cause. Causes include:

- unusual presentations of common diseases: UTI, upper respiratory tract infection (sinusitis, otitis, tonsillitis), pneumonia, chronic mastoiditis, CMV, EBV (infectious mononucleosis), meningitis, allergic disorders, dehydration, rheumatic fever
- infectious diseases: osteomyelitis, septic arthritis, occult abscesses (dental, liver, pelvic, abdominal), pyelonephritis, hepatitis (chronic active), endocarditis, tuberculosis, salmonellosis, brucellosis, spirochetes (leptospirosis, relapsing fever, syphilis, Lyme disease), malaria, rickettsial infections (Q fever, RMSF)
- collagen vascular diseases: juvenile rheumatoid arthritis, SLE
- malignancies: leukemia, lymphoma, neuroblastoma
- miscellaneous: Crohn's disease, drug fever, serum sickness, factitious fever, sarcoidosis, ectodermal dysplasia

Prognosis

The prognosis is generally better than for adults but there is still 5–10% mortality rate

Approach

The diagnostic evaluation depends on a meticulous history and physical examination (see section on 'fever in children under 3 years old'):

- history:
  - complete travel history (any prophylactic treatment)
  - contacts with ill individuals (especially TB) or animals (pets or wild)
  - insect contact (ticks and mosquitoes)
  - diet (unpasteurized milk, water supply, raw fish or game)
  - medications (including topical or nonprescription drugs, including ethnic/herbal remedies)
  - ethnic or genetic background
- examination:
  - growth parameters
  - anomalous dentition or alopecia
  - ophthalmological anomalies
  - nasal discharge, sinus tenderness
  - thorough skin examination
  - careful examination of bones, muscles, joints
  - rectal examination imperative in all ages
  - pelvic examination in sexually active adolescents

Investigations

Investigations are guided by history and physical examination and by prior screening data: divide the investigations in two phases: phase 1 is a broad screen for all patients, and phase 2 includes invasive procedures which are done sequentially as indicated.

- *phase 1*: CBC, ESR, urinalysis and culture, chest X-ray, blood culture, antistreptolysin-O-titre, ANA, EBV serology, TB skin test (test also for anergy), lumbar puncture (young infant)
- *phase 2*: hospitalize, repeat blood cultures, sinus and mastoid X-rays, ophthalmological examination, serology (CMV, toxoplasmosis, hepatitis, brucella, leptospirosis), liver enzymes, abdominal ultrasound or CT scan, upper gastrointestinal, X-ray with follow-through, bone scan, gallium scan, biopsy (lymph node, liver where indicated), bone marrow (histology and cultures—bacteria, tuberculosis and fungal—where indicated)

RASHES

Table 2.7.2 gives differential diagnoses for rashes associated with fever; Table 2.7.3 gives the prodrome, key features and useful laboratory studies in common diseases with rashes, and Table 2.7.4 outlines the clinical disease states and specimens required for laboratory study in specific viral illnesses.

✔ KEY POINTS

- ➤ In critical illness due to presumed sepsis, therapy tends to be broad rather than specific in the first instance. The aims are: (a) to intervene early to support life; (b) to anticipate and treat system failure; and (c) to treat the likely underlying cause
- ➤ Any febrile child under 3 years old requires prompt careful evaluation and stabilization, and comprehensive measures to identify the cause of an infectious illness. The choice of antibiotics is based on the likely organism considering the child's age, history and physical signs, and local knowledge of possible unique pathogens or patterns of drug resistance
- ➤ Any child with sepsis and a degree of hemo-dynamic compromise that does not respond readily to basic treatment should be transferred to a pediatric ICU for support.
- ➤ Physicians must have a high level of suspicion and low threshold for presumptive treatment of infection (particularly group B streptococcus and *E. coli* in neonates).

✗ COMMON ERRORS

- ➤ Failure to recognize the potential for abrupt deterioration/complication in a sick febrile child
- ➤ Delay in recognizing and treating inadequate perfusion and in regularly reassessing circulatory status once symptoms occur
- ➤ Failure to start antipyretic management measures early in small children with high or rapidly rising temperature

TABLE 2.7.2 Differential diganoses for rashes with fever

Lesion	Pathogen or associated factor
Maculopapular or macular rash	• Viruses: measles, rubella, roseola, fifth disease (parvovirus), Epstein-Barr virus, enteroviruses, hepatitis B virus (papular acrodermatitis or Gianotti–Crosti syndrome) • Bacteria: rheumatic fever (group A streptococcus), scarlet fever, *Corynebacterium haemolyticum*, secondary syphilis, leptospirosis, *Pseudomonas*, meningococcal infection (early), *Salmonella*, Lyme disease • Rickettsia: early Rocky Mountain spotted fever, typhus (scrub, endemic) • Other: Kawasaki's disease
Diffuse erythroderma	• Bacteria: scarlet fever (group A streptococcus), toxic shock syndrome (*Staphylococcus aureus*) • Fungi: *Candida albicans*
Urticarial rash	• Viruses: EBV, hepatitis B • Bacteria: *Mycoplasma pneumoniae*, group A streptococcus
Vesicular, bullous, pustular	• Viruses: herpes simplex, varicella-zoster, coxsackie virus • Bacteria: staphylococcal scalded skin syndrome, staphylococcal bullous impetigo, group A streptococcal crusted impetigo • Other: toxic epidermal necrolysis, erythema multiforme (Stevens–Johnson syndrome), rickettsial pox
Petechial or purpuric	• Viruses: atypical measles, congenital rubella, CMV and enterovirus infection • Bacteria: sepsis (meningococcal, gonococcal), endocarditis • Rickettsia: early RMSF, epidemic typhus • Other: vasculitis, thrombocytopenia, Henoch–Schönlein purpura
Erythema nodosum	• Viruses: EBV, hepatitis B • Bacteria: group A streptococcus, tuberculosis, *Yersinia*, cat-scratch disease • Fungi: coccidioidomycosis, histoplasmosis • Other: sarcoidosis, inflammatory bowel disease, estrogen-containing oral contraceptives
Distinctive rashes (ecthyma grangrenosum, erythema chronicum migrans, necrotic eschar)	• *Pseudomonas aeruginosa*, Lyme disease, aspergillosis, mucormycosis

Modified from Forbes J. and Dobson S. Infectious Diseases. In: The Pocket Pediatrician. Seear M. (ed) Cambridge University Press, 1996.

➤ Failure to assess the safety of doing a lumbar puncture in a child with possible meningitis
➤ Failure to consider fungi as possible infectious agents in neutropenic children, especially in those on broad-spectrum antibiotics or with invasive lines
➤ Failure to recognize that there are no hard and fast diagnostic criteria for sepsis in the neonate
➤ Failure to recognize noninfectious causes for fever, e.g. drug fever
➤ Failure to view fever in the immunocompromised child as a serious clinical sign

FURTHER READING

1. Shulman ST, MacKendrick WP, Stamos JK. Handbook of pediatric infectious disease and antimicrobial therapy. St Louis: Mosby; 1993
   – (*An excellent concise and practical pediatric infectious disease resource, with emphasis on the principles of pathogenesis and therapy*)

2. Nizet V, Vinci RJ, Lovejoy FH. Fever in children. Pediatr Rev 1994; 15(4): 127–135
   – (*2 comprehensive and logical reviews including acute fever with bacteremia and fever of unknown origin*)

3. Talan DA. Infectious disease issues in the Emergency department. Clinical Infectious Diseases 1996; 23: 1–14

4. Baraff LJ, Bass JW, Fleisher GR et al. Practice guideline for the management of infants and children 0–36 months of age with fever without cause. Pediatr 1993; 92: 1–12

5. Jafari HS, McCracken GH. Sepsis and septic shock: a review for clinicians. Pediatr Infect Dis J 1992; 11: 739–748
   (*Three papers from leaders in the field with excellent practical advice*)

6. Cronin L, Cook DJ, Carlet J et al. Cortocosteroid treatment for sepsis: a critical appraisal and meta analysis of the literature. Crit Care Med 1995; 23: 1430–1439
   – (*Analyses suggest possible benefit from steroid with Gram-negative sepsis*)

7. Baltodano A. Septic shock. In: Gillis J, editor. Paediatric intensive care. Ballière's Clinical Paediatrics 1998; 6(1): 95–110
   – (*Comprehensive review in an excellent text*)

8. Ahmed A, Brito F, Goto C et al. Clinical utility of the polymerase chain reaction for diagnosis of enteroviral meningitis in infancy. J Pediatr 1997; 131: 393–397
   – (*PCR is useful, rapid and reliable for this diagnosis*)

TABLE 2.7.3 Prodrome key features and useful laboratory studies in common childhood diseases with rashes

Disease	Prodrome	Rash	Key features	Laboratory
Maculopapular eruptions				
Atypical measles	2–4 days fever, cough, headache, myalgia	Mainly limbs, may be vesicular	Frequent pleural effusion	As in measles
Drug eruptions	None	Variable, usually widespread, pruritic, sudden onset, may be systemic effects	Circumstantial	None
Enteroviral infections	Variable	Rubella-like; hand, foot and mouth disease; discrete and nonpruritic	Summer and fall months; may have aseptic meningitis	Viral culture; stool CSF, nasopharyngeal washing
Erythema infectiosum (parvovirus B19)	None	Slapped cheek: lace pattern; evanescent, lasts about 2 weeks	Typical rash in well child; may be pruritic	None
Erythema subitum (herpesvirus 6)	3–4 days high fever with rapid resolution and then rash	Discrete rose-red, trunk to face and limbs, disappears in 1–2 days	Rash appears as fever wanes	None
Infectious mononucleosis	1–2 days	Triad: tonsillitis, lymphadenopathy, hepatosplenomegaly; enanthem in 50%, exanthem in 15%	Incubation period 30–50 days; exanthem with ampicillin therapy in 80% of cases	Atypical lymphocytes; monospot; serology
Kawasaki's disease	4–6 days fever; sore throat, lymphadenopathy	Generalized rash; palms and soles progress to desquamation, cracked red lips, strawberry tongue, conjunctivitis	Constellation of features	None
Measles	3–4 days fever conjunctivitis, coryza, cough	Reddish brown; face to trunk to limbs; confluent on trunk; fades day 5 brawny desquamation	Koplik's spots; incubation period 10–12 days	Serology culture in special circumstances
Meningococcemia	Variable but usually < 24 h; fever, irritable, ± meningism	Transient maculopapular rash rapid progression to petechial, purpuric rash; no regular distribution	Irregular distribution of petechiae; short incubation period	Cultures blood CSF or petechiae
Rubella	0–4 days malaise, low fever, lymphadenopathy (occipital)	Pink; face to limbs within 48 h; discrete; disappears day 3–4; no desquamation	Postauricular or posterior occipital nodes; incubation period 14–21 days	As in measles

TABLE 2.7.3 *continued*

Disease	Prodrome	Rash	Key features	Laboratory
Scarlet fever	12 h to 2 days fever, sore throat, vomiting	Erythematous and blanches 'sandpaper'; oral pallor; flexor surfaces to generalized 24 h; desquamation in 1–2 weeks	Strawberry tongue, membranous tonsillitis	Culture, anti streptolysin O titre
Staphylococcal toxic shock (*S. aureus*)	None; fever, headaches, confusion, vomiting and diarrhea, shock	Scarlatiniform mainly on trunk and limbs, edema face, desquamation	Fever, toxicity, shock	Culture; phage typing
Papulovesicular lesions				
Coxsackievirus	Variable	Hand, foot and mouth disease	Summer and fall months; may have aseptic meningitis	Viral culture; stool, CSF, naso-pharyngeal washing
Herpes simplex	None	Primary mostly subclinical; may be generalized Reactivation: localized, thin-walled vesicles which rupture or heal in 10 days	Skin or genitalia (usually HSV-2); incubation period 6 days	Same as varicella
Herpes zoster	None	Unilateral and along dermatome; vesicles grouped together and become confluent	Dermatome distribution painful	Same as varicella
Impetigo	None	Vesicles become confluent and rapidly progress to pustules and crust; not in crops and not on mucous membrane	Yellow crusting; contagious	Culture (group A streptococcus); *Staphylococcus aureus* secondary agent
Papular urticaria (insect bites)	None	Hypersensitivity reaction; urticarial eruption ± vesicles; may later form persistent papules	Preceding insect exposure; exposed areas; pruritic	None
Pediculosis (lice)	None	Scalp, body and pubic lice; pruritic excoriation	Nits on hair shaft	Microscope exam for nits
Scabies (*Sarcoptes scabiei*)	None	Discrete 'burrows' ± vesicle or excoriated papule which may become generalized	Pruritic; contagious common in 'webs' between fingers	Burrow scraping microscopy
Staphylococcus aureus toxic shock	None; fever and irritability with rash	Generalized; tender, bullae 1–2 days to moist desquamation	Nikolsky's sign (skin lysis)	Cultures
Varicella	1–2 days fever, malaise	Rapid evolution of macules to papules to vesicles to crusted; lesions; central; crops; mucous membranes; all stages present	Incubation period 14–21 days; 'teardrop' vesicles pruritic	Vesicle scraping for immuno-fluorescence serology

Modified from Forbes J. and Dobson S. Infectious Diseases. In: The Pocket Pediatrician. Seear M. (ed) Cambridge University Press, 1996.

TABLE 2.7.4 Clinical disease states and specimens required for diagnosis in common viral illnesses

Virus	Clinical disease states commonly associated	Specimens[a]
Adenovirus	Acute respiratory disease, pneumonia, pharyngoconjunctival fever, keratoconjunctivitis, etc.	Throat swab, rectal swab, stool, eye swab
Cytomegalovirus	Mononucleosis, hepatitis, pneumonia	Buffy coat, urine, throat swab, serology
Enterovirus	Aseptic meningitis, pleurodynia, myocarditis, pericarditis, herpangina, poliomyelitis	Stool, rectal swab, throat swab, CSF (consider PCR assay on CSF)
Epstein–Barr virus	Mononucleosis, chronic, mononucleosis syndrome	Serology
Hepatitis A virus	Jaundice	Serology
Herpes simplex virus	Gingivostomatitis, keratoconjunctivitis, herpes labialis, genital herpes, encephalitis	Vesicle fluid, throat swab or mouthwashing, vaginal swab, brain biopsy, serology
Influenza and parainfluenza viruses	Pharyngitis, croup, bronchiolitis, pneumonia, urinary tract infection	Nasopharyngeal washing, nasal swab, throat swab, blood, urine
Measles virus	Measles, subacute sclerosing pan-encephalitis, encephalitis	Throat swab, CSF, serology, urine
Mumps virus	Parotitis, orchitis, aseptic meningitis	Throat swab, serology, urine, CSF
Respiratory syncytial virus	Croup, bronchiolitis, pneumonia	Nasopharyngeal aspirate
Rhinovirus	Nonspecific febrile illness, common cold	Nasopharyngeal washing
Rotavirus	Gastroenteritis	Stool
Rubella virus	Congenital rubella rash, lymphadenopathy	Throat swab, rectal swab, urine, serology
Varicella-zoster virus	Chickenpox, herpes zoster	Vesicle fluid, lesion swab, serology

[a]For antibody determinations, acute-phase serum should be collected immediately after onset; convalescent serum should be collected 10–14 days later. Modified from Forbes J. and Dobson S. Infectious Diseases. In: The Pocket Pediatrician. Seear M. (ed) Cambridge University Press, 1996.

2.8 Bleeding

Stephen Keeley

In normal circumstances there is a balance between factors leading to clot formation and factors that inhibit it or lyse thrombus. Vessel injury or exposure of subendothelial collagen leads to platelet adherence (facilitated by von Willebrand factor, vWF). Adherent platelets release factors that promote vessel constriction, adherence of other platelets and fibrin formation. Fibrin stabilizes the platelet plug and bleeding is stopped by the combination of vasoconstriction, plugging of the defect with platelets and fibrin, and compression (externally applied or due to local tamponade). In the absence of surgical or traumatic vessel injury, bleeding is due to defects in formation of the platelet plug (primary hemostasis), stabilization of the platelet plug (coagulation) or vessel function.

Apart from trauma, the most common causes of bleeding in childhood are:

- an isolated decrease in platelet number, usually immune-mediated, e.g. idiopathic thrombocytopenic purpura (ITP)
- a single (usually hereditary) coagulation factor deficiency, e.g. hemophilia A.

Among children who become critically ill, bleeding is rarely a primary presenting feature but is often secondary to a serious underlying disorder such as asphyxia, burns, sepsis or liver failure, which leads to a combination of deficiencies of multiple clotting factors with thrombocytopenia and vessel injury (Table 2.8.1).

DIAGNOSIS

CONGENITAL DISORDERS

Early onset of bleeding after minor injury or surgery.

DISORDERS OF PRIMARY HEMOSTASIS

Disorders of primary hemostasis (platelets) are characterized by:

TABLE 2.8.1 **Classification of bleeding disorders**

Abnormalities of primary hemostasis
- Thrombocytopenia
  - immune (ITP)
  - non-immune (e.g. dilution)
  - marrow failure (e.g. leukemia)
- Thrombocytopathy
  - aspirin ingestion
  - von Willebrand's disease

Coagulation
- Single factor deficiencies (e.g. factor VIII)
- Multiple factor deficiencies (e.g. vitamin K deficiency)
  - complex coagulopathy (e.g. liver failure or DIC)

Blood vessels
- Trauma
- Endothelial damage (e.g. heatstroke)

- bleeding immediately after injury
- spontaneous bleeding of the gums, nose or gastrointestinal tract
- petechiae and small, superficial bruises

DISORDERS OF COAGULATION

Characterized by:

- delayed (1–2 days) severe bleeding after trauma
- bleeding into soft tissues and joints
- minimal bleeding after cuts and abrasions

DISSEMINATED INTRAVASCULAR COAGULOPATHY

Antecedent causes of disseminated intravascular coagulation (DIC) are shock, sepsis, asphyxia, pancreatitis, severe brain injury, and snakebite. It is sometimes associated with the hemolytic-uremic syndrome.

Clinical features include:

- bleeding from puncture sites
- prolonged PT and APTT (see below)
- low levels of fibrinogen and platelets

- raised levels of fibrin split products (D-dimers or X-linked degradation products)

DILUTION

Dilutional coagulopathy is associated with a history of large-volume (> 30 ml/kg) fluid resuscitation, usually after fluid loss or bleeding. Signs include:

- prolonged PT and APTT
- low levels of fibrinogen and platelets
- absent or low fibrin split products

HEPARIN-INDUCED THROMBOSIS– THROMBOCYTOPENIA SYNDROME (HITTS)

Clinical features of heparin-induced thrombosis–thrombocytopenia syndrome are:

- immune-mediated thrombosis in arteries, veins or capillaries
- thrombocytopenia with consequent bleeding
- resistance to platelet transfusion
- occurs after 7 days of heparin therapy (even at very low dose, e.g. 1–2 units/h to maintain catheter patency)
- less common with low molecular weight (LMW) heparin
- test: heparin-induced platelet aggregation

Treat by changing to LMW heparin; occasionally it is necessary to eliminate heparin completely from all infusions

INVESTIGATION

The following investigations will help to identify the cause of bleeding (Table 2.8.2):

- full blood count including platelets (normal 150–450 × 10⁹/L)
- prothrombin time (normal 11–15 s; INR 0.8–1.3)
- activated partial thromboplastin time (normal 25–40 s)
- fibrinogen (normal 1.5–4.0 g/L)
- Ivy bleeding time (normal 2–7 min)

A low platelet count should prompt examination of the cellular elements in a blood film to rule out marrow suppression, fragmentation of red cells (due to microangiopathy, e.g. hemolytic–uremic syndrome) or abnormality of platelet size. Rapid destruction of platelets, typically seen in ITP, leads to the release of large immature platelets.

The prothrombin time is not affected by heparin but reflects activity of factors II, V, VII and X. The International Normalized Ratio (INR) is the ratio of the measured prothrombin time to an international standard.

Abnormalities of PT and APPT provide a clue to the diagnosis:

- prolonged PT:
  - means factor concentrations < 30–40% of normal
  - very sensitive to deficiency of factor VII because of its short half-life
  - usual cause is multiple factor deficiencies (e.g. in vitamin K deficiency) or a low fibrinogen.
- Prolonged APPT:
  - the APPT measures activity of factors VIII, IX, XI and XII
  - prolonged APTT means the concentration of these factors is < 30% normal
  - an isolated prolongation of APPT usually means factor VIII or XI deficiency
- Prolongation of both PT and APTT:
  - means multiple factor deficiencies (e.g. liver impairment, shock, sepsis, DIC, dilution after severe hemorrhage) or abnormalities of fibrinolysis
  - measure fibrinogen and its breakdown products (fibrin split products)

Restoration of the circulating blood volume using crystalloid, colloid or blood products inevitably causes dilutional deficiencies of platelets and clotting factors. Bleeding is rare when the platelet count exceeds 300 × 10⁹/L and when the PT or APTT is less than 1.5 times normal.

If the history and examination suggest a disorder of primary hemostasis but the platelet count is normal, measure the bleeding time. If it is prolonged, a vessel abnormality or defective platelet function is likely to be present.

TABLE 2.8.2 Diagnostic signs in bleeding disorders

	Vitamin K deficiency	von Willebrand's disease	Hemophilia A	DIC	Liver disease	ITP	Dilution
PT	↑	N	N	↑	↑	N	↑
APPT	N/↑	↑	↑	↑	↑	N	↑
Bleeding time	N	↑	N	↑	N/↑	↑	↑
Fibrinogen	N	N	N	↓	N/↓	N	N/↓
Fibrin split products (normal < 10 mg/L)	N	N	N	↑	N/↓	N	N
Platelets	N	N	N	↓	N/↓	↓	↓

N, normal range; ↑, elevated; ↓, depressed.

MANAGEMENT

Look for the bleeding vessel. This may be in skin, subcutaneous tissue, or deeper tissues cut during surgery. Bleeding increases as the blood volume is restored by resuscitation. Apply pressure to bleeding points when possible. In general, treatment should aim to replace the deficient product. Nonselective use of blood products such as fresh frozen plasma to treat 'oozing' is not warranted. Avoid aspirin and intramuscular injections.

FACTOR VIII DEFICIENCY (HEMOPHILIA A)

1. Increase the factor VIII level to 30–50% of normal using 15–25 units/kg factor VIII concentrate.
2. For *any* head injury (even minor), raise the factor VIII level to 100% using 50 units/kg factor VIII, concentrate, and observe the child in hospital.
3. Consider using ε-aminocaproic acid (EACA) or tranexamic acid for oral bleeding.

VON WILLEBRAND'S DISEASE

1. Give cryoprecipitate (see below). Repeat after 48 hours if necessary.
2. May require desmopressin (0.3 µg/kg i.v. slowly 12–24 hourly).

FACTOR IX DEFICIENCY (CHRISTMAS DISEASE)

Give prothrombin concentrate 1–1.5 ml/kg (equivalent to 20–30 units of factor IX per kg) daily until bleeding stops.

DIC

1. Remove the precipitating cause (e.g. treat the sepsis or shock).
2. If bleeding continues, give FFP 20 ml/kg (a diuretic may be needed to prevent fluid overload). Repeat if necessary.
3. Give cryoprecipitate 0.2 units/kg for low fibrinogen.
4. Platelets (10 ml/kg: repeat if necessary) are required in very severe thrombocytopenia. This may give little benefit early, and unless the cause of the DIC is treated.
5. Heparin (10 units/kg·h after a bolus of 50 units/kg) is only used if vascular thrombosis is a prominent aspect of the DIC (e.g. after incompatible blood transfusion).

DILUTIONAL COAGULOPATHY

1. Treat the cause of bleeding or hypovolemia.
2. Top up the diluted components: FFP alone is usually sufficient.
3. Platelets and cryoprecipitate may be required.

BLOOD PRODUCTS

Products available for treatment of acute bleeding are summarized below (see also Ch. 3.6).

FRESH FROZEN PLASMA

Each unit (250 ml) of fresh frozen plasma is produced from a single unit of blood. It is stored at –30°C, and once thawed should be used within 6 hours.

It contains all clotting factors, antithrombin III, protein C, plasminogen, complement components and inhibitors in concentrations similar to those in plasma. Infusion of 15–20 ml/kg of FFP should produce clotting factor levels at least 30% of normal and be sufficient to control bleeding:

- indications:
  - correction of multiple factor abnormalities associated with a PT or APPT more than 1.5 times normal
  - correction of a single factor deficiency for which no factor concentrate is available
- blood group compatibility is given in Table 2.8.3
- there is a risk of transfusion-acquired infection

CRYOPRECIPITATE

One unit (10–15 ml) of cryoprecipitate contains 250 mg fibrinogen, 100 units factor VIII, 80 units vWF and 40–60 units factor XIII. Its shelf life is 6 months. One unit per 5 kg body weight increases plasma fibrinogen by 0.5 g/L. Stored frozen at –30°C, it requires approximately 45 minutes to thaw and must be used within 6 hours of thawing:

- indications:
  - bleeding with fibrinogen levels below 1 g/L (usually due to DIC, dilution or severe liver disease)
  - bleeding in hemophilia A where factor concentrate is not available: 1 unit/kg increases factor VIII by 2%
  - bleeding in von Willebrand's disease
- there is a risk of transfusion-acquired infection

PLATELETS

One unit, derived from a unit of blood, contains approximately 60 ml and 4×10^8 platelets. Platelets should be stored at 22°C with gentle mechanical agitation, and have a shelf life of 5 days:

- risks:
  - graft-versus-host disease (in newborns and immunocompromised children)
  - transfusion-acquired infection
- indications:
  - bleeding associated with a platelet count below 50×10^9/L (Ch. 3.6)
  - platelet count below 10×10^9/L without bleeding

The usual dose is 10 ml/kg, repeated daily if necessary. Aim for a platelet count above 50×10^9/L in the presence of active bleeding.

VITAMIN K

Acutely ill patients become vitamin K deficient in 7–10 days. Deficiency is more likely in those with liver injury (e.g. shock or sepsis) or on broad-spectrum antibiotics. Deficiency reduces plasma levels of factors II, VII, IX, X and proteins C and S; it causes prolonged PT and, later, prolonged APTT. Treat with vitamin K as follows:

- administration of vitamin K (10 mg i.m. or very slowly i.v.) restores clotting factor production to normal in 8–10 hours; give FFP if faster restoration is needed
- use in multifactorial coagulopathy (e.g. in shock, sepsis or asphyxia)

TABLE 2.8.3 **Compatibility of blood products with patient blood groups: Rh group is irrelevant; group O cryoprecipitate is used when no other groups are available**

Patient blood group	Fresh frozen plasma	Cryoprecipitate
O	Any	O or A
A	A or AB	A (or O)
B	B or AB	B (or O)
AB	AB	A (or O)

ANTIFIBRINOLYTIC AGENTS

Excessive fibrinolysis occasionally causes bleeding, e.g. after trauma or surgery with large, raw bleeding surfaces. Signs include low fibrinogen levels with normal PT, APTT and platelet counts. Appropriate treatment is FFP plus an antifibrinolytic agent such as EACA:

- dosage of EACA is 100 mg/kg (maximum 5 g) i.v. bolus, then 30 mg/kg·h (maximum 1.25 g/h)
- oral EACA (same dose) is used for mouth bleeding in hemophilia A
- EACA should not be used if DIC is present or suspected, as it can cause fatal intra-vascular thrombosis

GUIDELINES FOR INVASIVE PROCEDURES

Invasive procedures are often required in patients with a known bleeding disorder. The following guidelines are suggested:

1. Document the severity of the coagulopathy and the treatment used.
2. Document the indication for the proposed procedure.
3. Obtain informed consent.
4. Choose the most appropriate site for incision or needling (e.g. where local pressure can be applied in the event of bleeding).
5. Perform procedures within 30–60 minutes of blood product administration.

✔ KEY POINTS

➤ Bleeding in a critically ill child is usually due to a complex coagulopathy
➤ Give FFP if the PT and APPT are more than 1.5 times normal

➤ An isolated increase in PT is best treated with vitamin K
➤ Single factor deficiencies are unusual in the absence of a history of bleeding
➤ HITTS is rare in children and usually presents with thromboses

✗ COMMON ERRORS

➤ Indiscriminate use of blood products, e.g. FFP as a volume expander
➤ Failure to recognize the importance of hypothermia as a contributor to any complex coagulopathy: warm the patient and warm the blood
➤ Treating a number (e.g. transfusing purely on the basis of an abnormal test)
➤ Failure to recognize surgical bleeding: persisting signs of hemorrhagic shock despite transfusion of platelets and clotting factors or the need for more than a blood volume replacement suggest that surgical exploration is required

FURTHER READING

1. Luban NLC, DePalma L. Use and administration of blood and components. In: Chernow B, editor. The pharmacologic approach to the critically ill patient, 3rd ed. Baltimore: Williams & Wilkins; 1994
   – (*Overview of blood product therapy in adults and children*)

2. Manco-Johnson MJ. Hemostasis and bleeding disorders. In: Rudolph AM, Hoffman JIE, Rudolph CD, editors. Rudolph's Pediatrics, 20th ed. Stamford: Appleton & Lange; 1996
   – (*Review of congenital and acquired bleeding disorders in childhood*)

3. Eskanazi AE, Bernstein ML, Gordon JB. Hematologic disorders in the pediatric intensive care unit. In: Rogers MC, editor. Textbook of pediatric intensive care, 3rd ed. Baltimore: Williams & Wilkins; 1996
   – (*Reviews coagulopathy in the critically ill child*)

2.9 Metabolic failure

John Christodoulou

Many inborn errors of metabolism present in the first days or weeks of life, often as acute metabolic decompensation, but as the young infant has a limited repertoire of nonspecific responses to severe illness (which can include lethargy, vomiting, poor sucking reflex, hypotonia, respiratory distress, apnea, poor weight gain, altered state of consciousness or unexplained seizures), the clinical features in the neonate may not indicate the precise diagnosis. Up to one-third of children with so-called 'small molecule' disorders first present in late infancy or beyond.

Because the presenting features of genetic metabolic disorders are often nonspecific and can mimic other more common pediatric conditions such as sepsis, congenital heart disease, or intestinal obstruction, inborn errors are often only considered after all other disorders have been excluded. The development of permanent physical or neurological damage can only be reduced or prevented if the condition is diagnosed early and emergency treatment is implemented rapidly. Accurate diagnosis, aided by early consultation with the metabolic team, is needed for genetic counseling. Counseling is of crucial importance—particularly discussion of prognosis, and options for treatment and future reproduction.

DIAGNOSIS

When should a genetic metabolic disorder be considered?

Inborn errors of metabolism may present in the following ways:

- unexplained cardiorespiratory collapse (e.g. respiratory chain defects)
- acute encephalopathy (e.g. maple syrup urine disease)
- acute liver failure (e.g. tyrosinemia type I)
- hypoglycemia (e.g. medium-chain acyl-CoA dehydrogenase deficiency)
- metabolic acidosis with or without ketosis (e.g. methylmalonic aciduria)

- lactic acidemia (e.g. pyruvate dehydrogenase deficiency)
- hyperammonemia (e.g. ornithine transcarbamylase deficiency)

CLINICAL EVALUATION

A rapid clinical evaluation including specific questioning (as relevant points are often not volunteered), and physical examination (Table 2.9.1), can usually give enough information to indicate the appropriate urgent investigations and treatment. Most disorders that present with acute metabolic decompensation are 'small molecule' disorders (Table 2.9.2). Small molecules are water-soluble substances such as ammonia, amino acids and keto acids found in virtually all body fluids. In some of these disorders, the small molecules may accumulate in body fluids in toxic concentrations several orders of magnitude greater than normal. Examples of this type of disorder include the aminoacidopathies (e.g. maple syrup urine disease), the organic acidopathies (e.g. methylmalonic acidemia), and the urea cycle defects (e.g. ornithine transcarbamylase deficiency). In other

---

TABLE 2.9.1 Clinical evaluation of a child suspected of having a genetic metabolic disorder

History
- Family history (similar illnesses in siblings, unexplained deaths, stillbirths, etc.)
- Consanguinity (most inborn errors of metabolism are autosomal recessive in their inheritance)
- Intercurrent illnesses
- Dietary history (especially any recent changes to the diet, or periods of fasting)

Physical examination
(Often unhelpful in determining the precise diagnosis)
- Level of consciousness (Glasgow coma scale)
- Hepatomegaly
- Focal neurological signs
- Unusual odor (urine should be kept in a sealed, sterile container for at least 5 min at room temperature before testing)

> ### TABLE 2.9.2 Genetic metabolic diseases causing acute metabolic failure
>
> - Aminoacidopathies (e.g. maple syrup urine disease)
> - Organic acidopathies (e.g. methylmalonic acidemia)
> - Fatty acid oxidation defects (e.g. medium-chain acyl-CoA dehydrogenase deficiency)
> - Urea cycle defects (e.g. ornithine transcarbamylase deficiency)
> - Primary lactic acidosis disorders (including defects of the Krebs cycle, pyruvate metabolism and the mitochondrial respiratory chain)
> - Disorders causing acute liver failure (including galactosemia, tyrosinemia type I and hereditary fructose intolerance)

small molecule disorders such as the fatty acid oxidation defects (e.g. medium-chain acyl-CoA dehydrogenase deficiency) and the primary lactic acidosis disorders (e.g. pyruvate dehydrogenase deficiency), while some metabolites accumulate, the main problem is a defect of energy production.

SCREENING TESTS

To diagnose a specific genetic metabolic disorder, specific investigations such as enzyme assays must be performed. However, as the clinical presentations for many of these disorders overlap, a few investigations will screen for most of these disorders (Table 2.9.3).

To obtain meaningful results, many of these samples require special handling (especially for measurement of lactate, pyruvate, ammonia, and amino acids), and the biochemical geneticist or biochemist on call should be consulted before the samples are collected.

Table 2.9.4 lists clinical and biochemical clues to the common inborn errors of metabolism that can present as acute metabolic emergencies.

TREATMENT

ACUTE METABOLIC EMERGENCY

Emergency room

Initial resuscitation to preserve life and to minimize or prevent permanent damage is undertaken in parallel with the diagnostic investigations. Hypoventilation (Chs 2.1, 6.4), circulatory failure

> ### TABLE 2.9.3 Screening tests for genetic metabolic disorders. Tests in bold type are mandatory in any child suspected of having a small molecule disorder. Other tests are indicated in specific clinical circumstances, e.g. blood and CSF amino acids if nonketotic hyperglycinemia is suspected
>
> **Urine**
> - Dipstick tests
>   - **ketones**
>   - **reducing substances** (also test using reagent tablets)
> - Specific studies
>   - **amino and organic acid screens**[a]
>
> **Blood**
> - Routine investigations
>   - full blood count and film
>   - **urea, electrolytes and creatinine**
>   - **glucose**
>   - calcium
>   - **blood gases**
>   - **liver enzymes**
> - Specific studies
>   - **ammonia**
>   - **lactate and pyruvate**
>   - amino acids[a]
>   - carnitine[a]
>
> **Cerebrospinal fluid**
>   - lactate and pyruvate
>   - amino acids[a]
>
> **Hypoglycemia**
> The following additional blood tests should be performed at the time of hypoglycemia:
>   - growth hormone
>   - cortisol
>   - insulin
>   - free fatty acids
>   - β-hydroxybutyrate
>
> [a]These investigations are expensive and time-consuming: discussion with the laboratory is recommended.

(Ch. 2.3), brain swelling and seizures (Chs 2.5, 3.3) must be treated urgently. Important components of resuscitation include:

1. Correction of dehydration, electrolyte imbalance and hypoglycemia: a glucose intake of around 9 mg/kg·min, supplemented with the daily potassium requirement, maintains a blood glucose concentration of 5–10 mmol/L and reduces the endogenous catabolic release of the offending small molecule. If cerebral

TABLE 2.9.4 Clinical and biochemical clues to small molecule disorders

Disorder	Ketosis	Metabolic acidosis	Anion gap	Blood lactate	Blood glucose	Blood ammonium	Other clinical clues	Confirmatory tests
Aminoacidopathies	No to ++	No or +	Normal	Normal	Normal or ↑	Normal	Relationship to dietary protein intake and catabolic episodes	Urine and plasma amino acids
Organic acidopathies	++	+++	↑ or ↑↑	Normal or ↑	Normal or ↓	↑ or ↑↑	Relationship to dietary protein intake and catabolic episodes	Urine organic acids
Fatty acid oxidation defects	No or +	No or +	Normal or ↑	Normal or ↑	↓↓	↑ or ↑↑	Often precipitated by fasting or catabolic illness	Skin fibroblast enzyme studies Mutation analysis
Urea cycle defects	No	No	Normal	Normal	Normal	↑ to ↑↑↑	Relationship to dietary protein intake and catabolic episodes Respiratory alkalosis	Urine and plasma amino acids Urine orotic acid
Primary lactic acidosis (incl. PDH, PC, TCA, ETC and gluconeogenesis)[a]	No to ++	No to ++	Normal to ↑↑	Normal to ↑↑	Normal or ↓	Normal or ↑	May have multisystem disease	Muscle or liver enzyme and histochemistry studies Mutation analysis in specific instances

[a]PDH, pyruvate dehydrogenase deficiency; PC, pyruvate carboxylase deficiency; TCA, tricarboxylic acid (Krebs) cycle; ETC, defects of the mitochondrial electron transport chain; gluconeogenesis, defects of gluconeogenesis.

edema is suspected, all intravenous fluids should contain 0.9% saline (as well as glucose) and hyponatremia should be avoided. A high glucose intake is contraindicated when pyruvate dehydrogenase deficiency is suspected.

2. Correction of metabolic acidosis: intravenous sodium bicarbonate administration should be considered if the serum bicarbonate level is below 15 mmo/L. For example, give (15–patient's HCO_3) × 0.3 mmol $NaHCO_3$ over 30–60 min. Aim to increase the serum bicarbonate level to 15 mmol/L but avoid overcorrection. Dangerous iatrogenic hypernatremia may sometimes be unavoidable and may require gradual correction (Ch. 3.5).

Intensive care unit

Hemofiltration, hemodialysis, or peritoneal dialysis (Ch. 2.10) may be needed to remove small water-soluble molecules such as ammonium in the urea cycle defects or leucine in maple syrup urine disease if there is a rapid clinical or biochemical deterioration despite appropriate initial resuscitation.

Specific therapy for individual diseases

Specific treatments include:

- nutritional modifications (e.g. intravenous lipid emulsions, specific amino acid supplements)
- cofactor administration (such as pharmacological doses of specific vitamins which can be given orally)
- specific therapeutic agents (such as sodium benzoate for hyperammonemia)

LONG-TERM DIETARY THERAPY

The aim is to provide nutrients in sufficient amounts to allow normal growth, but not in excess

leading to accumulation of toxic metabolites. Supplements of specific amino acid mixtures, fatty acids, and specific vitamins such as thiamine, minerals and other micronutrients, may be needed.

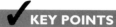
KEY POINTS

➤ Consider an inborn error of metabolism if a child has unexplained shock, encephalopathy, liver failure, metabolic acidosis, hypoglycemia or hyperammonemia

➤ Rapid clinical assessment including specific questioning usually indicates the appropriate investigations and emergency treatment

➤ Stabilize the airway, breathing and circulation and treat seizures

➤ Correct dehydration, electrolyte imbalance, hypoglycemia and metabolic acidosis

➤ Consider cofactor administration

➤ Consider blood purification techniques

FURTHER READING

1. Christodoulou J, McInnes RR. A clinical approach to inborn errors of metabolism. In: Rudolph AM, Kamei R, editors. Rudolph's fundamentals of pediatrics (2nd ed). Stamford: Appleton & Lange 1998; pp 181–208
   – (*Practical approach to diagnosis and management*)

2. Fernandes J, Saudubray JM, Van den Berghe G, editors. Inborn metabolic diseases: diagnosis and treatment. 2nd ed Berlin: Springer-Verlag 1994
   – (*See chapters entitled: clinical approach to inherited metabolic diseases (pp 3–39), diagnostic procedures: function tests and postmortem protocol (pp 41–46), emergency treatments (pp 47–55)*)

3. Saudubray JM, Charpentier C. Clinical phenotypes: diagnosis/algorithms. In: Scriver CR, Beaudet AL, Sly WS, Valle D, editors. The metabolic and molecular bases of inherited disease, 7th ed. New York: McGraw-Hill; 1995; pp 327–400
   – (*Comprehensive discussion of the diagnosis of inborn errors according to their clinical and biochemical mode of presentation*)

2.10 Water, electrolyte and acid-based disorders and acute renal failure

Barry Wilkins, Chula Goonasekera and Michael Dillon

INVESTIGATIONS

The following biochemical investigations are suggested for critically ill children:

- On presentation:
  - *Plasma* sodium, potassium, bicarbonate, urea, creatinine, glucose, lactate, calcium, magnesium, phosphate, liver function tests, albumin, osmolality
  - *Urine* sodium, potassium, urea, creatinine, osmolality, glucose.
- Twice daily:
  - *Plasma* sodium, potassium, bicarbonate, glucose blood gases.
- Daily:
  - *Plasma* calcium, magnesium, phosphate, urea, creatinine, liver function tests, albumin, osmolality
  - *Urine* sodium, potassium, urea, creatinine, osmolality, glucose/ketones

Urine creatinine measurement is useful if you cannot measure urine output. A level of less than 1000 μmol/L in babies or 2000 μmol/L in older children usually indicates polyuria, i.e. urine volume greater than 100 ml/kg per day, and a level of more than 4000 μmol/L in babies or 8000 μmol/L in older children usually indicates oliguria, i.e. less than 25 ml/kg per day, so long as the glomerular filtration rate is stable. If GFR is decreasing rapidly, then this formula overestimates the urine volume.

The fractional sodium excretion (FE_{Na}) can be calculated as in Formula 1 below.

FORMULA 1 Calculation of fractional sodium excretion

$$FE_{Na} = \frac{urine\ Na^+}{urine\ creatinine} \times \frac{plasma\ Creatinine}{plasma\ Na^+}$$

This formula is accurate even if the renal function (GFR) is changing rapidly. In health it is below 1%

or 0.01. A high fractional sodium excretion (natriuresis) suggests:

- a renal salt-wasting disorder (including tubular injury in acute renal failure)
- diuretics (including osmotic diuresis)
- volume overload (mediated by natriuretic hormones)

The osmolal gap is the difference between the measured osmolality and calculated osmolality (Formula 2).

FORMULA 2 Calculation of plasma osmolality

$$osmolality\ (mosmol/kg) = 1.86([Na^+] + [K^+]) + [glucose] + [urea] + 10\ (all\ in\ mmol/L)$$

If the osmolal gap is greater than 5 mosmol/kg, then another unusual substance, not normally measured, may be present such as *ethanol, mannitol* or *ethylene glycol.*

PRESCRIBING WATER, SODIUM AND POTASSIUM

The protocols for prescribing water and electrolytes given here are based on those used by the pediatric intensive care unit at the Royal Alexandra Hospital for Children, Sydney

A suitable starting figure for water input can be calculated easily using Formula 3. Often called 'maintenance' water, it is likely to be unsuitable for many critically ill children.

FORMULA 3 Calculation of 'maintenance' water

For the first 10 kg of body weight:
    100 mL/kg per day or 4 mL/kg per hr
For the second 10 kg of body weight:
    50 mL/kg per day or 2 mL/kg per hr
For any subsequent kg of body weight:
    25 mL/kg per day or 1 mL/kg per hr

Give a lesser amount when water retention may occur, or where a positive water balance is undesirable, such as in severe respiratory disease or brain injury (one-half to two-thirds maintenance). Other situations where water input may be reduced include heart failure (half maintenance), syndrome of inappropriate antiduiretic hormone (SIADH) (one-third), high humidity, e.g. an infant in a head box (two-thirds), and renal failure (one-third maintenance plus urine output). In renal failure the one-third maintenance is for transepidermal water loss based on 7.2 ml/100kJ (30 ml per 100 kcal). In mechanically ventilated patients water should be reduced to about two-thirds maintenance because respiratory water loss of 3.6 ml/100kJ (15 ml per 100 kcal) energy expenditure is abolished and there is further water gain because artificial ventilation is generally at a higher minute volume than normal spontaneous breathing. Give a greater quantity of water if dehydration exists or is expected, e.g. fever (add 12% for each 1°C above 37°C), burns, hyperventilation or radiant heat. See Table 2.10.1 for other adjustments in specific situations.

Always consider water, sodium and other electrolytes separately. A suitable maintenance intravenous fluid is 0.18% sodium chloride if the quantity given is derived using formula 3 above, because this provides approximately 3 mmol/kg per day of sodium in infants and 1 mmol/kg per day in adults. If a smaller quantity of water is prescribed then 0.45% NaCl is more appropriate. Addition of 40 mmol/L potassium also provides 1–3 mmol/kg per day of potassium.

OLIGURIA

Oliguria is defined as a urine output below 0.5 ml/kg·hr (< 1.0 ml/kg·h in infants). Beware of urine retention or a blocked bladder catheter before assuming true oliguria.

DIFFERENTIATING THE CAUSE

Hyperosmolar urine with low urine sodium (fractional sodium excretion < 0.5%, see formula 1 above) and high urine creatinine (> 4000 mol/L) suggest a 'prerenal' cause. A shocked child with poor peripheral perfusion is suggestive of hypovolemia. High urine sodium (fractional sodium excretion > 3%) suggests that oliguria is due to acute 'renal' renal failure (renal failure due to established renal parenchymal damage). In SIADH there is hyperosmolar urine with a high urine sodium plus hemodilution causing hyponatremia. (Table 2.10.2). The kidney is functioning well if the fractional sodium excretion is low.

HYPOVOLEMIA

Hypovolemia, as opposed to dehydration, should be treated urgently. Irrespective of the cause (hemorrhage, sepsis, burns, systemic inflammatory response syndrome, diabetic ketoacidosis), give colloid (e.g. 5% albumin) or crystalloid (e.g. 0.9% saline) in 10–20 ml/kg boluses until circulation is adequate on clinical examination. Assess heart rate, peripheral skin perfusion, capillary

TABLE 2.10.1 **Suggested initial adjustments to water input**	
Disorder	**Suggested adjustment**
Fever	+13% per °C > 37°C
High humidity (e.g. infant in head box)	0.7 × 'maintenance'
Radiant heat	1.5 × 'maintenance' for infants
Hyperventilation (spontaneous)	1.2 × 'maintenance'
Mechanical ventilation with humidifier	0.7 × 'maintenance'[a]
Brain injury	0.5–0.7 × 'maintenance'[a]
Renal failure	0.3 × 'maintenance'[b] + urine output
SIADH[c]	0.3 × 'maintenance'[b]
Congestive heart failure	0.5 × 'maintenance'

[a]This reduction is because respiratory water loss of 3.6 ml/100kJ (15 ml/100 kcal) energy expenditure is abolished and there is further water gain because artificial ventilation is generally at a higher minute volume than normal spontaneous breathing.
[b]The figure 0.3 × 'maintenance' is transepidermal water loss based on 7.2 ml/100kJ (30 mL/100 kcal).
[c]SIADH, syndrome of inappropriate ADH secretion.
Modified from Shann, F., Royal Children's Hospital, Melbourne. Principles and practice of children's emergency care. Sydney: MacLennan & Petty; 1997.

refill time (normal < 2 s), blood pressure, level of consciousness, urine output.

Giving 20% human albumin in 5 ml/kg boluses may be appropriate when there is hypoalbuminemia, especially where there is overall water and sodium retention (e.g. in patients with capillary leak syndrome).

DEHYDRATION

In many situations the degree of dehydration is easily overestimated, e.g. in diabetic ketoacidosis, but it may be underestimated in hypernatremic dehydration. Naked weight allows the degree of dehydration to be calculated if the premorbid weight is known.

1. *Mild dehydration* (< 5% body weight) causes oliguria with hyperosmolar urine (up to 600 mosmol/kg) and dry mucous membranes, but no hypotension or altered consciousness.
2. *Moderate dehydration* (5–10%) causes tachycardia, decreased skin turgor, prolonged capillary refill (> 3 s), depressed fontanelle in infants, mildly sunken eyes, and marked oliguria (except in diabetic ketoacidosis) with hyperosmolality (up to 800 mosmol/kg). The child looks unwell. There may be mildly depressed level of consciousness or apathy and a mild metabolic acidosis.
3. *Severe dehydration* (> 10%) causes shock with tachycardia, hypotension, hyperventilation, very poor peripheral perfusion, sunken eyes, sunken fontanelle, inelastic skin folds, very hyperosmolar urine (> 800 mosmol/kg), severe metabolic acidosis (pH may be < 7.0) and moderate to severe coma.
4. *Extreme dehydration* (> 15%) causes a severely ill, shocked, comatose child.

In hypernatremic dehydration neurological symptoms are noticeable, especially if acute, including lethargy, coma, irritability, hypertonicity and seizures.

DIFFERENTIATING THE CAUSE

There are many possible causes of a dehydrated child. Attention to the history and the biochemical investigations listed at the start of this chapter may identify one of the following causes:

- gastrointestinal loss, e.g. diarrhea, obstructive vomiting, nonobstructive vomiting
- renal loss, e.g. chronic renal disease, renal tubular diseases
- osmotic diuresis, e.g. diabetic ketoacidosis
- diabetes insipidus, central or nephrogenic
- salt-losing congenital adrenal hyperplasia, hypoaldosteronism and acute adrenal failure
- diuretics
- insensible loss, e.g. burns, sweating, fever, hyperventilation, especially with reduced intake (e.g. asthma)
- hyperthyroidism
- loss into body compartments where fluid does not normally accumulate ('third space'), e.g. ascites, interstitial edema
- it is unusual for decreased water intake alone to cause dehydration except when there is an abnormal loss, e.g. respiratory water loss in asthma.

Calculating potassium and sodium deficits in moderate or severe dehydration

Basic sodium deficit is approximately 0.8 mmol/kg for every 1% of dehydration (1.0 mmol/kg if rapid onset) on the basis that 60% of the dehydration is extracellular (80% if rapid onset), and extracellular sodium is 140 mmol/l. In addition, in hyponatremic dehydration, for every 10 mmol/L of hyponatremia there is 6 mmol/kg sodium deficit.

In hypernatremic dehydration, think of there being a water deficit in addition to the basic sodium deficit. Potassium deficit is approximately 0.6 mmol/kg for every 1% of dehydration (0.3 mmol/kg if rapid onset) on the basis that 40% of the dehydration is intracellular (20% if rapid onset), and intracellular potassium is 150 mmol/L.

MANAGEMENT OF THE OLIGURIC CHILD

Dehydration

Treat shock with intravenous colloid (e.g. 5% albumin) or crystalloid (e.g. 0.9% saline); see 'Hypovolemia' above. There is no urgency in treating

TABLE 2.10.2 Biochemistry in different causes of oliguria

	Plasma [Na$^+$] and osmolality	Plasma urea	Plasma creatinine	Urine [Na$^+$]	FE$_{Na}$[a]	Urine creatinine	Urine osmolality
Low cardiac output (inadequate renal perfusion, avid salt and water retention)	Normal[b]	Moderate increase	Moderate increase	Very low, usually < 10 mmol/L	< 0.5%	High, > 4000 μmol/L	High, > 400 mosmol/kg
Hypovolemia (mildly inadequate renal perfusion, avid salt and water retention)	Normal	Slight–moderate increase	Normal–moderate increase	Very low, usually < 10 mmol/L	< 0.5%	High, > 4000 μmol/L	High, > 400 mosmol/kg
Renal vasoconstriction (e.g. cyclosporin toxicity)	Normal	Slight–marked increase	Slight–marked increase	Very low, usually < 10 mmol/L	< 0.5%	High, > 4000 μmol/L,	High, > 400 mosmol/kg
Dehydration (avid water retention)	Normal, low or high	Mild–moderate increase	Normal–mild increase	Usually low, < 10 mmol/L	< 0.5%	High, > 4000 μmol/L	High, > 400 mosmol/kg
Acute renal failure (vasomotor nephropathy)	Usually normal or slightly low	High	High, but only slightly on day 1	High, > 20 mmol/L	> 3% [c]	Low, < 1000 μmol/L	(approx. = plasma)
Inappropriate ADH	Low	Normal or low	Normal or low	Very high, often 100–200 mmol/L	> 1%	Very high, often > 10 000 μmol/L	High to very high, often > 800 mosmol/kg

[a]Fractional sodium excretion.
[b]May be low owing to Na$^+$ and water retention, but more water retained than Na$^+$.
[c]A high FE$_{Na}$ does not necessarily indicate ARF if the patient is not oliguric.

mild dehydration if perfusion is adequate. Treat the underlying disease. Aggressive fluid administration may lead to overhydration or sudden osmolar changes. Aim to replace water deficit (note it is easy to overestimate the deficit) over 48 hours. For example, 10% dehydration needs only 50 ml/kg per day for 2 days in addition to normal maintenance. Usually renal compensation ensures that the child rehydrates more rapidly than this, unless water loss continues.

For the fluid repair, prescribe 0.45% sodium chloride (77 mmol/L) with 5–10% glucose (add 10–40 mmol/L potassium chloride as required, once urine output is established), on the basis that dehydration is usually shared by the extracellular and intracellular compartments in approximately a two-thirds to one-third proportion. If there is hyponatremia then there may be relatively more sodium depletion, so 0.9% sodium chloride should be chosen for part of the replacement.

A more sophisticated calculation of the composition of the repair fluid can be performed (see the calculations of potassium and sodium deficits given above), but probably does not improve the speed of recovery.

Hypernatremic dehydration

Give colloid, Hartmann's solution or Ringer-lactate solution, or 0.9% sodium chloride until the child is hemodynamically stable. Then give 0.225%–0.45% sodium chloride in dextrose 2.5%, with potassium as needed (usually 20 mmol/L), aiming to correct the estimated dehydration over 48 hours. Normal 'maintenance' water (without electrolytes, but slowly) may be given in addition. Monitor sodium and potassium, urea, glucose, and blood count every 6 hours. Plasma sodium concentration should fall slowly, preferably at no more than 0.6 mmol/L per hour. An encephalopathy or CNS vascular insult may occur, especially if there are rapid changes in plasma chemistry or circulating volume with potential for neurological deficit. Consider obtaining a cranial ultrasound or CT scan.

Low cardiac output

Support with inotropes, including dopamine at 3 μg/kg·min for its arguable effect of increasing renal blood flow. If salt and water retention exists clinically then try gentle diuresis, for example furosemide (frusemide) 0.5 mg/kg, 1 mg/kg, and then 5 mg/kg if poor response. Give no more if there is no response. Refer for renal substitution therapy early if there is existing water overload.

Renal vasoconstriction

Renal vasoconstriction is not uncommon in critically ill patients. The kidney behaves as though the patient is hypovolemic. The kidney itself is usually in good health and diuretics are indicated if water needs to be removed. Dopamine at 3–5 μg/kg·min may improve renal blood flow, but this is a matter of controversy. Refer for renal substitution therapy early if water overloaded.

Acute renal failure

Water restriction and a trial of diuretic-furosemide (frusemide) 1 mg/kg, then 5 mg/kg)—is the initial approach. Refer for renal substitution therapy early if poor response or existing water overload. Mannitol is not recommended as it may worsen the situation by acute expansion of the intravascular volume, especially if there was no diuretic response.

POLYURIA

Polyuria is defined as a urine output exceeding > 4 mL/kg·hr for more than 2 consecutive hours.

DIFFERENTIATING THE CAUSE

Polyuria may be caused by:

- water overload, including psychogenic polydipsia
- osmotic diuresis, especially hyperglycemia
- diuretic drugs
- diabetes insipidus
- ARF (polyuric phase)
- renal tubular disease
- hypercalcemia
- cerebral salt wasting – a condition not yet well defined where there is natriuresis associated with high blood levels of natriuretic peptides in the absence of water overload or other causes of diuresis.

A low urine osmolality (< 200 mosmol/kg) with a normal or high plasma osmolality suggests diabetes insipidus. A high urine fractional sodium excretion (> 1%) suggests otherwise. An osmolal gap suggests an unmeasured solute causing osmotic diuresis. Measure urine sodium and potassium on 4-hourly urine collections, in order to estimate losses for replacement, if polyuria persists for more than 4 hours.

MANAGEMENT OF THE POLYURIC CHILD

Treat the underlying condition. Replace urine water loss (and other losses, e.g. gastrointestinal) hour by hour intravenously, adding 15–25 ml/kg per day for insensible losses. Replace measured sodium and potassium losses. Calculate 4-hourly urine sodium and potassium loss and replace in next 4 hours of intravenous fluid.

Diabetes insipidus (DI) should be treated by giving 0.225% sodium chloride with 3.75% glucose, replacing the previous hour's urine volume plus 15–25 ml/kg per day for insensible losses. Desmopressin (DDAVP) or vasopressin may be prescribed in acute central DI, but not until water balance is being controlled successfully by replacement of losses. Patients may be extremely sensitive to exogenous vasopressins and severe water retention may result. Beware of hyperglycemia from the glucose load.

Special treatment is required in cases of diabetes insipidus in a brain-dead patient awaiting organ retrieval. An intravenous infusion of vasopressin both controls the polyuria of the DI and has a vasopressor effect treating the hypotension that accompanies loss of sympathetic tone. Larger doses of vasopressin are required than are used in managing other forms of central DI. Put 1 unit/kg in 50 ml 5% glucose or 0.9% sodium chloride. A dosage rate of 1 ml/h gives 18 milliunit/kg·hr of vasopressin. Start at 0.5 ml/h. Add an inotrope, e.g. epinephrine (adrenaline) at 0.1–0.2 µg/kg·min.

EDEMA, WATER OVERLOAD AND PULMONARY EDEMA

DIFFERENTIATING THE CAUSE

Causes of edema or water retention include:

- congestive heart failure (congenital or acquired structural heart disease, tachyarrhythmias, pericardial effusion) suggested by tachycardia, hypotension, elevated jugular pressure, hepatomegaly and lung crepitations
- renal disease, suggested by oliguria, hypertension or hematuria
- liver disease (cirrhosis, metabolic disease)
- other causes of hypoproteinemia (e.g. protein-losing enteropathy)
- inappropriate ADH secretion or administration (rarely causes edema)
- excess sodium plus water intake

MANAGEMENT

Water and sodium input should be reduced. Diuretics should be used carefully and in small doses initially, because acute hypovolemia can occur (especially in nephrotic syndrome where there is already hypovolemia). Refer early for renal substitution therapy if diuretics are ineffective. Hemofiltration can remove water very rapidly if there is refractory pulmonary edema, cardiac failure or hypertensive encephalopathy.

Pulmonary edema complicating acute respiratory disease, such as after near-drowning or relief of acute upper airway obstruction, may be treated by continuous positive airway pressure (CPAP), 5–10 cmH$_2$O.

HYPONATREMIA

Clinical features of hyponatremia include nausea, lethargy, altered consciousness, and seizures. Symptoms may be more marked if the hyponatremia has developed rapidly.

DIFFERENTIATING THE CAUSE

In cases of water overload without sodium, e.g. water intoxication (deliberate, psychogenic or iatrogenic) or inappropriate ADH syndrome, edema is rare. The FE$_{Na}$ is high. Urine osmolality is high (urine sodium concentration up to 300 mmol/L) in inappropriate ADH because of natriuresis induced by the hypervolemia. Urine osmolality will usually be low in water intoxication, but it can be elevated for the same reason as in SIADH.

Salt and water retention (water > sodium) occurs in nephrotic syndrome, heart failure, renal failure and liver failure. Edema is possible. The FE_{Na} is usually low.

In cases of dehydration where there is more sodium than water depletion, including third space 'losses', think of hypoadrenalism, e.g. congenital adrenal hyperplasia and acute adrenal failure. The FE_{Na} is usually low, but is high when the cause is 'renal'. Plasma urea and urine osmolality are likely to be high in dehydration (Table 2.10.2).

The presence of an abnormal solute in the extracellular fluid, e.g. glucose in diabetes mellitus, causes a water shift from the intracellular to the extracellular space. There may be an osmolal gap if the cause is not glucose.

The causes of hyponatremia (serum Na+ concentration below 130 mmol/L) include:

- dilution:
  - water excess (ingestion or administration)
  - edema
    - congestive heart failure
    - nephrotic syndrome
    - renal failure (fall in GFR)
    - pancuronium (paralysis)
    - hepatic failure
  - ADH excess
  - hyperglycemia
  - altered osmostat
  - drugs: barbiturates, cyclo-phosphamide, narcotics, NSAIDs, phencyclidine, vincristine
  - infection: respiratory syncytial virus
- depletion:
  - salt wasting: renal disease (Fanconi's syndrome), adrenal disease
  - glucosuria
  - diuretics
  - hypotonic replacement of body fluids (vomiting or diarrhea)
  - excess loss in sweat (e.g. fibrocystic disease)
- Pseudohyponatremia:
  - severe proteinuria
  - severe hyperlipidemia

MANAGEMENT

Treat shock with 20 ml/kg of 5% albumin. Manage dehydration by replacing extracellular fluid loss with 0.9% sodium chloride or Ringer-lactate solution slowly over 48 hours. Hyponatremia will correct slowly. In water intoxication restrict water to half maintenance or less, with sodium supplements if there is natriuresis (see above). The use of hypertonic (3% = 500 mmol/L) sodium chloride is controversial. It should be restricted to children with water overload and hyponatremia which is severe (< 120 mmol/L) and symptomatic (i.e. seizures or coma). Only correct to a plasma sodium concentration of 125 mmol/L, aiming for an increase of no more than 2 mmol/L per hour, i.e. no more than 1.2 mmol/kg·h. For severe acute symptoms or impending cerebral herniation it may be safe to give the first 2–3 mmol/kg over 30–60 minutes, then continue with 0.9% sodium chloride as above. With lesser cerebral symptoms, e.g. irritability or lethargy, aim to correct plasma sodium by 0.5 mmol/L·h up to 125 mmol/L.

FORMULA 4 Calculation of sodium dose for correction to 125 mmol/L

Sodium dose (mmol) = $(125 - \text{Plasma } [Na^+]) \times 0.6 \times (\text{Weight in kg})$

In SIADH the child is water overloaded but sodium depleted, so management is to restrict water, giving it as 0.9% sodium chloride. In edematous states restrict water and sodium input. Hypotension, convulsions and decreasing level of consciousness may occur at any time during treatment, especially if there are rapid changes in circulating volume or plasma chemistry. Some neurological deficit may result from the encephalopathy of severe hyponatremia.

HYPERNATREMIA

Hypernatremia is usually caused by water loss rather than sodium accumulation and in dehydration states may be accompanied by sodium depletion.

DIFFERENTIATING THE CAUSE

Causes of hypernatremia include:

- gastrointestinal water loss (diarrhea is the most common cause)

- increased insensible water loss
- diabetes insipidus—central or nephrogenic
- water deprivation
- osmotic diuresis including diabetic ketoacidosis
- loop diuretics (very rare unless with excess Na$^+$ supplementation)
- obstructive uropathy
- salt poisoning (rare)

The clinical features of hypernatremia are usually those of dehydration. If plasma sodium concentration exceeds 160 mmol/L then there may be seizures and depressed consciousness.

Fractional sodium excretion is high (> 1%) if there is sodium excess or if the cause is an osmotic diuresis.

Fractional sodium excretion is low (< 0.5%) if the cause is water loss, for example with high insensible loss, other nonrenal water loss, or water deprivation. Urine osmolality is high (> 600 mosmol/kg) except in diabetes insipidus unless the water depletion of DI is extreme.

MANAGEMENT

The management of diabetes insipidus is described above in the section on polyuria.

The management of hypernatremic dehydration is described in the section on dehydration.

Restrict water, with minimal sodium input, if there is salt excess without dehydration, aiming for a very slow correction of plasma sodium levels (< 15 mmol/L per day). Diuretic administration may be considered, and hemodialysis may be required in extreme cases.

HYPOKALEMIA

DIFFERENTIATING THE CAUSE

Usually there is potassium depletion, but hypokalemia may occur by shift of the cation from the extracellular to the intracellular space with normal total body potassium levels:

- potassium depletion may be caused by:
  - inadequate intake
  - excessive renal loss: diuretics, tubular disease (drug-induced or other), steroids (primary or secondary hyperaldosteronism, glucocorticoids), nonresorbable anions (e.g. penicillins, bicarbonate), diabetic ketoacidosis
  - gastrointestinal loss: vomiting, diarrhea, laxatives
  - skin losses: excessive sweating, burns
- shift from extracellular to intracellular compartments may be caused by:
  - alkalosis
  - insulin
  - β_2-adrenergic agonists

The clinical picture may depend on whether the potassium depletion is acute or chronic. Symptoms and signs may include skeletal muscle weakness, decreased contractility of smooth muscle (usually manifesting as ileus, especially in acute hypokalemia). Chronic cases can be asymptomatic.

Electrocardiographic findings include depression of the ST segment, decrease in T wave amplitude and appearance of a U wave. Automaticity is increased, arrhythmias may occur, including varying degrees of heart block, ventricular tachycardia, bigeminy or ventricular fibrillation. Hypokalemia increases the cardiac toxicity of digoxin.

Estimate current or recent potassium intake. Obtain a drug history, especially of previous potentially nephrotoxic agents. Check acid–base status and urine potassium concentration. Other investigations (such as aldosterone and plasma magnesium estimation) may be indicated.

TREATMENT

Oral replacement is often adequate. Intravenous therapy should be considered in the presence of:

- cardiac arrhythmias
- neuromuscular features
- 'nil by mouth' or vomiting
- severe potassium depletion

Total deficit is difficult to estimate because potassium is principally an intracellular ion. If there is hypochloremic alkalosis, the hypokalemia may not be corrected until the chloride deficit is replaced. Cardiac monitoring is essential, and potassium input should be reviewed frequently, especially if renal function is changing. Note that 0.1 mmol/kg·h of potassium will supply normal daily maintenance requirements. Add 10 mmol, 15 mmol or 20 mmol potassium chloride to every 500 ml of intravenous fluid (usually 0.225% sodium chloride with 3.75% glucose), depending on the severity of hypokalemia. Concentrated potassium solutions are not usually needed unless there is risk of life-threatening arrhythmias (e.g. patients with congenital heart disease with a history of dysrhythmias), or there is high continuing renal loss (e.g. tubular injury from chemotherapy). Concentrated potassium infusions are usually administered through a central line at a rate in the range 0.1–0.4 mmol/kg·h. Potassium levels should be checked frequently during infusion.

> KEEP POTASSIUM INFUSIONS PROMINENTLY LABELED AND WELL AWAY FROM OTHER SOLUTIONS TO AVOID ANY ACCIDENTAL ADMINISTRATION

HYPERKALEMIA

Hyperkalemia (plasma potassium (K^+) levels in excess of 5.5 mmol/L) is an emergency in critically ill children, caused by renal failure or catabolism (including hemolysis, tumor lysis) and continued potassium intake, including blood products. Moderate hyperkalemia (< 6.0 mmol/L) may be asymptomatic, but higher levels may cause cardiac dysrhythmia, including ventricular tachycardia, ventricular fibrillation and asystole. The ECG is a sensitive indicator of the effect on the heart (Table 2.10.3). However, potassium levels at which specific ECG abnormalities are seen vary widely between patients. Hypocalcemia can turn a 'safe' plasma potassium level into a toxic one. The risks of a modest increase in plasma potassium ions in the presence of hypocalcemia are much greater than if calcium levels are normal.

DIFFERENTIATING THE CAUSE

A full list of causes is given in Table 2.10.4.

Increased total body potassium

An increase in total body potassium content may be caused by:

- increased intake:
  - intravenous fluids
  - potassium-containing drugs (penicillins)
  - blood transfusions
- decreased renal excretion:
  - renal failure
  - adrenal insufficiency (Addison's disease), or aldosterone deficient or resistant states
  - potassium-sparing diuretics (spironolactone, amiloride)
  - drugs: cyclosporin, NSAID's, ACE inhibitors

Shift from intracellular to extracellular compartments

A shift in potassium to the extracellular compartment without overall change in total body potassium concentration may be due to:

- acidosis
- rhabdomyolysis or other cell lysis (crush injury, burns, tumor lysis, tissue necrosis)
- drugs: succinylcholine (suxamethonium), beta-blockers

Pseudohyperkalemia

Pseudohyperkalemia may be due to hemolysis of drawn blood (difficulty with sampling, especially with use of a tourniquet).

TABLE 2.10.3 **Electrocardiographic manifestations of hyperkalemia**	
Plasma K+ (mmol/L)	**ECG manifestations**
5.5–6.5	Tall, peaked T waves, normal or decreased QT interval, short PR interval
6.5–7.5	Widening of QRS complex, increased PR interval
7.5–8.0	Broad, low-amplitude P waves, broad T waves, ST segment elevation or depression
> 8.0	P waves disappear, marked widening of QRS, 'sine wave' pattern, high risk of VF or asystole

TABLE 2.10.4 **Causes of hyperkalemia**

High intake
- Potassium supplements
- Potassium salts of antibiotics (penicillin)
- Salt substitutes
- High-potassium diet: bananas, orange juice, carrots, celery, broccoli
- Transfusion of stored blood

Decreased renal excretion
- Drugs:
  - ACE inhibitors
  - β-adrenergic blockers
  - cyclosporin
  - KCl, K$^+$-sparing diuretics
  - NSAIDs
  - spironolactone
  - triamterene
- Renal failure
- Mineralocorticoid deficiency
- Hyporeninemic hypoaldosteronism (diabetes mellitus)
- Tubular unresponsiveness to aldosterone (e.g. sickle cell disease, SLE)
- Heparin administration

Abnormal distribution (excessive cellular release)
- Acidosis (each 0.1 decrease in pH, results in a 0.4–0.6 mmol/L increase in K$^+$)
- Hypoxic cell death
- Insulin deficiency
- Hypertonicity
- Intravascular hemolysis
- Tissue necrosis, rhabdomyolysis, burns, acute tumor lysis
- Hyperkalemic periodic paralysis

Pseudohyperkalemia
- Local release due to muscular contraction (strenuous exercise)
- Hemolyzed specimen (particularly capillary samples collected following heel stab)
- Severe thrombocytosis (platelets > 10^9/ml)
- Severe leukocytosis (WBC > 10^8/ml)

TREATMENT

Estimate potassium intake. Other investigations are dictated by the possible cause.

A wide QRS complex or a plasma potassium concentration in excess of 7.0 mmol/L demands emergency treatment. Commence cardiopulmonary resuscitation if no or low output, stop all exogenous sources of potassium, and give calcium, bicarbonate and salbutamol as outlined in Table 2.10.5.

General principles of treatment include cessation of all exogenous sources of potassium (intravenous and oral supplements), changing the cell membrane threshold potential (e.g. give calcium), shifting potassium from extracellular to intracellular compartments (e.g. alkalinize), and promoting potassium loss from the body.

METABOLIC ACIDOSIS

In metabolic acidosis the plasma bicarbonate level is low. There is either hyperchloremia (plasma chloride concentration in excess of 105 mmol/L, normal anion gap < 16 mEq/L), or normochloremia (chloride 105 mmol/L, high anion gap > 20 mEq/L). The excess anion gap consists of unmeasured anions such as inorganic acids (e.g. sulfate, phosphate) or organic acids (e.g. lactate, ketoacids, drugs).

FORMULA 5 **Calculation of the anion gap**

Anion gap (mEq/L) =
plasma [Na$^+$ + K$^+$] − [Cl$^-$ + HCO$_3^-$] (all in mmol/L)

TABLE 2.10.5 An outline for treatment of hyperkalemia

Treatment	Onset	Duration	Benefit
Calcium gluconate 10% (0.5 ml/kg slow i.v.). Monitor the results of calcium infusion by measuring plasma ionized calcium	Immediate	Brief	Stabilizes myocardium by increasing threshold potential
Sodium bicarbonate (1 mmol/kg slow i.v.) or hyperventilate if intubated	20–60 min	Few hours	Shifts K^+ into cells
Salbutamol 2.5–5 mg (nebulized) or 4 μg/kg i.v. over 15–20 min	30–60 min	1–2 h	Shifts K^+ into cells
Glucose 50% (1 ml/kg) over 15–20 min possibly with insulin (0.1 units/kg), but monitor for hypoglycemia	20–60 min	Few hours	Shifts K^+ into cells
Potassium exchange resins (calcium polystyrene sulfonate 0.5–1 g/kg rectally)	1–4 h	Few hours	Removal of K^+
Consider a loop diuretic, e.g. furosemide (frusemide) 1 mg/kg in nonanuric patients (not in salt-depleted subjects)	Depends on urine output, usually within 1 h	Few hours	Increased K^+ loss in urine
Hemodialysis, hemofiltration or rapid cycling peritoneal dialysis may be indicated if hyperkalemia is refractory to above management	2–3 h	Several hours	Removal of K^+

Note—to maintain electrical neutrality, the cations and anions in plasma are equivalent. Plasma sodium and potassium ions are largely balanced by chloride and bicarbonate, but other unmeasured, polyvalent anions such as phosphate, sulfate, organic acids and proteins represent the anion gap; which should therefore be expressed in milliequivalents and not millimoles.

DIFFERENTIATING THE CAUSE

High anion gap

Acidosis with a high anion gap may be caused by:

- diarrhea (starvation, ketosis)
- sepsis
- diabetic ketoacidosis
- renal failure
- hepatic failure
- drugs (e.g. salicylates, ethanol, methanol, ethylene glycol)
- inborn errors of metabolism (especially in babies)
- hypoxia
- circulatory failure

Normal anion gap

Causes of acidosis with a normal anion gap include:

- dehydration
- renal tubular acidosis
- intestinal fistulas or enterostomies

A plasma lactate estimation should be performed if there is a significant base deficit or high anion gap. Urine for drug screening may be indicated. For suspected inborn errors of metabolism if the anion gap exceeds 20 mEq/L, send urine for metabolic screening.

MANAGEMENT

First treat the underlying disease, including general management of renal, hepatic and cardiac failure, shock and hypovolemia. Alkali is not usually needed for mild acidosis (pH > 7.2) because the acidosis itself does not cause any compromise. Sudden changes in acid-base status should be avoided. Bicarbonate therapy may be useful but avoid large boluses which may cause a sudden hyperosmolality, hypocalcemic tetany, or late alkalosis.

In high anion gap acidosis (lactic acidosis) be careful in giving bicarbonate if the patient is not depleted of sodium. Enough bicarbonate to correct the acidosis may cause sodium overload. Consider a bicarbonate-based dialysis technique instead (e.g. hemofiltration with bicarbonate-based replacement fluid). Consider hemodialysis, or hemofiltration with bicarbonate-based replacement fluid, in severe metabolic acidosis (pH < 7.2), especially if caused by inherited metabolic disease.

A bicarbonate infusion may be given in normal anion gap acidosis because excessive chloride therapy would exacerbate hyperchloremia. A suggested approach is to correct the bicarbonate deficit over 6 hours (Formula 6), then at a rate of 2 mmol/kg per day. Chronic metabolic acidosis with hypocapnia should not be treated with bicarbonate.

Correct hypoglycemia. If an inborn error of metabolism is suspected give glucose at a dosage of at least 8 mg/kg·min, correct electrolyte imbalance, and partially correct acidosis with bicarbonate, giving this over at least 1 hour (see above).

If there is a risk of sodium overload from sodium bicarbonate, then tromethamine, also known as tris(hydroxymethyl)aminomethane, trometamol or THAM, is a useful alternative. The dose for correction (in mmol) is as for bicarbonate. It is given as a 300 mmol/L solution. It has the advantage of being a mild osmotic diuretic; the salt, THAM-H$^+$Cl$^-$, is excreted by glomerular filtration.

FORMULA 6 Calculation of dose of bicarbonate or THAM for full correction

Dose (mmol) = weight (kg) × base deficit (mmol/L) ÷ 3

METABOLIC ALKALOSIS

Metabolic alkalosis is usually caused by chronic potassium and/or chloride depletion, e.g. gastric (accompanied by volume depletion) or renal (including diuretic use). It may be compensatory (chronic renal bicarbonate retention) in chronic respiratory failure, in which case it should not be treated. Alkalosis can cause tetany by lowering plasma ionized calcium.

MANAGEMENT

Correct acute chloride deficit (approximately 6 mmol/kg for every 10 mmol/L fall in plasma chloride) by rehydration with 0.45% sodium chloride (77 mmol/L) plus 40 mmol/L potassium chloride with added glucose. Hypotonic solutions, which may exacerbate hyponatremia, should not be used. Intravenous hydrochloric acid (or arginine hydrochloride) is indicated in rare severe cases when alkalosis may be depressing respiratory drive, and when the chloride deficit is not accompanied by sodium deficit. Give hydrochloric acid (150 mmol/L solution) by central intravenous catheter. Give half-correction over at least 1 hour.

FORMULA 7 Dose of HCl for full correction

Dose (mmol) = weight (kg) ×
base excess (mmol/L) ÷ 3

FORMULA 8 Dose of arginine hydrochloride for full correction

Dose (mg) = weight (kg) ×
base excess (mmol/L) × 70

Acidifying diuretics such as acetazolamide, spironolactone and amiloride may be indicated in metabolic alkalosis where there is sodium and water retention (but relatively less chloride retention).

HYPOCALCEMIA

Most hypocalcemia is caused by total body calcium depletion. Alkalosis may cause symptoms of hypocalcemia with a normal total plasma calcium, but low ionized calcium levels. Symptoms—which may be absent—include weakness, tetany, laryngospasm, hypotension and seizures. Seizures are usually accompanied by other signs of hypocalcemia. An X-ray or clinical examination may detect rickets. The QT interval may be prolonged on the ECG.

DIFFERENTIATING THE CAUSE

Hypocalcemia may be due to:

- reduced calcium intake
- vitamin D deficiency

- hypoparathyroidism or pseudo-hypoparathyroidism
- renal tubular disorders
- diuretics
- phosphate intoxication
- magnesium deficiency

Consider assessing serum parathyroid hormone and vitamin D levels if refractory. Other investigations include blood gas analysis, urine calcium creatinine ratio (normal < 0.7,) $FE_{phosphate}$ (normal is < 30%), ECG, and radiography of wrist or knee.

MANAGEMENT

If the cause is acute alkalosis due to hyperventilation then the latter should be treated. An intravenous calcium infusion should only be given slowly, and if the condition is symptomatic, into a central venous catheter. Give calcium 0.1 mmol/kg at a time until symptoms subside. Follow if necessary with an infusion of 2 mmol/kg per day. If the plasma calcium does not correct, or if seizures are unresponsive to calcium, then magnesium deficiency may be a cause, even if plasma magnesium concentration is normal. The treatment for hypomagnesemia is given below. Vitamin D therapy may need to be considered. If the patient is hyperphosphatemic consider using diuretics, enteral phosphate binders or dialysis.

HYPOMAGNESEMIA

Hypomagnesemia usually indicates magnesium depletion and is common in critically ill children. The clinical features are similar to hypocalcemia. Note that hypomagnesemia is arrhythmogenic, and shares its etiology with—and may coexist with—hypokalemia.

CAUSES

Causes of hypomagnesemia are:

- diarrhea and vomiting
- diuretics and osmotic diuresis
- renal tubular disease (including some cytotoxic drug effects)
- diabetic ketoacidosis

TREATMENT

Prescribe magnesium chloride or sulfate 0.4 mmol/kg by slow intravenous injection and repeat every 12 hours until plasma concentration is normal.

HYPOPHOSPHATEMIA

Hypophosphatemia is common in critically ill children, especially in diabetic ketoacidosis. It indicates phosphate depletion, but represents this poorly. Any cause of diuresis, renal tubulopathies such as Fanconi's syndrome, cystinosis, vitamin D resistant rickets, and tubular damage following drugs such as Ifosfamide can cause hyperphosphaturia. Most phosphate is immobile in bone. The rest is nearly all intracellular (50–55 mmol/L compared with 2 mmol/L extracellular). It is important in enzyme regulation and energy transfer processes. Measures that promote entry of potassium into cells also promote phosphate entry (e.g. insulin, glucose, β_2-adrenergics). A relative hypophosphatemic state may also be seen in the presence of hypercalcemia.

Clinical features include:

- skeletal muscle weakness
- respiratory depression
- hemolytic anemia
- rhabdomyolysis
- cardiac dysfunction
- insulin resistance in diabetic patients
- shift of oxyhemoglobin dissociation curve to the left (2,3-DPG depletion), with resultant decreased oxygen delivery to tissues

Correction of acidosis may acutely unmask these effects, and exacerbate the hypophosphatemia.

INVESTIGATION

Urine for phosphate, measurement of $FE_{phosphate}$ (or tubular reabsorption of phosphate i.e. $1-FE_{phosphate}$), and urinary tubular protein excretion (such as retinol binding protein, N-acetylglucosaminidase, β_2-microglobulin) may be useful if a primary renal tubular disease is suspected.

TREATMENT

First, treat the underlying disease causing the phosphate loss (e.g. manage acute diabetic keto-acidosis).

Rapid or excessive correction of phosphate depletion may cause hypocalcemia or hypomagnesemia. Boluses should not be given. As phosphate depletion is often accompanied by potassium depletion, especially in diabetic ketoacidosis, a useful formula is to give one-third of potassium as phosphate (potassium dihydrogen phosphate). There is risk of diarrhea with oral administration. Always monitor treatment with repeated plasma phosphate, calcium and magnesium levels. The effect of a given dose on plasma phosphate levels is unpredictable. Continuous intravenous infusion of up to 3 mmol/kg per day is safe and effective. Frequent phosphate supplements may be needed in conditions with continuing losses.

ACUTE RENAL FAILURE

Acute renal failure (ARF) is rapid loss of renal function with oliguria or anuria (< 0.5 ml/kg·h in children or < 1 ml/kg·h in infants) and a rise in plasma creatinine concentration. It may present with gastrointestinal (anorexia, nausea, vomiting, hemorrhage, hiccups), cardiovascular (fluid overload, hypertension, arrhythmias, pericarditis), respiratory (tachypnea, pulmonary edema) and neuropsychiatric (confusion, agitation, seizures) manifestations. In catabolic states (e.g. acute trauma, tumor lysis, rhabdomyolysis), a clinical picture similar to ARF may arise.

DIFFERENTIATING THE CAUSES

Renal failure can be 'prerenal' (inadequate blood flow), 'renal' (intrinsic renal cell injury) or 'postrenal' (urine outflow obstruction) in origin (Ch. 3.5). In Western countries hemolytic–uremic syndrome is the most common cause, whereas in tropical countries 'prerenal' causes predominate outside the hospital environment. In hospital, renal failure is a common complication in critically ill children (e.g. following bypass surgery).

Clinical history and examination is usually helpful in identification of the 'prerenal' and 'renal' causes. However, especially in the very young, renal ultrasound imaging is essential for the diagnosis of obstructive causes.

Subjects with 'prerenal' or 'postrenal' renal failure may suffer renal damage if the condition is prolonged; therefore identify and correct treatable disorders urgently.

Table 2.10.6 summarizes the investigations useful in ARF. It is important to differentiate between causes of oliguria. Plasma and urine biochemistry can be useful tools for this (see Table 2.10.2).

MANAGEMENT

Recognize and treat life-threatening complications first. Establish adequate airway and oxygenation and then treat hyperkalemia, hypovolemia, pulmonary edema and hypertensive crises (Tables 2.10.7 and 2.10.8).

The investigations listed in Table 2.10.6 will help to identify complications, give clues to the etiology of renal failure and help monitor progress. The frequency of biochemical and other investigations (Ch. 3.5) depends very much on individual need.

HYPERTENSION

Blood pressure in children should be interpreted against nomograms based on age, weight or height (Ch. 7.3). High blood pressure in children could be a consequence of a reflex increase in peripheral resistance, such as in hypovolemia (nephrotic syndrome), low cardiac output states and pain, where treatment would be correction of the volume status (colloid or crystalloid), inotropes and analgesics respectively. In acute renal failure hypertension is often related to salt and water overload.

DIFFERENTIATING THE CAUSE

Causes of hypertension are as follows:

- reflex increase in blood pressure:
  - raised intracranial pressure (intracranial tumors, bleed)
  - postictal
  - encephalitis, stroke

TABLE 2.10.6. **Basic investigations in acute renal failure**

Investigation	Points of interest
Blood	
Hemoglobin, WBC, platelets, blood film	Anemia, thrombocytopenia, neutrophilia, hemolysis, fragmented red cells
Coagulation screen	
Na^+, K^+, HCO_3^-, Ca^{2+}, Mg^{2+}, PO_4, albumin	Electrolyte disturbances, acidosis, baseline to assess progress
Urea, creatinine	
Uric acid, glucose	
Blood culture	Exclude sepsis
Liver function tests	
Blood lactate, amino acids, ammonia	Assess these if metabolic causes suspected, especially in babies
Urine	
Dipstick—protein, blood	Negative in prerenal and postrenal states
Microscopy cells, sediment	
Electrolytes (Na^+, K^+, urea, creatinine)	Electrolytes helpful to elucidate cause
Osmolality	
Culture—urine (clean catch)	Exclude infection routinely
Imaging	
Ultrasound—abdominal, renal	Exclude urinary obstruction, especially in neonates; may also give clues in other cases, e.g. enlarged kidneys may suggest acute intrinsic renal injury
Renal isotope scans (DTPA, MAG3)	Perform urgently if no identifiable cause. Assesses functioning renal tubular mass and renal blood flow. Useful in distinguishing acute tubular necrosis from other causes of ARF
Chest X-ray	Pulmonary edema, effusions ± cardiomegaly
Echocardiography (2D)	Useful in assessing myocardial function, hypertension. Exclude bacterial endocarditis

---

TABLE 2.10.7 Basic principles of management of acute renal failure

Basic principles of management	Common aspects needing attention
Treat established complications Minimize further damage Remove the precipitating cause	Treat life-threatening complications (hypoxia, hyperkalemia) Correct hypotension, hypovolemia Treat sepsis Remove agents of nephrotoxicity (drugs, poisons, metabolic products) Relieve obstruction Give dopamine (renal dose), furosemide (frusemide)
Minimize load on the kidney	Do not administer excessive fluids Do not administer excessive electrolytes (especially Na^+ and K^+) Reduce catabolism (supply adequate energy) Avoid or reduce dose of renally excreted drugs
Remove accumulated load and/or balance biochemical parameters to physiological limits	Phosphate Water and electrolytes Urea and creatinine Drugs, toxins

---

- with salt and water overload:
  - renal parenchymal disease
  - mineralocorticoid excess or apparent mineralocorticoid excess (e.g. 11 β-hydroxydehydrogenase deficiency)
  - corticosteroid excess (e.g. Cushing's syndrome)
  - salt-retaining syndromes (e.g. Liddle's syndrome)
- without salt and water overload
  - hypercalcemia
  - coarctation of aorta
  - catecholamine excess (pheochromocytoma)
  - hyperreninemia (e.g. renovascular disease)

Hypertension in children is often secondary and at least in two-thirds of cases renal causes predominate. Renovascular disease is a common cause, particularly in the very young. Some may present in a crisis state, i.e. with encephalopathy (convulsions, cranial nerve palsies, altered level of consciousness), raised intracranial pressure, heart failure, pulmonary edema, or even in renal failure as a consequence. These subjects should be initially treated in a pediatric intensive care unit.

MANAGEMENT

Reflex increases in blood pressure (for example in the presence of an intracranial space-occupying lesion, hypovolemia, postictal states) may not always be treated, as this may be harmful. If the primary cause of hypertension is fluid overload, this should be corrected by fluid restriction, and even dialysis if necessary. In any case, antihypertensive therapy should be commenced with the aim of reducing blood pressure very slowly, particularly if there are associated neurological complications. Reduce blood pressure only by a third towards the target over the first 24–48 hours. Intravenous sodium nitroprusside or labetalol (in the absence of heart failure), are recommended, with direct arterial blood pressure monitoring.

Other hypertensive patients may be treated with oral or sublingual antihypertensive drugs (e.g. nifedipine). Investigate to elucidate the cause. Remember, severely hypertensive subjects may be relatively hypovolemic owing to pressure natriuresis, so be cautious with the use of diuretics.

RENAL SUBSTITUTION THERAPY

INDICATIONS

Renal substitution therapy is indicated for complications of acute renal failure, especially with oliguria, or a severe metabolic or other disorder without oliguria:

- indications in ARF:
  - hyperkalemia unresponsive to conservative measures

TABLE 2.10.8 Management issues in acute renal failure

Clinical problem	Etiology	Risks	Treatment
Electrolytes			
Hyperkalemia	Reduced excretion Excessive intake Excessive catabolism	Cardiac arrhythmia or arrest (in the presence of hypocalcemia cardiac arrhythmias can occur with relatively normal levels of potassium)	Calcium gluconate i.v. Salbutamol i.v./inhalation Ca^{2+} exchange resins oral/NG/pr Diuretics i.v. Dialysis (if refractory) Minimize K^+ intake Reduce catabolism
Hyperphosphatemia	Decreased phosphate excretion or excess catabolism (e.g. lymphoma when treated)	Hypocalcemia-associated complications	Oral phosphate binders Reduce intake Reduce catabolism Hemodialysis or peritoneal dialysis
Hypocalcemia	Often associated with hyperphosphatemia	Tetany, convulsions (especially if the associated acidemia is corrected aggressively)	Rarely may need Ca^{2+} supplements, especially in hypercatabolic states with very high phosphate levels Deal with hyperphosphatemia before correction of acidosis
Hyponatremia	Usually a problem of salt and water excess (but more water than salt); rarely due to extrarenal loss of Na^+	Neurological damage, seizures	Water restriction Rarely may need salt supplements, particularly if renal failure was of prerenal origin Dialysis/filtration
Hypernatremia	Excessive water loss (nephrogenic or extra-renal) or excess salt administration (e.g. parenteral nutrition)	Neurological damage	Reduce salt intake Correct slowly May need peritoneal or hemodialysis—initially with hypertonic (i.e. high Na^+) solutions
Water			
Overload, intoxication	Reduced excretion Excessive administration	Edema (uncommon unless Na^+ also involved) Pulmonary edema, neurological features, seizures myocardial dysfunction, hypotension	Water restriction Dialysis
Blood pressure			
Hypertension	Salt and water retention Vasoconstriction	Encephalopathy Cardiac failure Pulmonary edema Target organ damage	Reduce BP slowly over 48–72 h especially if associated with encephalopathy Control convulsions (e.g. phenytoin i.v.), correct hypoglycemia and hypocalcemia May need IPPV Reduce salt and water intake Improve excretion of salt and water (diuretics, dialysis) Vasodilators (intravenous sodium nitroprusside, or sublingual nifedipine). Labetalol (give i.v. beta-blockers cautiously in the presence of heart failure) Beta-blockers (oral)
Acidosis			
Acidemia	Accumulation of organic acids due to loss of H^+ excretion pathway	Poor cardiac function and effects on other biological systems, especially with hyperketonemia	Correction by administration of bicarbonate or THAM (sodium bicarbonate increases Na^+ input, hence may need dialysis to offset this) Can be corrected by ordinary dialysis but if severe needs bicarbonate dialysis

TABLE 2.10.8 Management issues in acute renal failure *continued*

Uremia			
	Accumulation of urea, creatinine and other metabolic products	Clouding of consciousness Pericarditis Bleeding tendency Vomiting Itching	Supply adequate energy Dialysis (slow correction as risk of reverse osmosis leading to encephalopathy)
Problems of the primary disease	Burns	Fluid and protein loss Hypercatabolism Infection	Adequate nutrition (may need dialysis to create space) protein replacement antibiotics
	Septicemia	Shock	Circulating volume/blood transfusion Antibiotics Gram-negative shock may require vasodilators, large volumes of colloid/crystalloids and continuous dialysis/filtration Inotropes may be needed
	Hemolytic-uremic syndrome	Extrarenal manifestations	Dialysis Blood transfusion Plasma exchange

- fluid overload associated with hypertensive encephalopathy, pulmonary edema or cardiac failure
- fluid overload unresponsive to conventional treatment, with continuing marked acidemia
- symptomatic uremia with altered mentation, lethargy, nausea, vomiting
- severe hyponatremia or hypernatremia
- prolonged oliguria with inability to provide adequate nutrition
- indications in the absence of renal failure:
  - severe acidemia especially in inherited metabolic disease
  - sodium and water overload
  - tumor lysis syndrome
  - systemic inflammatory response syndrome (cytokine clearance)
  - drug overdose

AIMS

The principles of all forms of renal substitution therapy are similar—to remove excess water, electrolytes or other solutes by filtration (the movement is called convection) or dialysis (called diffusion). The filtration is sometimes called 'ultrafiltration' when it is done by artificially increasing hydrostatic pressure across the dialysis membrane. More detailed applications are listed in Table 2.10.9.

MODE

The best mode of renal substitution therapy to choose depends upon the individual patient's needs (see above). The patient's hemodynamic status, indication for dialysis therapy, speed of correction needed, catabolic state, availability of vascular access, and the anticipated fluid volume load that must be given should also be considered. The availability of equipment and expertise are also important. Various modes of dialysis therapy include conventional peritoneal dialysis, crossflow peritoneal dialysis (continuous flow of dialysate across the peritoneal cavity using separate in and out lines, thus avoiding respiratory compromise), intermittent hemodialysis, and continuous venovenous hemofiltration or hemodiafiltration (CVVH or CVVHDF). The last two have now generally replaced earlier modes of continuous arteriovenous hemofiltration or hemodialysis.

Peritoneal dialysis

Peritoneal dialysis uses the peritoneum as a semipermeable membrane for water removal down an osmotic gradient, and solute removal by diffusion down a concentration gradient. It is a continuous procedure which corrects abnormalities slowly. Rapid cycling with no dwell time, however, can be an extremely effective semifast procedure correcting chemical imbalances, especially in young chil-

TABLE 2.10.9 **Aims of renal substitution therapy**

Aim	Mode	Intermittent or continuous	Slow or fast	Rate determinants
Fluid removal (water and solute)	Ultrafiltration (hemodialysis)	Intermittent	Fast	Hydrostatic pressure gradient
	Filtration (hemofiltration)	Continuous	Fast	Filtration rate minus replacement rate
Water removal	Osmotic (peritoneal dialysis)	Continuous	Slow	Osmotic gradient, cycle volume, dwell time, cycle frequency
Solute removal	Diffusion (hemodialysis)	Intermittent	Fast	Size of pores, thickness of membrane, blood and dialysate flow rate, dialysate potassium concentration
	Diffusion (peritoneal dialysis)	Continuous	Slow	Cycle volume, dwell time, cycle frequency, dialysate potassium concentration
	Filtration (hemofiltration)	Continuous	Slow[a]	Filtration rate, replacement fluid potassium concentration

[a]*Continuous dialysis can be added to hemofiltration (hemodiafiltration) to increase solute clearance.*

dren. It is simple, rapidly instituted and effective for long-term treatment. In children, peritoneal dialysis is particularly effective because of the relatively large peritoneal surface area. Gut or peritoneal disease, pulmonary edema and heart failure are relative contraindications for the use of peritoneal route.

Technique

The first step is insertion of a peritoneal dialysis catheter. The preferred method is to insert a silicone, single-cuff catheter percutaneously using a sheath/dilator over a wire (Seldinger technique) after initially filling the peritoneal cavity with a suitable fluid (e.g. saline) to displace bowel, which also works as a sump to ensure a 'siphon' effect. The procedure is performed under local anesthesia and sedation, although in the very young general anesthesia may be needed. Aim to place the tip of the catheter in the pelvis to ensure efficient drainage. Start dialysis with a 1.5% dextrose-based dialysis fluid and small volumes initially (10 ml/kg). Add 200 units/L heparin to the dialysate, as during the initial period fibrin deposition can block catheters.

Frequent (hourly) cycles and increased cycle volume up to 35 ml/kg improves solute removal, and increasing dextrose concentration in the dialysate improves water removal. Add potassium 3.5 mmol/L if there is no evidence of total body potas-

sium retention. The dialysate should be warmed with a blood warmer.

Prophylactic antibiotics are not needed.

Continuous hemofiltration

Hemodialysis or hemofiltration is more suitable for subjects with metabolic disorders (e.g. branched-chain aminoacidemia, hyperammonemia), tumor lysis syndrome (especially hyperphosphatemia, hyperuricemia), and poisoning. Continuous venovenous hemofiltration is a demanding and technically complex intervention which, if performed properly, provides a very smooth treatment of ARF and certain severe metabolic derangements such as inborn errors of metabolism. It can only be performed in a dedicated PICU with established hemofiltration facilities and developed protocols for setting up, running and troubleshooting the system. It is never a first line of treatment but can be established within 1–2 hours if needed, although not before admission of the patient to the PICU. There is no single correct way to do it, there being many options for machines, filters, priming of circuits, anticoagulation, pre- or post-filter replacement fluid, etc. In general a blood flow of 3–6 ml/kg·min and a filtrate of 30–70 ml/kg·h provide adequate clearances. Filtration rate is only about half of a normal GFR, so hemofiltration cannot be relied on to achieve rapid removal of retained solute, e.g. in the emergency management of severe hyperkalemia. Water overload (excess extracellular fluid), however, can be treated rapidly by slow continuous ultrafiltration. If water overload is the only problem then this can be achieved with a lower blood flow and a much lower filtration rate, avoiding some of the problems of high blood flow, such as hypothermia and catheter-related problems.

Technique

A double-lumen central venous catheter is inserted into the internal jugular, subclavian or femoral vein (size 6–7 FG for children weighing < 10 kg, 8–10 FG for 10–20 kg, 11–12 FG for > 20 kg). Heparinize the lumens until connection to the hemofiltration circuit.

Set up the circuit and hemofilter. Flush with at least 2 litres of 0.9% saline with 5000 units/L of heparin.

Choose the blood flow, filtration rate and replacement fluid rate. In general a blood flow of 3–6 ml/kg·min and a filtrate of 30–70 ml/kg·h provide adequate clearances. Replacement fluid rate depends on the overall negative hourly balance desired. A very low filtration rate without replacement fluid can be chosen if fluid overload is the only problem.

Heparinize the patient with 10–20 units/kg·h continuous infusion. Maintain activated clotting time at 150–200 s. Prostacyclin 5 nanograms/kg·min can be used in place of heparin if there is frequent filter clotting, or heparin-induced thrombocytopenia.

Connect circuit to patient and begin blood flow and filtration. Initially connect the venous take-off line to the distal lumen and the venous return line to the proximal lumen. Interchange them only if there are problems with obtaining adequate venous take-off at the set blood pump rate.

Beware of heat loss. Replacement fluid should be warmed with a blood warmer. Replacement fluid can be pumped into the line before the filter or into the bubble trap after the filter, according to the preference of the unit. Prefilter dilution of the blood by the replacement fluid reduces solute clearance but may prolong filter life and permit slightly reduced blood flow in pump-controlled CVVH.

Standard commercial replacement fluid is suitable for most purposes. This usually contains lactate as buffer, and a bicarbonate-based solution may be preferable in the presence of hyperlactatemia.

Filtrate flow should be controlled by using a peristaltic intravenous pump or other pump. In this case the pump is used in an unusual way such that it 'sucks' filtrate out of the filter rather than pumping into a line with supraatmospheric pressure. The subatmospheric pressure upstream (in the filtrate compartment) may cause the pump to deliver less than the set amount. The filtrate should therefore be measured hourly by weighing, and the pump settings for filtrate and replacement fluid adjusted frequently to achieve the desired fluid balance in the patient.

Reassess fluid status and monitor chemistry frequently until stable.

Intermittent hemodialysis

Intermittent hemodialysis can only be undertaken if there is a hemodialysis service and the patient is in an ICU or other area that is plumbed for hemodialysis. It can be performed daily or more frequently initially, especially in situations such as tumor lysis, or three or four times a week in a stabilized patient. Hemodialysis can remove solute more rapidly than hemofiltration.

Technique

Vascular access sites are the same as for CVVH. In neonates, umbilical artery and venous catheters have been used. Insert either a double-lumen venous catheter or two single-lumen catheters. Higher blood flow is needed than for CVVH (10 ml/kg·min) so a larger catheter is desirable. This may need surgical placement under general anesthesia.

FURTHER READING

See Chapter 3.5.

2.11   Liver failure

Julie McEniery

Severe liver failure, acute or chronic, is rare in childhood. Acute fulminant liver failure is a potentially reversible condition in which the onset of encephalopathy occurs within 8 weeks of the first symptoms. Its mortality rate exceeds 60% and that of stage 4 encephalopathy is 80%. If the child survives, the liver can rapidly regenerate. In the neonatal period, the cause of severe liver failure (usually metabolic disease) is often elusive, transplantation is generally unavailable, and the prognosis is very poor. Accurate diagnosis is essential for genetic counseling.

PHYSIOLOGY

The functions of the liver are summarized in Table 2.11.1.

CAUSES

Disorders causing severe liver failure are listed in Table 2.11.2. In up to 30% of cases no cause can be identified.

VIRAL INFECTION

Hepatitis A accounts for 20% of viral causes of fulminant hepatitis but rarely progresses to liver failure (< 0.5% of cases). Hepatitis B accounts for more than half of viral causes of fulminant disease and progresses to liver failure in 1% of cases. Serology or viral culture may distinguish viral acute liver failure from other causes, but histological findings are rarely specific.

DRUGS

Acetaminophen (paracetamol) metabolites cause dose-dependent liver injury, especially in overdose. Even high therapeutic doses of acetaminophen (15 mg/kg × 6 doses per day) may precipitate liver injury when other risks factors (fasting, viral illness or ischemia) are present.

Sodium valproate may unmask an underlying mitochondrial cytopathy (e.g. Alpers' disease) and precipitate liver failure.

TABLE 2.11.1 Liver function and its derangement in liver failure

Function	Derangement
Intermediate carbohydrate metabolism; glycogen stores	Hypoglycemia
Amino acid and ammonia metabolism	Hyperammonemia
	Decreased urea synthesis
	Encephalopathy
Protein synthesis	Decreased albumin synthesis
	(long half-life: late effect)
	Clotting factors
	(short half-life: early effect)
	Complement reduced
Detoxification	Drug and hormone accumulation
Biliary excretion	Jaundice
Hormone metabolism: insulin, glucagon	Hyperinsulinemia
	Hyperglucagonemia: muscle protein catabolism
	Anaerobic metabolism and lactic acid generation
Regulation of inflammatory mediators:	Profound microcirculatory effects:
– control of the microcirculation	– pulmonary shunt; hepatorenal syndrome
– maintenance of the cell membrane (Na^+-K^+)-ATPase	– encephalopathy
Reticuloendothelial function	Gut-derived bacteremia and endotoxemia

---

TABLE 2.11.2 Causes of severe acute liver failure (in order of frequency)

Viral hepatitis (50–60%)
  Hepatitis B
  Hepatitis A, C, Epstein–Barr virus
  Especially in young infants: herpes virus, echovirus, adenovirus
Unknown (30%)
Drugs and toxins (10%)
  Acetaminophen (paracetamol) overdose
  Idiosyncratic reactions to sodium valproate, isoniazid, methyldopa, tetracycline, halothane, actinomycin D,
    azathioprine, rifampicin, flucloxacillin, methotrexate
  Bone marrow transplant: ablative preconditioning (venoocclusive disease)
  Anticonvulsant medications (particularly phenytoin, carbamazepine): especially in protracted status epilepticus in
    a child with chronic epilepsy
  Carbon tetrachloride, phosphorus, arsenic, trichloroethylene (glue sniffers), vitamin A (in overdose), some herbal
    teas, death cap mushroom (*Amanita phalloides*)
Metabolic disease
  Neonatal: tyrosinemia, neonatal hemochromatosis, neonatal Neimann–Pick disease
  Later: Wilson's disease (often first presentation), galactosemia, hereditary fructose intolerance
  Mitochondrial cytopathies, e.g. Reye's syndrome, Alpers' syndrome
  Global hypoxic–ischemic insult, severe shock

METABOLIC DISEASE

In Wilson's disease, asymptomatic liver disease may precede the onset of acute liver failure. Reye's syndrome (acute fatty liver with encephalopathy) and mitochondrial hepatopathies (e.g. Alpers' disease) are characterized by hepatic failure with disproportionately low serum aminotransferase and bilirubin levels.

DIAGNOSIS

Liver failure is heralded by anorexia, vomiting, easy bruisability and altered behavior. Hyperventilation, jaundice, and the onset of encephalopathy (Table 2.11.3) then ensue. Seizures may be induced by hypoglycemia, hyponatremia or cerebral edema. The liver is typically enlarged and may be tender. Ascites may develop early. The mean and diastolic blood pressures are typically low with bounding pulses reflecting a low peripheral vascular resistance and increased cardiac output.

Serum aminotransferases are usually increased 10-fold to 100-fold. Hypoglycemia (< 3 mmol/L) is usual and the prothrombin time is prolonged (often > 100 s). A conjugated hyperbilirubinemia is common but not invariable. Hyperammonemia and lactic acidosis occur frequently. Many children have a marked hyponatremia ($Na^+ < 130$ mmol/L) and hypokalemia ($K^+ < 3.0$ mmol/L). A modest neutrophil leukocytosis with left shift reflects hepatic necrosis. Thrombocytopenia due to intravascular consumption or marrow depression is often found.

ENCEPHALOPATHY

Encephalopathy is the most common cause of death in acute liver failure. Its causes include:

- accumulation of neuroinhibitory compounds
- altered function of the sodium pump in the nerve cell membrane
- altered blood-brain barrier permeability
- altered brain microcirculation causing ischemia

GASTROINTESTINAL BLEEDING

Gastrointestinal bleeding due to stress ulceration and coagulopathy worsens the encephalopathy and may cause death. Variceal bleeding is not seen in acute liver failure but may precipitate acute decompensation in a child with chronic liver failure.

COAGULATION

The following disturbances of coagulation occur:

- hepatic synthesis of clotting factors I, II, VII, IX and X fails

TABLE 2.11.3 **Stages in hepatic encephalopathy**	
Stage	**Clinical features**
1	Normal conscious level, periods of lethargy, reversal of day-night sleep pattern
	Asterixis EEG normal
2	Increased drowsiness, disorientation, agitation
	Asterixis and fetor hepaticus present
	EEG slowing
3	Sleeping most of the time although rousable to noxious stimuli
	Markedly confused, incoherent speech
	Equates to a Glasgow coma score of 5 or more
	Hyperreflexic
	EEG slowing further: triphasic waves appear
4	Unconscious and unresponsive to noxious stimuli, may have an extensor or flaccid posture
	Equates to a GCS below 5

- production of factor VIII by vascular endothelial cells is increased
- profoundly low levels of coagulation inhibitors such antithrombin III and protein C occur

SEPSIS

Sepsis causes 10% of deaths in acute liver failure. In health, the gut mucosal barrier prevents escape of most microorganisms from the gut lumen into the portal circulation, and those that do enter portal blood are removed by liver reticuloendothelial cells. In liver failure, the loss of gut barrier function due to fasting and splanchnic hypoperfusion, and ineffective clearance by Kupffer cells allows microorganisms and endotoxin to reach the lung, causing acute lung injury and multiorgan failure.

ELECTROLYTE DISTURBANCES

Electrolyte disturbances occur commonly. Failure to degrade aldosterone causes sodium and water retention and profound hypokalemia. Accumulation of antidiuretic hormone and a low level of serum albumin impair free water excretion, causing dilutional hyponatremia.

OLIGURIC RENAL FAILURE

Intravascular volume depletion from vasodilatation, gastrointestinal bleeding, capillary leak and ascites reduces the renal blood flow.

The hepatorenal syndrome occurs in severe liver failure and usually progresses rapidly to refractory oliguria.

Intense renal cortical vasoconstriction reduces the glomerular filtration rate.

Microcirculatory derangements involving vasodilatation and vasoconstriction in various organs are common in liver failure. Inappropriate vasodilatation in many vascular beds causes relative hypovolemia.

LUNGS

Hypoxia is common in acute liver failure, due to intrapulmonary shunt, lung fluid overload and the development of acute respiratory distress syndrome.

The hepatopulmonary syndrome can develop acutely and consists of marked pulmonary capillary vasodilatation and hemoglobin desaturation which responds to increasing the inspired oxygen concentration (FIO_2).

Inappropriate vasoconstriction causes cellular hypoxia in other organs.

MANAGEMENT

The aim of supportive therapy is to maintain a near-normal metabolic milieu to promote liver recovery. Early discussion with a pediatric liver transplantation service (certainly as soon as intensive care support is needed for liver failure) should lead to transfer to a tertiary referral center before the child's condition deteriorates further.

Investigations for diagnosis, monitoring severity and detecting complications are presented in Tables 2.11.4 and 2.11.5. Occasionally, known poisoning or metabolic disease can be managed by antidote or specific therapy, e.g. chelation therapy for Wilson's disease, and acetylcysteine for acetaminophen (paracetamol) poisoning. The decision to perform a liver biopsy must balance the risk of severe hemorrhage with possible diagnostic gains which may affect management. Better hemostasis may be achieved by mini-incision open biopsy than by needle biopsy. Management is summarized in Table 2.11.6.

IMMEDIATE CARE

Diagnosis and resuscitation proceed simultaneously, when the cause of acute liver failure is unknown. In a child who presents with severe liver failure, the Airway (Ch. 6.3), Breathing (Ch. 6.4) and Circulation (Ch. 2.3) should immediately be assessed and secured. A 10% glucose solution is infused intravenously. The cause and severity of liver failure should be established clinically and by laboratory tests. In particular, the heart rate, blood pressure, respiratory rate, core temperature, hemoglobin saturation (by pulse oximetry), pupil size and response and the conscious state are monitored half-hourly until the child is stable. Blood glucose levels should be monitored 4-hourly and blood gases and serum electrolytes 8-hourly (or more often if unstable). Accurate fluid balance requires the insertion of an indwelling urinary catheter. A nasogastric tube should be inserted for drug administration. Enteral intake of food and fluid should stop until the child has been stabilized.

TABLE 2.11.4 Investigation of underlying diagnosis in acute liver failure

Plasma and urine for toxic screens, drug levels
Serology for hepatitis and other viruses
Throat swab, urine, feces for viral culture
Serum ceruloplasmin level (may be low in fulminant presentation of Wilson's disease)
Metabolic studies (urine amino acid, organic acid profiles); skin fibroblast culture for later studies; mitochondrial DNA studies
Liver biopsy (frequently cannot be done safely when coagulopathy severe)

TABLE 2.11.5 Investigations for monitoring of severity and complications

Serum electrolytes, blood glucose, ionized calcium, magnesium, urea, creatinine
Serum indicators of liver function (albumin, AST, ALT, γ-glutamyl transferase, serum amyloid P-component, bilirubin conjugated and total, LDH)
Serum ammonia, lactate, amylase, creatine kinase
Arterial blood gases
Hemoglobin, white cell count, platelet count
Prothrombin time, partial thromboplastin time, fibrinogen, fibrin degradation products
Chest X-ray

INTRAVENOUS FLUID THERAPY

Glucose solution (10%) should be infused continuously to maintain a normal blood glucose concentration. The total intake of fluid is restricted to 50–70% of maintenance requirements (Ch. 2.10), as sodium and water excretion is impaired.

SYMPTOMATIC COAGULOPATHY

Symptomatic coagulopathy (Ch. 2.8) requires administration of frozen plasma, platelets and red cell concentrate. Cryoprecipitate may be needed to correct hypofibrinogenemia. Vitamin K should be given by slow intravenous infusion. Control of bleeding rather than a normal prothrombin time should be the goal. Frozen plasma will also restore thrombolytic factors such as antithrombin III. Hypoalbuminemia should be corrected using 20% albumin infusion. Repeated bolus administration of colloid including these blood products may be needed to improve poor tissue perfusion. The need for supplemental potassium may be high but close monitoring of serum potassium levels is essential as oliguria may supervene.

A multilumen central venous catheter is required:

- if hypertonic concentrations of glucose (more than 10%) or inotropes are necessary
- to secure venous access in sick, edematous infants and young children
- to monitor central venous pressure

Insertion in the femoral vein is safer when the coagulopathy is severe (Ch 6.1).

> **TABLE 2.11.6 Management**
>
> **General supportive therapy**
> - Cardiorespiratory monitoring: pulse oximetry, ECG monitoring, regular blood pressure measurement
> - Monitor conscious state
> - Blood glucose levels 4-hourly
> - Strict fluid balance; indwelling urinary catheter
> - Nasogastric tube; stop feeds until stable
> - Maintain serum glucose levels (5–10 mmol/L) using 10% glucose
> - Restrict sodium and water intake
> - Frozen plasma, platelet concentrates, and cryoprecipitate for symptomatic coagulopathy
> - 20% albumin infusion
> - Supplemental K^+
> - Supplemental oxygen
>
> **Intensive care supportive therapy**
> - Multilumen central venous catheter (consider femoral vein)
> - Indwelling arterial catheter
> - Elective endotracheal intubation and mechanical ventilation to normal blood gases
> - Maintain adequate intravascular volume
> - Inotropic and/or vasopressor support as needed
> - Enteral lactulose and neomycin
> - CT head scanning
> - Osmotherapy with mannitol for cerebral edema
> - Anticipation of and treatment for seizures and hyperthermia

RESPIRATORY AND CARDIOVASCULAR SUPPORT

When hypoxemia and pulmonary edema appear, elective endotracheal intubation and mechanical ventilation should be undertaken early, rather than delayed until an emergency develops. For endotracheal intubation, adequate intravenous anesthesia is essential to prevent any reflex rise in intracranial pressure. Ventilation with PEEP is necessary to overcome atelectasis (Ch. 2.1), hypoxia being a more serious risk to liver recovery than theoretical concerns about impairment of venous return by positive intrathoracic pressure. Hypovolemia must be corrected urgently, preferably using colloid or blood. Inotropic and vasopressor support (Ch. 2.3) may be needed to maintain an adequate blood pressure and to preserve organ perfusion. The use of vasoconstrictors such as vasopressin, norepinephrine (noradrenaline) or high dose (> 7.5 μg/kg·min) dopamine reduces liver blood flow and exacerbates liver injury.

SUPPORTIVE THERAPY FOR ENCEPHALOPATHY

Reduction in serum ammonia may help in controlling encephalopathy. Lactulose, administered enterally, is metabolized by bacteria and lowers colonic pH. This reduces absorption of ammonia from the gut by favouring its conversion to ammonium ion, and leaches ammonia from blood to the bowel lumen. Neomycin given by nasogastric tube reduces the concentration of colonic bacteria and may have a beneficial additive effect to lactulose. Aggressive management of gastrointestinal hemorrhage prevents further accumulation of metabolites from the breakdown of blood in the gut. Elective mechanical ventilation is indicated for stage 3 encephalopathy (see Table 2.11.3). There is no evidence that hyperventilation improves outcome and it may aggravate cerebral ischemia.

MANAGEMENT OF RAISED INTRACRANIAL PRESSURE

Cerebral swelling is difficult to diagnose clinically (Ch. 2.4). The most useful indicator is bedside assessment of the level of consciousness, posture, respiratory pattern and brain-stem reflexes (oculovestibular, e.g. doll's eye, and pupillary response). Sedation is necessary for the ventilated child but the dose should be minimized to avoid obscuring clinical signs. Papilledema is rarely seen, as brain swelling develops too rapidly. A cerebral CT scan is a sensitive test of brain edema but the risks of moving a child receiving intensive supportive care may not be justified.

Management of a child with raised intracranial pressure (Ch. 2.6) depends on:

- maintenance of an adequate cerebral perfusion pressure (by ensuring an adequate preload and blood pressure)
- maintenance fluids given as 0.9% saline containing 5–10% dextrose (i.e. a hypertonic solution)
- maintaining the serum sodium level at a minimum of 145 mmol/L
- osmotherapy with mannitol 0.3 g/kg i.v. every 6–8 hours
- elevation of the head 15° to improve cerebral venous drainage
- maintenance normal blood gases— Pao_2 > 13 kPa (100 mmHg) and $Paco_2$ 4.7–5.3 kPa (35–40 mmHg).
- prevention of hyperthermia by using a cooling blanket if necessary

SEIZURES

Seizures must be detected and treated (Ch. 2.5). Detection requires close observation and an unparalyzed child. Benzodiazepines are used for short-term treatment of seizures, and phenytoin or phenobarbital (phenobarbitone) with close drug monitoring (Ch. 5.1) for longer-term treatment.

RENAL SUPPORT

Diuretic therapy with furosemide (frusemide) and mannitol may temporarily prevent progression to oliguric renal failure. Furosemide in frequent small doses or by continuous infusion is preferable to infrequent large doses which may cause hypovolemia. Severe fluid overload resulting from refractory oliguria requires peritoneal dialysis or continuous venovenous hemofiltration, both of which may be complicated by bleeding, cardiorespiratory instability and sepsis.

MANAGEMENT OF GASTROINTESTINAL BLEEDING

Prophylaxis or treatment of stress ulceration is recommended, using a cytoprotective agent (e.g.

sucralfate) and by suppression of gastric acid secretion (by a histamine-2 receptor antagonist or proton pump inhibitor).

TRANSPORT CARE

The airway, breathing and circulation should be stabilized before departure. The child's heart rate, blood pressure, respiratory rate and oxygen saturation and blood glucose levels are monitored before departure and half-hourly during the retrieval (glucometer or point of care assay device). Glucose solution (50%) should be available for administration by i.v. bolus (1 ml/kg) or infusion (start at 0.5 ml/kg·h and adjust according to frequently measured blood glucose concentration). Oxygen is given by mask and a nasogastric tube inserted and left on free drainage. When significant encephalopathy is present (see above), the child should be intubated and mechanically ventilated to $Paco_2$ 4.5–5.0 kPa (35–40 mmHg). Mannitol 0.3 g/kg is given i.v. if the child's conscious state deteriorates before or during transfer.

NOSOCOMIAL INFECTION

Nosocomial pneumonia, bacteremia and urinary tract infection occur frequently. Gram-positive infections, especially of vascular catheters and usually with staphylococci, are common. Gut-derived Gram-negative infections also occur. Fungal infections—particularly with *Candida* spp.—are difficult to detect, but are often found postmortem. Prophylactic antibiotics have not been shown to improve outcome, but a low index of suspicion of infection is needed. The total and differential white cell count are monitored carefully; cultures of blood, urine and tracheal aspirate should be taken at the slightest suspicion of infection and broad-spectrum antibiotic cover provided if indicated.

NUTRITION

Provision of adequate nutrition (Ch. 5.3) is difficult when fulminant liver failure is complicated by severe encephalopathy and renal failure. Enteral or parenteral nutrition is commenced as soon as cardiorespiratory resuscitation is complete, aiming for a high-carbohydrate, low-protein intake.

CONTROVERSIES IN CARE

The benzodiazepine antagonist flumazenil may temporarily improve the conscious level in hepatic encephalopathy.

Acetylcysteine may improve acute liver failure from any cause by detoxifying metabolites and improving microcirculation by formation of nitrosoacetylcysteine.

Prostaglandin E_1 may improve the renal cortical, cerebral, hepatic and gastric mucosal microcirculation.

Prostacyclin may improve microcirculation by its vasodilatory and antiplatelet aggregation effects but should not be used in the presence of cerebral edema as it reduces the cerebral perfusion pressure.

Emergency orthotopic liver transplantation has an increasing role in acute liver failure.

Human hepatocyte growth factor may accelerate regeneration.

The following are of debatable benefit:

- measurement of intracranial pressure and jugular venous bulb oximetry
- prophylactic antibiotics
- branched-chain amino acid infusion
- plasma exchange
- charcoal hemoperfusion

✔ KEY POINTS

➤ Secure the airway, breathing and circulation
➤ Infuse 10% glucose solution and monitor the blood glucose level closely

➤ Anticipate and investigate the potentially fatal complications of brain swelling, gastrointestinal hemorrhage, nosocomial infection, renal failure, metabolic derangements, respiratory and cardiovascular instability
➤ Oxygen by mask and gastric drainage by nasogastric tube is necessary before and during transport

✗ COMMON ERRORS

➤ Inadequate monitoring and control of blood glucose concentration
➤ Inadequate treatment of cerebral edema and raised intracranial pressure
➤ Inadequate monitoring of electrolyte abnormalities, especially hyponatremia
➤ Use of prophylactic antibiotics
➤ Inadequate surveillance for sepsis

FURTHER READING

1. Lee WM. Acute liver failure. New Engl J Med 1993; 329: 1862–1872
2. Fingerote RJ, Bain VG. Fulminant hepatic failure. Am J Gastroenterol 1993; 88: 1000–1010
3. Peters M, Meyer zum Buschenfelde KH, Gerken G. Acute hepatic failure: limitations of medical treatment and indications for liver transplantation. J Clin Invest 1993; 71: 875–881
4. Mowatt AP. Hepatic encephalopathy: acute and chronic. In Eyre JA (ed). Coma. Clinical Paediatrics. International practice and research; 1994; 2(1): 81–108
– (*Four papers providing a general review of pathophysiology and management of acute liver failure*)

2.12   Multiple organ failure

Michael D. Seear

Multiple organ failure (MOF) can be defined as functional failure of two or more organ systems following a major illness or injury. The criteria for failure of individual organ systems have been defined by Wilkinson. It would be unfair to call multiple organ failure an iatrogenic disease. Following major insult, a patient needs to live for about 3 days before the complication known as acute (formerly adult) respiratory distress syndrome starts to develop. The first descriptions of hemorrhagic lung failure complicating battlefield injuries were published about 1920. Subsequently terms such as 'shock lung', 'transfusion lung' and 'Da Nang lung' were in common use until the term 'acute respiratory distress syndrome' (ARDS) was applied to the condition of noncardiogenic pulmonary edema. The term was prompted by histologic similarities to infant respiratory distress syndrome (Ch. 3.1).

As techniques of respiratory support improved, some patients with ARDS were able to survive, but a high percentage went on to develop progressive failure in other organs. By the mid-1970s, the term 'multiple organ failure' was introduced to describe the sequential failure of major organ systems following an initial inciting event. The first prospective study of this condition in children was only performed in the late 1980s and there is still little information that is specific to the pediatric population. Sepsis was the initial factor blamed for the steady deterioration found in MOF and there are still those who champion the central role of sepsis (particularly unnoticed abdominal sepsis) as the 'motor' that drives continuing inflammation. However, the most popular current explanation for MOF is the unregulated inflammatory cascade set in progress by an initial shock-inducing event. Increasing knowledge about the inflammatory response has led to a better understanding of the causes of MOF, but little useful therapy.

PATHOPHYSIOLOGY

Conditions that commonly precede or initiate MOF are listed in Table 2.12.1.

TABLE 2.12.1 Conditions that precede or initiate MOF

- Shock
- Sepsis
- Trauma (multiple, neurological)
- Burns
- Surgery (extensive, prolonged abdominal, complicated by infection)
- Gastrointestinal bleeding
- Multiple transfusions
- Diabetic ketoacidosis
- Renal failure
- Pancreatic or liver failure
- Malignancy
- Steroid therapy

It has become increasingly clear that an interaction between activated leukocytes and injured endothelial cells is the final common pathway of injury in a wide range of diseases. Leukocyte-endothelial adhesion with subsequent release of toxic products is an endlessly complex system of interrelated inflammatory cascades that is the basis of a range of diseases including MOF and transplant rejection. Ehrlich coined the term 'horror autotoxicus' to describe the fear of autodestruction that could occur from the then newly discovered system of antibodies. The term is sometimes applied to MOF but is more reasonably reserved for diseases caused by the development of specific autoantibodies. In MOF, the tissues are damaged by the dysregulated activation of the immune system. Specific autoantibodies are not produced; tissues are simply damaged as 'innocent bystanders' during the inflammatory process.

Following a state of shock, leukocytes and endothelial cells are activated by circulating inflammatory mediators which include tumor necrosis factor and interleukin-1. Interaction between L selectin expressed on neutrophils and both E selectin and P selectin expressed by endothelial cells forms the first weak adhesion. Subsequent firm binding and transendothelial migration is stimulated by interactions between the CD18-CD11 integrin on neutrophils and the endothelial ICAM-1 receptor. Neutrophils produce a range of toxic substances including oxygen radicals and proteases that do not seem to be able to distinguish between host and foreign antigens.

Cascade reactions such as coagulation and inflammation are controlled by a complex system of feedback loops. Knowledge of the control mechanisms for inflammation is limited because many of the mediators of inflammation have only been discovered in recent years. Acute-phase proteins such as α_2-macroglobulin and heat shock proteins are produced by any major stress and probably have an important role in the control of inflammation and subsequent repair. Research in this area may offer one avenue of future treatment. For instance, it has been shown that animals stressed by exposure to heat subsequently survive a septic insult better than controls.

CLINICAL PICTURE

Despite extensive research into multiple organ failure in adults, differences in definition and local management have led to wide differences in quoted frequencies and outcome. A typical adult case will develop respiratory failure within 3 days of the initial insult, subsequently followed by progressive failure in other organs. There is no reliable order for the subsequent failure of kidney, liver and heart, and individual patients vary widely. The mortality rate in adults is correlated with the number of organs failed and, in particular, the presence of sepsis. Quoted mortality rates range from 30% to over 60%. The predicted incidence of MOF depends on definition, but a study of over 5000 adult ICU patients quoted an incidence of 15%.

An attempt at consistency in pediatric studies has been made by the development of age-adjusted organ system failure criteria by Wilkinson et al. Using these definitions, a study of 777 critically ill children showed that MOF in this age group mostly, but not always, follows the adult experience. The incidence of at least two organ system failures was 10.9% with an overall mortality of 50.9%. Compared with adults, children developed MOF more rapidly after admission to an ICU and the condition was also more rapidly fatal. Indicators of poor outcome were:

- age < 12 months
- poor pediatric risk of mortality (PRISM) score on day of admission
- number of organ systems failing

The presence of sepsis was not an independent risk factor for death.

TREATMENT

Shock, the development of ARDS, and the subsequent autolysis of other organs is a continuum that begins with an initial severe insult. The increasing understanding of the inflammatory cascade will probably lead to the development of therapies aimed at several aspects of this complex system. However, there is at present no specific therapy for MOF except early intervention with conventional supportive therapy to restore oxygenation, perfusion and metabolism.

Considerable debate has surrounded the issue of resuscitation. One school of thought maintains that in order to reverse the peripheral endothelial damage it is necessary to drive the patient with inotropes to supranormal hemodynamic levels. This approach has come under much criticism, both theoretical and methodological, and there is still no evidence to suggest that any benefit is obtained from it. This leaves the question, 'What is normal resuscitation?' Unfortunately, there is no absolute guide. Urine output, blood pressure, pulse, subjective assessments of peripheral perfusion and even invasive hemodynamic measurements can all only be a guide to the patient's condition. Widely accepted normal values have been developed but the final decision on whether a patient is fully resuscitated from an inciting event is still a subjective clinical judgment. Apart from treatment of the initiating cause and vigorous resuscitation, subsequent therapy relies entirely on careful conservative management.

Increasing understanding of the underlying mechanism of inflammation has led to numerous exotic therapies that aim to inhibit the inflammatory cascade at various levels. These have ranged from passive immunization against Gram-negative bacteria to the use of monoclonal antibodies against different receptors involved in leukocyte adhesion. Manipulation of repair and immunological control has also been tried with prosta-glandin blockade, thymopentin and manipulation of heat shock proteins. A number of these approaches have been tried in human studies. An earlier trial of monoclonal antibodies directed against the lipid A region of Gram-negative endotoxins was initially thought to show useful results, but subsequent study failed to bear this out. More recent trials of IL-1 receptor antagonists or monoclonal antibodies to a TNF-α also failed to show any benefit.

Although the theory of inflammatory cascade sounds attractive, it is quite possible that manipulation of poorly understood biological systems might even make the patient worse. The rare syndrome of leukocyte adherence failure leads to serious bacterial and fungal infections, suggesting that inhibition of leukocyte adhesion is not necessarily beneficial. We are playing with a machine whose workings are only dimly understood.

✔ **KEY POINTS**

➤ MOF is a syndrome of progressive organ failure that results from a wide range of systemic insults

➤ The most common inciting agents are major trauma and septicemia. Mortality rates vary but are on average about 50%

➤ Immune modulatory therapies have, so far, been of no value. Therapy consists of meticulous conventional systemic support and aggressive therapy for the causative insult

FURTHER READING

1. Pinsky M. Organ-specific therapy in critical illness: interfacing molecular mechanisms with physiological interventions. J Crit Care 1996; 11: 95–107

2. Vincent J. Prevention and therapy of multiple organ failure. World J Surg 1996; 20: 465–470

– (*These two references provide pathophysiological justification for the available therapies in multiple organ failure*)

3. Wilkinson JD, Pollack MM, Glass NI, Kanter KK, Katz RW, Steinhart CM. Mortality associated with multiple organ system failure and sepsis in pediatric intensive care units. J Pediatr 1987; 111: 324–328

– (*This paper gives criteria for failure of specific organ systems*)

Organ system disease

3

3.1 Respiratory system

David Wensley, Michael South, Anthony Slater and Michael Yung

Severe disorders of the respiratory system, alone or combined with abnormalities of other organ systems, account for a large proportion of critical illness in childhood. Interventions to support an inadequate airway (Ch. 6.3), or inadequate breathing or gas exchange (Chs 6.4, 6.7), are a large part of the care of the critically ill.

DEVELOPMENTAL PHYSIOLOGY

LUNG GROWTH AND DEVELOPMENT

There are four stages of prenatal lung growth and development, outlined in Table 3.1.1. Surfactant storage is present in type II alveolar cells at 24 weeks gestation, and in terminal air sacs at 30 weeks. The presence of adequate surfactant is one of the major factors determining independent survival in infants born prematurely.

Following birth, immediate changes occur within the lungs to adapt to extrauterine life. The thorax is compressed by passage of the infant through the birth canal and initiation of extrauterine breathing results in negative pleural pressures of 40–70 mmHg during the first few breaths. This helps clearance of lung fluid from the alveoli into the interstitium and lymphatics and establishes a volume of gas in the lung at the end of tidal expiration of approximately 30 ml/kg. This is the functional residual capacity (FRC) which acts as a buffer against changing alveolar gas composition. The structural alteration of the pulmonary vascular bed by lung inflation and the increase in alveolar oxygen tension and blood pH all reduce the pulmonary vascular resistance (Fig. 3.1.1). However, the pulmonary vasculature retains the ability to react to vasoconstrictor stimuli until remodeling of the arteriolar musculature has occurred, several weeks after birth. This ability is less in premature infants. Hence, infants with cardiac disease resulting in an unrestricted left-to-right shunt (i.e. ventricular septal defect) generally present in cardiac failure at 3–4 weeks of age when the pulmonary vascular tone has relaxed sufficiently to allow high pulmonary blood flow. Premature infants with a patent ductus arteriosus generally develop cardiac failure at 1–2 weeks of age. Lung expansion and the maintenance of lung volume depend on the presence of surfactant, as the elastic recoil of the chest wall is reduced in infants. The drop in pulmonary vascular resistance, removal of the placental circulation with the

TABLE 3.1.1 **Phases of development of the lung**

Phase (gestation)	Airways	Vasculature	Clinical comments
Embryonic (3–5 weeks)	The lung develops as an outgrowth of the foregut, beginning at about 3 weeks gestation, and divides into two mainstem bronchial buds	The pulmonary arteries develop from the 6th branchial arches and connect to a vascular plexus which develops from the surrounding mesenchyme	
Pseudoglandular (5–16 weeks)	The conducting airways develop as far as the terminal bronchioles. No further increase in the number of cartilaginous airways occurs after this time. The trachea separates from the esophagus and the diaphragm is formed	The pulmonary arteries develop and branch with the airways	Conditions that interfere with lung growth at this stage, such as a diaphragmatic hernia, cause pulmonary hypoplasia
Cannalicular (16–24 weeks)	Type II alveolar cells which produce surfactant appear at 24 weeks gestation	Intraacinar arteries develop and branch with the respiratory bronchioles. Alveolar capillaries proliferate and grow closer to the air spaces	Gas exchange and ventilation are possible at the end of this period although mechanical ventilation causes chronic lung disease
Saccular (6–9 months)	Respiratory bronchioles and terminal saccules appear	For a given size of muscular preacinar pulmonary artery, the wall thickness is double that of the adult	The vasoconstrictor response to hypoxia increases with advancing gestation
Postnatal growth	Airways increase in size. Alveoli increase in number until 3 years. After this, growth results from increase in alveolar size. Adult lung size is reached by late childhood	Vascular remodeling causes an initial reduction of the muscle wall in preacinar arteries during infancy	Gradual reduction in vasoconstrictor response as remodeling occurs

consequent closure of the foramen ovale and eventually the closure of the ductus arteriosus change the circulation from that of the fetus to that of the adult (Fig. 3.1.1).

CONTROL OF VENTILATION

The respiratory pump resembles a feedback loop (Fig. 3.1.2), consisting of effectors (respiratory muscles), controllers (brain stem), and sensors (chemoreceptors and lung receptors). The chest wall is more compliant in the young infant, resulting in wasted diaphragmatic effort, particularly if there is increased work of breathing or increased oxygen requirements. The diaphragm may also fatigue more quickly in infants because of imma-ture muscle development. In the adult, hypoxia causes increased ventilation. In newborn infants, hypoxia may cause an initial increase in ventilation, soon followed by depression of ventilation, periodic breathing and apnea. The central chemoreceptors (medulla) respond to changes in cerebrospinal fluid pH which is mainly affected by blood CO_2 levels. The newborn's CO_2 response curve (Fig. 3.1.3) is shifted to the left, resulting in a lower resting P_{CO_2} 4.4 kPa (33 mmHg). The more premature an infant, the flatter the CO_2 response curve.

Periodic breathing is commonly seen in premature infants and although this is thought to be a benign phenomenon, it may be associated with apnea (cessation of ventilation for > 20 s). Apnea

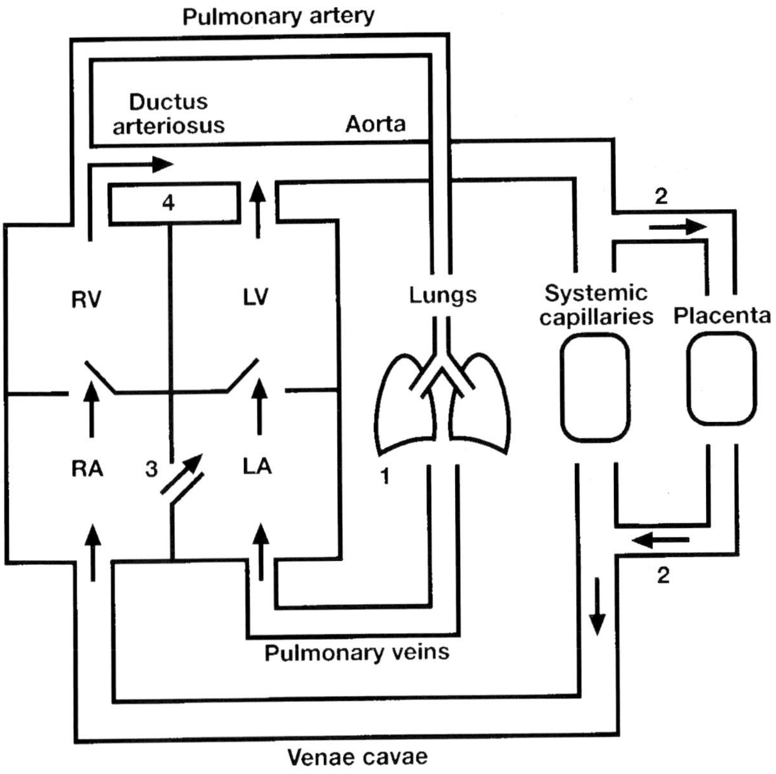

Figure 3.1.1 The circulation at birth, showing the pulmonary circulation (1); the placental circulation (2); the foramen ovale (3) and the ductus arteriosus (4). LA, left atrium; LV, left ventricle; RA, right atrium; RV, right ventricle

is caused by failure of one or more parts of the respiratory pump as outlined above, and is commonly seen in premature infants. Obstructive sleep apnea occurs in infants and older children usually because of pharyngeal obstruction by adenoidal tissue or structural anomalies of the airway, compounded by the loss of pharyngeal tone during sleep. Central control of breathing may also be abnormal in these children, placing them at increased risk of apnea following anesthesia and surgery for relief of the obstruction.

LUNG VOLUMES AND MECHANICS

Lung volumes in infants and adults are compared in Table 3.1.2; mechanics are listed in Table 3.1.3. The closing volume is the lung volume at which some small airways close during tidal expiration, causing intrapulmonary shunting (see 'oxygen delivery' below). The development of the supporting elastic tissue after birth causes the ratio of

closing volume to FRC to fall steadily with age, to a minimum at around 10 years. The high closing volume in the first 6 years of life may encroach upon FRC, causing regional hypoventilation and may increase ventilation–perfusion mismatch.

The respiratory pump produces air movement between the atmosphere and the alveoli in order to maintain O_2 and CO_2 gradients for gas exchange between alveoli and blood. Contraction of the inspiratory muscles generates a pressure gradient between the mouth and alveolus to achieve this gas movement. Part of the inspiratory work is required to overcome the resistance to air flow and tissue movement. The rest is used to overcome the elastic recoil of the lung and chest wall and is stored to provide energy for expiration in a similar way to stretching an elastic band. The compliance (volume change/pressure difference) is used to describe the elastic properties of the lung or respiratory system, while the resistance (pressure difference/flow) is used to describe the

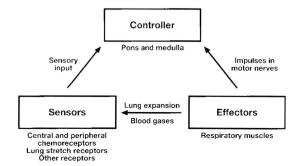

Figure 3.1.2 Respiratory control of blood gases by a negative feedback loop

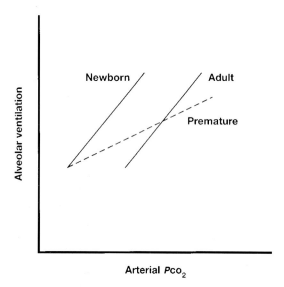

Figure 3.1.3 The ventilatory response to arterial P_{CO_2} in the adult, the term newborn and the premature newborn

TABLE 3.1.2 **Lung volumes of the infant and adult**		
Volume	**Infant**	**Adult**
VC (ml/kg)	35–40	50–60
FRC (ml/kg)	27–30	30–40
V_t (ml/kg)	6–8	5–7
V_a (ml/kg·min)	100–150	60

VC, vital capacity; FRC, functional residual capacity; V_t, tidal volume; V_a = alveolar ventilation.

elastic properties of the lung or respiratory system, while the resistance (pressure difference/flow) is used to describe the resistive properties. The shape of the pressure–volume curve (Fig. 3.1.4) is sigmoid if measurements are taken throughout vital capacity, but during tidal breathing (E to F), it is generally assumed that the relationship is linear, and thus a single value for compliance ([A–B] ÷ [C–D]) is often given.

During laminar flow, airways resistance is inversely proportional to the 4th power of the radius (Poiseuille's law). Since children have smaller airways than adults, resistance is greater and diseases such as bronchiolitis and croup, which reduce airway diameter, cause a proportionally greater increase in resistance in young children. Compliance (Table 3.1.3) varies with lung volume, and conditions that reduce the lung volume by causing atelectasis (such as respiratory distress syndrome) reduce compliance, making the lung stiffer and more difficult to ventilate.

OXYGEN DELIVERY

Oxygen delivery to the tissues consists of arterial oxygenation and oxygen transport by the blood.

Arterial oxygenation

Arterial oxygenation depends on adequate gas movement from the atmosphere to the alveoli and transfer into the blood. Hypoventilation reduces the alveolar oxygen tension, but this is easily corrected by increasing the inspired oxygen concentration. Reduced diffusion across the alveolar capillary membrane rarely causes arterial hypoxemia. The most common causes of arterial hypoxemia are ventilation–perfusion (V/Q) mismatch and right-to-left shunting. When desaturated pulmonary arterial blood passes through the lungs without coming into contact with ventilated alveoli, the blood remains desaturated. This is termed 'pulmonary shunting'. If there is a communication outside the lungs (i.e. congenital heart disease with right-to-left shunting) which allows passage of desaturated systemic venous blood into the systemic arterial circulation, then this is termed 'extra pulmonary shunting' (usually cardiac). When pulmonary arterial blood passes poorly ventilated

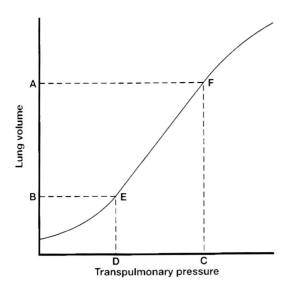

Figure 3.1.4 Static lung compliance curve: the change in lung volume as transpulmonary pressure changes. Points E and F represent the range of tidal breathing

alveoli the pulmonary venous blood will be less saturated than blood passing normally ventilated alveoli, and this results in V/Q mismatch. Regional variation of pulmonary blood flow occurs within the normal lung as a result of gravity and is affected by the position of the child. If a child has disease involving only one lung, the child's saturation will be higher and dyspnea less when the normal lung is uppermost. The reverse is true in adults.

Oxygen delivery by the blood

Oxygen delivery by the blood to the tissues depends on hemoglobin concentration, cardiac output and tissue perfusion.

TABLE 3.1.3 **Lung mechanics in infants and adults**

Variable	Neonate	Adult
C_L (ml/cmH$_2$O)	4–6	150–200
C_L (ml/cmH$_2$O·kg)	1–2	2–3
C_L/FRC	0.04–0.08	0.04–0.07
R_{aw} (cmH$_2$O/L·s)	26–40	3–5
f (/min)	40–60	10–15

C_L, lung compliance; FRC, functional residual capacity; R_{aw}, airway resistance; f, frequency (respiratory rate)

RESPIRATORY SYSTEM DEFENCES AGAINST INFECTION

The interface between the respiratory system and the environment is large and effective defences against invading microorganisms are crucial. These can be categorized as mechanical, phagocytic and immune (Table 3.1.4).

Mechanical

Mechanical defences (e.g. nasal vibrissae, an intact airway mucosa, normal mucus secretion and ciliary activity) prevent entry of particles into the lung or aid the clearance of those entering the lung. Diseases involving these defences cause significant lung disease (chronic pulmonary aspiration, cystic fibrosis, cilial dyskinesia).

Phagocytic

The phagocytic defences act in a nonspecific fashion to ingest, neutralize and remove particles that breach the mechanical defences.

Immune

The immune defences include specific recognition of antigens, their neutralization with antibodies and the amplification of the inflammatory process in response to the presence of the antigen. Cellular (T cell) and antibody-mediated (B cell or humoral) immunity is present in the lung as elsewhere in the body. However, secretory immunoglobulin A (IgA) is specific to the respiratory and gastrointestinal tracts and provides a unique function of immune exclusion by neutralizing and preventing adhesion of bacterial and viral pathogens to the respiratory mucosa, thus limiting penetration of these pathogens. The newborn infant has good mechanical defences, and after birth the air spaces are rapidly populated by phagocytic cells. The immune defences mature more slowly, with normal T cell function established by 6–12 months of age, and although antibodies have been detected at 20 weeks gestation, antibody levels including secretory IgA do not reach those of the adult until 5 years of age. Passive transfer of maternal immunoglobulins both prenatally (IgG) and postnatally (secretory IgA in breast milk) are important immune defences for the infant.

TABLE 3.1.4 **Defences against infection**

Mechanical	Phagocytic	Immune
Filtration	Pulmonary macrophages	Antigen sampling cells
Airway reflexes	Polymorphonuclear leukocytes	Humoral immunity
Mucous/epithelial barrier		Cellular immunity
Mucociliary transport		

UPPER AIRWAY OBSTRUCTION

Upper airway obstruction is relatively common in children. Causes include:

- choanal stenosis or atresia
- adenotonsillar hypertrophy: acute or chronic
- retropharyngeal abscess
- thyroglossal cyst
- congenital anomalies:
  - macroglossia
  - retrognathia
  - midface hypoplasia
- epiglottitis
- angioneurotic edema
- airway burns
- laryngospasm
- vocal cord paresis
- inhaled foreign body
- laryngeal web
- subglottic stenosis
- laryngotracheobronchitis (croup)

DIAGNOSIS OF THE CAUSE OF OBSTRUCTION

The characteristic sign of upper airway obstruction is stridor. Intrathoracic lesions cause most obstruction in expiration, while lesions in the extrathoracic airways cause most obstruction in inspiration. The cause can often be established from the clinical features:

- time course (age and rapidity of onset and change in severity with time)
- quality and pitch of the stridor (e.g. high-pitched in croup; low-pitched inspiratory and expiratory snore in epiglottitis; high-pitched inspiratory and expiratory stridor in tracheal lesions)
- influence of posture, sleep, crying and feeding on the degree of obstruction

- presence of fever, difficulty in swallowing or pain on movement of the larynx
- presence and character of cough (e.g. 'barking' in croup, muffled or absent in laryngeal edema)

SIGNS OF SEVERITY OF OBSTRUCTION

The severity of obstruction is best assessed by clinical signs rather than specific investigations. As obstruction increases, so does the amount of recession: from intercostal recession in mild cases to suprasternal or costal recession and finally significant sternal recession in severe obstruction. A severely obstructed child is pale, anxious, apprehensive and restless, unable to settle or sleep and has increasing tachycardia and tachypnea.

Blood gas analysis and pulse oximetry are less useful than clinical signs in assessing the severity of obstruction. Arterial CO_2 tension may be normal in a severely obstructed child and the stress caused to the child in obtaining the blood specimen may be dangerous. Hypoxia does not occur until airway obstruction is severe, so its absence should not be reassuring. Conversely, hypoxia may be present in mild upper airway obstruction if there is associated lung disease.

LARYNGOTRACHEOBRONCHITIS OR CROUP

Several respiratory viruses can cause viral croup, the most common being parainfluenza virus. Croup can occur at any age, although significant airway obstruction is most likely to occur in infants and young children (see above).

Diagnosis

The diagnosis of croup is made clinically. There is usually a history of a prodromal upper respiratory infection and mild fever for 24 hours before the onset of respiratory difficulty. Stridor and a 'barking' cough are frequently worse at night. The stridor is characteristically harsh, dry, high-pitched and inspiratory. Laryngitis causes a hoarse voice and there is no restriction to head and neck movement or swallowing. There are usually signs of upper airway obstruction (see above) that may vary in severity with time.

Management

Most children with croup do not have significant upper airway obstruction and can be safely managed at home. Children with stridor or recession at rest should be observed in hospital, while those with severe obstruction should be observed in a pediatric intensive care unit (PICU). Investigation is not usually necessary unless an associated disease process is suspected.

Steroids

Corticosteroid use in croup has reduced the number of children requiring intubation. Steroids shorten the duration of intubation and make successful extubation more likely. In mild to moderate croup, a single dose of inhaled budesonide 2 mg = 4 ml of 5% solution) in the emergency department reduces the number of children who require hospital admission. Hospitalized children with severe croup should receive a short course of oral or intravenous steroids, e.g. dexamethasone 0.6 mg/kg (maximum 10 mg) as an initial dose followed if necessary by 0.15 mg/kg every 6 hours.

Nebulized epinephrine (adrenaline)

In severe obstruction, inhaled nebulized epinephrine (adrenaline) 1:1000 (0.5 ml/kg; maximum 4 ml) reduces the severity of obstruction and of respiratory distress. Its effect lasts from 30 minutes to several hours. The dose may be repeated as required. Side-effects are minimal. Although virtually all children with severe croup respond initially, a few subsequently fail to sustain this response. If severe obstruction does not respond to epinephrine, or the effect lasts less than 30–60 minutes, the trachea should be intubated (Ch. 6.3).

Tracheal intubation

Intubated children with croup require expert nursing care by experienced PICU nurses. The endotracheal tubes are 0.5–1.5 mm smaller in internal diameter than usual for the child's age and are prone to obstruction with mucus (maintain optimal humidity of inspired gases). These children more than any other group are at risk of accidental extubation because of their young age, mobility and the difficulty of taping tubes to the face in the presence of copious nasal secretions. The risk can be minimized by constant bedside nursing surveillance, by splinting the arms to prevent elbow flexion and by extreme care with tube position and fixation (Ch. 6.2). Low-dose sedation (e.g. chloral hydrate 30–60 mg/kg per dose) may be useful, but mechanical ventilation and muscle relaxants or high-dose sedation are not necessary.

EPIGLOTTITIS

Epiglottitis, a bacterial infection of the laryngeal inlet, is usually caused by *Haemophilus influenzae* type b (Hib). Since the introduction of Hib vaccine the incidence of epiglottitis has fallen dramatically, but the vaccine does not offer complete protection and the disease can occur in immunized children. Other cases are still seen, caused by miscellaneous organisms, including *Pneumococcus*, group A *Streptococcus* and *Staphylococcus aureus*.

Diagnosis

The following signs are characteristic of epiglottitis:

- a few hours of high fever and difficulty with breathing and swallowing
- usually no prodrome
- the child looks ill (because of septicemia)
- severity of upper airway obstruction varies from minimal to severe
- the stridor is typically a soft, muffled inspiratory and expiratory snore
- reluctance to speak or swallow because of pain
- lying down often increases the degree of obstruction, so children with epiglottitis adopt a characteristic posture: sitting forward and drooling, with minimal head and neck movement

The diagnosis of epiglottitis can usually be made clinically and confirmed by visualizing an inflamed, swollen epiglottis under general anesthesia before intubation. A lateral radiograph of the neck may confirm a swollen epiglottis, but radiographs are not usually required and should not be obtained routinely. If the diagnosis is in doubt and airway obstruction is not severe, a lateral neck radiograph taken in ICU or the operating room (not the radiology department) may help clarify the diagnosis. If the airway obstruction is severe, the child should be intubated under general anesthesia (inhalation, e.g. halothane, with child in sitting position) without waiting for radiography: the diagnosis is made by inspection during intubation. Hib can be isolated from blood cultures in or from a swab of the epiglottis taken during intubation. Bacterial antigens may also be detected in urine.

Management

In a child thought likely on clinical grounds to have epiglottitis:

- do not upset the child (e.g. by sending the parents from the room)
- do not examine the mouth or make the child lie down
- do not insert an i.v. cannula until the child is anesthetized
- any child with significant airway obstruction and possible epiglottitis needs examination under anesthesia and tracheal intubation, not a radiograph
- the intubation should be performed by an anesthesiologist experienced in anesthesia of children with severe airway obstruction (Ch. 6.3).
- care of the endotracheal tube, including positioning, fixation, humidification, suction and arm splinting are vital to the safe care of a child with epiglottitis
- an i.v. cannula is inserted, blood cultures taken and antibiotics given once the child is anesthetized
- third-generation cephalosporins (e.g. cefotaxime) are the drugs of choice

If the diagnosis of epiglottitis is established but there is no significant airway obstruction, most hospitals still regard intubation as essential, although a few hospitals observe unobstructed children expectantly in the PICU (while giving i.v. antibiotics), provided that equipment and staff capable of anesthetizing and intubating a child with epiglottitis are immediately available around the clock at the child's bedside. Most, if not all, children with epiglottitis can be extubated safely within 24 hours of intubation. Families with siblings under 6 years of age should receive chemoprophylaxis with rifampicin.

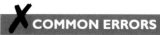

COMMON ERRORS

- ➤ Obtaining neck radiographs unnecessarily and in the radiology department
- ➤ Performing an oral examination
- ➤ Upsetting the child
- ➤ Using nebulized epinephrine (adrenaline)
- ➤ Using steroids
- ➤ Transporting a child with epiglottitis or symptomatic respiratory burn injury between hospitals unintubated

FOREIGN BODY

In 80% of cases of foreign body (FB) inhalation, the child is less than 3 years old. Infants usually inhale radiolucent food items (peanuts, seeds, pieces of carrot), whereas toddlers inhale radio-opaque items (coins, teeth, metal or plastic toy parts). Foreign bodies lodge at or above the larynx, in the trachea or a bronchus (usually the right).

Esophageal foreign bodies cause stridor or wheeze, dysphagia and drooling. Bronchial FBs cause unilateral wheeze. Laryngeal or tracheal FBs cause inspiratory or expiratory stridor. Dysphonia or dysphagia implies an FB in or above the larynx.

Radiography

The following radiographs may be helpful:

- anteroposterior and lateral neck radiograph for a suspected extrathoracic FB
- inspiratory and expiratory chest radiographs may show ipsilateral hyperlucency of the lung with a bronchial FB

Tracheal foreign bodies can rotate, causing sudden complete obstruction. Any FB in a child should be removed by an expert pediatric bronchoscopist and a pediatric anesthesiologist, as the child's tracheal mucosa is easily lacerated. If the child is stable though mildly obstructed, oxygen (10 L/min by mask) is given and the child transported to a pediatric hospital without intubation. If the airway is severely obstructed or deteriorating, the most experienced available bronchoscopist and anesthesiologist should travel to the child and perform bronchoscopy at the child's hospital. For imminent complete obstruction:

1. Open the airway using chin lift or jaw thrust.
2. Manually remove a visible FB but do not use blind finger sweeps, which cause impaction of the FB and mucosal laceration in children.
3. Back blows with 60° head-down tilt or sternal thrusts in infants, supine side-to-side chest compression, abdominal thrusts or the Heimlich maneuver in older children may dislodge the FB in an extreme emergency.
4. Bag-and-mask ventilation with oxygen may sustain life despite severe obstruction. Obtain optimal seal (mask to face) consider two-person technique (one to bag, one to manage the mask).

If the child is moribund with an obstructive tracheal FB, passage of an endotracheal tube may displace the FB into a bronchus, permitting ventilation of the opposite lung. Severe wheezing or stridor after bronchoscopy may be due to mucosal edema or a residual foreign body, requiring a trial of i.v. steroid, nebulized epinephrine (adrenaline), and possibly repeat bronchoscopy.

✗ COMMON ERRORS

➤ Attempting to intubate a stable child with an FB
➤ Performing blind finger sweeps of the mouth to remove the FB

RETROPHARYNGEAL ABSCESS

Clinical features:

- mostly in children less than 6 years old
- several days of fever and sore throat
- ill-looking, febrile child with dysphagia, drooling, muffled voice, respiratory distress
- lateral neck radiograph on inspiration shows a wide soft tissue shadow between the vertebrae and the pharynx (normal is half to one-third of width of third vertebra; films in expiration or with neck flexion can artificially widen the soft tissue image up to 3-fold)

Treatment:

- surgical drainage with the trachea intubated to prevent lung soiling
- give antibiotics: intravenous flucloxacillin and metronidazole (causative bacteria usually *Staphylococcus aureus* and anaerobic streptococci)

PERITONSILLAR ABSCESS (QUINSY)

Clinical features:

- usually occurs in an older child or teenager
- clinical signs are similar to those of epiglottitis with the addition of trismus

Treatment:

- needs surgical drainage under anesthesia
- antibiotic: intravenous penicillin G (benzylpenicillin) 60 mg/kg 6-hourly

✓ KEY POINTS

➤ In upper airway obstruction, the diagnosis and severity of obstruction are determined clinically, not by investigations
➤ Children with stridor at rest of recent onset should be admitted to hospital
➤ Corticosteroids reduce the duration and severity of croup
➤ Endotracheal tube care including fixation, humidification and suction are critically important to the safety of children intubated for upper airway obstruction
➤ Children with epiglottitis look sick and rarely if ever cough
➤ A lateral neck radiograph is only needed if the diagnosis of epiglottitis is uncertain and there is minimal obstruction

➤ An escort capable of intubation must be with the child throughout if X-rays have to be done in radiology (rather than the OR or PICU)

UPPER AIRWAY INJURY IN BURNED CHILDREN

See Chapter 4.2.

MEDIASTINAL MASSES

The usual cause is malignant lymphadenopathy: often a T cell lymphoma. Compression of the trachea and bronchi may increase over hours. Compression of the superior vena cava (SVC) causes conjunctival edema, distention of the neck veins and edema of the tracheal mucosa. Compression of the SVC and trachea is worse on lying down, and usually increases in the first 48 hours after chemotherapy commences.

Treatment:

- obtain early advice from an expert intensive care pediatrician or anesthesiologist
- intubate the trachea if respiratory distress is severe or is increasing rapidly
- an armored endotracheal tube (Ch. 6.3) may be needed
- be prepared for severe difficulty with intubation and ventilation

TRANSPORT

All children with epiglottitis or symptomatic upper airway burns (Ch. 4.2) should be intubated before transport. In children with other forms of upper airway obstruction, the decision to intubate before departure depends on:

- the cause and severity of upper airway obstruction
- the expected response to treatment
- the expected time course of progression relative to the time required for transport

If it is possible that severe obstruction may occur during transport, then the child should be intubated. On the other hand, if a child with severe croup requires transport for a short distance, it will often be appropriate to evaluate the response to inhaled epinephrine (adrenaline) before making a decision. Following a good response it may be appropriate to transport without intubation. Before transporting an intubated child it is essential to check that the tube is secure, that it is in good position on chest X-ray (tip of the tube sited level with the medial end of the clavicles), and that the child's hands cannot reach the tube. Accidental extubation during transport of a child with upper airway obstruction, particularly if the child is sedated, can easily lead to disaster.

ASTHMA

Asthma frequently begins in childhood, and is more prevalent in children (7–19%) than in adults (< 5%). Since the 1970s the lifetime prevalence of asthma in children has more than doubled. There is a familial association among asthma, allergic rhinitis and atopic dermatitis, suggesting a common genetic basis. The onset of asthmatic symptoms in childhood often follows a viral upper respiratory tract infection (URTI), especially that caused by respiratory syncytial virus (RSV).

PHYSIOLOGY

Air flow limitation in asthma is caused by mucosal edema, contraction of bronchial smooth muscle and mucous plugging. Small airways close prematurely during expiration, causing air trapping and hyperinflation. Although pulmonary overdistention helps to maintain airway patency, the strongly negative pleural pressure required to maintain high lung volumes increases the work of breathing, and lung hyperinflation places the diaphragm and other respiratory muscles at a mechanical disadvantage.

Hypoxemia occurs early in acute asthma, because of ventilation–perfusion mismatching and intrapulmonary right-to-left shunting. On admission to hospital, the degree of hypoxemia is related to clinical and spirometric (FEV_1) severity (Fig. 3.1.5). Carbon dioxide tension is usually low in mild or early acute asthma, rises with increasing severity, and is elevated in severe acute asthma (Fig. 3.1.6). Oxygenation (and ventilation–perfusion matching) improves (over days to weeks)

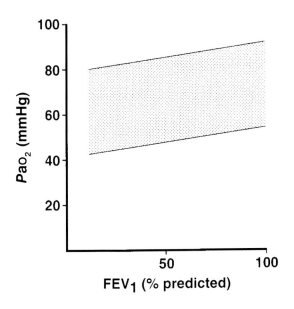

Figure 3.1.5 Relationship of Pao_2 to FEV_1 on presentation in acute asthma

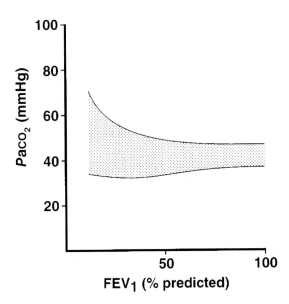

Figure 3.1.6 Relationship of $Paco_2$ to FEV_1 on presentation in acute asthma

during recovery from severe acute asthma, but more slowly than airway function (hours to days), so measures of oxygenation do not correlate with FEV_1 or peak expiratory flow rate during convalescence. The combination of hypoxemia, hypercapnia and acidosis may cause cardiovascular depression and cardiorespiratory arrest.

CLINICAL ASSESSMENT OF SEVERITY

Clinical pointers to the severity of the attack include:

- accessory muscle use and retraction of the chest wall
- dyspnea impairing speech or feeding
- impaired alertness

Children able to concentrate on tasks other than breathing (e.g. reading or watching television) are seldom severely ill. Pulsus paradoxus (a reduction in systemic blood pressure during inspiration) greater than 20 mmHg is a useful sign of severe asthma in adults and older children, but can be difficult to measure in small children. Increased respiratory rate (> 50 breath/min) correlates with severity, but is very variable. Almost all patients have a tachycardia, due to the disease or its treatment. Cyanosis, fatigue and unconsciousness are late signs indicating very

severe asthma. Loudness of wheeze is an unreliable sign of asthma severity. Absence of breath sounds may indicate severe asthma or occasionally a pneumothorax.

Few investigations are necessary in children admitted to the ICU with asthma.

Pulse oximetry and arterial blood gas analysis

Hemoglobin saturation is easily increased to 95–100% by supplemental oxygen despite severely impaired or deteriorating gas exchange, so pulse oximetry is useful for monitoring gas exchange in asthma only if the patient is breathing room air.

Arterial puncture is often difficult and distressing for small and sick children. Clinical estimation of severity is a more useful indicator of severity and need for mechanical ventilation than arterial blood gas analysis, but rapidly rising $Paco_2$ (> 1.5 kPa/h, 10 mmHg/h) is sometimes used as an indication for intubation. Arterial blood gases (ABG) monitored via an indwelling arterial cannula are essential in the assessment and adjustment of mechanical ventilation. Metabolic acidosis (e.g. due to excessive β-sympathomimetic dosage) and hypoxemia may also be detected by ABG monitoring.

A chest radiograph rarely yields useful information in nonintubated asthmatic children, but all intubated patients should have a chest radiograph to confirm endotracheal tube position and exclude pneumothorax.

Spirometry

Spirometry during forced expiration is useful for assessing patients with mild to moderate acute asthma, but is difficult or impossible for young or sick children. Forced expiratory volume in 1 second (FEV_1) is reproducible and can detect acute responses to bronchodilator. An FEV_1 value below 50% of predicted is considered severe, and below 35% very severe.

MANAGEMENT

Oxygen should be given by mask: 8–10 L/min to keep the hemoglobin saturation above 95%. Beta-2-sympathomimetics are the mainstay of treatment. The most commonly used drugs are salbutamol (albuterol), terbutaline and orciprenaline, of which the drug of choice is salbutamol.

Nebulized salbutamol

Nebulized salbutamol (albuterol) is given diluted (5 mg per dose, or 1 ml of 0.5% solution diluted to 4 ml with 0.9% saline) or undiluted (20 mg per dose), regardless of weight, through a jet nebulizer driven by 8–10 L/min of oxygen. The large volume and high gas flow through the nebulizer produce a small aerosol particle size, maximizing deposition of the drug in small airways.

Drug delivery to the lungs through a metered dose inhaler (MDI) and holding chamber with a mouthpiece or mask is at least as effective as nebulization and is less cumbersome. One puff is given per three breaths for a total of six puffs (child < 25 kg) or 12 puffs (> 25 kg), repeated as often as needed. Frequent (every 20 min) doses of salbutamol have been shown to be more effective than hourly doses. For very severe asthma, continuous nebulized salbutamol can be used safely in children, and is more effective than intermittent doses. Such therapy warrants PICU care.

Nebulizers and metered dose inhalers are used to deliver aerosol medication to the lungs during mechanical ventilation, although only 3–10% of the nebulized dose is deposited in the lungs of ventilated patients.

- use a volume of 4 ml in the nebulizer
- insert the nebulizer into the inspiratory limb of the circuit at least 45 cm from the Y-piece
- use intermittent (inspiratory) flow from the ventilator if possible; if not, use a continuous flow of 8 L/min from the ventilator
- bypass the heated humidification system which reduces aerosol delivery by 50%
- for those on volume-limited ventilators, readjust the tidal volume control to maintain a constant tidal volume

Metered dose inhalers

An in-line spacer should be used with a metered dose inhaler to maximize delivery. The smaller the endotracheal tube, the less drug is delivered to the lung. The technique is as follows:

- use a dose of 10–20 puffs (i.e. more than would be used in a nonintubated patient)
- insert the spacer into the inspiratory limb of the circuit, 18 cm from the Y-piece
- bypass the heated humidifier
- actuate the MDI at end-expiration
- apply a 2 s inspiratory pause hold on the ventilator, if not contraindicated

Intravenous salbutamol

Intravenous β_2-agonists are used when the child's tidal volume is so reduced that it limits aerosol drug delivery to the small airways. The intravenous route appears to be as effective as the inhaled route, but it is not certain that i.v. infusion offers extra benefit in a child already receiving a maximal inhaled dose. Hypoxemia due to the abolition of hypoxic pulmonary vasoconstriction is more common with β_2-agonists given i.v. than by the inhaled route.

The dose of i.v. salbutamol in children is higher than that used in adults, and is limited by its adverse effects: tachycardia (stop if heart rate > 200/min) and lactic acidosis. A suggested starting dose is 15 µg/kg i.v. over 10 minutes. This is followed by infusion of 2–10 µg/kg·min in children but in teenagers, a much lower dose is then used: 2–5 µg/min (not per kg).

Ipratropium bromide

Inhaled ipratropium bromide, a quaternary ammonium derivative of atropine, has a useful bronchodilator effect in children (including those younger than 2 years) with severe acute asthma who are already receiving an inhaled β_2-sympathomimetic drug. Three 250 µg doses of ipratropium are given in the first hour unless there is a contraindication to anticholinergics (e.g. glaucoma). Thereafter, 250 µg should be given 4-hourly. Ipratropium can be mixed with salbutamol in the nebulizer.

Corticosteroids

The use of corticosteriod drugs can:

- reduce the severity of acute severe asthma in controlled trials in children
- reduce the inflammation in bronchial mucosa
- potentiate the relaxation of bronchial smooth muscle by β_2-agonists
- reduce mucus production

Hydrocortisone (4 mg/kg), methylprednisolone (1 mg/kg) or dexamethasone (0.2 mg/kg) is given every 6 hours i.v. Oral corticosteroids are given when the patient's condition has improved.

Aminophylline

Aminophylline is a standard therapy for severe acute asthma, although the evidence for its effectiveness is conflicting. Of five controlled trials in children, one showed that aminophylline improved FEV_1, but used outmoded sympathomimetic agents. Four showed no benefit, but all excluded intensive care patients. Aminophylline may have beneficial nonbronchodilator effects, such as improvement in respiratory muscle strength, but this is controversial. Theophylline may also have an antiinflammatory effect, but its onset is probably delayed, and may not be additive to that of corticosteroids.

Aminophylline may have a place in the treatment of children whose asthma is severe enough to need ICU admission and who are at risk of respiratory muscle fatigue requiring intubation and mechanical ventilation despite the use of β_2-sympathomimetics (nebulized and i.v.), steroids and ipratropium. Because of its adverse effects, particularly nausea and vomiting, and rarely seizures, aminophylline should not be used routinely in all asthmatic children admitted to an ICU. If it is used, a loading dose of 10 mg/kg, followed by an infusion of 1.0 mg/kg·h in children 1–9 years of age, or 0.7 mg/kg·h in those aged 10 years or older, should be used. Plasma levels must be monitored, and kept in the range 55–110 µmol/L.

Other agents

Magnesium is not standard therapy for severe acute asthma, and in the absence of convincing evidence of its efficacy in controlled trials in adults or children it cannot be recommended. It is sometimes given as magnesium sulfate in a dose of 25–40 mg/kg (maximum 1.2 g) i.v. over 30 minutes once, when the child is deteriorating and appears likely to need mechanical ventilation despite all the treatments already mentioned.

Other therapies

Calcium channel blockers, inhalational agents (halothane, isoflurane, ether), helium-oxygen mixtures and extracorporeal membrane oxygenation (ECMO) have all been used for severe acute asthma. None has undergone a controlled trial.

Fluids

Mild dehydration is common on admission, and may be harmful because of increased viscosity of lower airways secretions and impaired mucociliary clearance. Overhydration is also harmful, because the highly negative intra-thoracic pressures and increased AD Hormone secretion found in severe acute asthma may lead to pulmonary edema.

Seventy per cent of calculated maintenance fluid needs (Ch. 3.5) should be provided (60% if the patient is ventilated with humidified gases). Hypokalemia and glycosuria, due to salbutamol, are common in severe acute asthma.

MECHANICAL VENTILATION

See also Chapter 6.4. Indications for medical ventilation include:

- cardiorespiratory arrest
- fatigue, with decreased respiratory effort
- altered conscious state
- arrhythmia
- rising Pa_{CO_2} level is a less useful criterion in children because of the difficulty of obtaining serial blood gas measurements.

Technique

A rapid sequence induction (Ch. 6.3) should be used. Ketamine has sedative, analgesic and bronchodilator effects and can be used to induce anesthesia and as an infusion (4 µg/kg·min) with midazolam for sedation. Pancuronium, which amplifies preexisting tachycardia, should be avoided if possible.

During mechanical ventilation the patient should be sedated and paralyzed initially, to eliminate patient-ventilator asynchrony, to improve chest wall compliance, to provide a period of respiratory muscle rest, and to enable a controlled hypoventilation strategy to be employed.

Dynamic hyperinflation

Inadequate exhalation time during IPPV causes gas trapping and positive alveolar pressure at the end of expiration, termed 'intrinsic PEEP' or 'auto-PEEP', which is directly related to tidal volume. This increases the risk of barotrauma and impairment of venous return. A 'controlled hypoventilation' strategy (Ch. 6.4), the deliberate tolerance of relatively high carbon dioxide tensions ('permissive hypercapnia'), should be used to limit barotrauma and volutrauma. Controlled (i.e. nontriggered) ventilation is used for paralyzed and sedated children and triggered ventilation (e.g. pressure support) is started as the attack resolves. The F_{IO_2} is adjusted to maintain normal saturation, but should preferably be kept below 0.5.

Volume-limited ventilation

Volume-limited ventilation ensures consistent minute ventilation despite variable lung resistance and compliance:

- start with tidal volume below 10 ml/kg and adjust to keep the peak inflation pressure (PIP) below 35 cmH$_2$O
- a high inspiratory gas flow rate (100 ml/min) causes high peak inspiratory pressures, but allows more time for expiration at a given tidal volume and breathing rate
- rate less than 10–15 breath/min

Pressure-limited ventilation

Pressure-limited ventilation (PIP 35 cmH$_2$O or less):

- minimizes barotrauma and volutrauma
- the tidal volume and Pa_{CO_2} vary as lung compliance changes
- high inspiratory flow rate reduces the tidal volume at any given PIP
- reduce the PIP when the attack is resolving and the Pa_{CO_2} is falling.

Positive end-expiratory pressure is usually best avoided, as it often increases gas trapping.

Assessment and monitoring of ventilation

Ventilation is assessed by:

- pulse oximetry
- ECG
- blood pressure

Arterial blood gases are measured 4-hourly. If pulmonary hyperinflation (assessed by physical examination and by chest radiograph) increases, the peak airway pressure or the tidal volume must be reduced, regardless of the Pa_{CO_2}.

A falling mean arterial blood pressure indicates hyperinflation with impaired venous return. This can be confirmed by disconnecting the patient from the ventilator and allowing the lungs to empty over 30–60 seconds. The mean arterial pressure will rise if hyperinflation is impairing venous return.

Weaning from mechanical ventilation

Muscle relaxant drugs can be stopped and weaning commenced when the PIP needed to keep the Pa_{CO_2} below 8 kPa (60 mmHg), falls to 25 cm H$_2$O.

COMPLICATIONS OF TREATMENT

Complications include:

- pneumothorax, pneumomediastinum and subcutaneous emphysema
- tachycardia, lactic acidosis and hemoglobin desaturation caused by β_2-sympathomimetics
- hypokalemia, metabolic alkalosis and hyperglycemia due to steroids
- upper gastrointestinal bleeding due to steroids
- profound muscle weakness requiring prolonged mechanical ventilation, possibly due to steroids or muscle relaxants in high dose for long periods
- theophylline toxicity

Because of substantial interindividual variation in theophylline pharmacokinetics, theophylline levels must be monitored carefully. In patients receiving oral theophylline, a level should be obtained before any additional aminophylline is given. Levels should be obtained 1 hour after a loading dose, again during the continuous infusion and if a suspected adverse reaction occurs. Adverse reactions can occur with levels within the therapeutic range.

COMMON ERRORS

- ➤ Underestimation of severity by the patient and physicians, before hospitalization, is a frequent cause of death. Measurement of peak expiratory flow rate is relatively insensitive to deterioration and reliance on PEFR alone may cause underestimation of severity.
- ➤ Overestimation of severity: wheeze is an unreliable measure of severity. Pulse oximetry, used in isolation, may be misleading if interpreted as a measure of ventilation. Salbutamol can worsen ventilation–perfusion mismatching, causing hypoxemia despite improving airway constriction and reducing dyspnea. If this occurs, a chest radiograph should be obtained to exclude a pneumothorax, but if dyspnea remains severe, the salbutamol dose should not be reduced, even if the drug appears to worsen the hypoxemia.
- ➤ inadequate therapy in severely ill patients: inadequate dosage and nebulizer volume for

salbutamol. Ipratropium is frequently omitted, despite good evidence of its efficacy in severe acute asthma
- ➤ Attempting to achieve normal blood gases: failure to recognize progressive lung hyperinflation

✓ KEY POINTS

- ➤ Not everything that wheezes is asthma. Consider vascular ring, mediastinal masses, tracheal or broncheal stenoses or malacia, foreign body, bronchiolitis, pertussis and *Mycoplasma* infection
- ➤ Chest radiographs are not useful in asthma except to exclude pneumothorax and to check the position of an endotracheal tube
- ➤ Radiographic evidence of atelectasis is common in acute asthma but does not imply infection. Antibiotics are very rarely indicated in acute asthma
- ➤ Oxygen administration *never* suppresses the respiratory drive in childhood asthma
- ➤ Mechanical ventilation does not cure asthma; it only sustains life. The lowest airway pressures needed to maintain the pH above 7.15 and PaO_2 above 7 kPa (50 mmHg) are sufficient

PNEUMOTHORAX

Air can enter the pleural space either following a tear in the lung or via penetration of the chest wall. A pneumothorax (air in the pleural space) can cause lung collapse. When under pressure a pneumothorax may cause the mediastinum to shift, placing pressure on the opposite lung.

DIAGNOSIS

Most air leaks are evident on AP chest X-ray but lateral views can be helpful.

Physical signs of pneumothorax are:

- reduced or absent breath sounds over the site of the pneumothorax
- reduced chest movement on the affected side
- a shift of the mediastinum (cardiac apex and trachea) away from the affected side

- hyperresonance and appearance of hyperinflation on the affected side
- subcutaneous emphysema

MANAGEMENT

Needle thoracentesis and/or chest tube drainage are required for life-threatening pneumothorax; stable air leaks in spontaneous breathing children free of significant respiratory difficulty can be observed and followed radiologically

Needle thoracentesis

Needle thoracentesis is an effective emergency procedure:

- equipment:
  - materials for sterile procedure
  - lidocaine (lignocaine) without epinephrine (adrenaline)
  - 16–20 gauge needle with catheter
  - three-way stopcock
  - 20 ml syringe
- Procedure:
  - prepare skin
  - drape appropriately
  - achieve analgesia at second intercostal space in midclavicular line
  - introduce needle/catheter to achieve drainage of air
  - aspirate
  - consider chest tube insertion
- Technique:
  - site of insertion should be immediately above the inferior rib
  - aspirate gradually (sudden removal can cause pain and nausea)
  - reaccumulation is likely

Chest tube insertion

Effective treatment of pneumothorax often requires a chest tube insertion:

- indications:
  - pneumothorax (tension); spontaneous exceeding 20% of thoracic volume or traumatic
  - hemothorax

- pleural effusion
- chylothorax
- Equipment:
  - lidocaine (lignocaine) 1%, without epinephrine (adrenaline)
  - 25 or 27 gauge needle
  - 3 ml syringe
  - scalpel
  - Kelly forceps
  - sutures
  - chest tube (no. 12 newborn, no. 16 infant, no. 22 small child)
  - closed drainage system or Heimlich valve or equivalent
- Procedure:
  - consider premedication (e.g. morphine or midazolam)
  - restrain infant or young child (to decrease the risk of lung injury)
  - prepare skin with antiseptic solution; drape area
  - identify the fifth or sixth intercostal space in the mid or anterior axillary line
  - achieve analgesia by infiltration under the skin through the intercostal muscle to the rib (to include periosteum) up to the pleura
  - make the skin incision with a scalpel 1–1.5 cm long over the bottom edge of the rib
  - using Kelly forceps and blunt dissection, create an oblique passage from the skin incision up over the top of the rib; take care to spread the forceps adequately to create an appropriate passage for the size of chest tube to be inserted
  - with the forceps closed (tips together) enter the pleural space just above the ribs (this procedure requires moderate force). The index finger should be used to avoid excessive penetration causing secondary damage to the lungs; place the index finger firmly against the forceps approximately 1 cm from the tip
  - grasp the tip of the chest tube in the forceps and guide the tube through the passage into the pleural space

- clamp the tube with forceps
- advance the tube to its optimal position
- release the clamp to allow gradual rather than sudden drainage
- suture the chest tube to the chest wall and apply a dressing
- connect to a drainage system
- Radiograph the chest to confirm correct placement
- Technique:
  - avoid the intercostal neurovascular bundle below the inferior aspect of the rib
  - direct the tube anteriorly for optimal drainage of air and posteriorly for fluid
  - ensure all side holes are within the pleural space
  - tape all connections in the drainage system
  - clamp the chest drain with a hemostat if the drainage system has to be elevated above the site of insertion
  - alter the child's position to remedy incomplete drainage
  - consider applying suction to the drainage system if air remains under tension
  - ensure the tip of the catheter is not compressing the aorta in small infants developing hypotension
- Complications:
  - lung puncture causing additional air leak or hemorrhage
  - subcutaneous emphysema (check proximal drain holes on chest tube are within the pleural cavity)
  - trauma to the intercostal neurovascular bundle
  - incorrect placement (can cause injury to liver, spleen, kidney or aorta)
  - infection where sterile technique is deficient

BRONCHIOLITIS

Bronchiolitis is a seasonal viral infection that affects infants. Respiratory syncytial virus is the usual cause, although bronchiolitis may also be caused by adenovirus, influenza or parainfluenza viruses. Infants who were preterm at birth and those with preexisting chronic lung disease, congenital heart disease or immunodeficiency are at increased risk of severe infection.

Children with bronchiolitis have fever, a wheezy cough, audible wheezing and difficulty in feeding. Physical signs include tachypnea, tachycardia, intercostal and sternal retraction and chest hyperinflation. Expiration is prolonged and involves contraction of the abdominal muscles. Auscultation of the chest reveals fine inspiratory crackles or expiratory wheeze. Hypoxia is prominent, and hypercarbia is also relatively common. Central apnea may occur before the development of significant lung disease, especially in ex-premature and very young infants. A liver palpable several centimeters below the costal margin is almost always lowered by lung overinflation, rather than enlarged by right heart failure.

PHYSIOLOGY

The small airways are obstructed by inflammation, edema, increased mucus production and bronchoconstriction. Chest X-rays reveal hyperinflation with areas of atelectasis.

MANAGEMENT

Infants with respiratory distress, inability to feed, hypoxia or apnea require hospital admission. Oxygen therapy should be adjusted according to pulse oximetry. Infants at risk of apnea (ex-premature infants, the very young and the severely ill) require continuous monitoring and nursing staff trained and equipped to provide bag-and-mask ventilation.

Fluids

Infants with bronchiolitis are often too breathless to feed. Nasogastric feeding is only appropriate in an infant with sufficient respiratory reserve and airway reflexes to deal with vomiting or regurgitation of feeds. A lethargic infant with a weak cry and cough should be treated with i.v. fluids without nasogastric feeding. Fluid intake should be tailored to the child's state of hydration. A few infants with bronchiolitis develop hyponatremia secondary to the syndrome of inappropriate antidiuretic hormone (SIADH): fluids should then be restricted to 30% of maintenance (Ch. 2.10). In the absence of dehydration or SIADH, a fluid intake of 80% of maintenance is appropriate.

Drugs

Bronchodilators such as salbutamol, ipratropium bromide or epinephrine (adrenaline) have been shown to improve lung function in some but not all patients. Routine use of bronchodilators is not recommended in bronchiolitis, but the response to a single dose of nebulized bronchodilator such as salbutamol should be evaluated and therapy continued if benefit is demonstrated.

Ribavirin, a specific antiviral agent, has not been shown conclusively to improve the outcome of bronchiolitis and most centers do not use it routinely. Ribavirin has significant disadvantages: it is delivered by small particle aerosol, and its environmental safety and teratogenicity in health care workers remains controversial. In ventilated children, close attention is required to prevent endotracheal tube or expiratory valve occlusion from ribavirin build-up.

Respiratory support

Indications for respiratory support (Chs 2.1, 6.4) include:

- apnea or irregular respiratory effort
- refractory hypoxia (SpO_2 < 90% despite an inspired oxygen concentration above 60%)
- exhaustion secondary to increased work of breathing, e.g.
  - paucity of spontaneous movement
  - handling causes tachypnea and rapid desaturation
  - inability to settle due to marked respiratory distress

In some infants, apnea and respiratory failure respond to i.v. aminophylline or nasopharyngeal CPAP, while others require intubation and mechanical ventilation.

Up to 70% of infants requiring support can be satisfactorily managed with nasopharyngeal CPAP alone, delivered via a short 'endotracheal' tube inserted to the level of the soft palate (6–8 cm from the nares depending on the size of the child). The CPAP of 5 cm is applied and increased to 12 cmH_2O if necessary. The major problem with the technique is tube obstruction with nasal secretions. The aim of nasopharyngeal CPAP is to reduce the work of breathing and improve oxygenation. The concern that CPAP (or PEEP) will exacerbate hyperinflation is unfounded. If nasopharyngeal CPAP does achieve the desired effect then intubation and ventilation (Ch. 6.4) are appropriate.

Guidelines for respiratory care in bronchiolitis are:

- intubation is usually required for several days
- tracheal mucus is copious in bronchiolitis and may precipitate the need for intubation
- tracheal suction may be needed as frequently as every 20 minutes, to keep the airways clear of mucus
- inadequate humidification and tracheal suction cause atelectasis followed by increasing oxygen and ventilation requirements
- the child's own respiratory and coughing efforts assist secretion clearance, so the best ventilation strategy is to assist spontaneous respiratory efforts (i.e. triggered ventilation; Chapter 6.4) rather than to control ventilation
- PEEP or CPAP (5–12 cmH_2O) may reduce the infant's respiratory work
- small airway obstruction slows expiration and causes lung hyperinflation, so a slow ventilator rate and long expiratory time are important to allow adequate expiration (short inspiratory times should also be avoided, as they cause lung units supplied by narrowed airways to be underventilated)
- hypercapnia should be tolerated ($PaCO_2$ < 11 kPa or 80 mmHg; pH > 7.15) both before and during ventilation; hypercapnia on its own is not an indication for respiratory support, and attempts to ventilate to normocapnia will cause iatrogenic lung injury

- suggested initial ventilator settings are:
  - pressure-limited synchronized intermittent mandatory ventilation (SIMV)
  - peak pressure 25 cmH$_2$O adjusted to achieve visible chest excursion
  - PEEP 6–8 cmH$_2$O
  - rate 20–25 breath/min
  - inspiratory time 0.7–1.0 s
- blood gases are measured after 30 minutes, and ventilator settings adjusted according to the results
- pulse oximetry and transcutaneous PCO$_2$ monitoring are useful for adjusting ventilation

✓ **KEY POINTS**

➤ Nasopharyngeal CPAP frequently improves apnea and respiratory failure in bronchiolitis and avoids the need for mechanical ventilation
➤ Handling and gavage feeding are best avoided in bronchiolitis

PNEUMONIA

Most inflammatory parenchymal lung disease in children is caused by infection. Pneumonia always involves alveolar consolidation, but interstitial lung tissue and pleura may also be inflamed.

DIAGNOSIS

The signs and symptoms may be typical or atypical. Features of *typical* pneumonia (e.g. due to *Streptococcus pneumoniae* or *Haemophilus influenzae*) include:

- sudden onset (over 24 hours) of fever, cough, dyspnea, rigors
- in older children, production of purulent sputum
- tachycardia, tachypnea and an expiratory grunt
- dullness to percussion and bronchial breathing are often absent

Features of atypical pneumonia (e.g. due to *Pneumocystis carinii* or influenza virus) include:

- gradual onset (over 3–5 days)
- malaise, fever, myalgia, arthralgia and headache may precede respiratory symptoms
- the cough may not appear for several days and is usually nonproductive
- disparity between clinical and radiological signs is characteristic: there may be bilateral inter-stitial and alveolar opacity with minimal chest signs

INVESTIGATION

In typical bacterial pneumonia it is unusual to identify the causative agent in blood cultures, tracheal aspirates or urine antigens. Empirical antibiotic therapy is usually required. If the patient deteriorates despite empirical therapy or if there are atypical features, a number of investigations are indicated. Table 3.1.5 shows the tests most likely to reveal common respiratory pathogens. In severely ill patients, a bronchoalveolar lavage (BAL), through the ET tube or a bronchoscope, with bacterial and viral cultures and specific staining of the smear may reveal tubercle bacillus, *Pneumocystis carinii*, fungi or other atypical pathogens. If the BAL is negative, an open lung biopsy should be performed, especially if a noninfectious cause of inter-stitial lung disease is suspected.

Streptococcus pneumoniae is the most common cause of typical pneumonia. The drug of choice in community-acquired lobar pneumonia is penicillin G (benzyl penicillin). In some countries a third-generation cephalosporin or vancomycin may be required because of the prevalence of penicillin-resistant pneumococci.

Staphylococcal pneumonia is often preceded by a viral respiratory infection. It should be considered in severe pneumonia or if there is severe systemic illness or pneumatoceles or cavitation on chest X-ray. Initial treatment is usually flucloxacillin plus an aminoglycoside and is modified according to sensitivity testing of bacterial isolates.

Gram-negative pneumonia in children usually occurs only in those with underlying lung disease, immune compromise, or long-term tracheal intubation. The appropriate antibiotic is an aminoglycoside, with or without a third-generation cephalosporin.

Mycoplasma pneumoniae is the most common cause of community-acquired pneumonia in

TABLE 3.1.5 **The most appropriate test for a suspected respiratory pathogen**

Pathogen	Test
Streptococcus pneumoniae; Haemophilus influenzae; Gram-negative bacilli	Blood culture
Gram-positive bacteria; Gram-negative bacteria; fungi	Microscopy and culture of sputum or tracheal aspirate
S. pneumoniae; H. influenzae	Urine bacterial antigens
Respiratory viruses	Nasopharyngeal aspirate + viral culture
RSV; adenovirus; influenza and parainfluenza viruses; Bordetella pertussis; Chlamydia; Pneumocystis carinii	Immunofluorescence; polymerase chain reaction
CMV	Viral culture of urine and saliva
Chlamydia	Conjunctival scraping: immunofluorescence and tissue culture
Mycoplasma; Legionella; CMV	Acute serology (IgM)
Influenza and parainfluenza viruses; adenovirus; CMV; varicella; Mycoplasma; Legionella	Acute and convalescent serology
Pneumocystis carinii; Mycobacterium; fungi; Legionella	BAL + specific stains + microscopy and culture + rapid identification tests (as for NPA)
Pneumocystis carinii; Mycobacterium; fungi; Legionella	Lung biopsy + specific stains + microscopy and culture + rapid identification tests + culture of lung homogenate + histology of frozen and fixed sections

BAL, bronchoalveolar lavage; CMV, cytomegalovirus; NPA, nasopharyngeal aspirate; RSV, respiratory syncytial virus.

children. The highest infection rate occurs in children of 5–9 years of age. It presents as atypical pneumonia and is rarely life-threatening. The diagnosis is confirmed with serology. The drug of choice in children is erythromycin.

Exposure and seroconversion to *Legionella* is common in childhood but severe pneumonia is uncommon. Early diagnosis is established if a high IgM titer is demonstrated. The drug of choice is erythromycin.

Viruses are responsible for most respiratory infections in children and adults, although most infections are mild and self-limiting. Adenovirus, influenza, measles and RSV can all result in fatal pneumonia or permanent respiratory sequelae. Secondary infection with *Staphylococcus aureus* (see above) can cause severe deterioration. With the possible exception of ganciclovir in CMV pneumonitis in the immunocompromised, antiviral agents are of little benefit in viral pneumonia.

Pneumocystis carinii pneumonia (PCP) is the most common cause of atypical pneumonia in immunocompromised children. Although it only occurs in this group of patients, it may be the presenting feature of the immune defect, especially in infants. Patients at risk include children with AIDS; congenital defects in cell-mediated immunity; oncology

patients with drug-induced immune deficiency, and organ transplant patients. The diagnosis of PCP should be considered whenever pneumonia is progressing despite treatment. Other suggestive features include marked tachypnea, a significant oxygen requirement, and a dry, nonproductive cough. In the early stages, chest auscultation is usually normal. The chest X-ray may initially show a unilateral, soft alveolar opacity which subsequently becomes bilateral. The diagnosis is usually established by silver staining or, more recently, polymerase chain reaction (PCR) testing of BAL fluid. The drug treatment of choice is high-dose trimethoprim and sulfamethoxazole (co-trimoxazole)—i.v. trimethoprim 250 mg/m^2 immediately, then 150 mg/m^2 8-hourly in children < 11 years or 12-hourly (> 11 years). Adjuvant corticosteroids have proved to be beneficial (methylprednisolone 0.5 mg/kg i.v. 6-hourly) especially in HIV-associated PCP. Response to treatment is slow and may not occur for several days. The hypoxia may become more severe after treatment is commenced.

Aspiration pneumonia is common in children. The prognosis is far better in children than in adults. Not every child that aspirates saliva, food or gastric contents develops pneumonia. There is no benefit from prophylactic antibiotics or steroids. If the child is intubated, a tracheal aspirate should be sent for culture and if signs of infection develop (fever, neutrophilia, etc.), antibiotic choice should be based on culture results. Secondary infection is usually caused by mixed aerobes and anaerobes, either oral flora (mostly Gram-positive) or bowel-derived (Gram-negative) bacilli.

For ventilator management of pneumonia, see ARDS below and Chapters 2.1 and 6.4.

✓ **KEY POINTS**

➤ Blood culture frequently fails to reveal the infecting organism in pneumonia. Tracheal aspirate and—more reliably—BAL or lung biopsy are often required

➤ *Streptococcus pneumoniae* is the most common cause of typical pneumonia

➤ *Pneumocystis carinii* is the most common cause of atypical pneumonia in immunocompromised children

ACUTE RESPIRATORY DISTRESS SYNDROME

Acute respiratory distress syndrome (ARDS) is characterized by:

- tachypnea
- rapidly progressive hypoxia (PaO_2/FIO_2 ratio < 150 without PEEP)
- noncardiogenic pulmonary edema
- loss of lung volume
- reduced pulmonary compliance
- diffuse pulmonary infiltrates on chest X-ray

Many different insults may precipitate ARDS (Table 3.1.6). The triggering process may cause direct lung injury (e.g. pulmonary aspiration or viral pneumonia) or it may be part of a systemic process where indirect lung injury is part of a multisystem disease (e.g. sepsis or nonthoracic trauma). Although insertion of a pulmonary artery occlusion catheter is no longer regarded as essential to confirm the diagnosis, cardiac disease should be excluded by clinical and echocardiographic examination before the diagnosis is made.

TABLE 3.1.6 Conditions associated with the development of ARDS

Direct lung injury
- Pneumonia
- Aspiration of saliva or gastric contents
- Inhalation of smoke and other toxic gases (Ch. 4.2)
- Near-drowning (Ch. 4.9)

Indirect lung injury
- Sepsis
- Multiple trauma
- Fat embolism
- Disseminated intravascular coagulation
- Reperfusion following shock or cardiac arrest
- Pancreatitis
- Cardiopulmonary bypass
- Drugs and toxins
- Massive transfusion
- Burns
- Ionizing radiation
- High altitude

PHYSIOLOGY

The host inflammatory response to a variety of insults (Table 3.1.6) plays a central role in the pathogenesis of ARDS. Inflammatory mediators implicated in the process include cytokines, free oxygen radicals, complement, kinins, coagulation products, arachidonic acid metabolites and proteases. Sources of these mediators include platelets, endothelial cells and neutrophils, although ARDS may also occur in neutropenic patients. Endothelial cell injury causes pulmonary edema due to vascular permeability, leading to inhibition of surfactant production and function, hyaline membrane formation, reduced lung compliance, intrapulmonary shunt and ventilation–perfusion mismatch. The result is impaired gas exchange, especially hypoxemia.

Superimposed on this inflammatory tissue damage are the adverse effects of mechanical ventilation. Overstretching the lung, particularly at the interface of collapsed and open areas, subjects the terminal airways to significant shear forces, especially if large ventilator tidal volumes are used in a disease characterized by low lung volumes. This form of injury is now known as 'volutrauma'. In ARDS, the closing volume is usually above the functional residual capacity (FRC), so with each tidal breath, small airways close and reopen, amplifying the damaging shear forces. Volutrauma and pulmonary oxygen toxicity contribute to the progression of lung injury during mechanical ventilation by potentiating the inflammatory stimulus and causing air leaks from alveoli and small airways. The air leaks produce pneumothorax, pneumomediastinum, subcutaneous emphysema or pulmonary interstitial emphysema.

TREATMENT

1. Find and treat the cause of ARDS
2. Assess tissue oxygenation by monitoring end-organ function (conscious state, urine output, peripheral perfusion), and monitoring metabolic or lactic acidosis.
3. Optimize the hemoglobin concentration and cardiac output by titrating 10 ml/kg boluses of blood (if Hb < 120 g/L, 12 g/dl) or colloid against the above indicators of organ perfusion and against the CVP.
4. Inotropes such as dobutamine or dopamine may improve gas exchange by improving the cardiac output.
5. Restrict the intake of nonresuscitation fluids to 60% of maintenance to minimize pulmonary edema formation.
6. Diuretics are used cautiously to achieve negative fluid balance once the circulation is stable. Specific measures (including corticosteroids) aimed at attenuating the inflammatory response have been tried but none is of proven benefit.

RESPIRATORY SUPPORT

The ventilation strategy used for respiratory support (Chs 2.1, 6.4) must keep the child alive while minimizing further lung injury. Lung volume is recruited with sustained inflations after suction or circuit disconnections and maintained using PEEP and prolonged inspiratory times. Attempts to normalize blood gases can cause significant lung injury. The FIO_2 is restricted to 0.6 or less by using PEEP (up to 15 cmH_2O). Provided the other components of oxygen delivery (cardiac output and hemoglobin concentration) are not compromised, arterial oxygen saturation of 85–90% is sufficient for tissue oxygenation. Small tidal volumes (3–8 ml/kg) are used to avoid overexpansion of compli-

ant parts of the lung and peak inflation pressures should remain below 35 cmH_2O. If this approach results in hypercapnia, this should be allowed ('permissive hypercapnia'). Although it is not certain that any particular level of $PaCO_2$ is harmful, it is generally recommended that $PaCO_2$ is maintained below 10.5 kPa (80 mmHg) and the pH above 7.15, provided oxygenation and hemodynamic stability are maintained. Central nervous system pathology (e.g. trauma or ischemia) is a contraindication to permissive hypercapnia. If the oxygenation target cannot be achieved, the mean airway pressure should be increased by increasing PEEP or prolonging the inspiratory time (and therefore increasing the I:E ratio). The limit to increasing mean airway pressure is overinflation either on chest X-ray or detected by observing a fall in compliance as mean airway pressure increases.

If conventional ventilation fails, consider:

- high-frequency oscillation
- inhaled nitric oxide
- ECMO
- surfactant therapy
- perfluorocarbon-associated gas exchange (partial liquid ventilation)

With the possible exception of one study suggesting benefit with high-frequency oscillation, these therapies have not been shown to improve outcome from pediatric ARDS.

NEUROLOGICAL AND NEUROMUSCULAR CAUSES OF RESPIRATORY FAILURE

PHYSIOLOGY

Periodic contraction and relaxation of the muscles of the diaphragm and chest wall provide the power of the respiratory pump. Other muscle groups help to keep the airways patent, either by holding them open (e.g. the pharyngeal and laryngeal muscles), or in clearing secretions by coughing and swallowing. If the function of any of these muscle groups is impaired, gas movement and exchange is reduced and respiratory failure can occur. Atelectasis, aspiration, and pulmonary infection may also complicate respiratory muscle dysfunction.

Respiratory muscle contraction is the final event in a process that starts in the cerebral cortex or brain stem, and passes via the spinal cord, peripheral motor nerves, across the neuromuscular junction to the muscle unit. A wide range of disorders (Table 3.1.7) can affect this process, at a single site (e.g. spinal cord trauma) or at several sites (e.g. some drug intoxications).

Since ventilatory support for children with neurological and neuromuscular disorders may be needed for many days or weeks, such children should be transferred to a tertiary PICU as soon as the airway and breathing have been secured. Many of these conditions can lead to respiratory failure by themselves (e.g. spinal cord trauma or botulism), but others usually cause respiratory failure only in association with other factors (e.g. spinal muscular atrophy plus acute viral bronchiolitis, or Duchenne's muscular dystrophy plus orthopedic surgery).

CENTRAL ALVEOLAR HYPOVENTILATION

Malfunction of the brain-stem respiratory control centers responsible for the automatic control of breathing causes deficient ventilatory and arousal responses to hypoxia and hypercapnia. The condition can be due to acquired brain-stem lesions such as trauma, infection, tumor or hemorrhage, or to congenital abnormalities such as Leigh syndrome or the Arnold–Chiari malformation. The most common form (Ondine's curse) is a primary congenital abnormality of control center responsiveness, of which the anatomical or physiological cause is unknown.

The syndrome mainly affects the control of respiration during sleep, but in all cases, the ventilatory response to CO_2 is subnormal day and night, and in the most severe cases, awake respiration may also be inadequate. Congenital central alveolar hypoventilation syndrome usually presents in the neonatal period or early infancy, but a few cases present later in childhood. Some babies who die during sleep, apparently from the sudden infant death syndrome, may have this condition. The usual features are cyanosis and hypoventilation during sleep. Polysomnographic evaluation shows reduced tidal volume, especially in non-REM sleep. The consequent hypercapnia and hypoxia lead to neither an increase in ventilation nor arousal.

TABLE 3.1.7 Neurologic and neuromuscular causes of respiratory failure

Brain and brain stem
Hypoxic ischemic encephalopathy
Trauma
Seizures
Raised intracranial pressure
Tumor
Drugs
Sedatives
Narcotics
Poisons
Central alveolar hypoventilation syndrome
Infection
    Meningitis
    Encephalitis
    Poliomyelitis (bulbar)
    Tetanus
Arnold-Chiari malformation
Achondroplasia
Osteogenesis imperfecta
Leigh syndrome

Spinal cord
Tumor
Trauma
Tetanus
Transverse myelopathy
Poliomyelitis
Spinal muscular atrophy

Neuromuscular junction
Myasthenia gravis
Botulism
Organophosphate poisoning
Snakebite
Spider bite
Muscle relaxants

Peripheral nerve
Guillain–Barré syndrome
Phrenic nerve injury
Vocal cord palsy
Porphyria
Tick paralysis
Heavy metal intoxication
Organic solvent poisoning
Cytotoxic therapy
Nitrofurantoin
Critical illness polyneuropathy
Diphtheria

Muscle unit
Muscular dystrophies
Mitochondrial myopathies
Carnitine palmitoyltransferase deficiency
Nemaline myopathy
Acid maltase deficiency
Uremia
Starvation
Hypermagnesemia
Hypophosphatemia
Hypokalemia
Fatigue
Polymyositis/dermatomyositis
Critical illness myopathy

Note that some conditions affect more than one site in the nervous system.

Various associated abnormalities of the autonomic nervous system have also been described, including constipation, Hirschsprung's disease, dry mouth and eyes, and sinus bradycardia.

SPINAL CORD TRAUMA

The respiratory effects of spinal cord trauma depend on the level of the injury:

- high cervical (C-1 to C-2):
  - innervate accessory muscles, diaphragm, intercostals, abdominals
  - lesions lead to early death from apnea
- Mid cervical (C-3 to C-5):
  - innervate diaphragm, intercostal and abdominal muscles
  - lesions lead to early hypoventilation, which is worse in young children because their accessory muscles of respiration are inefficient
- Low cervical (C-6 to C-7):
  - innervate intercostal and abdominal muscles
  - low cervical lesions lead to chest wall instability, again more marked in the young child
- thoracolumbar (T-1 down):
  - innervate abdominal muscles
  - thoracolumbar lesions reduce the ability to cough and clear secretions effectively

Spinal cord trauma is often accompanied by severe head trauma and other injuries. The diagnosis of cord injury is sometimes missed in this setting because the respiratory abnormalities are attributed to the brain or other injuries. Clues to spinal cord injury include loss of sympathetic tone with peripheral vasodilatation and hypotension, and urinary retention.

Spinal cord injury can also affect respiration indirectly via pulmonary edema (fluid overload from treatment of hypotension) and aspiration of stomach contents (secondary to ileus).

POLIOMYELITIS

Immunization has greatly reduced the incidence of poliomyelitis, but sporadic cases are still seen in immunocompromised hosts, those who are unimmunized and travel overseas, and in countries where poliomyelitis remains common. Direct infection of the central nervous system by the poliomyelitis virus particularly involves the anterior horn cells in the spinal cord, and the brain stem nuclei of the cranial nerves.

Most infections with poliovirus are asymptomatic or only produce a short-lived febrile illness. Fewer than 1% of cases go on to a paralytic phase which may involve the respiratory muscles.

Flaccid paresis involving the muscles of the eyes, face and pharynx, as well as respiratory and limb muscles, leads to hypoventilation, pharyngeal incoordination and aspiration of secretions or gastric contents. Involvement of the cerebral cortex can produce an encephalitis-like illness with impairment of consciousness. The diagnosis may be confirmed by isolation of poliomyelitis virus from stool specimens or throat swabs, and subsequently by serology.

The duration of respiratory muscle paralysis is variable, with some patients making a good recovery in a few weeks, and others needing mechanical support of ventilation for life.

TETANUS

Immunization has also reduced the incidence of tetanus, but sporadic cases continue to occur in unimmunized children.

Wound infection with *Clostridium tetani* is followed by the production of a neurotoxin which binds to the inhibitory neurons in the spinal cord. Loss of inhibitory neuron function leads to spasms in many muscle groups including those of the face, spine and limbs. There are also spasms of the respiratory pump muscles and the muscles of the pharynx and larynx. Trismus (lockjaw) occurs in about 75% of children and adults but is a much less prominent feature in the neonatal form of tetanus.

In neonates, contamination of the umbilical cord stump is the usual portal of entry. In 75% of older children the wound can usually be identified but in other cases it may not be found and this can lead to a delay in diagnosis.

Complications include exhaustion, asphyxia, aspiration pneumonia, pneumothorax, hypertension, vertebral fractures and urinary retention.

The diagnosis of tetanus is predominantly clinical, based on the combination of muscle rigidity and spasms, trismus, presence of a wound, and exclusion of other causes of muscle spasm including seizures. Laboratory investigations are generally unhelpful.

For treatment, see below.

GUILLAIN–BARRÉ SYNDROME

More informatively known as 'acute inflammatory polyradiculoneuropathy', Guillain–Barré syndrome is characterized by widespread demyelination of peripheral nerves leading to abnormalities in motor and sensory function (Ch. 3.3). Involvement of nerves supplying the respiratory pump muscles and those of the pharynx and larynx often leads to respiratory failure, atelectasis and aspiration of saliva.

Classically the abnormalities start in the distal limb motor and sensory nerves and 'ascend' to involve other regions; other patterns of involvement, however, are quite common. Muscle weakness, areflexia and 'glove and stocking' sensory deficits are characteristic findings. Autonomic dysfunction (especially constipation and labile heart rate and blood pressure) is also common. The CSF protein level is usually raised without significant leukocytosis. The speed of onset of symptoms varies from days to weeks. Some patients become very weak over 6–12 hours. Respiratory function (particularly vital capacity) and tests of bulbar function (cough and swallow) should be monitored frequently.

BOTULISM

Clostridium botulinum produces a toxin which disrupts transmission at the neuromuscular junction, causing generalized muscle weakness which can affect all respiratory muscles. Synaptic transmission in the autonomic nervous system is also disturbed, and autonomic disturbances may be the presenting features.

The classical form of botulism, usually seen in adults and older children, follows ingestion of the toxin, when food (often home-processed food) is contaminated with *C. botulinum* and then canned or bottled under anerobic conditions. The organism multiplies and produces large amounts of toxin. Within 1–2 days of ingestion, symptoms of parasympathetic dysfunction appear: nausea, vomiting, constipation, and dry mouth and eyes are followed by weakness of the facial and bulbar muscles with progress to the skeletal and respiratory muscles.

The infantile form of botulism is the most common form of botulism to affect children and is most usually seen in those less than about 8 months of age. It follows ingestion of the *C. botulinum* organism. Several foods, especially honey, have been shown to contain the organism, which, once ingested, multiplies in the gut and releases toxin which is then absorbed. The presenting features are similar to the classical form: lethargy, hypotonia, poor feeding, and facial weakness being the most prominent. Botulinum toxin may be found in the stool, and *C. botulinum* may be isolated from the stool in some cases. A characteristic EMG finding has been described and electrophysiological studies may be helpful. Paralysis may last from a few days to several months, but complete recovery is usual.

MYASTHENIA GRAVIS

Myasthenia gravis is caused by autoantibodies which bind to acetylcholine receptors on the postsynaptic membrane of muscles. There are several different presentations. The classical form typically affects older children, teenagers and adults, but can occur in children as young as 2 years of age. Respiratory muscle involvement may follow a protracted course of motor weakness. Alternatively, it may be part of the initial presentation of myasthenia gravis, which may be precipitated by stresses such as viral infection or surgery. Features of this form include variable weakness (often worse later in the day), more marked involvement of ocular, facial, and bulbar muscles, and a remitting and relapsing course.

Myasthenia gravis can present in the neonatal period. This is usually obvious when the mother is known to have myasthenia gravis, but there are forms where this is not the case. Features of the neonatal form vary from ophthalmoplegia, poor feeding, and hypotonia, to severe paralysis and apnea.

The diagnosis of myasthenia gravis is made by a combination of:

- clinical features
- electrophysiological studies (decreasing amplitude of EMG potentials following repetitive nerve stimulation)
- response to short-acting anticholinesterases (edrophonium)
- the presence of antiacetylcholine receptor antibodies in blood

CRITICAL ILLNESS POLYNEUROPATHY AND MYOPATHY

Several syndromes of polyneuropathy and myopathy have been described following severe illness. Important factors may include:

- sepsis
- use of corticosteroids
- use of neuromuscular blocking agents

The clinical, electrophysiological, and biochemical features of these conditions vary and there appears to be a spectrum from pure neuropathy to pure myopathy but often with overlap of features. These conditions should be considered when a child continues to be weak and to need respiratory support despite apparent recovery from a primary severe illness.

TREATMENT OF RESPIRATORY FAILURE DUE TO A SUSPECTED NEUROLOGIC OR NEUROMUSCULAR CAUSE

In many of these children, the underlying neurological diagnosis is known by the time they present. Respiratory failure may be part of the inevitable progression of the condition (e.g. Duchenne's muscular dystrophy), or triggered by some other stress (e.g. following surgery in a patient with known myasthenia gravis). Chapter 2.1 discusses the signs of progress of respiratory failure in these children. If a neurologic cause of respiratory failure is suspected, investigation as discussed in Chapter 3.3 is undertaken.

Investigative approach

The diagnostic approach includes the following:

- history:
  - age
  - previous health
  - time course and pattern of illness
  - family history
  - previous similar episodes
  - medications
  - access to drugs or poisons
  - exposure to snakes or ticks
  - contact with illness
  - immunization status
- examination:
  - involvement of respiratory pump and bulbar muscles (cough, gag, swallow)
  - pattern of skeletal muscle involvement (proximal or distal, craniofacial)
  - conscious state
  - presence and level of sensory involvement
  - tendon jerks
  - anal tone
  - urinary retention
  - pupillary response
  - presence of sweating, and dry mouth or eyes
  - hypersalivation
  - bronchorrhea
  - observation during sleep
- investigations to consider:
  - bedside evaluation of respiratory function (oximetry, forced vital capacity, tidal volume, maximal inspiratory/expiratory pressures)
  - bedside evaluation of neuromuscular transmission (nerve stimulator: train of four or tetany)
  - blood tests: urea; sodium; potassium; magnesium; calcium; phosphate; creatinine kinase; ESR
  - EMG and nerve conduction studies
  - EEG
  - muscle biopsy
  - edrophonium test
  - *C. botulinum* (toxin and culture from stool)
  - poliovirus culture (stool, throat swab) and serology
  - CT or MRI scan of brain and spinal cord

- polysomnography
- CSF protein, cytology, culture, viral studies
- blood or urine toxicology screen
- venom detection tests
- response to naloxone and flumazenil
- urine metabolic screen

Intubation (airway protection)

Indications include:

- failure of bulbar function with inadequate gag and swallow reflexes to prevent aspiration of saliva
- poor cough with secretion retention and atelectasis or consolidation on chest X-ray

Ventilation

Indications for ventilation are:

- loss of bellows function
- FVC < 15–20 ml/kg
- maximum inspiratory pressure < 20–30 cmH$_2$O
- $Pa\text{CO}_2$ > 6.5–8.0 kPa (50–60 mmHg)

None of these indications is absolute, and some are difficult to measure in sick young children. The rapidity of deterioration is as important as any individual measurement. When a patient with a neurological or neuromuscular condition for which the prognosis is poor presents with respiratory failure, careful discussion should take place with the family and other medical attendants before proceeding to intubation and mechanical ventilation. Options for treatment in this situation include:

- palliative care only
- noninvasive mechanical ventilation (e.g. face mask BiPAP/CPAP)
- short or long-term intubation and mechanical ventilation

The aims of mechanical ventilation in neurologic illness (Ch. 6.4) are:

- to maintain life until an acute reversible condition resolves
- in a few cases, to maintain life in the longer term, even in the absence of

reversibility, provided that this can give the child a tolerable existence
- to achieve normal blood gas levels for that child, or levels that will prevent symptoms of hypoxemia or hypercapnia
- to maintain respiratory muscle strength using a triggered mode of ventilation whenever possible

If there is no improvement in vital capacity or bulbar function after 2 weeks of intubation, consider tracheostomy.

Drug considerations

Many drugs commonly used in the critically ill can exacerbate respiratory failure secondary to neurologic or neuromuscular disorders. In myasthenia gravis, for example, weakness and fatiguability are worsened by neuromuscular blocking agents, both depolarizing, e.g. succinylcholine (suxamethonium) and nondepolarizing (e.g. pancuronium, curare, vecuronium), aminoglycoside antibiotics (e.g. gentamicin, amikacin, neomycin, streptomycin, and tobramycin), other antibiotics (e.g. tetracycline, co-trimoxazole, ciprofloxacin), quinidine, beta-blockers, calcium channel blockers, chloroquine, phenothiazines, and phenytoin.

Ideally all muscle relaxants should be avoided in patients with neuromuscular disease, but if one is needed for tracheal intubation, a short-acting nondepolarizing agent (e.g. vecuronium) is used.

TRANSPORT OF CHILDREN WITH LUNG DISEASE

The child must be stabilized before departure, as transport will usually cause some deterioration owing to movement and handling or to the reduced partial pressure of oxygen at altitude during air transport (Ch. 1.5). If there is any possibility that the child will need respiratory support, the trachea should be intubated before transport. Close attention should be paid to tube size, position, fixation, humidification and suction (Ch. 6.3). The stomach should be drained with a nasogastric tube in all children with respiratory distress as gastric distention may limit diaphragmatic excursion. It is now possible to pressurize many fixed-wing aircraft used for long-distance interhospital transport of critically ill patients. This has alleviated some of the problems of reduced oxygen tension in a nonintubated child and of expanding gas cavities within the body; however, every pneumothorax should be evaluated carefully. Those under tension must be drained and virtually all require chest tube insertion prior to transport.

FURTHER READING

1. Chernick V, Mellins RB. Basic mechanisms of pediatric respiratory disease: cellular and integrative. Philadelphia: BC Decker; 1991
 – (*Extensive discussion of developmental respiratory physiology*)

2. Nunn JF. Applied respiratory physiology, 4th ed. Boston: Butterworths; 1993
 – (*Detailed textbook of respiratory physiology*)

3. West JB. Respiratory physiology–the essentials, 4th ed. Baltimore: Williams & Wilkins; 1990
 – (*Easy to read and contains all the respiratory physiology that is needed for most purposes*)

4. Enright P, Lebowitz M, Cockcroft D. Physiologic measures: pulmonary function tests. Asthma outcome. Am J Crit Care Med 1994; 149: S9–S18
 – (*Reviews the role and accuracy of the various lung function tests in asthma management*)

5. Papo MC, Frank J, Thompson AE. A prospective, randomized study of continuous versus intermittent nebulized albuterol for severe status asthmaticus in children. Crit Care Med 1993; 21(10): 1479–1486
 – (*Study of the efficacy of continuous albuterol dosing*)

6. Gross N, Jenne J, Hess D. Bronchodilator therapy. In: Tobin M, editor. Principles and practice of mechanical ventilation. New York: McGraw-Hill, 1994; pp. 1077–1123
 – (*Review of administration techniques and efficacy of bronchodilators in ventilated patients*)

7. Tuxen D, Oh T. Acute severe asthma. In: Oh TE, editor. Intensive care manual, 4th ed. Oxford: Butterworth Heinemann; 1997; pp. 297–307
 – (*Review of pathophysiology and management, including mechanical ventilation, of very severe asthma in adults and children*)

8. Paulson RH, Spear RM, Peterson BM. New concepts in the treatment of children with acute respiratory distress syndrome. J Pediatr 1995; 127: 163–175
 – (*A comprehensive review of pediatric ARDS with emphasis on treatment including strategies of ventilation and new treatments, for example surfactant and nitric oxide*)

9. Rakshi K, Couriel JM. Management of acute bronchiolitis. Arch Dis Child 1994; 71: 463–469
 – (*Review of the management of bronchiolitis from the British perspective: covers the controversial areas from feeding to ribavirin*)

10. Landau LI, Geelhoed GC. Aerosolized steroids for croup. N Engl J Med 1994; 331: 322–323
 – (*This editorial accompanied one of the steroid trials in croup. It succinctly reviews the management of croup from mist tents to various steroids options*)

11. Masur H. Prevention and treatment of pneumocystis pneumonia. N Engl J Med 1992; 327: 1853–1860
 – (*A useful source of information about chemotherapy and adjuvant therapy for Pneumocystis pneumonia*)

12. Shaffner DH. Neuromuscular disease and respiratory failure. In: Rogers MC, editor. Textbook of pediatric intensive care, 3rd ed. Baltimore: Williams & Wilkins; 1996; pp. 234–261
 – (*Review of neuromuscular causes of severe respiratory failure in children*)

13. Haddad GG, Bazzy-Asaad AR. Respiratory muscle function: implications for respiratory failure. In: Chernick V, Mellins RB, editors. Basic mechanisms of pediatric respiratory disease: cellular and integrative. Philadelphia: BC Decker; 1991; pp. 100–113
 – (*Review of the pathophysiology of respiratory muscle fatigue and failure in infants and children*)

3.2   Cardiovascular system

Margrid Schindler

Congenital heart disease occurs in 0.8% of live births and many critically ill children have cardiac abnormalities. In this chapter, key diagnostic and general management issues relating to the child with heart disease are reviewed. In addition, the management of common cardiovascular problems likely to be encountered during the care of the critically ill child is discussed (see also Chs 2.2, 2.3).

FETAL AND NEONATAL CIRCULATIONS

Knowledge of the fetal circulation and the changes that occur after birth assists with understanding the circulatory changes that occur in congenital heart disease. In the adult circulation there are no intracardiac communications between the systemic and pulmonary circuits, resistances are in series, the systemic circuit is high pressure, and the pulmonary circuit is low pressure. The fetal circulation has intercardiac communications, the pulmonary circuit is high pressure owing to the collapsed lungs and is connected in parallel with the systemic circuit which is at low pressure owing to the low resistance placenta (see Figure 3.1.1). Oxygenated blood from the placenta enters the inferior vena cava (IVC) via the umbilical vein and the ductus venosus in the liver. Blood is then shunted across the right atrium and the foramen ovale to the left atrium (because the free margin of the septum secundum overrides the IVC), and mixes with the pulmonary venous blood. It then enters the left ventricle and is pumped into the ascending aorta supplying the coronary arteries, brain and upper body. Blood returns via the superior vena cava (SVC) to the right atrium and then the right ventricle. From here it is pumped into the pulmonary artery and then across the ductus arteriosus to the descending aorta (only a small proportion of blood enters the lungs because of the high pulmonary vascular resistance of the collapsed lungs). This deoxygenated blood goes to the lower body and the placenta. Prostaglandin E2

is produced in the placenta and helps to keep the ductus arteriosus patent. The oxygen saturation of blood in the ascending aorta is 65% and in the descending aorta it is 55–60%.

At birth the placenta is eliminated, resulting in elevated systemic vascular resistance. A marked decrease in pulmonary vascular resistance occurs after the first breath resulting in increased pulmonary blood flow. The increased pulmonary blood flow elevates left atrial pressure, and removal of the placenta decreases IVC flow which decreases right atrial pressure. This reversal of atrial pressures causes flap closure of the foramen ovale within a few hours of birth. Any factors resulting in high right atrial pressure will cause the foramen ovale to remain open with marked interatrial shunting. Anatomical closure of the foramen ovale usually occurs at 3 months of age; however, 20% of children and adults will have a patent foramen ovale for life. The ductus venosus closes soon after birth, and with the arrival of oxygenated blood from the lungs, the arterial duct constricts and is usually obliterated by 3 weeks of age.

The fetal parallel circulation permits survival with a wide variety of complex congenital heart defects, e.g. obstructed total anomalous pulmonary venous return where survival occurs as only 7% of the cardiac output crosses the lungs, and transposition of the great arteries where intracardiac shunts allow survival. The fetal oxygen saturation of 60–65% and the high levels of fetal hemoglobin explain the relative comfort of a cyanosed baby with transposition of the great arteries (unless the child is profoundly hypoxic and acidotic). The right ventricle performs two-thirds of the total work in the fetal circulation, which explains the right ventricular dominance seen in neonatal ECGs and the relative sparing of obstructed right heart lesions from acute collapse. However, the postnatal circulatory changes may have a marked effect on congenital heart defects resulting in cyanosis, heart failure or circulatory collapse soon after birth. Ductus arteriosus-dependent cardiac lesions include hypoplastic left heart syndrome, transposition of the great arteries, coarctation of the aorta, pulmonary atresia, and total anomalous pulmonary venous connection.

The pulmonary vascular resistance continues to fall with time after birth. In infants with ventricular septal defects or single ventricle physiology, an increasing proportion of the combined ventricular output is committed to the low resistance lungs resulting in increased left-to-right shunting. Initially, to improve systemic output, there is an increase in stroke volume and heart rate. However, eventually cardiac failure and pulmonary edema result during the first few weeks (4–12 weeks) after birth.

PRESENTATIONS OF CARDIAC DISEASE

Presentations of cardiac disease in children vary widely from incidental detection of a heart murmur to acute cardiopulmonary collapse. Common presentations include:

- cyanosis
- shock
- congestive heart failure
- chest pain

CYANOSIS

The important causes of cyanosis in neonates are respiratory and cardiac disease.

Respiratory causes include:

- respiratory distress syndrome (RDS)
- pneumonia
- meconium aspiration syndrome
- persistent pulmonary hypertension of the newborn (PPHN)
- sepsis and central nervous system depression resulting in hypoventilation

Cardiac causes include:

- transposition of the great arteries
- right-to-left shunting due to right ventricular outflow tract obstruction (pulmonary atresia or stenosis, tricuspid atresia)

A guide to differentiating between respiratory and cardiac disease is given in Table 3.2.1.

TABLE 3.2.1 An approach to the 'blue baby': differentiating between cardiac and pulmonary disease

- Is the infant in respiratory distress?
  YES—think pulmonary or severe cardiac failure
  NO—think cardiac

- Are the lung fields on the CXR oligemic?
  YES—think right-sided outflow obstruction
  NO—think pulmonary, transposition of the great arteries or total anomalous pulmonary venous connection

- Does the oxygenation improve when breathing 100% oxygen?
  YES—think pulmonary (PaO_2 > 15 kPa or 110 mmHg excludes cardiac cause)
  NO—think cardiac (transposition of the great arteries) or PPHN
  SMALL INCREASE—think cardiac or pulmonary

Management

Infants with cardiac causes of cyanosis often improve with prostaglandin E_1 infusion 10–50 ng/kg·min to maintain a patent ductus arteriosus to allow systemic to pulmonary flow. This should be commenced prior to transfer to a pediatric cardiac center for further management such as a balloon atrial septostomy, palliative systemic-to-pulmonary shunt or a definitive surgical repair.

Possible side-effects of prostaglandin E_1 include:

- apnea (usually in neonates weighing < 2 kg, and usually appears during the first hour of drug infusion when higher doses are used)
- fever (usually low-grade)
- hypotension (rare)
- cutaneous vasodilatation
- jitteriness, seizures
- gastric outlet obstruction due to antral hyperplasia

The side-effects can be minimized by using the lowest effective dose.

SHOCK AND POOR PERIPHERAL PERFUSION

The three main causes of shock and poor peripheral perfusion in infants are:

- Sepsis:
  - Gram-negative sepsis (*Escherichia coli, Klebsiella, Enterobacter*)
  - Gram-positive sepsis (B-haemolytic streptococcus, *Staphylococcus, Listeria*)
  - viral (cytomegalovirus, herpes simplex virus, coxsackie virus)
- cardiac disease:
  - left heart obstruction: critical aortic stenosis, coarctation of the aorta, hypoplastic left heart syndrome
  - myocardial failure: cardiomyopathy, anomalous left coronary artery (from pulmonary artery), arrhythmias (especially ectopic atrial tachycardia), high-output cardiac failure due to an arteriovenous malformation, obstructed total anomalous pulmonary venous connection
- metabolic disease:
  - lactic acidosis
  - urea cycle disorders
  - effects of birth asphyxia

Careful examination of the pulses and measurement of four limb blood pressures help to differentiate the causes of shock. If the pulses are uneven or very poor, then cardiac causes need to be excluded. A chest X-ray showing cardiomegaly or prominent pulmonary vasculature would also indicate cardiac causes.

Shocked infants require immediate resuscitation with ventilatory support, volume expansion and inotropic support, and this should not await a definitive diagnosis. Antibiotic treatment should be commenced without waiting for culture results. These infants also usually require dextrose infusions for hypoglycemia and correction of metabolic acidosis. If left heart obstruction is suspected, then prostaglandin E_1 infusion 10–50 nanogram/kg·min (0.01–0.05 μg/kg·min) to maintain a patent ductus arteriosus to allow pulmonary to systemic flow is required prior to transfer to a pediatric cardiac center for further management.

CONGESTIVE HEART FAILURE

The symptoms and signs of congestive heart failure in children are tachypnea with costal and subcostal recession, poor feeding, sweating, hepatomegaly and gallop rhythm. The management involves identification and treatment of the underlying cause. Symptomatic management includes salt and water restriction, supplemental oxygen, and diuretic drugs—furosemide (frusemide) and a potassium-sparing diuretic such as spironolactone or amiloride. Cardiac glycosides such as digoxin are still widely used. Angiotensin converting enzyme inhibitors such as captopril are increasingly being used in infants and children with heart failure; however, their role in left-to-right shunts is debated. They are undoubtedly useful in conditions associated with valvular regurgitation and dilated cardiomyopathies.

For the management of severe heart failure, see the section on low cardiac output.

HYPERCYANOTIC EPISODES

In patients with tetralogy of Fallot or severe pulmonary stenosis, the right ventricular outflow tract (RVOT) is very muscular and hyperreactive to stimuli. Acute life-threatening RVOT obstruction may occur with resultant right-to-left shunting and inadequate pulmonary blood flow causing marked cyanosis.

The aim of the initial management is to increase systemic vascular resistance and decrease pulmonary vascular resistance. Systemic vascular resistance is increased acutely by:

- squatting (placing the child in a knee-to-chest position)
- correcting hypovolemia with intravenous fluids (5% albumin 10 ml/kg i.v.)
- vasoconstrictors such as phenylephrine 10–20 μg/kg, metaraminol 10 μg/kg i.v. or norepinephrine (noradrenaline) by infusion

Pulmonary vascular resistance is decreased by administering 100% oxygen via a face mask or endotracheal tube, correcting any respiratory or metabolic acidosis, and giving intravenous morphine 0.1 mg/kg. Propranolol 10–100 μg/kg i.v. also decreases systolic infundibular narrowing of the RVOT. If cyanosis persists, urgent surgical correction of the right ventricular outflow tract obstruction or a systemic-to-pulmonary shunt is required.

CHEST PAIN

Unlike adults, chest pain in children and adolescents is rarely of cardiac origin and its cause is frequently unknown. Investigation initially involves a thorough history, physical examination, chest X-ray and ECG. Possible noncardiac causes of chest pain in children include:

- gastrointestinal reflux
- spontaneous pneumothorax
- pulmonary embolism
- pneumonia or pericarditis
- exercise-induced asthma
- sickle cell crises
- mediastinal masses
- familial Mediterranean fever
- psychiatric disturbances

Angina in infancy may occur due to coronary artery involvement in Kawasaki's disease, anomalous left coronary artery, and prolonged arrhythmias.

INVESTIGATION OF CARDIAC DISEASE

CHEST X-RAY

A chest X-ray (CXR) is a useful investigation in any infant or child with suspected heart disease. The cardiac silhouette is enlarged in most forms of congenital heart disease, and abnormalities in the shape of the cardiac silhouette may indicate specific heart chamber abnormalities. The pulmonary vascularity should be examined closely, as the pulmonary vascular markings are increased in lesions with left-to-right shunts, and decreased in cyanotic right-sided obstructive lesions such a tricuspid or pulmonary atresia. In cyanosed infants with increased pulmonary vascular markings, transposition of the great arteries and total anomalous pulmonary venous connection with obstruction of the pulmonary veins needs to be excluded (Table 3.2.2). There may be evidence of pulmonary edema, and congestive heart failure with Kerley's B lines and cardiomegaly indicating volume overload or poor cardiac contractility. Bronchial morphometric changes (bilateral left or right bronchial morphometry) may indicate anomalous position or transposition of organs. Other noncardiac diseases such as pneumothorax or pneumonia also need to be excluded.

ELECTROCARDIOGRAM

The ECG may be normal even in complex congenital heart disease, but certain patterns are associated with specific defects. The presence of left axis deviation may suggest tricuspid atresia if the infant is cyanotic, or an endocardial cushion defect if the child is not cyanotic. Right axis deviation, right ventricular hypertrophy or right bundle branch block may indicate right-sided lesions, and P wave changes may indicate left or right atrial enlargement. If there is evidence of ischemia, an anomalous origin of the left coronary artery needs to be excluded. The ECG may also show abnormalities of cardiac rhythm (Table 3.2.2).

ECHOCARDIOGRAPHY

The advent of cross-sectional echocardiography has revolutionized the approach to congenital heart disease and it is now the diagnostic technique of choice in experienced hands. It has, in many instances, replaced or obviated the need for invasive cardiac catheterization. Using cross-sectional echocardiography, most anatomical details can be defined, such as the position of the pulmonary veins, the relationship of the atria, ventricles and great vessels, and the presence of atrial or ventricular septal defects. With the addition of color flow mapping, small jets of blood flow across an atrial septal defect (ASD), ventricular septal defect (VSD) or patent ductus arteriosus (PDA) can be detected, and the direction, velocity and turbulence of blood flow can be determined. Doppler echocardiography can be used to estimate ventricular pressures as well as gradients across stenotic valves. Standard M-mode measurements of left ventricular dimensions are used to assess systolic ventricular function and ventricular wall thickness. The shortening fraction (difference between end-diastolic and end-systolic dimensions, divided by the end-diastolic dimensions) is used as an index of systolic ventricular function (normal > 35%).

Transesophageal echocardiography is a useful diagnostic technique in sedated, intubated children

TABLE 3.2.2 Characteristic chest X-ray and ECG changes in infants

CXR or ECG findings	Cardiac lesion
CXR	
Boot-shaped heart, oligemic lung fields	Tetralogy of Fallot or pulmonary atresia
Boot-shaped heart, normal or increased pulmonary vascularity	Pulmonary atresia with VSD and possible aortopulmonary collaterals
Normal cardiac silhouette; decreased, normal or increased pulmonary vascularity	Transposition of the great arteries or tricuspid atresia
Wall-to-wall heart	Ebstein's tricuspid valve anomaly
Small heart, 'ground glass' lungs	Obstructed total anomalous pulmonary venous connection
ECG	
Left axis deviation, left ventricular hypertrophy	Tricuspid atresia
Right axis deviation, left ventricular hypertrophy	Pulmonary atresia with intact ventricular septum
Right axis deviation, right ventricular hypertrophy	Normal heart
	Transposition of great arteries
	Pulmonary atresia with VSD
	Tetralogy of Fallot
	Ebstein's anomaly
Right atrial enlargement	Atrioventricular septal defect
Left and superior axis deviation, right ventricular hypertrophy	
Ischemic ECG changes	Anomalous left coronary artery (from pulmonary artery)
	Kawasaki's disease
ST segment changes	Pericarditis
Unexplained tachycardia	Atrial tachycardia
	Other arrhythmia

VSD, ventricular septal defect.

in the early postoperative period or in adolescents who have suboptimal transthoracic echocardiographic windows. It allows improved imaging of the aorta (to exclude dissection in Marfan's syndrome) and posterior cardiac structures such as the atrial appendages (to detect thrombus). It can provide assessment of ventricular function and adequacy of repair during procedures such as cardiac surgery and weaning from cardiac extracorporeal life support. It is contraindicated in infants less than 2 kg in weight. Significant compression of the airways by the transesophageal probe occurs in 4.5% of cases.

CARDIAC CATHETERIZATION

Cardiac catheterization is an invasive technique used to provide additional hemodynamic information not available from echocardiography, or to undertake interventional intracardiac or intravascular procedures. Cardiac catheterization is usually performed under general anesthesia, and allows improved assessment of hemodynamics. Pressure gradients may be measured using two catheters or rapid pullback of a single catheter from one structure to another. Flow measurements are made using thermodilution or the Fick method. Angiography is performed using nonionic contrast medium through a pressure injector. The major role of cardiac catheterization is in therapeutic options such as valve, artery or vein dilatation, stent implementation, transcatheter occlusions of small vessels, catheter closure of small ASDs, electrophysiologic studies and catheter ablation of accessory conduction pathways.

MAGNETIC RESONANCE IMAGING

Cardiovascular MRI can provide two-dimensional and three-dimensional images of the heart, in addition to blood flow measurements. Magnetic resonance imaging gives excellent delineation of the aorta, distal pulmonary arteries, abnormal venous connections, trachea and bronchi. Hemodynamic information is based on volume determinations of ventricular mass and lumen in systole and diastole and is independent of geometric assumptions used during angiography. This method of imaging and associated techniques such as spectroscopy are undergoing rapid development and will have an increasing role in the future.

LOW CARDIAC OUTPUT

ASSESSMENT OF CARDIAC OUTPUT

Cardiac output is difficult to measure in children. For clinical purposes indirect indicators of cardiac output are usually used (Table 3.2.3). Techniques used for direct measurement of cardiac output include thermodilution, dye dilution, and the Fick, Doppler and bioelectrical impedance methods. None of these methods is ideal, many are highly invasive, and all are subject to considerable variability.

Methods of cardiac monitoring are listed in Table 3.2.4.

MANAGEMENT OF LOW CARDIAC OUTPUT

The determinants of cardiac output are:

- preload
- contractility
- afterload
- heart rate and rhythm

Arterial blood pressure is determined by the cardiac output and the peripheral vascular resistance. Maintaining an adequate cardiac output is vital; however, a certain perfusion pressure is also required for myocardial, cerebral and renal perfusion.

Preload

Preload is the degree to which the myocardium is stretched before it contracts, or the end-diastolic volume of the ventricle. If preload is low, cardiac output improves with intravenous fluid administration to increase the end-diastolic volume; however, a point is eventually reached where the heart may become overdistended, putting it at a mechanical disadvantage, and the cardiac output begins to fall (Frank–Starling curve). Preload is assessed using jugular venous pressure, liver size, CVP, left atrial pressure (LAP), heart rate, and urine output. The current position on the Frank–Starling curve may be determined by giving a small fluid challenge (5 ml/kg colloid) and observing the response. If the LAP or CVP rises by 3–4 mmHg and lingers with minimal improvement in cardiac output, the patient is not hypovolemic and an increase in inotropic support is required. If preload is too high, diuretics and vasodilators may be required to decrease myocardial overdistention and thus improve myocardial contractility. Concomitant imaging with cross-sectional echocardiography may be helpful.

Contractility

Early inotropic support is beneficial in the child with low cardiac output, initially with

TABLE 3.2.3 **Clinical assessment of cardiac output**		
Clinical indicator	**Low cardiac output**	**Adequate cardiac output**
Peripheral perfusion	Poor capillary refill	Capillary refill < 3 s
Core–peripheral temperature gradient	> 3°C	< 3°C
Pulses	Impalpable or weak	Full peripheral pulses
Urine output	< 1ml/kg	> 1ml/kg
Mental status	Combative, disorientated	Cooperative
Arterial pressure wave form	Small area under curve	Large area under curve
Metabolic acidosis	Base excess > −5 mmol/L	Base excess < −5 mmol/L
Blood pressure	Normal or low	High, normal, or low and peripherally vasodilated
Respiratory muscle function	Poor	Good
Gut function	Poor	Absorbing feeds

TABLE 3.2.4 Cardiac monitoring

Method	Information gained
ECG	Heart rate and rhythm
Arterial blood pressure	Mean arterial and diastolic perfusion pressures
Central venous pressure	Right ventricular preload
Temperature: core (rectal) and peripheral (foot)	Hyper- and hypothermia, cardiac output via core/peripheral gradient
Pulse oximetry	Oxygenation
Urine output	Cardiac output and renal perfusion
Peripheral perfusion	Cardiac output
Base deficit and lactate	Metabolic acidosis due to low cardiac output
Pulmonary artery catheter	Pulmonary artery pressure measurement
Thermodilution and dye dilution	Cardiac output
Left atrial pressure	Left ventricular preload

catecholamines such as dopamine, or dobutamine, followed by epinephrine (adrenaline) and/or norepinephrine (noradrenaline) depending on the response to treatment (Table 3.2.5). Catecholamines increase myocardial contractility through their action on the cardiac β-adrenergic receptors which increases intracellular cyclic AMP, resulting in increased intracellular calcium concentrations during systole.

In addition to inotropic support, reversible causes of decreased myocardial contractility such as hypoxia, acidosis and myocardial depression due to drugs such as barbiturates and benzodiazepines should be corrected.

Possible side-effects of catecholamines include tachydysrhythmias and increased afterload from activation of α-adrenergic receptors resulting in vasoconstriction. Sustained use of catecholamines can also lead to downregulation of β-receptors and thus decrease their efficiency.

Phosphodiesterase inhibitors such as amrinone and enoximone inhibit the breakdown of cyclic AMP, and thus also increase myocardial contractility through increased intracellular calcium during systole, however, they cause less tachycardia and vasoconstriction as they do not stimulate the α-

and β-adrenergic receptors. They also have vasodilator properties and are lusitropic (improve diastolic relaxation by improving the clearance of intracellular calcium back into the sarcoplasmic reticulum during diastole), a useful characteristic in patients with impaired diastolic ventricular function.

Afterload

Increased afterload is poorly tolerated in patients with myocardial dysfunction. Afterload reduction may improve cardiac output by decreasing myocardial work and oxygen requirement, provided no fixed outflow tract obstruction (e.g. aortic stenosis) is present. Physiological causes of increased afterload such as hypothermia and pain should be corrected. Acutely, shorter-acting vasodilators such as nitroglycerin (glyceryl trinitrate) (venodilator and mild arteriolar dilator), sodium nitroprusside (potent arteriolar dilator), or amrinone or enoximone (phosphodiesterase inhibitors) are used. In more stable patients who are tolerating enteral feeding, angiotensin converting enzyme (ACE) inhibitors such as captopril may be used. Close monitoring of blood pressure

TABLE 3.2.5 A guide to choosing appropriate catecholamine support

Inotrope	Dose (μg/kg·min)	α Vasoconstriction	β_1 Inotropic	β_2 Vasodilator	DA Renal
Dopamine	3–20	++	++	±	++
Dobutamine	5–20	±	++	++	–
Dopexamine	1–6	±	±	++	++
Epinephrine (adrenaline)	0.05–1	++	++	++	–
Norepinephrine (noradrenaline)	0.05–1	+++	++	±	–
Isoproterenol (isoprenaline)	0.05–1	–	+++	+++	–

is essential and hypotension can be corrected with volume expansion.

Heart rate and rhythm

It is essential to maintain sinus rhythm or an atrioventricular rhythm using atrioventricular sequential pacing, as this preserves the 'atrial kick' which contributes approximately 10–25% to the cardiac output.

Tachycardia (especially over > 180 beats/min) may result in poor myocardial filling and perfusion. Treat the causes of tachycardia such as hypovolemia, fever, pain, excessive inotropic support, and arrhythmias whenever possible. A 12-lead ECG is essential to diagnose the presence of an arrhythmia and to document the response to agents such as adenosine.

Other contributory factors

Decrease oxygen consumption: avoid factors that increase metabolic demand, such as pyrexia, excessive respiratory effort or other skeletal muscle activity. Assisted ventilation and analgesics such as morphine decrease oxygen consumption.

Exclude tamponade and structural lesions: reversible causes of decreased cardiac output must be excluded (cardiac tamponade, tension pneumothorax, subaortic stenosis, coarctation of the aorta). Maintain a high clinical index of suspicion of cardiac tamponade in the early postoperative period. Cross-sectional echocardiography is very useful to exclude subaortic stenosis, coarctation of the aorta, and pericardial effusions causing tamponade.

Sternal opening and cardiac decompression

In the postoperative cardiac surgical patient whose cardiac output remains low despite the above measures, consider sternal opening (to relieve myocardial compression due to postoperative myocardial edema).

MECHANICAL CARDIAC SUPPORT

Venoarterial extracorporeal life support or a left ventricular assist device may benefit children with acute, severe, but rapidly reversible myocardial failure unresponsive to maximal conventional therapy.

Aortic balloon counterpulsation is not beneficial in small children owing to the distensibility of the aorta.

The normal range for heart rate and blood pressure in children is given in Table 3.2.6.

Mechanical ventilation in paediatric heart disease

Cardiovascular disease can often lead to respiratory failure, because of its effect on pulmonary blood flow and hydrostatic pressures, which influence gas exchange and pulmonary mechanics (e.g. to cause pulmonary edema). Certain cardiac lesions may also result in vascular compression of the airways. Conversely, important changes in hemodynamics can occur during respiratory-induced fluctuations in intrathoracic pressure, especially during positive pressure ventilation. Mechanical ventilation increases intrathoracic pressure, thus decreasing venous return and right atrial filling. This results in decreased cardiac output, especially if there is hypovolemia. Thus in right-sided lesions that are particularly preload-dependent (such as cavopulmonary shunts and the Fontan circulation), spontaneous respiration rather than positive pressure ventilation is preferable. Changes in intrathoracic pressure also affect left ventricular afterload, with negative inspiratory (pleural) pressure inhibiting left ventricular ejection by increasing the ventricular transmural pressure required to eject blood into the aorta

TABLE 3.2.6 **Normal range for heart rate and blood pressure at various ages**		
Age (years)	**Mean arterial blood pressure (95% range) (mmHg)**	**Heart rate (range) (beat/min)**
Term newborn	40–60	123 (95–145)
0.5–1	50–90	134 (110–175)
1–2	50–100	119 (105–170)
3–4	55–100	108 (80–140)
5–7	60–90	100 (70–120)
8–11	60–90	91 (60–110)
12–15	65–95	85 (60–100)

(which is at atmospheric pressure). This is particularly important in the failing heart, and is exacerbated by stiff lungs which result in increased negative intrathoracic pressures. In left ventricular failure, positive pressure ventilation reduces left ventricular afterload and may increase cardiac output by generating positive intrapleural pressure and decreasing left ventricular transmural pressure. Mechanical ventilation also decreases oxygen consumption by decreasing the work of breathing.

In the postoperative cardiac surgical patient, anesthesia and thoracic surgery reduce the functional residual capacity (FRC) of the lungs which may result in atelectasis, hypoxia, and respiratory failure. Mechanical ventilation postoperatively is beneficial as it increases FRC toward normal, increases oxygenation, reduces the work of breathing, allows control of $Paco_2$ and facilitates tracheal toilet. Postoperative mechanical ventilation is continued until there is hemostasis, and the patient is hemodynamically stable with acceptable cardiac performance on minimal cardiac support. Causes of failure to wean from ventilation postoperatively include:

- cardiac failure
- respiratory depression due to narcotics
- phrenic nerve palsy (especially if age < 6 months)
- pleural effusion, chylothorax
- pulmonary infection
- pericardial tamponade
- neurologic complications and poor cough
- recurrent laryngeal nerve paresis (failed extubation)

FLUID AND ELECTROLYTE MANAGEMENT IN THE CARDIAC PATIENT

In heart failure, or following cardiopulmonary bypass, children generally have sodium and total body water overloads, although intravascular fluid levels may be depleted. Renal regulation of sodium and water is poor and in intubated patients insensible water losses from the respiratory tract are reduced. Treat such patients with fluid restriction to 60–80% of normal maintenance fluids initially. Use appropriate fluid boluses with colloid to maintain intravascular volume. Start diuretics early, once the hemodynamics have stabilized. Restrict sodium intake to 1 mmol/kg per day. This may be provided in the arterial line flush solution alone in small infants. Hypokalemia, hypomagnesemia, and hypocalcemia are common and frequently cause arrhythmias. Total body potassium content is low and the patient is often in negative potassium balance. This can be corrected with boluses of potassium chloride 0.2–0.5 mmol/kg administered over 1 hour through a central line in addition to 2 mmol/kg per day of potassium in the maintenance fluid.

Ionized calcium measurements should guide calcium replacement (generally only required in unstable or symptomatic patients). Hypomagnesemia is corrected with a slow infusion of magnesium chloride 0.4 mmol/kg.

MANAGEMENT OF LOW URINE OUTPUT IN THE CARDIAC PATIENT

If the urine output is less than 0.5 ml/kg for longer than 2 hours, ensure catheter patency by irrigating the catheter, and optimize preload by giving aliquots of 10 ml/kg of colloid. Optimize cardiac output with inotropic support to improve renal blood flow. If filling pressures are high (CVP > 14 mmHg or LAP > 10 mmHg), give furosemide (frusemide) 1 mg/kg intravenously. A continuous infusion of furosemide (0.1–1.0 mg/kg·hr) may result in improved diuretic response, decreased dosage requirements, and fewer adverse effects. If there has been no response, a bolus of frusemide 5 mg/kg or ethacrynic acid 1 mg/kg may be effective. If the above measures are unsuccessful, consider early dialysis (peritoneal dialysis or continuous venovenous hemofiltration).

A diagnostic urinalysis should be performed in addition to a renal ultrasound scan to exclude obstruction and other reversible causes of renal failure.

ANALGESIA AND SEDATION

Analgesia should be provided, usually in the form of a morphine infusion at 10–40 µg/kg·h. In unstable ventilated patients, skeletal muscle relaxation is used initially to minimize oxygen consumption from muscle activity. Benzodiazepines and other sedatives should be used cautiously in unstable patients with low cardiac output, as boluses may cause profound hypotension. It is important to exclude reversible causes of the restlessness such as low cardiac output, hypoxia, inappropriate ventilator settings, pain, or a full bladder, before prescribing sedative drugs.

TEMPERATURE CONTROL

Hyperpyrexia increases oxygen consumption and the incidence of arrhythmias. Control of hyperpyrexia is achieved initially with nasogastric or rectal acetaminophen (paracetamol) and ice compresses to the head and trunk. If this is unsuccessful, then muscle paralysis (to prevent shivering) and a cooling blanket are used. The addition of a vasodilator may also facilitate cooling by promoting skin blood flow.

PROPHYLACTIC ANTIBIOTICS

In children with structural heart disease, adequate antimicrobial (especially staphylococcal) prophylaxis is required at the time of cardiac surgery or procedures, and should be continued for 24 hours. Flucloxacillin and an aminoglycoside are commonly used but specific therapy must be guided by the local flora. If sepsis is suspected clinically, appropriate antibiotics are used after the relevant cultures have been taken. Line- and catheter-related sepsis are common, thus all indwelling lines and catheters should be removed as early as possible.

NUTRITION

Early nutrition, preferably enteral nutrition, is beneficial to improve respiratory, myocardial and immune function.

CONGENITAL HEART DISEASE

RATIONALE FOR EARLY SURGICAL TREATMENT

Corrective cardiac surgery for congenital heart disease is now being performed earlier, before the onset of complications of the heart lesion. Untreated cyanotic heart lesions result in severe polycythemia with hyperviscosity, vascular sludging and thrombosis (especially cerebral thromboses), severe heart failure, decreased exercise tolerance and eventual death. Lesions with left-to-right shunting (ASD, VSD) result in pulmonary hypertension and pulmonary vascular remodeling with vascular smooth muscle hypertrophy and extension of the smooth muscle into smaller vessels. If these lesions are left untreated, progressive arterial fibrosis and obliteration of the pulmonary vascular bed occur, with irreversible severe pulmonary hypertension, right-to-left shunting, right heart failure and death (Eisenmenger's syndrome).

Palliative shunts and pulmonary artery banding can cause anatomical distortion of the pulmonary vasculature, and where possible full early corrective surgery should be performed (Table 3.2.7).

CARDIOPULMONARY BYPASS

Cardiopulmonary bypass (CPB) is used to facilitate cardiac surgical procedures that require direct 'open' access to the heart. Blood is drained from the right atrium (via a right atrial or superior and inferior vena cava cannula) and is passed through a membrane oxygenator to allow exchange of oxygen and carbon dioxide. The oxygenated blood is then warmed or cooled as required and returned to the aorta using a roller or centrifugal pump. The heart and lungs are isolated from the body through the use of snares and an aortic cross-clamp is placed just distal to the aortic valve, so that the surgeon can operate on a bloodless, motionless heart. The duration of aortic cross-clamping is the length of time the heart and the coronary arteries are isolated from the circulation of blood. To minimize ischemic injury to the heart, the heart is cooled (frequently to temperatures as low as 15–18°C) to drastically reduce myocardial oxygen consumption. In addition, asystole is artificially induced by infusing a high-potassium cardioplegia solution into the coronary arteries either directly or via the proximal aorta. Anticoagulation is required during CPB and is achieved using heparin. Hemodilution is used to counteract the increased blood viscosity that occurs during hypothermia.

TABLE 3.2.7 Types of surgical correction and outcome

Anomaly/operation	Acute mortality (%)	Outcome Immediate	Long-term
PDA	< 2	Total correction	
ASD	< 1	Total correction	
VSD	< 5	Total correction	
Tetralogy of Fallot	3–5	Low cardiac output due to restrictive RV physiology	Pulmonary regurgitation Subpulmonary restenosis
Arterial switch	5–10	Ventricular dysfunction	Coronary artery abnormalities
Coarctation of aorta	1–15	Residual abnormality	Recoarctation Aortic valve abnormalities
Atrioventricular septal defects	10	Valvar regurgitation	Valvar regurgitation (possible need for prosthetic valve replacement)
Total anomalous pulmonary venous connection (TAPVC)	5	Residual abnormality	Pulmonary vein restenosis Pulmonary hypertension
Glenn–Fontan procedure	8–12	Palliative	Cardiac failure Thrombosis Arrhythmia
Systemic-to-pulmonary shunts	5	Palliative	Shunt thrombosis Distortion of branch pulmonary arteries
Pulmonary artery banding	5	Palliative	Pulmonary stenosis Distortion of main pulmonary artery

In some small infants, profound hypothermic (15–18°C) circulatory arrest with no CPB is used to improve surgical exposure and allow a precise operative repair on a very small heart. Circulatory arrest time is usually limited to approximately 60 minutes to minimize organ dysfunction. Compared with low-flow cardiopulmonary bypass, circulatory arrest is associated with a higher likelihood of seizures and other neurological sequelae.

Despite the extensive steps taken to improve the biocompatibility of CPB, many components of the systemic inflammatory response are activated during this procedure, leading to increased capillary permeability and multiorgan dysfunction postoperatively. Modified ultrafiltration used immediately after CPB appears to decrease post-bypass organ dysfunction. The postoperative effects of CPB include:

- increased capillary permeability and edema
- decreased myocardial function
- decreased renal function
- decreased neurological function owing to emboli or low cerebral perfusion

- Abnormal platelet function and thrombocytopenia
- dilution of coagulation factors
- fever in first 24 hours after the procedure
- hyperglycemia

COAGULATION AND HEMOSTASIS AFTER CARDIAC SURGERY

Postoperative blood loss is abnormal if the mediastinal drain losses are greater than 3 ml/kg·h for longer than 3 hours or if blood loss is incessant despite attempts to normalize coagulation. Surgical bleeding is the most common cause of postoperative blood loss; however, a secondary coagulopathy may also develop. Coagulation studies—activated clotting time (ACT), prothrombin time (PT), activated partial thromboplastin time (APTT), fibrinogen and platelets—should be performed. Bleeding greater than 10 ml/kg·h requires urgent surgical review.

The 'rule of Ps' can be useful to guide the management of postoperative bleeding:

- if the ACT and APTT are prolonged and the PT is normal, consider residual or rebound heparin effect from CPB and give *protamine* 1 mg/kg slowly

- if the APTT, PT and fibrinogen are all abnormal, then dilution of coagulation factors on CPB, or consumption of clotting factors is the most likely cause, requiring 10 ml/kg fresh frozen *plasma* and review
- if bleeding continues, give *platelets* 10 ml/kg, as the number of platelets circulating is reduced by CPB, and those remaining have been activated and do not function normally
- if the coagulation profile is normal but bleeding still exceeds 3 ml/kg·h, surgical reexploration is required (*Prolene*)

If hypotension, low cardiac output, and tachycardia occur, with a rising CVP and LAP, consider *cardiac tamponade*, especially if the chest drain losses have decreased abruptly. Milk the chest drains, maintain the cardiac output with fluid boluses and inotropic support, and arrange urgent sternal opening and surgical evacuation of clot (echocardiographic diagnosis of the clot may be unreliable as the clot may be localized behind the heart and difficult to visualize).

If bleeding continues despite the above, the fibrinolysis inhibitors aminocaproic acid or tranexamic acid may be useful. Correction of hypothermia also improves coagulation. Desmopressin has not decreased transfusion requirements in children. Intraoperative and postoperative use of aprotinin, a protease inhibitor, reduces perioperative blood loss and the need for blood transfusion. It should be continued for the first 4–6 hours postoperatively, until the chest drain losses decrease.

STERNAL OPENING AND CARDIAC DECOMPRESSION

If the postoperative cardiac surgical patient still remains unstable and in low cardiac output despite the measures outlined earlier, consider sternal opening for relief of myocardial compression due to myocardial edema. Chest opening lowers left- and right-sided filling pressures, improves myocardial perfusion, and relieves compression from extracardiac conduits. The incidence of sternal wound infection from this procedure is relatively low.

CARDIAC SURGERY NOT REQUIRING CPB

Systemic arterial to pulmonary arterial shunts, pulmonary artery banding, repair of coarctation of the aorta and ligation of a patent ductus arteriosus are all performed without CPB. These procedures usually involve a thoracotomy with its inherent problems of pain and atelectasis. The patients all require good analgesia and chest physiotherapy postoperatively.

SYSTEMIC ARTERIAL TO PULMONARY ARTERIAL SHUNTS

Systemic arterial to pulmonary arterial shunts are designed to improve pulmonary blood flow in patients with right-sided obstructive lesions presenting with severe cyanosis in whom a definitive repair cannot be performed immediately. Usually a modified Blalock–Taussig (MBT) shunt is performed using a 3.5–4 mm Goretex shunt from the subclavian or innominate artery to the ipsilateral pulmonary artery. Occasionally a central shunt from the aorta to the pulmonary artery is created via a median sternotomy to avoid distortion of the branch pulmonary arteries.

Flow across the shunt depends on the systemic arterial pressure, the diameter and length of the subclavian artery, size of the shunt, and the pulmonary vascular resistance. The expected systemic oxygen saturation postoperatively is 70–80%, indicating approximately equal systemic and pulmonary flows. Unilateral (or bilateral) pulmonary edema may occur due to the sudden increase in pulmonary blood flow, and is managed with ventilation, fluid restriction and diuretics. Arterial blood pressure measurements in the arm on the same side as the shunt may be falsely low.

Inotropic support may be required to increase systemic arterial pressure and cardiac output to improve blood flow across a small shunt if the oxygen saturations are low. Also exclude pulmonary disorders (pneumothorax, atelectasis) with a CXR, and kinking or clotting of the shunt with an echocardiogram or cardiac catheter if the oxygen saturation remains low (echocardiography, even with color flow mapping, may not be helpful).

Small shunts may require initial heparinization to decrease the risk of clotting.

Signs of overshunting (excessive pulmonary blood flow) include high systemic oxygen saturations, persistent pulmonary edema, cardiac failure, and low systemic diastolic arterial pressures despite ventilation with $F_{IO_2} = 0.21$ and normocapnia. A residual patent ductus arteriosus or aortopulmonary window must be excluded. Surgical refashioning of the shunt may be required if mechanical ventilation and diuretics are unsuccessful (see also management of parallel circulation, stage 1 Norwood).

PULMONARY ARTERIAL BANDING

Pulmonary arterial banding is a palliative surgical procedure for patients with high pulmonary blood flow due to excessive left-to-right shunting. The aim is to reduce the flow of blood into the lungs, thus preventing the early onset of pulmonary hypertension. It involves placement of a ligature around the main pulmonary artery, to produce a circumferential narrowing. It is most commonly employed in small infants with high pulmonary blood flow secondary to multiple VSDs.

Pulmonary artery banding acutely increases right ventricular afterload, and inotropic support may be required if right ventricular failure develops. Acute bradycardia after banding indicates acute right heart failure and may necessitate urgent removal of the band. Systemic oxygen saturations are reduced to approximately 80% following banding, facilitating an improved balance between systemic and pulmonary blood flow. Oxygen saturations greater than 90% indicate excessive pulmonary blood flow and an ineffective band.

COARCTATION OF THE AORTA

Infants often present shortly after closure of the arterial duct, resulting typically in right upper limb hypertension, absent femoral pulses and grossly inadequate systemic perfusion. Severe metabolic acidosis and hypoglycemia are common. *Urgent resuscitation is required,* which must include an infusion of prostaglandin E_1 to reopen the arterial duct. Additional cardiac anomalies, such as a bicuspid aortic valve, are common in these infants. In older children, coarctation of the aorta causes upper limb hypertension and decreased or absent femoral pulses.

Postoperatively, ventilation and inotropic support may be required in young infants, especially if cardiac failure was present preoperatively. Older infants and children often develop postoperative paradoxical hypertension lasting 1–5 days, due to release of norepinephrine (noradrenaline), renin and angiotensin. An infusion of sodium nitroprusside is effective but may cause reflex tachycardia requiring the addition of a beta-blocker such as propranolol. A labetalol infusion (0.5–2 mg/kg·h) and later oral captopril are also effective.

Mesenteric arteritis may result from the introduction of pulsatile flow causing gut vessel reperfusion injury, and can lead to bowel ischemia and infarction. Spinal cord ischemia from intraoperative aortic cross-clamp may result in postoperative paraplegia.

Interrupted aortic arch represents the extreme form of coarctation of the aorta. It is often associated with DiGeorge syndrome, with associated cellular immune deficiency, and hypocalcemia due to hypoparathyroidism. Such infants require calcium supplementation and must only receive irradiated blood to prevent graft-versus-host disease.

PATENT DUCTUS ARTERIOSUS

Patency of the arterial duct is most frequently seen in infants with lung disease. Left-to-right shunting through the duct results in pulmonary plethora and heart failure.

Failure to induce duct closure medically with fluid restriction, diuretics and indomethacin is an indication for early surgical ligation in symptomatic neonates. An isolated PDA can also occur in older children and should be closed electively, either using a catheter-deployed occlusion device or surgically, as late pulmonary hypertension can occur. Postoperative problems include pulmonary atelectasis and pulmonary hypertension. Injury to other structures near the arch may occur, such as injury to the thoracic duct, recurrent laryngeal nerve and phrenic nerve. Recanalization of the duct can occur after simple suture ligation, and other vascular structures such as the pulmonary artery have been inadvertently ligated.

CARDIAC SURGERY REQUIRING CPB

ATRIAL SEPTAL DEFECT

An isolated atrial septal defect is usually asymptomatic in childhood. Congestive heart failure and pulmonary hypertension typically occur in the second or third decade of life. Atrial septal defects are usually repaired surgically with a pericardial patch, or stitch closure on CPB; however, some can be closed with endovascularly deployed clamshell devices. Postoperative complications are uncommon and the patients are usually extubated within a few hours of surgery. Postoperative pericardial effusions can occur.

ATRIOVENTRICULAR SEPTAL DEFECT, VENTRICULAR SEPTAL DEFECT

Atrioventricular and ventricular septal defects usually present with congestive cardiac failure and failure to gain weight at 1–2 months of age, owing to progressively increasing left-to-right shunting as the pulmonary vascular resistance falls postnatally. Complications of the excessive pulmonary blood flow include ventricular volume overload, cardiac failure and pulmonary hypertension. The repair, which involves patching the septal defects and reconstructing left and right atrioventricular (AV) valves from the common AV valve, is usually performed at 2–3 months of age.

Potential postoperative problems include decreased myocardial contractility, acute postoperative pulmonary hypertension leading to acute right ventricular failure (unusual with earlier repair), atrioventricular valvular dysfunction (following AVSD repair) resulting in high left atrial pressures, residual VSD patch leaks, and arrhythmias (see also maintenance of cardiac output, arrhythmia and pulmonary hypertension sections).

Severe preoperative heart failure and residual AV valve regurgitation are associated with delayed postoperative recovery. If inotropic support is required, agents such as dobutamine and enoximone or amrinone may be preferred as they provide inotropic support while also decreasing systemic and pulmonary vascular resistance.

TOTAL ANOMALOUS PULMONARY VENOUS RETURN

In this condition, the pulmonary veins drain to the right atrium, with systemic oxygenation only occurring if mixing takes place at atrial level. Infants present with cyanosis and respiratory distress, often with diffuse opacification of the lung fields on chest X-ray. Presentation occurs shortly after birth if the anomalous veins are obstructed, and later with cyanosis and cardiac failure if the veins are unobstructed. Urgent surgery is required. During surgery, the confluence where the pulmonary veins join is reimplanted into the posterior wall of the left atrium, and the ASD is closed. Potential postoperative problems include pulmonary hypertension, decreased myocardial function, arrhythmias, high left atrial pressures due to a small, noncompliant left atrium, and residual or late pulmonary vein restenosis. The prognosis is poor in patients with late pulmonary vein restenosis.

TETRALOGY OF FALLOT

Children with tetralogy of Fallot may be asymptomatic, or present with cyanosis and hypercyanotic episodes (spells). The surgical repair of tetralogy of Fallot requires patch closure of the VSD and enlargement of the right ventricular outflow tract. The RVOT enlargement involves resection of infundibular muscle and dilatation or incision of the pulmonary valve annulus. If there is severe pulmonary stenosis, a transannular pericardial patch is placed across the pulmonary valve resulting in free pulmonary valve regurgitation.

Common postoperative problems include decreased right ventricular function (both systolic and diastolic dysfunction) due to preexisting right ventricular hypertrophy, fibrosis, ventriculotomy and noncontractile VSD patch material in the ventricular septum. Right ventricular failure and low cardiac output may occur, especially if a transannular patch was necessary.

Arrhythmias (e.g. junctional ectopic tachycardia), residual RVOT obstruction, pulmonary regurgitation, and residual VSD patch leak may also occur (see also arrhythmia management and maintenance of cardiac output outline). Early evaluation by echocardiography can be valuable.

Postoperative management of the right heart failure includes adequate preload (these patients may require a high CVP, as the severe right ventricular diastolic dysfunction results in a 'restrictive physiology' with poor ventricular filling), inotropic support and measures to reduce pulmonary vascular resistance to reduce right ventricular afterload. Phosphodiesterase inhibitors such as enoximone or amrinone improve diastolic dysfunction and may be beneficial. Pleural effusions, ascites and pericardial effusions are common owing to the high CVP and frequently require drainage. Liver dysfunction may also complicate right heart failure resulting in hypoglycemia and coagulopathy.

ARTERIAL SWITCH FOR TRANSPOSITION OF GREAT ARTERIES

Infants with transposition of the great arteries (TGA) and intact ventricular septum usually present with profound hypoxia and cyanosis as there may be little mixing between the circulations. Initial management involves maintenance of ductal patency with infusions of prostaglandin E_1 and later a balloon atrial septostomy to improve mixing at atrial level. Previously, atrial switch (Senning or Mustard) procedures were performed for TGA, but late onset of arrhythmias, obstruction to the systemic or pulmonary venous pathways and systemic ventricular failure have led to the current preference for the arterial switch (Jatene) procedure. This procedure, performed in the first few weeks of life while the left ventricle is still adjusted to a relatively high pulmonary vascular resistance, appears to have improved long-term outcome. Surgical repair involves transecting the aorta from the right ventricle and the pulmonary artery from the left ventricle just distal to the valve commissures, and switching the aorta to the left ventricle and the pulmonary artery to the right ventricle. The coronary arteries are removed from above the pulmonary valve with a cuff of tissue and are reimplanted into the neoaorta.

Common postoperative problems include impaired ventricular function (the ejection fraction decreases by 30% or more in the first 6 hours postoperatively), and coronary artery kinking or obstruction causing myocardial ischemia. Other postoperative problems include arrhythmias and pulmonary hypertension. Postoperative management includes maintenance of cardiac output with adequate preload. Excessive volume is poorly tolerated as dilatation of the ventricles may cause distortion to the coronary artery anastomosis. Thus the left atrial pressure should be kept below 8–10 mmHg. An optimal coronary perfusion pressure should be maintained and nitroglycerin (glyceryl trinitrate) infusion may be useful as a coronary artery vasodilator. Inotrope support should be commenced early in addition to afterload reduction. Measures to reduce pulmonary vascular resistance are required to prevent postoperative pulmonary hypertension. Serial cross-sectional echocardiography is a useful adjunct to assess ventricular function and inotrope requirements.

TRUNCUS ARTERIOSUS

In truncus arteriosus a single ventricular outflow tract (truncus) feeds both the aorta and pulmonary arteries. A VSD is always present. These infants usually present with congestive heart failure within the first few weeks of life owing to high pulmonary blood flow. The preoperative circulation is similar to the stage 1 Norwood parallel circulation, and a careful balance between systemic and pulmonary blood flow must be maintained (see management of Norwood circulation). Surgical repair involves removing the pulmonary arteries from the truncus and implanting them into a pulmonary homograft which is attached to the right ventricle by a vertical ventriculotomy. The VSD is also closed, and the arterial trunk functions as the ascending aorta. Postoperative problems include impaired myocardial function due to the effects of CPB, preoperative myocardial ischemia (low diastolic perfusion pressures due to high pulmonary blood flow, and truncal valve regurgitation) and the ventriculotomy. Postoperative pulmonary hypertension is common (see pulmonary hypertension section). Possible residual anatomical problems include truncal (aortic) valve regurgitation, and distortion of the pulmonary arteries.

AORTIC STENOSIS

The presentation of aortic stenosis ranges from incidental detection in asymptomatic older children with mild stenosis, to presentation in the early neonatal period with shock, heart failure and duct-dependent systemic blood flow. When the infant is stabilized, either a transcatheter balloon valvoplasty or surgical valvotomy are performed. Surgical valvotomy is performed through a median sternotomy using CPB. The fused valve commissures are incised under direct vision. In older children therapeutic options include balloon aortic valvoplasty, aortic valve replacement or Ross procedure (pulmonary autograft to form the new aorta and a homograft to replace the original pulmonary valve). The advantage of the Ross procedure is that formal anticoagulation is unnecessary.

Postoperative problems include residual left ventricular dysfunction which occurs even after successful relief of obstruction. Function usually improves with time, but occasionally severe irreversible damage has been sustained. Residual aortic stenosis may occur and the valvotomy may create aortic regurgitation. Congenital aortic stenosis may also be associated with DiGeorge syndrome (see coarctation of the aorta).

PULMONARY STENOSIS OR ATRESIA

Critical pulmonary valve stenosis or atresia in the presence of an intact ventricular septum results in severe or complete obstruction of the RVOT with duct-dependent pulmonary blood flow. These infants usually present with severe cyanosis, right heart failure and acidosis when the duct closes. Some patients with severe hypoplasia of the right ventricle and tricuspid valve annulus may have a right ventricular-dependent coronary blood supply with coronary artery sinusoids and fistulas. Decompression of the right ventricle in these patients would lead to mycardial ischemia and infarction, so a palliative systemic to pulmonary shunt is performed, with a possible Fontan procedure later.

If a right ventricular-dependent coronary circulation is not present, a pulmonary valvotomy or transannular patch is performed to provide unobstructed pulmonary blood flow and allow regression of the right ventricular hypertrophy. Despite relief of the obstruction, the small, noncompliant right ventricle has a restrictive physiology and commonly results in elevated right ventricular end-diastolic pressure and persistent right-to-left shunting at atrial level with severe cyanosis requiring a modified Blalock–Taussig shunt. As the right ventricular function improves and right ventricular compliance increases, the right-to-left shunting decreases, and the shunt may then be taken down either surgically or coil embolized using a transcatheter approach.

Postoperative problems include possible myocardial ischemia from unrecognized right ventricular-dependent coronary circulation, right ventricular dysfunction, residual pulmonary stenosis and low cardiac output. Low cardiac output may also develop from 'circular shunt' where the transannular patch results in pulmonary and tricuspid regurgitation, and blood may flow backwards from the Blalock–Taussig shunt to the right atrium, resulting in inadequate systemic blood flow with oliguria, acidosis, and systemic hypotension. Measures to reduce pulmonary vascular resistance (increased oxygenation, alkalosis and pulmonary vasodilators) should be commenced, and correction of the tricuspid regurgitation or narrowing of the Blalock–Taussig shunt may also be required.

Some children with pulmonary atresia and VSD may develop an extensive bronchial collateral circulation (aortopulmonary collaterals) and relative hypoplasia of the distal pulmonary arteries. These children require staged repairs with systemic to pulmonary shunts and unifocalization of the aortopulmonary collaterals.

Mild pulmonary stenosis is usually an incidental finding on routine clinical examination, and is usually treated successfully by balloon valvoplasty.

FONTAN AND GLENN PROCEDURES

The Fontan operation was originally done for tricuspid atresia, but is now more widely used as extended palliation for children with complex congenital heart disease in whom a biventricular repair is not possible. It results in a circulation in series, with only a single systemic ventricle, and passive blood flow through the lungs directly from the superior and inferior vena cava (Fig. 3.2.1). Good ventricular function and low pulmonary vascular resistance are required for a successful Fontan repair. It is frequently performed in stages, initially only joining the superior vena cava to the pulmonary arteries (Glenn procedure) and then joining the IVC flow and completing the Fontan or total cavopulmonary connection (TCPC) at a subsequent operation. In infants less than 1 year of age the Glenn procedure results in two-thirds of the systemic venous return flowing through the lungs and an oxygen saturation of 70–80%. In older children this accounts for only one-third of the systemic venous return. The Glenn procedure allows more gradual adaptation to higher systemic venous pressures and results in less pleural effusions and lower mortality when the Fontan operation is completed. In higher-risk patients, a fenestrated Fontan repair may be performed, leaving a residual ASD to allow right-to-left atrial shunting, to maintain cardiac output at the expense of lower systemic oxygen saturations when right atrial pressures are high and blood flow through the lungs is suboptimal.

Common postoperative problems include decreased ventricular function from CPB, and inadequate pulmonary blood flow due to raised

pulmonary vascular resistance resulting in elevated systemic venous pressures, right atrial distention, pleural effusions, ascites and arrhythmias.

The normal transpulmonary gradient (CVP minus LAP) required for adequate flow through the lungs is 5 mmHg, resulting in a CVP of 10–15 mmHg and an LAP of 5–10 mmHg. A transpulmonary gradient greater than 10 mmHg and a CVP greater than 18–20 mmHg result in markedly increased postoperative morbidity and mortality.

Cardiac output depends entirely on pulmonary blood flow which in turn depends on the transpulmonary gradient divided by the pulmonary vascular resistance. Thus to increase cardiac output, maneuvers to increase the CVP, decrease LAP, and decrease pulmonary vascular resistance should be used:

1. Right atrial pressure is increased with intravenous fluids (5% albumin or blood) until the CVP reaches 12–15 mmHg; venous return may also be augmented by positioning the patient head up, flexing the hips and placing the feet up.
2. Left atrial pressure is decreased by improving systemic ventricular function using inotropes and afterload reduction. Inotropes that also decrease pulmonary and systemic vascular resistance such as dobutamine and amrinone or enoximone are beneficial.
3. A low pulmonary vascular resistance (see pulmonary hypertension management section) is maintained with alkalosis, good oxygenation, analgesia, optimum lung volume, and pulmonary vasodilators such as nitric oxide; early spontaneous ventilation may also improve pulmonary blood flow.

Pleural effusions, ascites and pericardial effusions are common owing to the high CVP and may require drainage and replacement with colloid. The low cardiac output and high CVP also results in low liver blood flow, liver dysfunction and hypoglycemia. Cerebral edema and cerebral irritability may also occur.

In the unstable Fontan patient, residual structural lesions such as mechanical obstructions to pulmonary blood flow, undiagnosed venous collaterals and subaortic stenosis (which may be

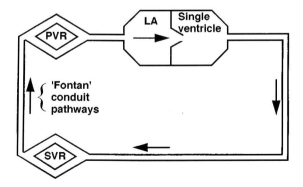

Figure 3.2.1 Fontan series circulation. The systemic vascular resistance (SVR) and the pulmonary vascular resistance (PVR) are in series; however, there is no right ventricle. LA, left atrium

unmasked by the reduced ventricular volume) need to be excluded with early cross-sectional echocardiography or cardiac catheterization.

The Fontan procedure reduces ventricular volume overload and decreases cyanosis; however, after 6–10 years the incidence of congestive heart failure and death increases again. Thus the Fontan operation is considered to be a palliative procedure.

HYPOPLASTIC LEFT HEART SYNDROME – 'NORWOOD' PHYSIOLOGY (PARALLEL SYSTEMIC AND PULMONARY CIRCULATION)

Hypoplastic left heart syndrome (HLHS) occurs when there is aortic valve stenosis or atresia, severe hypoplasia of the ascending aorta, and various degrees of left ventricular and mitral valve hypoplasia. These infants are duct-dependent, and without surgery the lesion is universally fatal. The stage 1 Norwood procedure involves formation of a new aorta using the rudimentary ascending aorta and the proximal pulmonary artery. Pulmonary blood flow is provided by a modified Blalock–Taussig shunt, and adequate mixing of oxygenated and deoxygenated blood is maintained through an atrial septectomy. Both before and after the operation it is important to maintain a good cardiac output and to 'balance' the systemic and pulmonary circulations, aiming for an oxygen saturation of 75%.

In patients with HLHS, and other patients with single ventricle physiology, the total ventricular output is divided between two competing parallel circuits. The relative proportions of the ventricular output to either the pulmonary or the systemic vascular beds, is determined by the relative resistances to flow in the two circuits (Fig. 3.2.2). The pulmonary and aortic saturations are equal in single-ventricle physiology. Resistance to pulmonary blood flow is determined by the pulmonary arteriolar resistance, pulmonary venous pressure, and left atrial pressure. Systemic flow is determined by the presence of anatomical obstructive lesions such as subaortic or aortic stenosis, arch hypoplasia or coarctation of the aorta, and the systemic arteriolar resistance. The aim is to maintain an acceptable balance between the systemic and pulmonary blood flows to provide enough pul-

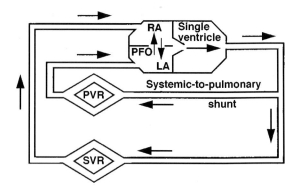

Figure 3.2.2 Norwood parallel circulation. The systemic vascular resistance (SVR) and the pulmonary vascular resistance (PVR) are in parallel, and the relative proportions of ventricular output to either the pulmonary or systemic vascular beds is determined by the relative resistances to flow in the two circuits. LA, left atrium, PFO, patent foramen ovale; RA, right atrium

monary flow for adequate oxygenation, and enough systemic flow to provide organ perfusion and prevent acidosis. This is best achieved when equal volumes of blood reach the systemic and pulmonary beds, resulting in a Qp/Qs ratio of 1. Assuming a pulmonary venous saturation of 95–100% and a mixed systemic venous saturation of 60–65%, a Qp/Qs ratio of 1 with equal flow to the pulmonary and systemic circulations would result in an arterial oxygen saturation of 75–80%. A Qp/Qs ratio of 2 means that twice as much blood is flowing through the lungs as through the systemic circulation, resulting in progressive ventricular volume overload, tricuspid regurgitation, cardiac failure, pulmonary congestion with decreased lung compliance, and an elevated systemic arterial oxygen saturation of approximately 85%. As pulmonary blood flow increases, there is a progressive 'steal' of the combined ventricular output into the lungs and inadequate systemic perfusion, with metabolic acidosis, renal dysfunction, hypotension, coronary hypoperfusion, acute myocardial ischemia and death. A number of ventilatory and pharmacological maneuvers are used to 'fine tune' the circulation, aiming for a Qp/Qs ratio of 1 and an oxygen saturation of 70–80% pre- and postoperatively (Table 3.2.8).

Inhaled carbon dioxide allows regulation of pulmonary vascular resistance, while avoiding the consequences of hypoventilation. It directly

TABLE 3.2.8 **Balancing systemic and pulmonary blood flow**

Management of excessive cyanosis (oxygen saturation < 70%)
- Exclude pulmonary cause (pneumothorax, atelectasis)
- Correct systemic venous desaturation (anemia, low cardiac output)
- Exclude mechanical obstruction to pulmonary blood flow
- Exclude inadequate mixing of pulmonary and systemic blood (restricted ASD)
- Decrease pulmonary vascular resistance
  - increase FIO_2
  - alkalosis (pH 7.45–7.5)
  - optimum lung volume
  - analgesia and sedation
  - pulmonary vasodilators (nitric oxide, enoximone, prostacyclin)
- Increase systemic arterial pressure to increase shunt flow
- Reduce left atrial pressure

Management of excessive oxygen saturation (oxygen saturation > 80%)
- Exclude left-sided obstructive lesions (arch obstruction)
- Increase pulmonary vascular resistance
  - decrease FIO_2 to 0.21
  - permissive hypercarbia (inhaled CO_2)
  - increase PEEP
  - hypoxic inspired gas mixture by addition of nitrogen
  - snare or clip to decrease size of systemic to pulmonary shunt
  - decrease systemic vascular resistance (dobutamine, enoximone)

increases pulmonary vascular resistance, and its effect is largely independent of pH and systemic vascular resistance. Postoperatively, an appropriately sized MBT shunt is of paramount importance in balancing the circulation. Myocardial function is decreased postoperatively and inotropic support will be required, but excessive systemic vasoconstriction should be avoided. As ventricular function improves and pulmonary vascular resistance becomes more stable, the 'balance' will be easier to maintain, especially with spontaneous respiration. At 6–12 months of age, the second stage of the repair, a Glenn anastomosis between the SVC and PA, is performed followed by diversion of the IVC blood to the PA, completing the Fontan repair at 2 years of age. The overall survival following the three stages is approximately 50%.

Norwood's operation can also provide satisfactory initial palliation for a wide variety of malformations characterized by ductal dependency of the systemic circulation, such as complex double-outlet right ventricle and subaortic stenosis.

CARDIAC TRANSPLANTATION

Cardiac transplantation is usually performed for end-stage cardiac failure secondary to dilated car-diomyopathy or congenital heart disease. The pulmonary vascular resistance must be less than 6–12 Wood's units. Postoperatively pulmonary hypertension must be avoided with good oxygenation, alkalosis and pulmonary vasodilators such as nitric oxide. Isoproterenol (isoprenaline) is infused to prevent bradycardia due to cardiac denervation. Inotropic support is usually required owing to decreased ventricular function from cold ischemia time and CPB. Other problems include acute rejection causing systolic and diastolic cardiac dysfunction, early coronary arteriosclerosis, and problems related to the immune suppression such as hypertension, renal impairment, opportunistic infections and lymphoproliferative disease. The overall 3-year survival is 66–71%. Heart-lung transplantation may be considered for children with high pulmonary vascular resistance who are unsuitable for an isolated heart transplant, although the long-term disease-free survival results are poor.

MANAGEMENT OF COMPLICATIONS

Common complications in cardiac intensive care include:

- pulmonary hypertension
- arrhythmias
- diaphragm paralysis
- traumatic chylothorax
- postpericardotomy syndrome
- mediastinitis, endocarditis (see cardiac infections)

PULMONARY HYPERTENSION

Postoperative pulmonary hypertension occurs when the mean pulmonary artery pressure (PAP) exceeds 50% of mean systemic arterial pressure. A pulmonary hypertensive crisis (PHC) is a sudden increase in pulmonary artery pressure which exceeds systemic arterial pressure leading to acute right ventricular failure, high CVP, low left-sided preload (low LAP), decreased cardiac output, hypotension, myocardial ischemia and cardiac arrest. Pulmonary hypertensive crises occur in children with excessive pulmonary blood flow preoperatively such as AVSD and VSD (especially also in cases of Down's syndrome or age > 6 months), mitral stenosis, obstructed pulmonary venous drainage, truncus arteriosus and transposition of the great arteries. Cardiopulmonary bypass leads to a temporary increase in reactivity of the pulmonary vascular bed, increasing the likelihood of PHC postoperatively. Pulmonary arterial catheters should be considered for postoperative monitoring in these patients, facilitating early detection of high PAP.

Pathophysiology

The pathophysiology of postoperative pulmonary hypertension is multifactorial, with preexisting hypertrophy and hyperreactivity of the pulmonary arterial smooth muscle owing to vascular remodeling caused by the underlying cardiac lesion, and impaired pulmonary vasodilatation. Endothelial cell dysfunction occurs with a decrease in the endogenous synthesis of nitric oxide, which is further exacerbated by CPB for 24–48 hours postoperatively. The sympathetic neural vasoconstrictor innervation to the lungs is increased, predisposing to sudden neurally mediated increases in pulmonary vascular tone. In addition, right ventricular function is decreased

following CPB and surgery, rendering the RV less able to tolerate the increased afterload. Acute bronchoconstriction may also occur during acute pulmonary hypertension, making the lungs stiff and more difficult to ventilate, predisposing to hypercarbia which may further exacerbate the pulmonary hypertension.

Management

The management of pulmonary hypertension involves manipulating factors that control pulmonary vascular resistance, which include alveolar oxygenation, blood pH, lung volume, and autonomic tone. Anesthesia is continued into the postoperative period to prevent neurally mediated acute increases in pulmonary vascular resistance in response to stimuli, using infusions of morphine 20–40 μg/kg·h or fentanyl 5–10 μg/kg·hr. Muscle relaxation is often continued in the initial postoperative period. Fentanyl boluses may be required before suctioning or procedures. Cardiac output is maintained with adequate preload, early inotropic support, and early afterload reduction. Strong α-vasoconstrictors such as norepinephrine (noradrenaline) should be avoided if possible, and above all, the following measures to reduce pulmonary vascular resistance should be used:

- maintain pH at 7.45–7.5 (mild hyperventilation and treat any metabolic acidosis)
- avoid hypoxia—aim for a PaO_2 of 10–14 kPa (80–100 mmHg)
- analgesia and sedation
- maintain optimal lung volume (avoid atelectasis and hyperinflation)
- maintain optimal blood viscosity— hematocrit 0.3, Hb 100–120 g/L (10–12 g/dl)
- vasodilators (inhaled nitric oxide, enoximone, prostacyclin)

Inhaled nitric oxide is the only selective pulmonary vasodilator. Nitroglycerin (glyceryl trinitrate), enoximone and prostacyclin are pulmonary and systemic vasodilators and hence may exacerbate systemic hypotension and ventilation–perfusion mismatching. Ventilation should be continued until the acute exacerbation of the pulmonary hypertension postoperatively resolves and right ventricular function has recovered.

ARRHYTHMIAS

The presenting symptoms of arrhythmias range from mild palpitations through to congestive cardiac failure and cardiogenic shock. For the diagnosis of arrhythmias, a 12-lead ECG is essential to give information on the rate and regularity of the rhythm, width of the QRS complex, presence or absence of P waves, and the P wave axis (normally positive in II, III and aVF). Information on hemodynamic stability during the arrhythmia also aids diagnosis. The presence or absence of a biphasic wave form on the LA or CVP trace also provides useful diagnostic information. In postoperative patients, an atrial electrogram is useful to gain more precise information on the relationship of the atrial activity to the QRS complex. An atrial electrogram may be performed using a 5-lead ECG. The four cutaneous limb leads are connected, and the atrial pacing wire is attached to lead V. A recording is then made on lead V_1. An atrial electrogram may also be performed in patients without pacing wires using an esophageal pacing wire as the atrial detector.

Tachyarrhythmias

If there is cardiovascular instability, initial resuscitation including ventilation, volume supplementation and cardiovascular support is required. Any reversible causes of tachyarrhythmias such as hypoxia, acidosis, fever, hypovolemia, electrolyte imbalance (especially hypokalemia, hypomagnesemia or hypocalcemia) or excessive inotropic support should be corrected.

Reentrant arrhythmias

Supraventricular tachycardia (SVT) is characterized by tachycardia (150–300 beats/min), with a regular R–R interval, narrow QRS complexes, and abnormal or difficult to define *P* waves. Atrioventricular reentry tachycardias are the most common form of SVT in childhood. They are usually associated with accessory pathways such as in Wolff–Parkinson–White syndrome, which is characterized by a short PR interval, widened QRS complexes and a slurred upstroke (delta waves). Reentrant arrhythmias respond to overdrive pacing (minimum 20 beats/min above the patient's

own rate) or cardioversion (0.5 J/kg). The management of SVT is as follows:

- vagal maneuvers (ice to face or Valsalva maneuver)
- i.v. adenosine for transient slowing of AV nodal conduction (0.05 mg/kg bolus, increasing by 0.05 mg/kg every 2 min to maximum of 0.3 mg/kg)
- overdrive pacing (minimum 20 beats/min above patient rate) using an esophageal, transvenous or epicardial electrode, *or cardioversion* (0.5–1 J/kg) if unstable
- amiodarone 25 μg/kg·min for 4 hours, then 5–15 μg/kg·min i.v.
- flecainide (has profound effects on AV node and accessory connection, but is negatively inotropic and can be proarrhythmic)
- digoxin may be used once Wolff–Parkinson–White syndrome has been excluded

Automatic focus tachyarrhythmia

Examples of automatic focus arrhythmias include postoperative junctional ectopic tachycardia (JET) and atrial ectopic tachycardia. Automatic focus arrhythmias do not respond to cardioversion or overdrive pacing, and therapies to reduce the automaticity of the irritable focus are used, such as cooling, decreasing adrenergic tone and giving amiodarone.

Junctional ectopic tachycardia (His bundle tachycardia) is caused by an ectopic irritable focus in the atrioventricular node or the bundle of His resulting in an incessant tachycardia with a heart rate greater than the 98th centile for age. The QRS complex is similar to that in sinus rhythm, the R–R interval is regular, and there is atrioventricular dissociation with a ventricular rate in excess of the atrial rate or retrograde 1:1 ventriculo atrial conduction giving rise to associated retrograde P waves in the QRS complex. A wide QRS complex may also occur in the presence of surgically induced bundle branch block. An atrial electrogram aids diagnosis by demonstrating the relationship of the P waves to the QRS complex (Fig. 3.2.3). This arrhythmia is relatively common following

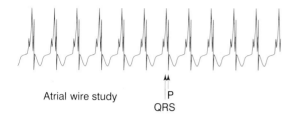

Atrial wire study

P
QRS

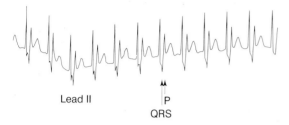

Lead II

P
QRS

Figure 3.2.3 Junctional ectopic tachycardia with retrograde conduction of P waves. More precise information on the relationship between the P and QRS complexes can be obtained with an atrial electrogram (upper trace)

tetralogy of Fallot repair, AVSD repair or the Fontan procedure. It usually occurs in young patients (< 6 months of age) who have had long CPB times and who require inotropic support. It is thought to be caused by traumatic injury or stretch to the His bundle during surgery resulting in an irritable focus. Hemodynamic compromise frequently occurs owing to loss of atrioventricular synchrony and a high tachycardia rate. It usually terminates spontaneously 3–8 days postoperatively. Management of JET is as follows:

- Correct reversible factors:
  - hypoxia
  - acidosis
  - hypovolemia
  - electrolyte abnormalities
- hypothermia (32–35°C) reduces automaticity of the cardiac pacemaker tissues, reduces heart rate, and improves systolic blood pressure
- decrease endogenous catecholamine release to slow the rate of discharge from the ectopic focus using analgesia and sedation
- decrease exogenous catecholamines— decrease the inotropic support where possible

- amiodarone reduces the tachycardia rate and improves systolic blood pressure (or give propafenone—may cause marked hypotension)
- atrial pacing—synchronizing to the R wave restores atrioventricular synchrony and thus increases cardiac output

Broad complex tachycardia

The two most common causes of broad complex tachycardia are ventricular tachycardia and SVT with aberrant conduction.

Ventricular tachycardia

Ventricular tachycardia (VT) may be difficult to differentiate from SVT in that they can both present as a wide complex, regular tachycardia associated with inadequate cardiac output. The presence of preexisting atrioventricular dissociation or fusion beats suggests VT. Adenosine is also helpful in differentiating, as it slows AV conduction temporarily and thus may allow ECG diagnosis. If hemodynamic compromise is present or drug therapy has been unsuccessful, cardioversion is the treatment of choice for VT. If the cardiac output is maintained, the drug of choice is lidocaine (lignocaine) 1 mg/kg bolus followed by infusion at 15–50 μg/kg·min. Amiodarone may be used in cases unresponsive to lidocaine. Phenytoin, procainamide and bretylium have also been used.

Ventricular pacing in addition to magnesium sulfate has been used for *torsade des pointes* and polymorphic VT.

Bradyarrhythmias

Sinus bradycardia

Sinus bradycardia in children is usually due to reversible causes such as hypoxia, acidosis, vagal stimulation, and raised intracranial pressure.

Atrioventricular conduction delay and blockade

Atrioventricular conduction delay and blockade results in loss of the atrial 'kick', slow ventricular rates and decreased cardiac output. The location and degree of conduction block will determine the type of arrhythmia (nodal, first-degree, second-degree or complete AV block). Management involves:

- treatment of reversible causes such as hypoxia, acidosis, hyperkalemia, hypothermia, and drugs (digoxin, amiodarone, beta-blockade)
- oxygenation and ventilation should be ensured and intravascular volume restored
- if hypotension and low cardiac output are present, then therapy is initiated to increase the heart rate
  - atropine 0.02 mg/kg is administered to decrease vagal tone
  - isoproterenol (isoprenaline) 0.1–1 μg/kg·min provides β_1 chronotropic activity, but may cause further hypotension through its β_2 vasodilating effect; if so, epinephrine (adrenaline) can be substituted
- as an alternative, cardiac pacing may be used to manage symptomatic bradycardia using transcutaneous, transesophageal, transvenous or epicardial pacing methods

DIAPHRAGM PARALYSIS

Diaphragm paralysis may occur when a cardiac or thoracic surgical procedure results in injury to the phrenic nerve. The nerve may be damaged by cold injury from topical cardiac hypothermia, surgical contusion or accidental surgical nerve division. Presentation includes radiological evidence of persistent left lower lobe collapse and/or an elevated hemidiaphragm, paradoxical respiration with indrawing of the abdomen during spontaneous inspiration on the affected side, and failure to wean from ventilation. The diagnosis can be confirmed by measuring phrenic nerve conduction time or using diaphragmatic screening, looking for paradoxical diaphragm motion during spontaneous respiration. Infants and young children have a compliant chest wall and are more dependent on diaphragm function for normal respiration, and unlike older children or adults, respiratory function is usually compromised when one or other hemidiaphragm is paralyzed. Diaphragm plication via a lateral thoracotomy prevents paradoxical motion of the paralyzed diaphragm and results in improved efficiency of the respiratory pump, with improved tidal volumes and decreased work of breathing. Phrenic nerve function recovers spontaneously in the majority of patients between 1 month and 2 years postoperatively.

TRAUMATIC CHYLOTHORAX

Postoperative chylothorax can complicate any cardiac or thoracic surgical procedure. Surgical division of the main thoracic duct can occur, and variations in lymphatic pathways account for chylous effusions resulting from operative approaches that do not expose the main thoracic duct. Patients with central venous hypertension will have a higher incidence of postoperative chylothorax owing to high levels of lymphatic flow (bidirectional cavopulmonary anastomosis has a 24% incidence of postoperative chylothorax). Superior vena caval obstruction or thrombosis should be excluded if chylothorax is diagnosed.

Initial management involves drainage of the pleural space. To confirm the diagnosis, a differential white cell count should be performed on the fluid, which will show an abundance of lymphocytes if it is chyle.

Enteral feed in which the fat is in the form of medium-chain triacylglycerides should be used, as medium-chain fatty acids pass directly into the portal system coupled to albumin, bypassing the lymphatic system and thus reducing the volume of chyle. If the chylous drainage continues then enteral rest using total parenteral nutrition is indicated, as even enteral water can increase chylous flow by 20%. Surgical intervention should be considered for unabated drainage lasting more than 2 weeks, especially if there is also raised venous pressure, or there is reason to suspect damage to a major lymphatic vessel such as the thoracic duct. Operations for persistent chylothorax include pleurodesis, ligation of leaking lymphatics, ligation of the main thoracic duct, and pleuroperitoneal shunting. Spontaneous resolution occurs within 20 days in 90% of patients. Complications of persistent drainage include lymphocyte depletion, poor nutritional status and respiratory compromise.

POSTPERICARDOTOMY SYNDROME

Postpericardotomy syndrome is characterized by fever beyond the first postoperative week, pericardial and pleural reaction with chest pain, effusions and occasional cardiac tamponade. The cause is thought to be autoimmune, in association with a viral infection. Management includes administration of aspirin and corticosteroids, and when indicated, drainage of the pericardial effusion.

CARDIAC INFECTIONS

Cardiac infections include:

- postoperative mediastinitis
- bacterial pericarditis
- infective endocarditis

Postoperative mediastinitis

Although the incidence of mediastinal wound infection in patients undergoing median sternotomy is approximately 0.9%, it is associated with high rates of morbidity and mortality. Risk factors predisposing to sternal wound infections include a long cardiopulmonary bypass time, excessive postoperative bleeding, low cardiac output for 24 hours or more postoperatively, and inadequate antimicrobial prophylaxis. Fever, leukocytosis and discharge from the sternal wound are common presentations. Stability of the sternum is a critical feature used to differentiate superficial from deep wound infections. *Staphylococcus aureus* and *S. epidermidis* are the most common causal organisms.

Management includes appropriate antibiotics and wound drainage. Deep mediastinitis requires wound debridement, and closed mediastinal catheter irrigation using dilute antibiotic or iodine solutions. For severe infections sternectomy and flap reconstructions may be required. Complications of mediastinitis include chronic sternal osteomyelitis and mycotic aneurysms.

Infectious pericarditis

The most common form of pericarditis is acute inflammation with no clearly identifiable cause. Such 'idiopathic' or 'aseptic' pericarditis is probably the result of unrecognized viral infection. The condition usually responds promptly to anti-inflammatory therapies.

Bacterial pericarditis should be suspected in patients with septicemia who have developed symptoms and signs of pericarditis (precordial pain, muffled heart sounds, pericardial friction rub and cardiomegaly). Echocardiography facilitates early diagnosis. The management includes appropriate antibiotic therapy and drainage of the pericardial space either surgically or using a percutaneous pericardial catheter.

Percutaneous pericardiocentesis

The indications for percutaneous pericardiocentesis include drainage of hemodynamically significant pericardial effusions. The patient is first stabilized with volume replacement and inotropic support. Afterload reduction is very poorly tolerated owing to the fixed cardiac output, and great care is required if sedation or anesthesia are to be administered. The ECG, arterial blood pressure and oxygen saturation should be monitored. Using a sterile technique, the operator introduces an 18 gauge needle at the left xiphocostal angle and advances it cephalad while aspirating continuously until fluid appears in the syringe. Possible complications include inadvertent puncture of the heart, arrhythmias, injury to coronary arteries and pneumothorax. Alternatives include formation of a surgical pericardial window. Acute postoperative pericardial tamponade requires urgent sternal opening and removal of clot.

Infective endocarditis

The diagnostic criteria for infective endocarditis (IE) include:

- positive blood cultures and vegetations demonstrated by echocardiography
- positive blood cultures, no demonstrable vegetations, but other evidence suggestive of endocarditis by history (joint pain, dental manipulations), laboratory data (positive ventilation–perfusion scan), or physical findings of fever, changing murmur, hepatosplenomegaly or cutaneous embolic phenomena

- fever and positive blood cultures in patients with congenital heart disease, and no other apparent source of infection
- fever and congenital heart disease with positive findings on an echocardiogram, embolic phenomena, or both, but no blood cultures positive for pathogens

Risk factors include structural heart disease, recent presence of central venous catheters (especially in premature infants) or transvenous pacing electrodes. Patients with congenital heart disease in whom foreign material is present such as Goretex shunts and patches, prosthetic valves, and homograft material, represent the largest group at risk. Only 50% of patients with endocarditis have demonstrable vegetations on echocardiography (lower in patients with complex congenital heart disease). In the cardiac surgical population, the most common pathogens associated with IE are *Staphylococcus aureus* and coagulase-negative staphylococci. Streptococci are the second most common pathogen in postsurgical patients and are the most common cause of IE in nonsurgical cases. *Candida* species, *Aspergillus*, and Gram-negative organisms can also cause IE. Serious morbidity can occur including valvular insufficiency, pulmonary emboli, and central nervous system complications such as cerebral emboli, seizures and meningitis. The mortality rate from pediatric endocarditis is approximately 10–20%. The American Heart Association guidelines for prevention of endocarditis are given in Table 3.2.9.

Management involves treatment with appropriate antibiotics for 4–6 weeks. Surgical intervention is required in 20% of patients and includes vegetectomies, debridement, valve reconstruction or replacement, and replacement of graft materials.

CARDIOMYOPATHY

Cardiomyopathy in children is classified into dilated, hypertrophic and restrictive types. Restrictive cardiomyopathy is rare in children and generally has a poor prognosis.

DILATED CARDIOMYOPATHY

Children with dilated cardiomyopathy present with cardiac failure, and cardiomegaly on CXR. A

TABLE 3.2.9 American Heart Association recommendations for prevention of endocarditis in patients with structural heart disease

Standard regimen
Amoxycillin 50 mg/kg orally 60 min prior to the procedure, then 25 mg/kg orally 6 h later

Standard regimen if allergic to penicillin
Erythromycin 20 mg/kg orally 2 h prior to the procedure, and 10 mg/kg orally 6 h later

OR

Clindamycin 10 mg/kg orally 60 min prior to the procedure and 5 mg/kg 6 h after the procedure

Alternative regimen for high-risk patients
Ampicillin 50 mg/kg i.v. and gentamicin 2 mg/kg i.v. 30 min prior to the procedure, then amoxycillin 25 mg/kg orally 6 h later

OR

Vancomycin 20 mg/kg i.v. over 1 h, starting 1 h before the procedure

Gastrointestinal or urogenital procedure
Add gentamicin 2 mg/kg i.v. or i.m. 30 min prior to the procedure to the above regimens

dilated, poorly contracting heart is seen on echocardiogram. Although the majority of cases are idiopathic, anomalous origin of the left coronary artery, arrhythmias, carnitine deficiency and other rare metabolic, endocrine, storage, mitochondrial, and connective tissue diseases must be excluded. Myocarditis due to viruses such as coxsackie, echo, influenza, parainfluenza, mumps, and rubella viruses may present with a dilated, poorly functioning heart; however, many improve spontaneously.

Management involves maintaining cardiac output with intravenous inotropes and vasodilators initially, and then oral ACE inhibitors and diuretics (see section on maintenance of cardiac output). Anticoagulation is advisable to prevent mural thrombi. Cardiac transplantation should be considered in children with progressive or end-stage cardiac failure. Five-year survival in children with dilated cardiomyopathy is 60%, with a slightly better outcome in younger children.

HYPERTROPHIC CARDIOMYOPATHY

The diagnosis of hypertrophic obstructive cardiomyopathy (HOCM) is based on the demonstration of a markedly hypertrophic, nondilated left ventricle in the absence of cardiac or systemic disorders capable of producing left ventricular hypertrophy. There is poor left ventricular filling, but systolic function is usually preserved. Left ventricular outflow tract obstruction may develop causing syncope and cardiovascular collapse. The obstruction may be intensified by hypovolemia, vasodilators, inotropes and digoxin. Causes of HOCM include Noonan's syndrome, familial hypertrophic cardiomyopathy, gestational diabetes, acromegaly, thyroid anomalies, lipodystrophy, and other metabolic conditions.

The management includes treatment with β-adrenergic blocking agents (usually propranolol), verapamil and surgical resection of the left ventricular outflow tract if obstruction persists. Myotomy with myectomy is beneficial for relief of symptoms but does not alter the natural history of the disease.

FURTHER READING

1. Rogers MC. Textbook of pediatric intensive care. 3rd ed. Baltimore: Williams & Wilkins; 1996
2. Kambam J. Cardiac anesthesia for infants and children. St Louis: Mosby-Year Book; 1994
3. Tunaoglu FS, Olgunturk R, Akcabay S et al. Chest pain in children referred to a cardiac clinic. Pediatr Cardiol 1995; 16: 69–72
4. Rice MJ, McDonald RW, Reller MD et al. Pediatric echocardiography: current role and review of technical advances. J Pediatr 1996; 128: 1–14
5. Beekman RP, Filippini LH, Meijboon EJ. Evolving usage of pediatric cardiac catheterization. Curr Opin Cardiol 1994; 9: 721–728
6. Newburger JW, Jonas RA, Wernovsky G et al. A comparison of the perioperative neurologic effects of hypothermic circulatory arrest versus low-flow cardiopulmonary bypass in infant heart surgery. N Engl J Med 1993; 329: 1057–1064
7. Elami A, Permut LC, Laks H et al. Cardiac decompression after operation for congenital heart disease in infancy. Ann Thorac Surg 1994; 58: 1392–1396
8. Mora GA, Pizarro C, Norwood WI et al. Experimental model of single ventricle. Influence of carbon dioxide on pulmonary vascular dynamics. Circulation 1994; 90: 1143–1146
9. Wessel DL, Adatia I, Giglia TM et al. Use of inhaled nitric oxide and acetylcholine in the evaluation of pulmonary hypertension and endothelial function after cardiopulmonary bypass. Circulation 1993; 88: 2128–2138
10. Bond SJ, Guzzetta PC, Snyder ML et al. Management of pediatric postoperative chylothorax. Ann Thorac Surg 1993; 56: 469–473
11. Till JA, Shinebourne EA. Supraventricular tachycardia: diagnosis and current acute management. Arch Dis Child 1991; 66: 647–652
12. Raja P, Hawker RE, Chaikitpinyo A et al. Amiodarone management of junctional ectopic tachycardia after cardiac surgery in children. Br Heart J 1994; 72: 261–265
13. Balaji S, Sullivan I, Deanfield J et al. Moderate hypothermia in the management of resistant automatic tachycardias in children. Br Heart J 1991; 66: 221–224
14. Till JA, Rowland E. Atrial pacing as an adjunct to the management of post-surgical His bundle tachycardia. Br Heart J 1991; 66: 225–229
15. El Oakley RM, Wright JE. Postoperative mediastinitis: classification and management. Ann Thorac Surg 1996; 61: 1030–1036
16. Zahn EM, Houde C, Benson L et al. Percutaneous pericardial catheter drainage in childhood. Am J Cardiol 1992; 70: 678–680
17. Saiman L, Prince A, Gersony WM. Pediatric infective endocarditis in the modern era. J Pediatr 1993; 122: 847–853
18. American Heart Association Committee on Rheumatic Fever, Endocarditis, and Kawasaki Disease. Prevention of bacterial endocarditis. JAMA 1990; 264: 2919
19. Burch M, Runciman M. Dilated cardiomyopathy. Arch Dis Child 1996; 74: 479–481
20. Zonis Z, Seear M. The effect of preoperative tranexamic acid on blood loss following cardiac surgery in children. J Thorac Cardiovasc Med 1996; 111: 902–907
– (*References addressing specific aspects of cardiac diagnosis, therapy and management in children*)

3.3   Central nervous system

Robert C. Tasker

The field of acute neurology holds an important place in the historical development of pediatric critical care. The management of poliomyelitis, Reye's syndrome and head trauma has shaped our present practice of emergency support and intervention in critical illness and injury. This chapter highlights aspects of the basic history, examination and investigation of acute neurological disease causing critical illness; central nervous system syndromes commonly seen that require intensive care; neurological complications of cardiac disease; and common neuromuscular disorders necessitating acute respiratory support.

CLINICAL ASSESSMENT

HISTORY

A careful history often provides clues to neurological diagnosis. Acute central deterioration is associated with metabolic disturbance, ingestions, cerebrovascular accidents or trauma. Cerebral deterioration over days or weeks is more compatible with infection, chronic intoxication or more slowly developing raised intracranial pressure. The presence of focal neurological abnormalities in the child prior to the onset of central disturbance suggests cerebrovascular disease, an intracranial mass or focal encephalitis. Toxic and metabolic encephalopathies cause diffuse neurological dysfunction. The medical history may provide vital clues of recurrent disorders such as seizures, migraine or sickle cell disease. A family history of epilepsy or tuberculosis may be discovered, or the report of previous stillbirths or deaths in infancy may indicate inherited metabolic disease. The social history may suggest nonaccidental injury, lead poisoning or brucellosis, or the family may recently have arrived from the tropics, introducing the possibility of a wide variety of intracranial infectious pathology.

GENERAL EXAMINATION

The general physical examination may provide signs of systemic disease, infection and trauma. The size and weight of the child may indicate failure to thrive, suggesting a long-standing metabolic disease, or emotional deprivation. The pulse, blood pressure and temperature should be measured and recorded and the breathing pattern observed. Hyperpyrexia may be central in origin, but is most likely to be due to infection. Hypothermia may result from shock, hypothalamic disturbance or inadequate measures for warming, possibly during transfer.

Hypertension may be the cause of acute neurological disease, but conversely may be neurogenic in origin. Hypertension and/or bradycardia may be a result of increased intracranial pressure. Hypotension may be due to shock or to central causes. Major vessels should be palpated and auscultation performed, especially over the neck. Breath odors may suggest diabetic ketoacidosis, solvent abuse, or one of the rare aminoacidopathies. Thorough inspection of the skin and scalp for evidence of bruises, abrasions or other trauma such as old cigarette burns should be carried out. The mouth should also be inspected for a torn frenulum. Fundal and subhyaloid hemorrhages should be specifically sought. Examination of the skin may suggest a neurocutaneous disorder or yield valuable clues of sepsis, such as the minor abrasion leading to staphylococcal toxic shock, the petechial hemorrhages of meningococcemia and, where prevalent, rickettsial disease. Bleeding into the skin or from any of the orifices suggests a bleeding diathesis.

HEAD AND NECK EXAMINATION

Examination of the head is important, particularly in infants and young children. The fontanelles and sutures should be palpated, and listening for bruits should not be forgotten. The head circumference should be measured and recorded and, if possible, comparison with earlier records made. In the infant, transillumination of the skull is occasionally helpful.

Distention of the neck veins should be observed and, where there is a ventricular shunt or reservoir in situ, assessment of ventricular cerebrospinal fluid pressure should be attempted if the child is obtunded. Evidence of dysraphism should be looked for, particularly in the lumbosacral and occipital regions, as a sinus here may well be a clue to the presence of meningitis. Signs of meningeal irritation must be sought, although these may be absent in the very young infant or in the critically ill child, even in the presence of subarachnoid hemorrhage or meningitis. Inspection of the eyes may reveal proptosis, lid swelling or unilateral exophthalmos. Examination of the nose and external auditory meatus might demonstrate cerebrospinal fluid rhinorrhea or otorrhea. Finally, the examination should be completed with a thorough examination of the mouth and pharynx.

NEUROLOGICAL EXAMINATION

Assessment of the eyes and examination of the neuromuscular system should also be carried out thoroughly.

Eyes

Ocular responses

The position of the eyes at rest is noted and any deviation, conjugate or dysconjugate, recorded. Spontaneous eye movements, including roving eye movements, ocular bobbing or nystagmus are looked for. Other noteworthy ocular phenomena are increased blinking, intermittent lid retraction, convergent or divergent spasms and monocular nystagmus, most of which imply brain-stem dysfunction. The corneal reflex should be tested since its presence does relate to the depth of coma.

Ocular motility should be assessed with the 'doll's eye' maneuver, but only if the cervical spine is known to be stable. This maneuver, eliciting the oculocephalic reflex, is accomplished by holding the child's eyelids open and briskly rotating the head first to one side and then the other (Fig. 3.3.1). A positive response indicating an intact pathway in the brain stem is obtained by full conjugate eye deviation to the opposite side (i.e. if the head is rotated to the right, the eyes deviate to the left). Vertical eye movements are tested by briskly flexing and extending the neck. A positive response is observed when the eyes deviate upward with neck flexion and downward with neck extension. Further assessment of brain-stem function by the 'caloric' or oculovestibular response (Fig. 3.3.2) may cause discomfort and should only be performed in the deeply unconscious child. It is important to ensure that the tympanic membranes are intact before starting to instil up to 80 ml of iced saline.

Pupillary responses

The pupillary size at rest should be noted and also the reaction to light (both direct and consensual). Pupillary responses like the corneal reflex show a close correlation with the severity of coma. Whenever a combination of impaired extraocular movements and preserved pupillary reflexes is found, disorders of neuromuscular transmission should be considered. Toxic levels of phenytoin may be associated with ophthalmoplegia. Unlike adults, pinpoint pupils due to pontine lesions are uncommon in comatose children, and when miotic pupils are present poisoning with opiates, phenothiazines, alcohol, barbiturates or sodium valproate should be considered. Asymmetrically reacting pupils do not have any specific diagnostic importance, but the occurrence of a unilaterally fixed and dilated pupil is a signal for urgent intervention as it strongly suggests transtentorial herniation. In children who have bilateral fixed and dilated pupils, administration of anticholinergics or sympathomimetic drugs given systemically or topically should be considered.

Fundoscopy

The fundi need careful examination and this is best left until other ocular signs and responses have been documented. Adequate fundal examination is important but on rare occasions it can only be achieved by the use of short-acting mydriatics. Consider this decision judiciously and when it is employed the patient must be prominently

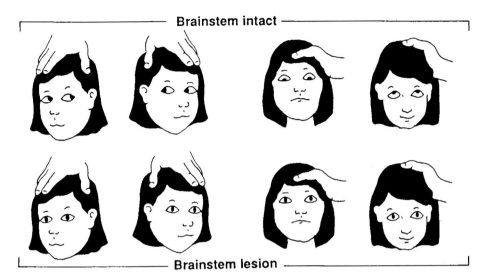

Figure 3.3.1 The doll's eye maneuver in the unconscious child, illustrating oculocephalic reflexes (From Brett E. (ed) Pediatric Neurology. London: Churchill Livingstone, 1997.)

labeled as having received these drugs and the fact clearly documented. Other intracranial hemorrhages should be strongly suspected if retinal hemorrhages are seen and the possibility of nonaccidental injury considered. Venous pulsations in the retinal vessels are a helpful sign as their presence precludes any significant increase in intracranial pressure. Papilledema is the single most reliable sign of intracranial hypertension. With acute elevations in intracranial pressure papilledema is rarely seen in the first 24–48 hours. However, its absence should not lull the attendant into a false sense of security.

Sometimes encephalitis (especially that due to varicella and mycoplasma) can be accompanied by a papillitis which is difficult to distinguish from papilledema on clinical grounds.

Neuromuscular

Examination of the peripheral nervous system and muscle strength is essential in the assessment of the weak or unconscious child.

Head and neck

Asymmetry of the face should be noted and the gag reflex elicited. Evidence of tongue wasting and fasciculation should also be sought. In the comatose child, assessment of power and response in the facial distribution is best achieved by observing movement in response to firm supraorbital or suprasternal pressure. Responses to stimulation of the limbs may be reflex and serve to confuse the picture, but focal weakness or laterality usually implies a structural lesion although it may rarely result from a metabolic disorder.

Limbs

Tone should be assessed in all four limbs. Extensor hypertonus should be closely observed for, since such spasms may be unilateral or bilateral, occur spontaneously or only after stimulation: they should not be mistaken for seizures. In infants, these episodes may be preceded by 'bicycling' movements of the upper and lower limbs. In extensor hypertonus the lower limbs are extended with internal rotation and often plantar flexion and scissoring. Positioning in the upper limbs may be one of two distinct types (Fig. 3.3.3). In *decorticate* rigidity the arms are flexed across the chest, while in *decerebrate* rigidity the elbows are extended. Such rigidity may result from structural lesions or metabolic dysfunction and is often as-sociated with a rise in intracranial pressure. The clinical picture of the two types of rigidity is quite distinctive, but from neither can an underlying pathological change in

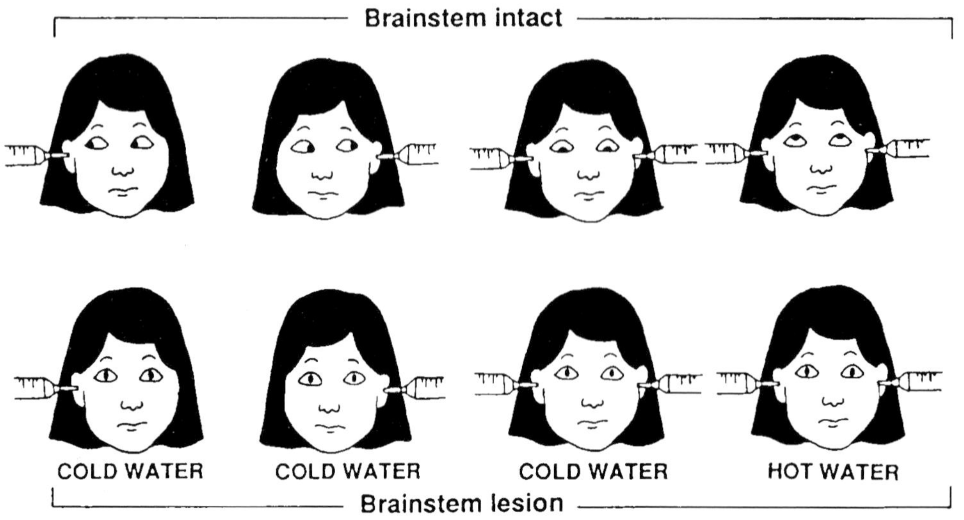

Figure 3.3.2 Oculovestibular reflexes in the unconscious child produced by instilling cold and hot water against the tympanic membranes (hot water should be no more than 44°C) (From Brett E. (ed) Pediatric Neurology. London: Churchill Livingstone, 1997.)

the brain be inferred. It is generally considered, however, that decorticate posturing is associated with cortical or hemisphere dysfunction, whereas the brain stem is more often damaged in children in whom the upper limbs show decerebrate patterns. Finally, wasting of muscle groups should be looked for, particularly in the small muscles of the hand, as this may represent evidence of 'critical illness' polyneuropathy or myopathy.

Movements

Extrapyramidal signs such as dystonia or dyskinesia may occur in both the conscious and the unconscious child, and should suggest the possibility of drug toxicity (e.g. phenothiazine poisoning). Repetitive or rhythmic movements suggest the possibility of seizures. The patient should be observed for obvious generalized tonic-clonic episodes or myoclonic jerks which are usually easily identified, but the more subtle seizure-related phenomena seen in infants, such as cyanosis from chest rigidity, chewing movements, or stiffening are less readily recognized.

Abdomen and chest wall

Synchrony and strength of chest and abdomen during breathing should be assessed. Paradoxical

movement, or posturing with preference for one particular side should alert the observer to the possibility of diaphragmatic weakness. In children receiving ventilatory assistance, the work of breathing with different levels of positive end-expiratory pressure is also a helpful guide to overall strength.

Deep tendon reflexes

The deep tendon reflexes should be elicited. Areflexia in combination with flaccidity is a grave portent in the unconscious child, provided a generalized peripheral neuropathy has been ruled out and muscle relaxants have not been administered.

NEUROLOGICAL INVESTIGATIONS

The initial investigation of the child with an acute neurological problem falls into two broad categories: investigations that may lead to or confirm a specific diagnosis, and those providing information that will help to give optimum supportive therapy during the child's illness. The investigations must be tailored to the individual child's history and examination. For instance, if a clear history of hypoxia has been recorded, a full skeletal survey will not only be unhelpful but may be detrimental, whereas in the child with retinal hemorrhages the investigation is essential. As a general rule, investi-

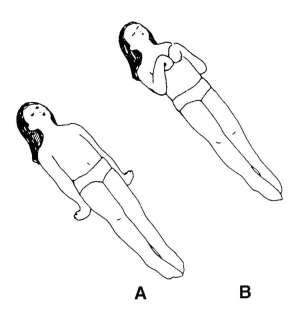

A　　　　　**B**

Figure 3.3.3 Motor responses to noxious stimulation in children with acute cerebral dysfunction. (A) Decerebrate posturing; (B) decorticate posturing (From Brett E. (ed) Pediatric Neurology. London: Churchill Livingstone, 1997.)

gations such as arterial blood gas analysis, blood glucose, urea, electrolytes and osmolality estimations should be carried out on admission.

Lumbar puncture

Bacterial meningitis is an important cause of childhood mortality and the need for urgent lumbar puncture (LP) if there is the slightest suspicion of this has been traditional teaching until very recently. A number of reports on transtentorial or transforaminal herniation following LP in children with meningitis have been published, however, and there is now debate about this policy. It is difficult to predict which children are at particular risk of tentorial herniation, but where the diagnosis of meningitis seems clear and there is impaired conscious- ness with fundoscopic signs of raised intracranial pressure, or focal signs or other signs of incipient coning, or when the child has been ill for several days, many physicians elect to treat the patient with antibiotics without obtaining confirmatory spinal fluid findings. A comprehensive report from the American College of Physicians in 1986 advocated withholding or delaying the LP where there is

evidence of raised intracranial pressure, serious cardiorespiratory disease, or where the skin over the planned puncture site is infected. Collective experience has shown that the great majority of children with pyogenic meningitis come to no harm from LP, but in the seriously ill child where consciousness is depressed, the decision is a difficult one and should be made only by the experienced clinician. Where a space-occupying lesion or severe cerebral edema is expected, this investigation is contraindicated.

Cranial imaging

Cranial imaging studies are indicated when the initial biochemical studies have failed to clarify the diagnosis, or if a structural lesion or poor cerebral function is suspected.

Cerebral ultrasonography is a sensitive tool for the detection of major intracranial abnormalities in young infants, but it is not as sensitive as cranial computed tomography (CT) in detecting smaller— though still clinically significant—lesions such as focal infarcts, subarachnoid hemorrhages, and small parenchymal hemorrhages. Magnetic resonance imaging has advantages over a CT scan, e.g. the absence of ionizing radiation; greater sensitivity to blood flow, edema, hemorrhage, and myelination; lack of beam-hardening artifacts; and easier differentiation between gray and white matter. In the comatose child cranial CT is invaluable for urgent assessment of potential underlying cerebral disorders and the need for surgical intervention. In the context of metabolic encephalopathy, the CT scan is particularly useful in the evaluation of cerebral edema and raised intracranial pressure. The likelihood of the latter can be determined by reviewing the presence or absence of cerebrospinal fluid (CSF) spaces both above and below the tentorium. Loss of spaces below the tentorium (i.e. the basal cisterns) is indicative of severe swelling. A grading system for worsening generalized loss of CSF spaces (Table 3.3.1) can be used in this context, and worsening loss of CSF spaces is associated with increasing levels of intracranial pressure.

Neurophysiological studies

Appropriately chosen clinical neurophysiological techniques have been used in combination with

TABLE 3.3.1 **Worsening severity of generalized loss of CSF spaces on cranial CT scan**

Grade	CT scan features
N	Normal CT scan
I	Loss of sulci cerebri and/or interhemispheric fissure and/or sylvian fissure and/or occlusion of body of lateral ventricle
II	Complete loss of sulci and fissures and/or chiasmatic cistern and/or quadrigeminal cistern and/or interpeduncular cistern
III	Complete loss of sulci, fissures, and all (perimesencephalic) cisterns

clinical assessment in a variety of neurological disorders in both infants and children. They are particularly useful in patients in whom clinical evaluation is unreliable because of administration of sedatives, hypnotics, or muscle relaxants. Although there may be difficulty in obtaining this type of testing at the time of admission, there is considerable information to be gained. During the acute phase of illness, electroencephalography (EEG) may provide information about the severity and distribution of altered cerebral function of the cortex, presence of discharges (seizure activity), and even on occasion a clue to the etiology.

Regardless of etiology, EEG during an acute encephalopathic process usually shows varying degrees of slow activity. The relationship between increasing severity of encephalopathy and worsening EEG changes in children can be incorporated in clinical staging with grading for degree of EEG abnormality between normal for age and electrocerebral silence (i.e. absence of all cerebral activity). The predominant abnormal background activity was classified as being:

1. Normal for age.
2. Borderline normal for age.
3. Abnormal for age—graded 1–5 according to frequency and amplitude of slow activity: (as patients deteriorated, predominant EEG activity became slower (4–6 cycles/s to 0.5–2 cycles/s) and of lower amplitude (less than 50 μV), then intermittent.
4. Electrocerebral silence.

Evoked potential studies have also been used in a similar manner to EEG for assessing the severity of brain injury in global insults as well as the potential cumulative detrimental effects of secondary cerebral injury. Other monitoring techniques using continuous signal-processed EEG have also been applied in the intensive care setting, with the supposition that early identification may result in early remedy and the avoidance of brain damage. There is, however, no clinical evidence that once a cerebral insult has occurred, monitoring of whatever form alters the eventual outcome—sadly, many of these techniques merely make us more sophisticated observers of events that usually have an unrelenting course. There is perhaps some benefit in that we may be able to evaluate prognosis or follow the effect of treatment such as anesthesia for refractory status epilepticus.

Postmortem protocol

In the event of a child dying, adequate diagnosis is important for family genetic counseling if an underlying neurometabolic disorder is suspected. A postmortem protocol which includes the taking of urine and serum samples, fibroblast culture, and muscle and liver biopsies (three or more specimens stored frozen on dry ice or in liquid nitrogen at –20°C) is outlined in Table 3.3.2. The details of such a protocol should be discussed locally, so that items such as biopsy needles (e.g. liver, kidney, and skin), dry ice, and culture media, can be made readily available and samples can be appropriately stored at any time.

CENTRAL NERVOUS SYSTEM SYNDROMES

The clinical patterns of presentation recognized by many practitioners seeing patients who require life support during an acute neurological illness, strictly speaking are not true syndromes, but are sufficiently consistent to enable a starting point for differential diagnosis. These syndromes are:

- Reye's syndrome and Reye-like illness
- raised intracranial pressure
- hepatic encephalopathy
- fulminant neonatal encephalopathy

TABLE 3.3.2 **Post-mortem diagnostic protocol for infants and children with encephalopathy of unknown etiology**

	Samples	Storage and usage
Body fluids		
Blood	Heparinized Unheparinized	Serum and plasma are separated then frozen at −20°C Chromosome analysis
	Whole blood in EDTA	Store at 4°C for up to 5 days Used to extract DNA
Urine	Centrifuge to remove blood and debris	Store at −20°C
Fibroblast culture		
Skin	Punch biopsy sample fully immersed in tissue culture media	Store at 4°C
Tissue enzyme activity		
Liver	Needle or open biopsy	Snap frozen: immerse immediately in liquid nitrogen
Muscle	Needle or open biopsy	Store at −70°C
Histology		
Liver	Needle or open biopsy	Tissue fixed in formalin for light microscopy and glutaraldehyde for electron microscopy
Muscle	Needle or open biopsy	Tissue fixed in formalin for light microscopy and glutaraldehyde for electron microscopy

EDTA, ethylenediamine tetraacetic acid

- postresuscitation disease
- profound biochemical derangement
- severe systemic disturbance or disease
- poisons and drug toxicities

REYE'S SYNDROME AND REYE-LIKE ILLNESS

Reye's syndrome is a disorder of unknown etiology and historically of high mortality. It is exemplified by the child who, while recovering from a viral prodrome, unexpectedly develops pernicious vomiting and subsequently a deteriorating level of consciousness. Abnormalities related to hepatic failure may occur, including enzyme elevations, coagulation disorders, and alterations of carbohydrate, amino acid, and lipid metabolism. Other accompaniments of multisystem failure may occur, including myocardial failure, dehydration and shock, acute renal failure, peptic ulcers, pancreatitis and sepsis. Patients who die have severe cerebral edema and fatty infiltration of the viscera, including the heart and kidneys. Although the usual cause of death is tentorial herniation secondary to intracranial hypertension, it may also result from myocardial failure, gastrointestinal bleeding, status epilepticus, renal failure, respiratory failure, or cardiovascular collapse.

The cause of Reye's syndrome has remained elusive. Since its original description in 1963 the syndrome has been seen both in large clusters as well as more sporadically during the 1970s. Over this time the debate about etiology has encompassed ideas concerning associated trigger factors and specific genetic-metabolic defects or some combined interaction. For example, some studies have documented an association between the use of aspirin in children with viral illnesses and the subsequent development of Reye's syndrome. In support of this, a campaign during the 1980s, aimed at reducing the use of aspirin in children, was linked with a subsequent decline in Reye's syndrome reports. This decline was seen at the same time as knowledge of metabolic diseases was rapidly expanding, and an alternative explanation may be that fewer patients with an underlying genetic-metabolic disease were being incorrectly labeled as having Reye's syndrome. Despite this, Reye's syndrome has not disappeared.

A 'Reye-like illness' or 'secondary' Reye's syndrome is the description given to patients who meet the standard clinical diagnostic criteria of Reye's syndrome (Table 3.3.3), but in whom a specific cause is identified from the large range of differential diagnoses which includes the spectrum of inflammatory encephalopathies, toxic ingestions, and primary infections of the liver. Multiple types of genetic metabolic disorders may look like Reye's syndrome, including ornithine transcarbamylase deficiency, arginosuccinic acid synthetase deficiency, pyruvate dehydrogenase and pyruvate carboxylase deficiencies, fatty acid oxidative abnormalities, and urea cycle abnormalities. Of these, the most common metabolic disorders that mimic Reye's syndrome are urea cycle disorders, organic acidemias, and disorders of fat oxidation.

Urea cycle enzyme disorders

Metabolic acidosis and hypoglycemia are not usually found but hyperammonemia is present and often severe. The plasma and urine amino acid profiles are abnormal and urinary orotic acid is elevated in the majority of these disorders. The most seriously affected patients present in the neonatal period but there is a wide spectrum of

severity and patients may present at any stage of childhood. The female carrier of the X-linked disorder ornithine carbamylase deficiency, as well as the homozygous male with partial enzyme deficiency, may present with mild episodic symptoms.

Organic acidemias

The main distinguishing feature in the organic acidemias is usually an overriding metabolic acidosis. Hyperammonemia, at times as dramatic as that associated with urea cycle disorders, is commonly seen in critically ill neonates, whereas it is less consistently observed in older children. These conditions arise from a defect in amino acid breakdown and the most common are propionic acidemia, methylmalonic acidemia and maple syrup urine disease. The plasma amino acid profile is diagnostic in the latter, but to establish the diagnosis in the majority of these disorders gas chromatography of plasma and urine organic acids is required.

Disorders of fat oxidation

Medium- and long-chain acyl-CoA dehydrogenase deficiency may resemble Reye's syndrome. Typically these patients have nonketotic hypoglycemia and hyperammonemia, but the metabolic acidosis is not striking. Episodes of encephalopathy are often associated with hepatomegaly (due to fatty infiltration) and tend to become less frequent with time. The serum carnitine level is low, which probably results from urinary losses of acyl carnitine. Some children may have a primary systemic carnitine deficiency and present with a Reye-like illness. The cause of this primary carnitine deficiency is unclear but is possibly due to a combination of impaired gastrointestinal absorption and renal tubular resorption.

RAISED INTRACRANIAL PRESSURE

In the absence of an intracranial space-occupying lesion or hydrocephalus, raised intracranial pressure can result from:

- increased venous pressure (as in dural sinus thrombosis)

TABLE 3.3.3 Centers for Disease Control case definition of Reye's syndrome

Acute noninflammatory encephalopathy
- Microvesicular fatty metamorphosis of the liver confirmed by biopsy or autopsy
- Serum glutamic oxaloacetic transaminase (SGOT), or serum pyruvic transaminase (SGPT), or serum ammonia greater than 3 times normal

Cerebrospinal fluid
- If obtained, there must be less than 9 leukocytes/mm³

Exclusion of other diagnoses
- There should be no other more reasonable explanation for the neurologic presentation of the hepatic abnormality

- increased resistance of arachnoid villi to resorption of cerebrospinal fluid (as in meningeal inflammation)
- hypersecretion of CSF (as seen in certain endocrine abnormalities)
- cerebral edema.

The toxic-metabolic causes of cerebral edema are listed in Table 3.3.4. Unfortunately in practice, the early symptoms and signs of raised intracranial pressure are relatively nonspecific (Table 3.3.5) and often this complication is identified only at a late stage of disease by signs of brain tissue herniation (Table 3.3.6).

The most common pathological finding is cerebral edema which is defined as an increase in brain volume due to an increase in its water content. When generalized, it will cause raised intracranial pressure. Localized edema, however, may result merely in an alteration in cerebral function with no change in bulk cerebral tissue and fluid dynamics. Cranial imaging will aid the diagnosis of cerebral edema: CT scanning may show diffuse or localized low attenuation as a result of high water content; T_2-weighted MRI will show an intense signal.

HEPATIC ENCEPHALOPATHY

Hepatic encephalopathy complicates both acute and chronic liver failure. This complex syndrome

TABLE 3.3.5 Early symptoms and signs of raised intracranial pressure

	Infant	Child
General state	Poor feeding Vomiting Irritability to coma Seizures	Anorexia and nausea Vomiting Lethargy to coma Seizures
Head/eyes	Full fontanelle Scalp vein distention False localizing signs	False localizing signs
Other	Altered vital signs Hypertension Pulmonary edema	Altered vital signs Hypertension Pulmonary edema

may be caused by potentially reversible metabolic abnormalities and in its extreme form can lead to coma and death. The differential diagnosis of the variety of possible etiologies includes:

- drugs:
  - sedatives
  - tranquilizers
  - narcotics
  - diuretics
- electrolyte imbalance:
  - hyponatremia
  - hypokalemic alkalosis
- excessive nitrogen load:
  - gastrointestinal hemorrhage
  - excessive dietary protein
  - azotemia
  - constipation
- other:
  - infection
  - hypoxia
  - hypovolemia

TABLE 3.3.4 Toxic-metabolic causes of cerebral edema

Inherited metabolic disease
- Aminoacidopathies
- Organic acidemias
- Hyperammonemia
- Porphyria
- Nonketotic hyperglycinemia

Organ failure
- Uremia
- Hepatic failure

Electrolytes, minerals and vitamins
- Hypercalcemia
- Hypernatremia
- Water intoxication
- Lead poisoning
- Vitamin A toxicity

Other
- Hypoglycemia
- Hypoxia–ischemia

FULMINANT NEONATAL ENCEPHALOPATHY

In the first postnatal month and early infantile period, the clinical presentation of metabolic disease may include a varied combination of biochemical derangement (e.g. glucose, acid–base, liver function), and hepatic failure. The most common etiologies associated with various constellations of

TABLE 3.3.6 Signs of brain downward herniation

	Tentorial	**Foramen magnum**
Mechanism	1. Diencephalon and hypothalamus move downward and caudally • optic chiasm stretched and twisted • infundibulum displaced • brain-stem torsion • vertebral arteries displaced 2. Compression of • cerebral peduncle • nerve VI • posterior cerebral artery 3. Secondary hemorrhage in the brain stem	1. Tentorial downward shift continues to the posterior fossa 2. Cerebellar tonsils herniate at the side of the cord, maybe down to C-5
Signs		
Consciousness	Decreased, tonic seizures	Comatose
Motor	Decerebrate responses	Hypotonia/spinal flexion Brisk flexor withdrawal Tongue fasciculation, bulbar palsy Erb's palsy
Eyes	III and VI nerve palsy 'Sunsetting' Cortical blindness	Absent caloric or doll's eye response Absent ciliospinal reflex
Respiration	Central neurogenic hyperventilation Cheyne–Stokes respiration	Bradypnea and apnea Laryngeal stridor
Other	Loss of temperature control Cardiac irregularity	Hypotension

metabolic derangement are discussed in Chapter 3.11). However, of particular note with respect to brain dysfunction are the neonatal sepsis syndrome and infantile seizure–myoclonic syndromes.

Neonatal sepsis syndrome

Nonspecific clinical signs and symptoms indistinguishable from the presentation of sepsis may be seen in the neonate presenting with one of a number of diseases of carbohydrate, fat, or protein metabolism. In some infants, a history of apparent normality in the early neo-natal period is deceptive, it may merely indicate that either the metabolic disturbances have taken time to accumulate to toxic levels or the toxic process has taken time to evolve. Although in general there are few pathognomonic findings during the neonatal period, many of the disorders presenting at this age are associated with an anion-gap acidosis, and some with hyperchloremic acidosis.

Infantile seizure–myoclonic syndromes

A variety of names have been given to the occurrence of repeated and intractable seizures, spasms, or 'subtle' episodes starting in the neonatal period. These 'syndromes' are of importance in that seizure control is poor and outcome is usually dismal. In some patients, there is the possibility that an inborn error of metabolism (e.g. pyridoxine-dependent seizures and nonketotic hyperglycinemia) may be responsible—particularly in the infant with truly no documented history of acute central nervous system insult. Two epileptic syndromes that fall into this category are the early myoclonic encephalopathy and the early infantile epileptic encephalopathy syndromes.

Early myoclonic encephalopathy is characterized clinically by the occurrence of erratic fragmentary myoclonus of early onset, usually in association with other types of seizures and, from EEG, by the intermittent or 'suppression-burst' pattern. This clinical picture may be seen in infants affected by various neurologic disorders. However, it has been suggested by some that specific metabolic disorders should be sought, such as glycine abnormalities. Early infantile epileptic encephalopathy may be a variant of West's syndrome with onset in early infancy, and typified by mainly intractable tonic spasms, invariant intermittent activity on EEG, severe neurodevelopmental deficits, and multiple causes, especially brain malformations.

POSTRESUSCITATION DISEASE

Acute neurological complications may occur after successful artificial cardiopulmonary resuscitation and support may have been carried out. Irrespective of the initiating cause of the life-threatening event, e.g. primary cardiorespiratory dysfunction or following severe head trauma, the postresuscitation neurological features and clinical problems encountered have many pathophysiological similarities with the other causes of coma and are described in other chapters (Chs 2.2, 4.9).

PROFOUND BIOCHEMICAL DERANGEMENT

A variety of biochemical disturbances, such as hypoglycemia and electrolyte abnormalities, may account for an altered level of consciousness as well as specific clinical signs or features. Many of these are discussed in other chapters, but are summarized briefly here.

Hypoglycemia

Hypoglycemia may result from a variety of disorders which can be categorized as deficient substrate provision, deranged endocrine balance; inborn errors of carbohydrate, lipid, or amino acid metabolism; drugs, hepatic failure, and systemic derangement.

Hyperammonemia

Hyperammonemia may in sufficient concentrations cause neurologic symptoms. In both neonates and older children, the acute presentation can be a catastrophic illness. The hyperammonemia can result from acquired diseases such as toxic or infectious hepatic failure or Reye's syndrome,

and from a number of inborn errors of metabolism that affect nitrogen metabolism. Less acute presentations of hyperammonemic disorders are more varied and coma may ensue only after significant stress, such as intercurrent illness, pregnancy, or augmented protein intake.

Electrolyte disturbance

Any central neurological disturbance in patients hydrated through intravenous or nasogastric tubes should prompt the search for an abnormal concentration of electrolytes, e.g. sodium, calcium, and magnesium.

Hypernatremia

Hypernatremia may produce varying degrees of impaired consciousness, fever, spasticity, and subdural hemorrhage. It can be due to severe dehydration, body water loss, diabetes insipidus, salt poisoning, or sodium retention seen in hyperaldosteronism or Cushing's disease.

Hyponatremia

Hyponatremia may produce an altered level of consciousness and seizures. Its causes include injudicious solute-poor intravenous fluid administration, water retention in cardiac or liver failure, the syndrome of inappropriate secretion of antidiuretic hormone, and drugs such as vincristine and carbamazepine.

Calcium and magnesium derangement

Calcium and magnesium metabolism is closely linked. When levels are profoundly low, focal or multifocal seizures may be observed. Hypermagnesemia can induce weakness, hypotonia, coma and respiratory failure.

ACUTE CENTRAL NEUROLOGY SEEN IN SYSTEMIC DISTURBANCE OR DISEASE

A variety of disease states are known to induce acute neurological features. Those that could be attributed to a 'metabolic' or toxic process are discussed briefly below.

Vitamin deficiency

Thiamine (vitamin B_1), pyridoxine (vitamin B_6), and vitamin A deficiencies may result in an alteration in level of consciousness, sometimes rather precipitously.

Thiamine

Thiamine has an important role in the decarboxylation of pyruvate and of α-ketoglutarate (two steps of the Krebs cycle), and the conversion of 5-carbon to 6-carbon sugars by means of the enzyme transketolase. Thiamine deficiency will therefore decrease energy available to the brain and increase the concentration of the two keto acids. In patients receiving total parenteral nutrition, chronic dialysis, or a high-carbohydrate diet during debilitating illness, Wernicke's encephalopathy may be observed. In these settings, the features are highly variable and may be manifested by sudden collapse and death or seizures, to the classic ataxia, confusion, and ocular abnormalities.

Pyridoxine

Pyridoxine in the form of pyridoxal 5-phosphate is essential for normal brain function. It is particularly necessary for the decarboxylation of glutamic acid to γ-aminobutyric acid, an essential inhibitory neurotransmitter. In deficiency states such as that seen in patients who are receiving isoniazid or penicillamine, seizures may be observed.

Vitamin A

Vitamin A deficiency can result in a rise in intracranial pressure, which may be reversed by replacement.

Diabetes mellitus

Coma may complicate various abnormal biochemical states associated with diabetes mellitus:

- diabetic ketoacidosis may result in a marked impairment in cerebral blood flow and oxygen uptake by the brain, cerebral edema, and focal neurological deficit
- nonketotic hyperosmolar coma does occur in children and results in generalized or focal seizures, ophthalmoplegia and hemiparesis
- hypoglycemia may result in a spectrum of clinical findings ranging from transient focal neurological signs to coma and focal or generalized seizures

Renal disease

The central nervous system problems associated with underlying renal disease are invariably multifactorial and may be attributable to electrolyte disturbance, hypertension, or specific disease toxins. Those that warrant specific mention are listed below.

Uremic encephalopathy

Uremic encephalopathy is characterized by obtundation, hypotonia, seizures, athetoid movements, nystagmus and ataxia; it is the main neurological complication of renal insufficiency. Focal cerebral symptoms, hemiparesis, and cortical blindness are more usually due to hypertensive encephalopathy.

Dialysis dyseqilibrium syndrome

Dialysis dysequilibrium syndrome is caused by a failure of urea to rapidly establish equilibrium between brain and blood during dialysis, thus resulting in a net shift of extracellular water into the brain.

Rejection encephalopathy

Rejection encephalopathy which is not due to electrolyte disturbance, hypertension, steroids, or fever, occurs in some renal transplant patients. More recently cyclosporin toxicity has been implicated. This produces a syndrome of coma, cortical blindness, quadriplegia, and seizures.

Sepsis syndrome-related encephalopathy

An encephalopathy seen in bacteremic patients, not due to meningitis, abscess, cerebritis, or emboli, has been described in critically ill adults. Mortality and morbidity rates are high. The conditions causing this state may include microabscesses in the cerebral cortex (appreciable only at postmortem), metabolic disturbance such as the ratio of branched-chain to unbranched and aromatic amino acids, cerebral microcirculatory dysfunction, cerebral edema, and drugs administered.

POISONS AND DRUGS

Drug intoxication is an important cause of abnormal neurology in children. Table 3.3.7 summarizes the findings in the more commonly seen episodes.

NEUROLOGICAL COMPLICATIONS OF CARDIAC DISEASE

Acute neurological insult as well as the sequelae of operative repair in children with cardiac disease remains a major concern to those involved with intensive care. Although such problems are thankfully infrequent, a significant number of children do suffer permanent neurologic sequelae, and neurodevelopmental dysfunction.

ACUTE NEUROLOGIC EVENTS

Episodic cyanosis and convulsions

Cyanotic attacks constitute a major complication of cyanotic heart disease, and may be seen in as many as 10–20% of such children. The episodes occur most frequently in children between 6 months and 3 years of age and are precipitated by exertion, feeding or defecation. They are marked by hyperpnea and a sudden increase in the previous level of cyanosis. Consciousness is usually decreased and acutely generalized convulsions commonly occur later in severe cases. Electroencephalography in the early stages and during these severe attacks shows large amplitude, slow activity and not spike discharges, indicating that such seizures result from anoxia rather than underlying epilepsy. In some cases, the cyanotic attack may be followed by the features of an acute cerebrovascular accident.

Cerebrovascular accidents

Cerebrovascular accidents occur during the first 20 months of life in 75% of cases, and tetralogy of Fallot and transposition of the great vessels

TABLE 3.3.7 **Drug intoxication and the effects on the CNS and other organ systems**				
Drug	**Neurology**	**Eyes**	**Cardiac**	**Other organ systems**
Amphetamines	Depressed consciousness Delirium Agitation Chorea Hyperreflexia	Mydriasis	Cardiac arrhythmia Tachycardia Hypertension	Hyperpyrexia Sweating
Tricyclic antidepressants	Agitation Muscle rigidity Seizures Coma	Mydriasis	Tachycardia Arrythmias: prolonged QRS conduction block Hypotension	Sweating Vomiting
Antihistamines	Depressed consciousness Hallucinations Tremor Seizures	Mydriasis	Hypotension	Dry mouth Urinary retention
Barbiturates	Ataxia Coma Areflexia	Miosis	Hypotension	Hypothermia Respiratory depression
Methadone	Depressed consciousness	Miosis	Hypotension	Urinary retention Respiratory depression

account for 90% of all cases. Infarcts may occur spontaneously, especially in children under 2 years of age, and often appear following an attack of cyanosis and dyspnea. Children with low hemoglobin concentrations are at particular risk for arterial accidents, whereas a high hematocrit is common in venous thrombosis. Overall venous thrombi are more common than arterial occlusions. They are particularly correlated with dehydration and a high hematocrit, whereas arterial infarcts are often observed in patients with iron-deficiency anemia. Both may be associated with increased blood viscosity.

The clinical features of *arterial infarction,* in most cases, do not differ whether they result from thrombosis or embolism, and are manifested by the sudden appearance of neurological deficit in the territory of one major cerebral vessel. In children with cyanotic congenital heart disease the majority of arterial infarcts are due to occlusions mainly located in the territory of the middle cerebral artery, but other large vessels may be involved. Hemiplegia of sudden onset is the usual clinical presentation but other focal deficits such as hemianopia or aphasia may be seen (Table 3.3.8). Weakness is maximal immediately after onset, and flaccidity is the rule. Spasticity and pyramidal tract signs appear later. The degree of recovery is extremely variable, with a substantial change being expected during the first 2–3 weeks of recovery. Subsequently, further slow progress may continue for several months. Seizures may also accompany the acute episode; in some 10% of children they can follow the attack after a latent period of 6 months to 5 years. About 20% of children, particularly those who incur a cerebrovascular accident during the early years of life, are left with permanent neurological sequelae.

Venous thrombosis is difficult to distinguish from stroke of arterial origin. The children most susceptible are those with cyanotic disease, especially during the first year of life. The child typically is polycythemic, but red blood cell indices show hypochromasia and microcytosis. The onset, often precipitated by dehydration, is calamitous, with headache, disturbance of consciousness, visual disturbances including papilledema, and focal signs such as seizures, hemiparesis, hemianopia and aphasia. A fluctuating course is not unusual

and the clinical evolution depends on the extent and location of parenchymal damage, which is usually hemorrhagic in type. If the venous infarction is extensive, the intracranial pressure will be raised, and the mortality rate high. Treatment is difficult, but should include general supportive measures such as correcting dehydration and treating any systemic infection that might be present. Overhydration should be avoided, as severe cerebral edema is usually present. The latter is treated, if necessary, with endotracheal intubation and the judicious use of mannitol.

Acute hemiplegia may also be the result of embolism due to bacterial endocarditis in patients with congenital left-to-right shunts. About half of such children develop emboli in the course of their illness. Most frequently, these emboli are to the lungs or the brain. Evidence for cerebral embolization can be a sudden disturbance of consciousness, hemiparesis, seizures or aphasia. Although most patients show hematuria because of embolization to the kidneys, cerebral embolization may rarely be the presenting clinical feature. The specific diagnosis and management of this condition relies on blood cultures and appropriate antibiotic treatment.

Mitral valve prolapse, a relatively common familial disorder, can also be a rare cause of recurrent *transient ischemic attacks* which may involve any territory, including the retinal vessels. Finally, thromboembolic complications may rarely be seen after cardiac catheterization, particularly in those investigated in the first few months of life.

Brain abscesses

Brain abscesses are rare before the age of 2 years, perhaps because they develop on previous small infarcts. With the increased longevity of children with cyanotic heart disease, the incidence of this complication has risen considerably. In a series reported in 1974, approximately 2% of patients with cyanotic congenital heart disease developed brain abscess. About 80% of the abscesses occurred in subjects with tetralogy of Fallot and transposition of the great vessels, and morbidity and mortality were related to the degree of cyanosis. The clinical presentation can be progressive, with initially minimal neurologic signs subsequently becoming readily

TABLE 3.3.8 **Main syndromes of supratentorial arterial occlusion**		
Arterial territory	**Region of ischemia**	**Clinical findings**
Internal carotid	Whole or part of territory of middle cerebral artery Rarely territories of both middle and anterior cerebral arteries	Hemiplegia Hemianopsia Unilateral sensory deficit Aphasia if dominant hemisphere Partial involvement with only incomplete hemiplegia is not rare
Middle cerebral	Convexity of hemisphere, except: paramedical aspect and occipital lobe, insula, part of temporal lobe, internal capsule and basal ganglia, and orbital aspect of frontal lobe	Hemiplegia with upper limb predominance Hemianopsia Aphasia if dominant hemisphere
Anterior cerebral	Medial aspect of hemisphere, and paramedial aspect of their convexity Anterior part of the internal capsule and basal ganglia	Hemiplegia predominating on the lower limb
Anterior choroidal	Optic tract, posterior limb of internal capsule, cerebral peduncle, and pallidum Variable involvement of thalamus, caudate, and lateral geniculate body	Hemiplegia Visual field defects Dysarthria Ataxia sometimes
Thalamostriate	Caudate, putamen, and internal capsule	Hemiplegia – motor, sensory, or mixed No hemianopia Language disturbances sometimes
Posterior cerebral	Lower part of temporal lobe, posterior part of thalamus, subthalamic nuclei, superior cerebellar peduncle, optic radiations, and occipital lobe	Homonymous hemianopia Ataxia Hemiparesis Vertigo

apparent (Table 3.3.9). Unfortunately papilledema is of little value in the diagnosis of brain abscess in patients with cyanotic heart disease, because their retinal vessels are frequently engorged and tortuous with blurring of the disc margins even in the 'normal' state.

Examination of the cerebrospinal fluid reveals an increased protein concentration and a variable pleocytosis. Cranial CT with contrast enhancement is the most effective technique to differentiate infarction from abscess. An acute infarction often is not demonstrated, whereas an abscess has the characteristic ring enhancement with surrounding cerebral edema. Multiple abscesses may be present in as many as 20% of such patients.

Management

Because it is often practically difficult to differentiate a brain abscess from an intracranial vascular accident, it has been suggested that systemic antibiotics be given to all patients with suspected 'stroke'. The initial treatment depends heavily on antibiotic therapy, which must cover a wide spectrum of organisms, as abscesses often have a mixed bacterial flora including some anaerobic organisms. If bacterial endocarditis is present, unusual organisms may be present. Formerly the initial antibiotic treatment comprised intravenous chloramphenicol, ampicillin or methicillin, and at times also an aminoglycoside. Now the third-generation cephalosporins are widely used, although when possible, all such therapy should be guided by available antibiotic sensitivities. Unfortunately many specimens are negative on culture. Antibiotics should be continued for 4–5 weeks and the therapeutic response can be monitored by serial cranial CT scans, which often continue to demonstrate ring enhancement for several weeks. Irrespective of surgical puncture, medical treatment can certainly achieve a complete cure, with disappearance of the capsule on cranial CT scan. In patients where the diagnosis of cerebral abscess is in doubt but antibiotics have been started, this therapy can be discontinued if the cranial CT scan fails to show any evidence of an abscess after 1 week.

Brain abscesses also produce severe cerebral edema, and management of this problem is of utmost importance. Seizures may also complicate the acute disease process and should be treated vigorously (Ch. 2.5). If the abscess causes significant mass effect that cannot be controlled with physiological and pharmacological treatment methods, surgery may be life-saving, although the mortality rate is high. Overall the mortality rate for brain abscess is now around 10%, with sequelae including epilepsy (30–40%), which is usually of the partial type; localized neurologic deficits; hydrocephalus; and mental retardation. The last may, however, be more related to the underlying congenital cardiac disorder rather than the abscess itself.

Intracranial arterial aneurysms

The association of coarctation of the aorta with intracranial arterial aneurysms has been well documented. Although they are only seen in a small proportion of children with coarctation, they account for about 25% of aneurysms in childhood, and they are located around the circle of Willis and its major branches. Hemorrhagic stroke is the presenting clinical manifestation in the majority of cases and this may be preceded by premonitory 'pseudotumoral' symptoms such as severe focal headache, meningeal signs, or transient neurological deficits. Seizures may also be the first clinical manifestation of aneurysm.

All children suspected of intracranial hemorrhage should undergo a cranial CT scan for

---

TABLE 3.3.9 Symptoms and signs of patients with brain abscess and congenital heart disease

Symptoms	Neurologic signs
Headache and/or vomiting	Lateralizing signs
Seizures	Papilledema
Fever	Hemiparesis
Listlessness	Increased deep tendon
Disorientation	reflexes
Neck pain	Extensor plantar responses
	Pupillary changes
	Stupor
	Neck stiffness
	Aphasia
	Homonymous hemianopia
	Localized percussion
	tenderness of skull

anatomical localization. Four-vessel angiography or MRI angiography will provide complete information on the circle of Willis and collateral circulation. Surgical treatment is the usual therapy, with a not insignificant mortality or residual morbidity.

SEQUELAE OF CARDIAC SURGERY

Complications of cardiac surgery are one of the major sources of neurodevelopmental sequelae of congenital heart disease. While studies in adults who have undergone open heart surgery suggest that permanent neurological sequelae, including strokes and seizure disorders, may occur in as many as 9–40% of survivors (with perhaps more less severe, but still disabling, cognitive and learning disorders), the overall incidence of neurological sequelae in children is generally unknown.

When cerebrovascular complications do occur, they are believed to result from impaired cerebral perfusion and from micro- and macroembolic phenomena, and are associated with marked EEG abnormalities. The clinical presentation and time course of these complications can be categorized into acute and chronic forms (Table 3.3.10). In children, the most prominent of the acute complications are focal and generalized seizures, intracranial hemorrhage, and spinal cord infarction. The chronic or late sequelae of cardiac surgery include developmental delay, cerebral palsy, gait disorders, seizures and learning disorders.

Acute problems

The acute neurological complications that can occur during or immediately after the operation include coma or lesser disturbances in the level of consciousness, seizures (generalized, focal, or multifocal), abnormalities in muscle tone, hemiparesis, organic mental syndromes, dyskinesias, gaze palsies, and personality changes. In the immediate postoperative period these problems may be difficult to assess, because of the confounding effects of anesthesia and pharmacological muscle relaxation.

Altered level of consciousness

When anoxic brain damage has been extensive, patients do not recover consciousness postoperatively. In general, persisting acute neurologic symptoms and signs reflect a period of impaired cerebral perfusion (local or generalized) or embolization during the time of bypass or postoperative period. In some of these patients focal cerebral infarction or diffuse cortical changes may be seen on cranial CT or MRI. In the perioperative period global cerebral hypoperfusion may result from a variety of problems, such as incorrect

---

TABLE 3.3.10 **The time course of CNS problems related to cardiac surgery**

Acute postoperative problems	Long-term sequelae
Seizures	Seizure disorders
Altered level of consciousness	Mental retardation
Focal neurologic signs	Cerebral palsy
hemiparesis	motor defects
gaze palsy	paraplegia
Altered muscle tone	Learning disorders
Movement disorders	Communication disorders
athetoid posturing	hearing loss
choreiform	language disorder
Behavior problems	Communicating hydrocephalus
irritability	
organic mental changes	
Spinal cord infarction	
Peripheral nervous system injury	
Horner's syndrome	
brachial plexus neuropathy	
vocal cord paralysis	

cannula placement, poor tolerance of circulatory changes because of native intracranial vascular disease, or inadequate perfusion pressure. Currently the most effective means of protecting the brain from injury induced by cardiopulmonary bypass or total circulatory arrest is hypothermia: it reduces cerebral blood flow and metabolism, and preserves cellular stores of high-energy phosphates. In the context of cardiopulmonary bypass (CPB), however, it should be remembered that in children, adequate cerebral perfusion pressure remains to be defined. It has been shown that regional cerebral blood flow autoregulation remains intact during hypothermia with mean arterial pressures in the 30–40 mmHg range, when so-called 'alpha-stat' management of CO_2 is used during the period of cardiopulmonary bypass. Autoregulation of cerebral blood flow, during hypothermia and CPB remains an area of controversy and extensive research, with some groups preferring the pH-stat (temperature-corrected) to alpha-stat (non-temperature-corrected) methods and vice versa. Currently, the 'alpha-stat' method is more widely used.

The method of hypothermia (either moderate, deep, or deep with total circulatory arrest) also has significant bearing on the potential for differing effects on cerebral physiology. In relation to clinical care, the periods or events of particular concern, when the brain is at increased risk of neurologic insult, are:

- the active cooling period
- the period of low-flow cardiopulmonary bypass or total circulatory arrest
- during weaning and separation from cardiopulmonary bypass

Seizures

In early studies, performed prior to the advent of cranial CT scanning, it was suggested that seizures were a not infrequent problem following surgery that involved profound hypothermia and circulatory arrest. In two-thirds of these patients there was no obvious cause for the seizures, which occurred 24–48 hours following surgery, and there was no relation to the type of cardiac lesion or to the duration of the hypothermia and circulatory arrest. These seizures responded to anticonvulsant therapy, and the children did not have seizures or neurological abnormalities on long-term follow-up. It is possible that some of these cases would have shown CT scan abnormalities and that some residual learning deficits might have been present if looked for. More recently, there have been reports that suggest a correlation between the duration of CPB and the occurrence of seizures. Some seizures, particularly if focal, may be difficult to control, despite the use of large doses of antiepileptic medication. In this context, it is noteworthy that CT scans of children with acute neurological symptoms following cardiac surgery may be normal or show diffuse or focal ischemic changes.

Spinal cord infarction

Ischemic spinal cord injury may occur not only following repair of coarctation of the aorta but also in open heart surgery, following vascular collapse. The presumptive causative factors included local spinal cord hypoperfusion, microemboli, and postoperative hypotension leading to ischemia.

Intracranial hemorrhage

Although a variety of intracranial hemorrhages and hematomas can occur following cardiac surgery, the incidence of this problem or the frequency of a particular lesion is not available from a large series of recently managed patients. The pathogenesis is not fully understood, but may be related to intraoperative anticoagulation, hypertonic perfusion, excessive diuresis, and venous and/or arterial hypertension during or after CPB.

Peripheral nerve lesions

A variety of peripheral nervous system lesions have been reported in adults following open heart surgery. These include brachial radiculoplexopathy; mononeuropathies of the saphenous, common peroneal, and ulnar nerves; singultus (secondary to phrenic nerve injury); unilateral vocal cord paralysis; Horner's syndrome; and facial neuropathy. The presumed causes include trauma associated with jugular venous cannulation, stretching of nerve roots due to positioning, trauma from cauterization, nerve compression at susceptible sites, or traction on nerves. Most of the deficits resolved in 6–8 weeks. Transient Horner's syndrome and brachial plexus neuropathies have been seen in children, particularly after difficult jugular vein cannulation in the small infant.

Long-term sequelae

In contrast to the early period following cardiac surgery, the exact incidence of long-term or delayed neurological sequelae of cardiac surgery, such as mental retardation, cerebral palsy, gait disorders, seizures, speech disorders, hearing loss, and learning disorders, is poorly documented.

Delayed choreoathetoid syndrome

The onset of acute chorea is both dramatic and profoundly disturbing. In the majority of children the clinical picture is rather stereotyped. It appears that the reported cases were all in early childhood, and the onset is 2–7 days after operation. Although it is possible that in some of these cases the onset may have been suppressed by necessarily heavy sedation in the immediate postoperative period, in most patients there was a clear period of normality beforehand. Generally the severity of the chorea progresses over 1–3 weeks, and affects the face, bulbar muscles, and all four limbs. The tone seems to be poor in both trunk and limbs, with reflexes either normal or suppressed. Some recovery seems to take place in all patients, with a few cases showing complete recovery — follow-up periods vary, however, and insufficient information is available on which to base a firm prognosis. The precise neuroanatomical localization and pathogenesis of this condition are unknown, but presumably the basal ganglia and deep subcortical structures are involved, with the following processes implicated: distortion of the microvascular bed and localized 'no-reflow phenomenon'; super-cooling of certain brain structures, perhaps due to alterations in cerebral blood flow; and the uncertain role of pH at profoundly hypothermic temperatures. Other variables also may be involved, including calcium and glucose homeostasis. Of interest is the delayed onset of neurologic deficits, which may be a reflection of altered neurotransmitter status.

Neuropsychologic sequelae

Surgery may be associated with impairment of cognitive function. On long-term follow-up the exact incidence of this problem is difficult to ascertain, mainly because of a general lack in neuropsychological studies with adequate pre- and postoperative assessments. Such studies are, however, fraught with methodological shortcomings.

Other late sequelae

A variety of other late neurologic sequelae are also seen complicating cardiac surgery. First, communicating hydrocephalus secondary to superior vena cava obstruction has been reported in infants following the Mustard operation for transposition of the great arteries. The SVC obstruction occurred secondary to obstruction of the superior limb of the intracardiac baffle. Clinically, facial swelling, plethora, and megaloencephaly were noted and the CT scan showed ventricular enlargement. Secondly, there is a surprisingly high incidence of hearing loss in children with congenital heart disease, which may or may not be related to surgery. As many as 25% of children aged 3 days to 12 years suffered hearing loss that was not associated with otitis media with effusion. Finally, vertebrobasilar ischemia after a Blalock–Taussig anastomosis can be the result of significant subclavian steal, but this is rare.

POSTOPERATIVE NEUROINTENSIVE CARE

Seizures, focal neurological signs, and an unexpected depressed level of consciousness may all be features of significant neurological insult. As discussed above, these features of an acute neurological process may be masked by concomitant pharmacological sedation and neuromuscular blockade. The priority in all patients having cardiac surgery must be good cardiopulmonary care, with meticulous attention to hemodynamic state (i.e. blood pressure, cardiac rhythm, cardiac output, and perfusion). Within this context, a concerted effort should be made to attend to a regular neurological examination. In patients in whom this is not possible because of the necessary drugs administered, attention should be given to the possibility of unappreciated (and uncontrolled) seizures or continuing cerebral insult from poor cerebral perfusion—factors which of themselves will contribute to any primary neurological injury.

Anticonvulsant therapy for seizures or treatment of any metabolic derangement causing seizures should be administered rapidly (Ch. 2.5, 3.2). Airway and ventilatory support with continued intubation may be necessary because of the seizures themselves or obtundation from anticonvulsant medications. Poor cerebral perfusion and the development of 'cytotoxic cerebral edema' with raised intracranial pressure will require the usual support for that problem. In this context, it should however be remembered that these acute problems require a coordinated approach between neurology and critical care specialists so that the right investigations and monitoring, when deemed necessary, are carried out.

NEUROMUSCULAR DISORDERS

A variety of disorders that affect the neuromuscular system may result in respiratory failure. Although it is beyond the scope of this chapter to catalog every disorder in the differential diagnosis of presenting problems such as 'apparent life-threatening life events' or the 'floppy infant' syndrome, a framework which is useful in the context of critical illness is shown in Tables 3.3.11–3.3.13. The final section of this chapter concentrates on intensive care aspects of the central hypoventilation syndrome, Guillain–Barré syndrome, myasthenia gravis and prolonged paralysis in intensive care unit patients.

CENTRAL HYPOVENTILATION SYNDROME

Central hypoventilation syndrome is characterized by respiratory depression during sleep, more marked during the non-REM state. It represents a more protracted form of central apnea which can progress to hypoventilation during all sleep and awake states. The syndrome may be congenital, with onset in the perinatal period, or acquired, when it is associated with conditions such as posterior fossa tumors, encephalitis, hypoxic-ischemic encephalopathy, pyruvate dehydrogenase defi-

TABLE 3.3.11 Known etiologies of 'apparent life-threatening events', defined as episodes that seem to occur during sleep, wakefulness or feeding, and consisting of some combination of apnea, color change (usually limpness, rarely rigidity), choking or gagging

Digestive
- Gastroesophageal reflux
- Infection
- Aspiration
- Malformation
- Dumping syndrome

Neurological
- Vasovagal syndrome
- Epilepsy
- Infection
- Subdural hematoma
- Malformation

Respiratory
- Infection
- Airway abnormality
- Alveolar hypoventilation

Cardiovascular
- Infection
- Cardiomyopathy
- Arrhythmia
- Malformation

Metabolic and endocrine
- Hypoglycemia
- Hypocalcemia
- Reye's syndrome
- Hypothyroidism
- Fatty acid metabolic disorder
- Leigh's disease
- Carnitine deficiency
- Menkes' syndrome
- Fructosemia

Miscellaneous
- Trauma
- Sepsis
- Drugs
- Munchausen syndrome by proxy

ciency and idiopathic hypothalamic dysfunction. Reversible disorders of hypoventilation and apnea, e.g. sepsis, hypothermia, hypocalcemia, hypoglycemia and seizures, should be excluded before embarking on the investigations listed in Table 3.3.12.

Infants with congenital central hypoventilation syndrome require long-term ventilatory support or equivalent alternative such as phrenic nerve

TABLE 3.3.12 Diagnostic procedures for 'apparent life-threatening events'

Initial studies	Potential diagnoses
History	
Full blood count	Infection, anemia
Urinalysis and culture	Infection, metabolic screen
CSF	Infection
EEG	Seizure, encephalopathic disorder
Chest X-ray	Infection, cardiomegaly
ECG	Arrhythmias, prolonged QT interval
Secondary studies	
Esophageal pH study	Gastroesophageal reflux
Barium esophagogram	Vascular ring
Microlaryngo-bronchoscopy	Airway abnormalities
Echocardiography	Cardiac abnormaility
Metabolic studies	Inherited metabolic disease
Cranial CT	Hematoma
Sleep study	Abnormality of respiratory control

pacing. This is best undertaken in centers where such children are frequently assessed and reviewed.

GUILLAIN–BARRÉ SYNDROME

The Guillain–Barré syndrome (GBS) is defined as a subacute symmetrical and progressive motor weakness with areflexia. The paresis is caused by inflammatory and demyelinating lesions scattered throughout the peripheral nervous system. Life-threatening complications which necessitate intensive care include:

- respiratory insufficiency due to ascending paralysis with inspiratory muscle involvement
- deep vein thrombosis
- autonomic disturbance

Respiratory failure

Respiratory failure is a complication that can be easily supported with mechanical ventilation; respiratory capacity should therefore be tested regularly with expiratory vital capacity measurements. Arterial blood gas values are less reliable indicators of when ventilatory support should be instituted: delaying intubation and assisted ventilation until hypercarbia occurs will lead to more frequent emergency intubations, a less than optimal approach to patients with potential autonomic disturbance. Mechanical ventilation should be started when the vital capacity falls below 15 ml/kg or if the patient is too fatigued to be tested. It is important to remember that succinylcholine (suxamethonium) is contraindicated since it is likely to cause ventricular dysrhythmias.

Autonomic dysfunction

Dysfunction of the autonomic nervous system is seen in children with GBS, especially in those who require mechanical ventilation. The problems encountered are summarized in Table 3.3.14. Each problem requires specific management:

TABLE 3.3.13 Neuromuscular disorders associated with respiratory muscle compromise and respiratory control abnormalities

Cerebral cortex
- Rett syndrome
- Leigh's disease
- Cerebral palsy
- Congenital central hypoventilation syndrome
- Joubert's syndrome

Brain stem and spinal cord
- Tumors
- Hemorrhage
- Infection and tetanus
- Brain-stem atrophy (Joseph disease)
- Trauma

Anterior horn cell disease
- Spinal muscular atrophy
- Poliomyelitis

Peripheral nerve
- Guillain–Barré syndrome
- Metachromatic leukodystrophy
- Phrenic nerve injury

Neuromuscular junction
- Infantile myasthenia gravis
- Infant botulism
- Critical illness disease

Primary muscle disease
- Myotonic dystrophy
- Duchenne's muscular dystrophy
- Nonprogressive myopathy — nemaline rod and central core disease, congenital muscular dystrophy
- Polymyositis and dermatomyositis
- Critical illness disease

TABLE 3.3.14 **Autonomic dysfunction in GBS**	
Dysfunction	**Clinical problem**
Sympathetic activity	
Excessive	Hypertension
	Sinus tachycardia
	Hyperhidrosis
Insufficient	Postural hypotension
Parasympathetic activity	
Excessive	Facial flushing
	Bradycardia
Insufficient	Tachycardia
	Sphincter disturbance

- *sphincter disturbance* requires catheterization of the bladder
- *hyperhidrosis* and *hypersalivation* can cause loss of fluid and electrolytes requiring changes in intravenous fluid therapy
- *ileus* is rare but can cause loss of large amounts of gastrointestinal secretions and inadequate enteral feeding
- *cardiac dysrhythmias* and *blood pressure disturbance* are characterized by periods of instability with hypo- or hypertensive episodes and tachy- or bradyarrhythmias; the administration of alpha- and beta-blockers and stimulators can therefore be dangerous. Episodes are frequently provoked by endotracheal tube toilet or physiotherapy with stimulation of the vagus nerve. Management of the susceptible child should if necessary include cardiac pacing.

Medical treatment

Children with mild cases of GBS who are able to walk can be managed without specific treatment. However, the child who loses the ability to walk or in whom respiratory compromise develops should receive intravenous immunoglobulin therapy or plasmapheresis. Remitting-relapsing or prolonged cases (longer than 1 month) should receive steroids provided other mechanisms of relapse have been excluded (e.g. lead toxicity, porphyria, hereditary motor sensory neuropathy).

MYASTHENIA GRAVIS

The cardinal clinical feature of myasthenia gravis is fatiguability. Exercise induces progressive, notable weakening of patients, with impairment increasing as the day advances. Difficulties range in severity from mild ptosis to respiratory difficulty. The latter may cause death despite optimum treatment. In most pediatric cases myasthenia gravis can be categorized as transient neonatal, persistent neonatal, or juvenile.

Transient neonatal myasthenia gravis

Transient neonatal myasthenia gravis is present in neonates of mothers with myasthenia gravis and is due to placental transfer of maternal antiacetylcholine receptor antibodies or maternal immunocytes which then compromise the infant's receptors. Impairment is usually evident within hours of birth but may be delayed for a few days. Early findings include weak suck, dysphagia, generalized muscle weakness, paucity of spontaneous movements, respiratory inadequacy and ptosis.

Persistent neonatal myasthenia gravis

Infants with persistent neonatal (congenital) myasthenia gravis have acquired the autoimmune or nonautoimmune hereditary type of disease. Their mothers do not have myasthenia gravis. Symptoms are usually evident on the first day of life, but as in the transient neonatal form of myasthenia gravis they may appear days later. Respiratory function may be so involved that ventilatory support is required and as the disease progresses bulbar dysfunction may become more obvious. Contractures similar to those associated with arthrogryposis may also be present.

Juvenile myasthenia gravis

Juvenile myasthenia gravis is very similar to the adult form of the disease. Features usually appear after the age of 10 years. It is more common in girls. The disease waxes and wanes with exacerbations that sometimes necessitate mechanical ventilation. Affected children have serum IgG antibody to nicotinic acetylcholine receptors less frequently than do adult patients.

Diagnosis

Diagnostic evaluation for probable myasthenia gravis in children consists of a trial of edrophonium chloride or neostigmine. Evaluation in infants is best done with oral neostigmine because of the difficulty in assessing weakness over a short period and because of poor cooperation. Peripheral neurophysiological investigation is also informative in the clinical assessment.

Treatment

Virtually all forms of myasthenia gravis are treated with one or more of the following agents: anticholinesterases, prednisolone, immunosuppressants, thymectomy and plasmapheresis. The specifics of when, what and how much to use are best left to consultation with pediatric neurology specialists.

Myasthenic crisis or cholinergic crisis?

Of particular importance to intensive care treatment of patients with myasthenia gravis is differentiating a myasthenic crisis from a cholinergic crisis. In such patients, despite seemingly optimal drug therapy, there is an inability to maintain basal ventilation needs or effective swallowing of oropharyngeal secretions. These problems may occur when the patient is receiving concurrent antibiotics, narcotics, barbiturates, tranquilizers, or antiarrhythmics such as lidocaine (lignocaine), quinidine, procainamide and propranolol. Hypokalemia may also cause similar symptoms.

Differentiating a myasthenic crisis from a cholinergic crisis can be difficult:

- *myasthenic crisis* is manifested by progressive and profound weakness and results from too little treatment
- *cholinergic crisis* looks similar to a myasthenic crisis but is accompanied by increased sweating, profuse formation of saliva, vomiting, abdominal colic and diarrhea; it results from excessive administration of anticholinesterase medication

If there is doubt, initially the patient should receive edrophonium chloride intravenously during the period when the optimal effect of the anti-cholinesterase therapy is anticipated. Attenuation of weakness indicates a myasthenic crisis and the need for larger doses of long-acting anticholinesterase drugs. For this test, the best indicator of a significant response is an increase in vital capacity. If the edrophonium injection is *not* effective then a cholinergic crisis is probably present: this condition requires the withdrawal of anticholinesterase therapy. Atropine may be required to reduce perspiration, vomiting, colic and diarrhea. Occasionally it is impossible to distinguish between the myasthenic and cholinergic crises. When this occurs, after appropriate specialist consultation, all medications should be withheld and ventilatory support provided if necessary for 48–72 hours until the underlying cause of the profound weakness becomes evident.

It is imperative when dealing with these problems that facilities for tracheostomy, ventilatory support and airway toilet are readily available and electively carried out when deemed necessary. If not, patients should be transferred to a hospital where these are available.

PROLONGED PARALYSIS IN INTENSIVE CARE PATIENTS

Reports of prolonged paralysis in intensive care unit patients predominantly refer to adult practice. However, a number of pediatric cases have been reported and so this topic does warrant special consideration (Table 3.3.15).

Neuromuscular blocking agents

Neuromuscular blocking agents are administered intermittently and by continuous infusion to selected mechanically ventilated, critically ill patients to promote better ventilatory management. Continuous infusion methods facilitate long-term drug administration and minimize the hemodynamic and ventilatory fluctuations due to rapidly changing drug concentrations which are associated with intermittent dosing. Of particular concern is the occurrence of prolonged neuromuscular blockade despite drug discontinuation. The causes of this problem can be divided into those based on drug pharmacokinetics and those based on neuromuscular function:

TABLE 3.3.15 Neuromuscular conditions in critical illness

Condition	Clinical features	Electromyography	Creatine phosphokinase	Muscle biopsy
Polyneuropathy				
Critical illness polyneuropathy	Seen with sepsis Flaccid limbs and respiratory weakness	Axonal degeneration of motor and sensory fibers	Near normal	Denervation atrophy
Motor neuropathy	Seen with NMBAs Flaccid limbs and respiratory weakness	Axonal degeneration of motor fibers	Near normal	Denervation atrophy
Neuromuscular transmission defect				
Transient neuromuscular blockade	Seen with NMBAs Flaccid limbs and respiratory weakness	Abnormal repetitive nerve stimulation studies	Normal	Normal
Myopathy				
Thick filament myopathy	Seen with steroids, NMBAs and asthma Flaccid limbs and respiratory weakness	Abnormal spontaneous activity	Elevated	Central loss of thick filaments
Disuse myopathy	Muscle wasting with illness	Normal	Normal	Normal, or type II fiber atrophy
Necrotizing myopathy of intensive care	Poor prognosis Flaccid weakness, myoglobinuria	Abnormal spontaneous activity	Markedly elevated	Panfascicular muscle fiber necrosis

NMBAs, neuromuscular blocking agents.

- *pharmacokinetic* problems are usually short term and are attributable to altered hepatic or renal clearance because of end-organ dysfunction; peripheral neurophysiology will confirm persistent neuromuscular blockade
- problems of *neuromuscular function* are usually manifested as prolonged paralysis in patients with normal end-organ function; electromyography will show neuromuscular defects.

Concomitant administration of several drugs alters the duration of action of neuromuscular blocking agents and can influence each of the above problems. Drugs thought to shorten the duration of action include furosemide (frusemide), methylxanthines, phenytoin (not with atracurium), carbamazepine and azathioprine. Drugs thought to potentiate blockade include other neuromuscular blocking agents; antibiotics (in particular aminoglycosides and clindamycin); antiarrhythmic agents; midazolam; β-adrenergic receptor block-

ers; calcium channel blockers; and cyclosporin. In addition, the combination of steroids and steroid-based neuromuscular blocking agents such as vecuronium and pancuronium have been implicated in prolonged blockade.

The aim for all those administering neuromuscular blocking agents must be to avoid the above problems. Proposed methods include peripheral nerve stimulation monitoring, periodic drug discontinuation, recognition of interacting drug therapy, and attention to electrolyte and acid–base management. Despite these approaches other peripheral neurological problems may still occur in certain high-risk groups such as people with asthma or sepsis syndrome (see below).

Critical illness polyneuropathy and related disorders

Symptoms of neuromuscular conditions seen in critically ill patients with either sepsis syndrome or multiple organ system dysfunction include failure to wean from mechanical ventilation in an expected time, limb weakness and impaired deep tendon reflexes. Sensory function often remains intact. Cerebrospinal fluid results are normal and electrophysiology shows a variety of findings. Interestingly, a number of the reported patients had not received neuromuscular blocking agents.

The treatment in these patients is essentially supportive once it has been recognized.

FURTHER READING

1. Plum F, Posner J. The diagnosis of stupor and coma. Philadelphia: FA Davis; 1980

2. Johnston MV, Trescher WH, Taylor GA. Hypoxic and ischemic central nervous system disorders in infants and children. Adv Pediatrics 1995; 42: 1–45
    –   (*Comprehensive reviews of recent advances in pathophysiology, diagnosis, imaging and management*)

3. Levin DL. In: Morriss (Ed) Essentials of Pediatric Intensive Care (2nd ed). London, New York: Churchill Livingstone 1997
    –   (*Detailed text on pediatric intensive care with comprehensive treatment recommendations re neurological issues*)

3.4 Endocrine emergencies

Glynis Price

DIABETIC KETOACIDOSIS

Diabetic ketoacidosis (DKA) is the most common cause of diabetes-related death in children and is always caused by an absolute or relative lack of insulin. It is defined as hyperglycemia in excess of 14 mmol/L (250 mg/dl), metabolic acidosis (pH < 7.3 or bicarbonate level below 15 mmol/L), and hyperketonemia or moderate to severe ketonuria.

PATHOPHYSIOLOGY

The pathophysiology of DKA is summarized in Figure 3.4.1.

CAUSES

The causes of diabetic ketoacidosis in children are:

- delayed diagnosis of insulin-dependent diabetes mellitus (IDDM): a high index of suspicion is needed in infants and toddlers

- omission of insulin—particularly in adolescents with recurrent DKA
- acute stress (infection, trauma, psychological) causing an increase in counter-regulatory hormones and decreased attention to diabetes care
- poor management of intercurrent illness: omission of insulin in a vomiting child or failure to increase the insulin dose appropriately

EVALUATION

History

The history should include:

- typical symptoms:
  - polyuria
  - polydipsia
  - significant weight loss

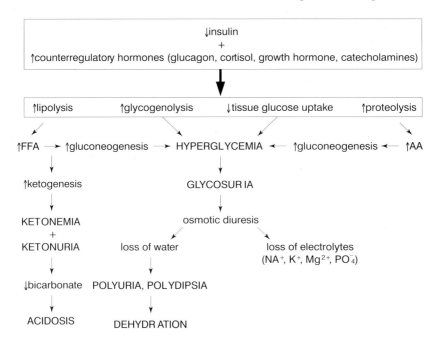

Figure 3.4.1 Pathophysiology of diabetic ketoacidosis. AA, amino acids; FFA, free fatty acids (Adapted from Annual Review of Medicine, 1979; 30: 347, Figure 3. With permission from the Annual Review of Medicine, C, © 1979, by Annual Reviews.)

- weakness and fatigue
- vomiting and abdominal pain
- precipitating causes (see above)

Physical examination

The following clinical features are characteristic of DKA:

- dehydration (estimate extent—see below)
- tachycardia, variable blood pressure (hypotension uncommmon)
- hypothermia (common)
- Kussmaul breathing or tachypnea
- altered level of consciousness (related to hyperosmolality)
- identify precipitating causes

Investigations

Investigations should include:

- blood glucose
- plasma urea and electrolytes
- serum osmolality: measured or calculated (see box)

$$serum\ osmolality = [Na^+] \times 2 + [glucose] + [urea]$$
$$(values\ in\ mmol/L)$$

- blood gas (arterial initially, then capillary or venous pH and bicarbonate)
- full blood count
- consider: urine culture, blood cultures and chest radiograph

Remember that: over-estimation of dehydration is common. Dehydration may be:

- mild (3–5%): decreased skin turgor just clinically detectable
- moderate (6–8%): easily detectable dehydration, e.g. markedly reduced skin turgor and poor capillary return
- severe (9–12%): poor skin perfusion, rapid pulse, reduced blood pressure
- to identify hypernatremia, compensate for the dilutional effect of hyperglycemia by calculating the corrected sodium value (see box)

$$corrected\ Na^+ =$$
$$[plasma\ Na^+] + 0.3\ ([plasma\ glucose] - 5.5)$$
$$(values\ in\ mmol/L)$$

- hypertriglyceridemia may also cause pseudohyponatremia
- whole-body potassium content is always depleted despite varying serum levels
- creatinine measurement can be falsely raised by interference of ketones

TREATMENT

If the child is mildly dehydrated and not vomiting, give oral fluids and rapidly acting insulin 0.25 unit/kg subcutaneously, 6-hourly before each meal until stable. If the condition is more severe; intravenous therapy is necessary using the following protocol. (For a treatment algorithm see Ch. 7.3, p. 597).

1. *Correct shock*: i.v. boluses of 0.9% saline (or colloid), 10 ml/kg, repeated as necessary.
2. *Fluid*: rehydration fluid (see box) plus maintenance fluids (Ch. 3.5) are given evenly over 48 hours. If the patient is hypernatremic or very hyperosmolar (serum osmolality > 340 mOsm/L), rehydrate over 72–96 hours. Saline (0.9%) is used for the first 6–12 hours, then 0.45% saline. Add 50% dextrose to the saline solution when the plasma glucose level is less than 15 mmol/L. Each 10 ml of 50% dextrose added to 500 ml of any solution adds 1% dextrose: 5% dextrose in saline is usually sufficient. Rehydration can be completed orally once the acidosis has resolved and the patient is tolerating feeds.

$$rehydration\ fluid\ (ml) =$$
$$10 \times dehydration\ (\%) \times body\ weight\ (kg)$$

3. *Potassium*: when the insulin infusion starts, add potassium chloride to all i.v. fluids (40 mmol/L for children weighing < 30 kg, 60 mmol/L if > 30 kg), provided the patient is not anuric and serum potassium concentration is no more than 5 mmol/L.

Half may be given as potassium phosphate, although the clinical benefit of the extra phosphate is unproven. Electro-cardiographic monitoring is recommended.

4. *Insulin*: Start after treatment for shock. Use regular crystalline insulin only (see below for details of insulin therapy).

Insulin

Continuous low-dose intravenous insulin infusion is used when syringe pumps and close nursing observation are available (i.e. after the child reaches the ward and is closely monitored). The starting dose is 0.1 units/kg·h. Hospitals vary in how they mix and run insulin infusions—*use the regimen your unit is familiar with. Either* 50 units of insulin in 500 ml of 0.9% saline run at 1 ml/kg·h *or* (50 units of rapid-acting insulin in 50 ml of 0.9% saline run at 0.1 ml/kg·h). The dose is only reduced to 0.05 units/kg:

- in a young child
- if insulin has already been administered
- when the plasma bicarbonate level is nearing 16 mmol/L and the glucose level is below 12 mmol/L

The rate should be doubled unless there is improvement in acidosis (increase in pH of at least 0.03 units/h or increase in bicarbonate) and blood glucose level within the first 2 hours of treatment. When the plasma glucose concentration falls below 10 mmol/L or less, the strength of dextrose solution added to the i.v. fluid should be increased, but the insulin infusion should *not* be reduced. Insulin should be continued until the glucose is controlled *and the acidosis and ketosis have completely cleared.* The first subcutaneous injection (0.25 units/kg 6-hourly) is then given provided that the child is well, and the insulin infusion is stopped 30 minutes later. *Insulin should not be mixed in the bag of rehydration fluid.* The insulin infusion should be run through a side line into the tubing carrying the rehydrating fluid, using a three-way tap and a volumetric or syringe pump.

Bolus intravenous or intramuscular insulin (never used in shock): give a bolus of 0.1 unit/kg of insulin i.v., then 0.1 units/kg i.m. or subcutaneously every hour.

General

General guidelines include:

- nurse the child in a 10° head-up position or in the coma position (Ch. 2.4)
- nil by mouth
- use a flow chart of biochemical test results (see appendix Ch. 7.3)
- hourly blood glucose measurement
- hourly BP, pulse and neurological observations for 24 hours
- assess blood gases and electrolytes every 2–4 hours until clearly improving, then 6-hourly
- strict fluid monitoring
- insert a nasogastric tube if vomiting (gastric atony is common) or decreased level of consciousness occurs
- routine catheterization is not necessary

Bicarbonate

Do not give bicarbonate without discussion with a pediatric endocrinologist. Increasingly $NaHCO_3$ is *not* recommended, regardless of pH. The acidosis of DKA is due to ketone bodies and lactic acid and resolves with fluid and insulin. No studies prove $NaHCO_3$ to be of benefit, but adverse effects include hypokalemia, alkalosis and delayed ketone clearance (see Ch. 3.5).

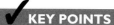
KEY POINTS

- ➤ Rehydration over 72 hours
- ➤ Give insulin
- ➤ Replace potassium
- ➤ Frequent monitoring of the patient's clinical, glucose, electrolyte and acid–base status is essential

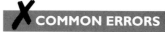
COMMON ERRORS

In diagnosis

- ➤ Acute abdomen: abdominal pain, tenderness and ileus are common in DKA
- ➤ Pancreatitis: amylase and lipase may be increased in DKA
- ➤ Infection

- check hidden sites of infection (urine, teeth, sinuses, injection sites)
- high white cell count and left shift are common in DKA but do not necessarily indicate infection
- fever suggests infection but the temperature of most infected patients is normal or low

In treatment

➤ Overestimation of dehydration

➤ Stopping or decreasing insulin because of falling glucose levels while acidosis is still present

➤ Stopping the insulin infusion before sub-cutaneous insulin has been given

➤ Persistent acidosis: inadequately treated ketoacidosis must be differentiated from nonanion gap hyperchloremic acidosis which can occur during recovery from DKA and which usually resolves spontaneously

TRANSPORT

Children with DKA should be managed in hospitals with expertise in the problem. If the patient is not very ill and the distance to a specialized center is short, give oral fluids only. If the patient is moderately or severely dehydrated, correct shock if present and start i.v. 0.9% saline (rehydration and maintenance calculated over 48 hours). Give iv insulin infusion at 0.1 unit/kg·h in severely acidotic and very hyperglycemic patients, but monitor blood glucose levels during transport and have dextrose available to treat hypoglycemia. A protocol/calculation flow sheet is included in Ch. 7.3.

DANGERS OF DKA AND ITS TREATMENT

Hypoglycemia (plasma glucose < 4 mmol/L)

Treat hypoglycemia with 0.5 g/kg dextrose (2 ml/kg of 25% dextrose) intravenously. Decrease insulin infusion *briefly* while returning blood glucose concentration to the normal range.

Cerebral edema

Cerebral edema is a particular danger in children, especially those under 5 years old, accounting for about 50% of mortality in pediatric DKA. Its cause is unknown but may be a reduction in extracellular fluid osmolality related to rapid correction of dehydration and hyperglycemia and the use of hypotonic fluids. This reduction in osmolality causes water to move into brain cells (i.e. cerebral edema). It occurs suddenly, usually 6–12 hours after starting treatment, when the patient's biochemical signs are improving.

Presentation

Cerebral edema presents with headache, vomiting, a change in behavior (increased irritability in infants, fighting or agitation) or altered level of consciousness, seizures, pupillary changes or ophthalmoplegia, and changes in vital signs. There is often rapid progression of neurological signs and respiratory arrest.

Treatment

Rapidly assess and secure airway, breathing and circulation. Intubate and ventilate to $Paco_2$ 4–5 kPa (30–40 mmHg). Give 0.5 g/kg 20% mannitol i.v. if cerebral edema is suspected; nurse the child head-up and decrease the fluid rate to rehydrate over 96 hours or longer. Monitor plasma glucose and sodium levels hourly and ensure that neither decreases until the child's conscious state returns to its pretreatment level. Do not wait for a confirmatory CT scan before treating.

Hypokalemia

Hypokalemia is most marked in the first few hours of insulin therapy and may cause arrhythmias and respiratory muscle weakness. Prevent by early potassium replacement, frequent monitoring and adjustment of supplementation, aiming to keep serum potassium levels above 4 mmol/L.

ADRENAL CRISIS

Adrenal crisis is caused by deficiency of glucocorticoid (cortisol) and/or mineralocorticoid (aldosterone). Cortisol secretion is controlled by ACTH from the pituitary gland and aldosterone by the renin–angiotensin system and by the serum potassium concentration. Conditions affecting ACTH production (secondary hypoadrenalism) therefore present with *cortisol deficiency* only, whereas those affecting the adrenal gland (primary hypoadrenalism) present with deficiencies of both *cortisol* and *mineralocorticoid*. Chronic hypoadrenalism may cause only fatigue and weakness. Adrenal crisis may then be precipitated by stress such as pyrexia, trauma or surgery, as the adrenal glands cannot increase cortisol production. Basal cortisol production is 12–15 mg/m^2 daily; this usually increases 2- to 5-fold in stress.

CAUSES

Primary adrenal disease

Primary hypoadrenalism may be caused by:

- congenital adrenal hyperplasia is the most common cause in neonates; it usually presents with salt-losing crisis on day 4 to 14
- chronic hypoadrenalism (Addison's disease): usually autoimmune
- adrenoleukodystrophy (X-linked)
- adrenal hemorrhage in the newborn: often involves large, male babies with traumatic delivery
- adrenal hemorrhage in acute infection (particularly meningococcal septicemia)

Secondary to ACTH deficiency

Secondary hypoadrenalism may be caused by:

- hypopituitarism:
  - congenital malformations of the brain, particularly midline defects, e.g. septo-optic dysplasia
  - cranial trauma, irradiation, surgery
  - pituitary/hypothalamic tumors, e.g. craniopharyngioma (deficiency of corticotropin releasing hormone— tertiary hypoadrenalism)
- abrupt withdrawal of steroids after chronic use
- removal of a unilateral cortisol-producing tumor

PREVENTION

Children considered to be at risk of an adrenal crisis should be given triple their normal oral maintenance steroid dose for 2–3 days during periods of stress. Give hydrocortisone i.m. to children with adrenal insufficiency when absorption of oral medication is doubtful, e.g. in vomiting or severe diarrhoea. Children at risk (see above) who present with vomiting but who are not otherwise unwell should be considered to have incipient adrenal crisis:

- check for hypotension (particularly postural)
- measure blood glucose and electrolytes
- administer i.m. hydrocortisone 2 mg/kg
- observe for 4–6 hours before considering sending home

ASSESSMENT

History and physical examination

The following signs may help to establish the etiology:

- *glucocorticoid deficiency*:
  - weakness; anorexia; nausea or vomiting; hypoglycemia; hypotension and shock
  - pigmentation and ambiguous genitalia may be present
- *mineralocorticoid deficiency*: dehydration; hyperkalemia; hyponatremia; acidosis and 'prerenal' renal failure
- precipitating causes should be searched for and treated

Investigations

Investigations should include:

- blood glucose
- electrolytes, in particular sodium and potassium
- urea and creatinine
- bicarbonate, P_{CO_2} and pH

When the underlying diagnosis is unknown, collect the following specimens if possible:

- plasma for cortisol and 17α-hydroxy-progesterone (17α-OHP) estimation

- urine for steroid gas–liquid chromatography (therapy should not be delayed to collect the urine specimen)
- plasma for aldosterone, ACTH and plasma renin activity (PRA) if laboratory facilities are available

TREATMENT

Fluids

In *shock, hypotension or severe dehydration* (10% or more), give 0.9% saline at 10–20 ml/kg over the first hour (a plasma expander such as polygeline or 5% albumin may also be used). Repeat until circulation is restored. Replacement and maintenance is then administered over 24 hours:

- deficit = 100 ml/kg (subtract initial bolus volume from this amount)
- maintenance:
  - 2 L/m^2 or 100 ml for first 10 kg body weight, 50 ml/kg next 10 kg, 25 ml/kg each successive 10 kg
  - adolescents will need 3–6 litres

Use 5% dextrose in 0.9% saline. After the first few hours, this may be reduced to 0.45% saline, depending on the plasma sodium level (> 130 mmol/L), while 10% dextrose may be needed to maintain euglycemia.

In *moderate dehydration* (6%), give 5% dextrose in 0.9% saline: 10 ml/kg in the first hour and then give maintenance (Ch. 2.10) and replace the deficit (60 ml/kg) over 24 hours.

In *mild* (3%) or *no dehydration*; give 1.5–2 times maintenance over 24 hours.

Hydrocortisone

Give hydrocortisone intravenously as hydrocortisone sodium succinate. In the absence of i.v. access, give i.m. while establishing an intravenous line. Dosage is based on 5–10 times the basal cortisol production (a minimum of 100 mg/m^2 per day):

- neonates: 25 mg at once and then 10 mg 6-hourly
- infants (1–12 months): 25 mg at once, then 25 mg 6–8-hourly
- toddlers (1–3 years): 50 mg at once, then 50 mg 6–8-hourly
- children (4–12 years): 75 mg at once, then 75 mg 6–8-hourly
- adolescents: 100 mg at once, then 100 mg 6–8-hourly

* Some centres give a continuous infusion of hydrocortisone at 100 mg/m^2 after the initial bolus as above.

Dose requirements may be variable and the dose should be adjusted according to the clinical response.

When the child is stable, reduce the i.v. hydrocortisone dose, then switch to triple dose oral hydrocortisone therapy, gradually reducing to maintenance levels (10–15 mg/m^2 per day).

In patients with mineralocorticoid deficiency, start fludrocortisone at maintenance doses (usually 0.1 mg daily) as soon as the patient can tolerate oral fluids.

Hypoglycemia

Hypoglycemia is common in infants and small children. Treat with an intravenous bolus of 2–3 ml/kg 10% dextrose (in neonates) or 1–2 ml/kg of 25% dextrose in an older child or adolescent. Maintenance fluids should contain 5–10% dextrose.

Hyperkalemia

Hyperkalemia usually normalizes with fluid and electrolyte replacement. Hyperkalemic patients should have an ECG and cardiac monitor as arrhythmias and cardiac arrest may occur. Treat hyperkalemia if potassium level is above 7 mmol/L with ECG changes (tall peaked T wave, wide QRS, decreased P wave). Use one or more of the following treatment alternatives:

- sodium bicarbonate at 1–2 mmol/kg i.v. infused over 5–10 minutes
- calcium gluconate 10% at 0.5 ml/kg i.v. infused over 10 minutes (adult maximum dose is 10–20 ml); monitor for bradycardia and hypotension; sodium bicarbonate and calcium gluconate are incompatible and will precipitate if given through same the i.v. line without flushing
- dextrose 25% 4 ml/kg and insulin 0.1 unit/kg i.v. Monitor blood glucose hourly
- nebulized salbutamol 0.5% solution 1 ml in 3 ml 0.9% saline

- cation exchange resins (sodium polystyrene sulfonate) may be given 6-hourly orally or by retention enema (may cause colitis in young infants); a dose of 0.3–0.6 g/kg 6-hourly lowers potassium by 1 mmol/L in infants and children.

General

Assess the following regularly and modify treatment if necessary:

- clinical signs: blood pressure, fluid balance, weight, hydration, ECG
- biochemical: electrolytes, glucose, acid–base; hourly bedside glucose testing is needed in infants and small children

✔ KEY POINTS

- ➤ Fluid replacement
- ➤ Give cortisol
- ➤ Correct hypoglycemia
- ➤ Treat hyperkalemia

✘ COMMON ERRORS

- ➤ Not thinking of adrenal crisis in a vomiting child with a history of secondary hypoadrenalism (no typical electrolyte changes)
- ➤ Overtreatment causing hypernatremia, hypokalemia, hyperglycemia, hypertension, pulmonary edema and congestive cardiac failure

PHEOCHROMOCYTOMA

Pheochromocytoma is rare is childhood but may present with acute hypertensive crisis, particularly during surgery in children with previously undiagnosed pheochromocytoma. Pheochromocytoma may be sporadic or familial. It may be part of the dominantly inherited multiple endocrine neoplasia (MEN) syndrome or associated with neuroectodermal dysplasias. The diagnosis should be considered in children with hypertension and paroxysmal symptoms of palpitations, headache, sweating and vomiting, and is confirmed by finding increased levels of:

- 24-hour urinary excretion of
  - total free catecholamines
  - metanephrine
- metanephrine in an overnight or spot urine sample
- plasma catecholamines (fasting and at rest): often difficult to interpret

Tumors are localized by:

- CT or MRI scan of adrenals (detects 90% of tumors)
- meta-iodobenzyl guanidine (MIBG) nuclear scan for extra-adrenal tumors (10%)
- selective venous sampling with catecholamine measurement

Hypertensive crisis is mediated by catecholamine-induced α-adrenergic receptor stimulation.

PREOPERATIVE MANAGEMENT

Hypertension

Hypertension (due to arteriolar constriction) and relative hypovolemia (due to venoconstriction) are controlled by adrenergic blockade started 7–10 days before surgery:

- phenoxybenzamine 0.2–1 mg/kg every 12–24 hours until blood pressure is controlled
- persistent tachycardia and arrhythmias can be controlled by beta-blockers *but only after adequate alpha-blockade*, to avoid precipitating a hypertensive crisis
- expand the extracellular fluid volume to prevent hypotension: use adequate hydration and liberal salt intake or i.v. boluses of 0.9% saline 10 ml/kg

Hyperglycemia

Control hyperglycemia with insulin:

- subcutaneously 0.125–0.25 units/kg 6-hourly before meals *or*
- i.v. infusion 0.05–0.1 units/kg.h in an emergency or in the operating room

Management of hypertensive crisis

Give sodium nitroprusside by i.v. infusion:

- 0.5–10 μg/kg·min (maximum of 4 μg kg·min if used for more than 24 hours)
- dilution 3 mg/kg in 50 ml 5% dextrose: 1 ml/h = 1μg/kg·min

or give phentolamine 0.1 mg/kg i.v. bolus then 5–50 μg/kg·min.

PROBLEMS DURING AND AFTER SURGERY

Hypotension is caused by excessive β-adrenergic stimulation or postoperatively by falling tumor-derived catecholamines, persistent α-receptor blockade, downregulation of adrenergic receptors and blood loss. Therapy is mainly volume expansion as there is little response to pressor amines. An infusion of norepinephrine (noradrenaline) (0.05–0.5 μg/kg·min or vasopressin 0.0005–0.005 units/kg·min) may be tried.

Monitor for *hypoglycemia*, irrespective of insulin use. Steroid cover (hydrocortisone 50–100 mg 6-hourly) is required if bilateral adrenalectomy is performed.

HYPOGLYCEMIA

Hypoglycemia caused by defective glucose production or increased glucose utilization occurs in diverse diseases which affect glucose homeostasis. Treatment is urgent, as the brain is the main consumer of glucose in fasting children, and both the duration and severity of hypoglycemia may contribute to morbidity. Hypoglycemia is a chemical finding and its presence should lead to a thorough search for the underlying disorder. Causes of hypoglycemia are shown in Table 3.4.1.

CLINICAL FINDINGS

Clinical signs are nonspecific and may be attributed to factors other than the chemical abnormality. A child with a temperature of 40°C as part of a viral syndrome may experience a seizure: this could be diagnosed as a 'febrile seizure', but if the child has not eaten for 48 hours, hypoglycemia could be the underlying, or a synergistic cause. The signs of hypoglycemia are due to both the decreased availability of glucose to the brain and adrenergic stimulation (caused by a low or falling

TABLE 3.4.1 **Causes of hypoglycemia**
Increased glucose utilization
• Hyperinsulinism
• Tumors:
– Wilms' tumor
• Drug ingestion:
– salicylates
– propranolol
– alcohol
Decreased glucose synthesis
• Inadequate glycogen stores
– defects of glycogen production
– glycogen synthetase deficiency
• Inability to mobilize glycogen
– glucagon deficiency
– defects in glycogenolysis
– debrancher deficiency
• Ineffective gluconeogenesis
– inadequate substrate
– ketotic hypoglycemia
– enzymatic defect
Diminished availability of fats
• Depleted fat stores
• Failure to mobilize fats
• Defective utilization of fats
– enzymatic defects in fatty acid oxidation
– long-chain or medium-chain acyl-CoA dehydrogenase deficiency
– carnitine transport defect
Decreased substrate stores
• Fasting
• Malnutrition
• Prolonged illness
• Malabsorption
Increased substrate requirements
• Fever
• Exercise
Inadequate counterregulatory hormones
• Growth hormone deficiency
• Cortisol deficiency
• Hypopituitarism

blood glucose level). Autoregulation of brain blood flow can also become disturbed. Symptoms include irritability, headache, confusion, unconsciousness, and seizure. Adrenergic signs include tachycardia, tremulousness, diaphoresis and hunger. Any combination of the above signs and symptoms requires prompt measurement of blood glucose; it is also required in any child presenting with seizure, coma, or a history of possible toxic ingestion (ethanol, propranolol or a hypoglycemic agent).

The endocrine causes of hypoglycemia are considered below. Nonendocrine causes are discussed in Chapter 2.9.

HYPERINSULINISM

Hyperinsulinism is the most common cause of persistent hypoglycemia in childhood, especially in the first year of life. Causes include:

- neonatal period:
  - infant of diabetic mother
  - Beckwith–Wiedemann syndrome (macrosomia, organomegaly, macroglossia, omphalocele)
  - Rh incompatibility
  - nesidioblastosis
- older infants and children:
  - exogenous insulin administration in children with IDDM (missed meal; deliberate or accidental overdose; exercise without appropriate snack)
  - nesidioblastosis
  - insulin adenoma (rare)

The following clinical features are characteristic:

- large, obese infant
- nonketotic hypoglycemia
- unusually high glucose requirement to maintain euglycemia
  - newborn > 10 mg/kg·min
  - young child > 5 mg/kg·min
  - adolescent > 3 mg/kg·min
- increased glucose utilization
- free fatty acids (FFA) and lactate levels not elevated

DEFICIENCY OF GROWTH HORMONE OR CORTISOL

The usual causes of growth hormone or cortisol deficiency are:

- hypopituitarism with growth hormone or ACTH deficiency (clinical pointers: micro-phallus and midline cephalic lesions, e.g. holoprosencephaly or central cleft lip and palate)
- adrenal failure; congenital adrenal hyperplasia (clinical pointers: ambiguous genitalia or skin pigmentation)

Clinical features include:

- ketotic hypoglycemia
- condition appears at any time after birth: often when 3-hourly feeds stop
- impaired glucose production and increased glucose utilization (because inadequate fat mobilization causes impaired ketogenesis)

Although glucometer readings are useful for screening, laboratory confirmation of hypoglycemia and investigation *at the time of hypoglycemia* are important in diagnosis.

INVESTIGATIONS

The following investigations are required:

- plasma glucose
- plasma insulin, cortisol and growth hormone
- plasma FFA, lactate and pH
- urine for ketones, organic acids and amino acids

The priorities are to measure the metabolic compounds associated with fasting and the hormones that regulate these processes. Blood obtained at the time the child is hypoglycemic is most helpful. Measurement of β-hydroxybutyrate and FFA (as markers of fatty acid metabolism), lactate, pyruvate, and alanine (as markers of the gluconeogenic pathways) and insulin, growth hormone, and cortisol (as the principal regulatory hormones) provide valuable clues to the cause of the hypoglycemia, e.g. low levels of ketones and FFA suggest that fat is not being appropriately mobilized (with ketones not formed by the liver). Hyperinsulinism could be the cause and would be confirmed by a high level of circulating insulin. Urine obtained at the time of hypoglycemia should be tested for ketones, evaluated for drugs and for metabolic by-products (organic acids, amino acids) associated with known causes of hypoglycemia.

TREATMENT OF HYPOGLYCEMIA

In critically ill children intravenous glucose is given initially. Later treatment depends on the underlying diagnosis.

If venous access cannot be achieved promptly, glucose can be given through a nasogastric tube (glucose is rapidly absorbed from the gut). The risk of prolonged hypoglycemia far outweighs the risk associated with the passage of a nasogastric tube in the obtunded child. Blood glucose levels should be monitored closely. Glucagon can effectively raise glucose levels under conditions where glycogen stores have not been depleted (promotes glycogen breakdown). Glucocorticoids are used primarily for cortisol deficiency.

Dosages for glucose administration are:

- neonate: 2–3 ml/kg of 10% dextrose (0.25 g/kg), followed by infusion of dextrose (5–10 mg/kg·min)
- older children: 1–2 ml/kg of 25% dextrose (0.5 g/kg dextrose or 12.5–25 g in a teenager), then 3–5 mg/kg·min until stable

Hyperinsulinism

Treat hyperinsulinism with glucagon 0.03 mg/kg i.m. or i.v. If hypoglycemia persists, start a glucagon infusion at 0.005–0.1 unit/kg·h (1 unit =1 mg). Give diazoxide 2–6 mg/kg 8-hourly orally.

Growth hormone or cortisol deficiency

If cortisol deficient, give hydrocortisone 25 mg/m^2 6-hourly i.v. – this is the minimum dose during stress. When the child is stable, switch to triple oral dose therapy (10–15 mg/m^2 hydrocortisone or cortisone acetate orally 8-hourly) and taper to a daily maintenance dose of 10–15 mg/m^2·day. In children with growth hormone deficiency, growth hormone is given at 2 units/m^2 daily subcutaneously (not usually urgent).

Diabetes mellitus

If the child is conscious, give a glucose drink or snack. If the child is unconscious or unable to cooperate:

- i.v. glucose bolus and infusion if child is severely symptomatic or blood glucose level very low
- i.m. glucagon (0.5 mg in children under 2 years old, 1 mg in older children) if not in hospital or i.v. access unavailable. Ensure

that the patient eats thereafter, or consider glucose infusion. Glucagon administration may be followed by headache and vomiting

DIABETES INSIPIDUS

Diabetes insipidus (DI) is characterized by hypotonic polyuria with increased serum osmolality resulting from deficiency of vasopressin (central DI) or poor renal response to vasopressin (nephrogenic DI). It is benign if the patient has adequate thirst and can respond by drinking, but otherwise becomes life-threatening.

CAUSES

Common causes of central DI are:

- head trauma
- cranial surgery, especially in the hypothalamic area
- tumors, e.g. craniopharyngioma
- infiltration, e.g. histiocytosis X
- idiopathic—may need repeated MRI to exclude underlying pathology
- birth trauma, asphyxia, intraventricular hemorrhage or severe infections (this should be suspected in a sick neonate with hypernatremia, weight loss and urine osmolality < 300 mOsm/kg)

Hypothalamic disturbance is often followed by a three-step sequence of

- transient DI
- excessive arginine vasopressin (AVP) release
- permanent DI

DIAGNOSIS

Hyperosmolar plasma (> 295 mOsm/kg or serum sodium >143 mmol/L) with inappropriately low urine osmolality (< 300 mOsm/kg in complete vasopressin deficiency) is diagnostic. Glycosuric osmotic diuresis must be excluded.

TREATMENT

Mild DI

Maintain fluid balance:

- if child is awake and thirst mechanism is intact: allow to drink freely
- if consciousness is depressed or the thirst mechanism impaired, replace output plus insensible loss (Ch. 3.5) i.v. or, if appropriate, orally; later intake is fixed to meet daily needs

Severe DI

Start desmopressin (DDAVP). Check urine osmolality and serum sodium levels every 6–12 hours initially then daily until stable. Strict monitoring of intake and output is essential, with frequent clinical examination to detect fluid overload, and twice-daily weighing to assess fluid balance.

Desmopressin or deamino-D-arginine vasopressin (DDAVP) is a synthetic analog of arginine vasopressin (AVP) with antidiuretic action of 6–24 hours. It can be given intranasally or parenterally:

- intranasal use:
  - buffered aqueous solution, 100 µg/ml, given by nasal catheter
  - nasal spray bottle delivering 100 µl (10 µg) per spray
- parenteral use: 5–20% of intranasal dose subcutaneously or i.v.

Start with a small *intranasal* dose: newborns 0.25 µg (0.1 µg/kg in preterm infants); infant 1 µg; young children 2.5 µg. Allow the polyuria to recur after the initial dose:

- dose can be increased if not achieving at least 8 hours control; 2.5–10 µg 12-hourly is usually sufficient.
- to establish the need for ongoing treatment (DI can be transient)

Continuous i.v. infusion of a dilute solution of L-arginine vasopressin at 1–3 mU/kg·h in a dextrose or saline solution can be used postoperatively or in ICU. The short half-life of vasopressin (10–20 min) means that its effects are rapidly terminated. Alternatively, replace the previous hour's urine output with an equal volume of 4% dextrose/0.15% saline containing 1–2 units of arginine vasopressin per litre.

✗ COMMON ERRORS

- ➤ The passage of dilute urine postoperatively may be normal excretion of excess intraoperative fluids—do not treat as DI unless hypernatremic
- ➤ Cortisol deficiency can mask underlying DI
- ➤ Suspect anterior pituitary dysfunction in any cranial trauma, surgery or tumor that causes DI and cover with hydrocortisone and thyroxine in an emergency
- ➤ Overtreatment—DDAVP leaves the patient unprotected against water overload: carefully monitor fluids, particularly intravenous and following cranial injury or surgery
- ➤ Hypernatremia in infants is commonly caused by vomiting or diarrhea: differentiate from DI by clinical symptoms and signs of dehydration (in extrarenal hypernatremia, urine sodium levels are below 10 mmol/L and potassium levels exceed 10 mmol/L)

FURTHER READING

1. Kitabchi AE, Wall BM. Diabetic ketoacidosis. Med Clin North Am 1995; 79(1): 9–37
- (*Comprehensive review of pathophysiology and management in adults and children*)

2. Rosenbloom AL, Schatz DA. Diabetic ketoacidosis in childhood. Pediatr Ann 1994; 23: 284–288
- (*Review of DKA in children, including discussion of cerebral edema, its pathogenesis and management*)

3. Urban MD, Kogut MD. Adrenocortical insufficiency in the child. Curr Ther Endocrinol Metab 1994; 5: 131–135

4. Pang S. Congenital adrenal hyperplasia. Curr Ther Endocrinol Metab 1994; 5: 157–166
- (*Two excellent brief reviews including management in health, during crises and in the perioperative period*)

5. Baker L, Stanley CA. Neonatal hypoglycemia. Curr Ther Endocrinol Metab 1997; 6: 409–413
- (*Good, brief review of diagnosis and treatment*)

3.5 Renal disease and disturbances of water and electrolytes

Chula Goonasekera, Barry Wilkins and Michael Dillon

ACUTE RENAL FAILURE

Acute renal failure (ARF) due to acquired intrinsic renal disease is rare among children (incidence 1 in 33000 children per year). However, it is commonly (~10% of cases) encountered in hospitalized critically ill children and is associated with significant mortality. The prognosis is more favorable if the ARF is nonoliguric. In a substantial proportion of cases ARF may be preventable and potentially totally reversible.

PHYSIOLOGY

Renal blood flow is 20–25% of cardiac output and remains relatively constant by autoregulation, under a wide arterial pressure range. Normally 20% of the renal plasma flow is filtered through the glomerulus, 100–120 ml/min per 1.73 m² body surface area. This glomerular filtration rate (GFR) is lower in infants and matures to above adult value by 2 years of age. The processes of tubular resorption and secretion significantly alter the volume and content of the filtrate before it is excreted as urine. Generally 99% of water, 99.5% of sodium, 100% of glucose and 50% of urea in the glomerular filtrate are resorbed. Creatinine is not resorbed, unlike urea, hence the plasma clearance is an indication of glomerular function.

Urine flow is higher in babies and small children because they drink more (for a higher energy input for growth). In health, the kidneys of all children are able to conserve or excrete water and salt over a wide range depending on intake and non-renal losses, but changes in total body water and sodium and other electrolytes are common in many diseases. Because critically ill patients may be hypercatabolic (rather than anabolic), solute load excreted by the kidneys may be higher than in health. Insensible water loss through skin may be high because of fever and the higher surface area to weight ratio in infants.

PATHOGENESIS OF ARF

Several mechanisms can impair glomerular filtration, for example a decrease in renal blood flow (hypovolemia), a decrease in efferent arteriolar tone (e.g. captopril administration) or an increase in afferent arteriolar tone (e.g. indomethacin administration). A rise in proximal tubular hydrostatic pressure, as occurs in acute tubular necrosis (as a result of intratubular obstruction due to brush border debris), and obstructive uropathy also decreases glomerular filtration.

Acute renal failure can be broadly categorized into three phases:

- an initiation phase in which ischemia or a toxin sets off injury to glomerular or tubular epithelial cells
- a maintenance phase where GFR remains relatively low for several days or weeks and
- a recovery phase characterized by gradual and progressive restoration of GFR and tubular function

The causes of ARF are summarized in Table 3.5.1.

In neonates, ARF is often related to perinatal events or congenital renal disease, such as birth asphyxia, renal parenchymal developmental abnormalities (dysplasia, hypoplasia, agenesis), posterior urethral valves, renal vein thrombosis, nephrotoxicity (commonly aminoglycosides) and sepsis.

CLINICAL AND LABORATORY FEATURES

Oliguria and edema are common presenting features. Vomiting, itching (a feature of uremia), respiratory distress (pulmonary edema), altered level of consciousness and convulsions (hypertensive encephalopathy) are generally late clinical signs. In hospital, a rise in blood urea and creatinine concentrations is the common presenting feature.

TABLE 3.5.1 Pathophysiology of acute renal failure

Pathophysiology	Etiology
Prerenal	
Mechanical occlusion of blood supply	Thrombotic occlusion (birth asphyxia, protein S, protein C deficiency)
	Coarctation
Volume depletion	Extracellular fluid loss (e.g. burns, blood loss)
	Extracellular fluid sequestration (pancreatitis, crush injury, nephrotic syndrome)
Altered renal hemodynamics	Hepatorenal syndrome
	Drugs (NSAIDs, ACE inhibitors)
	Sepsis (shock)
Hypoalbuminemia	Nephrosis
	Cirrhosis
Peripheral vasodilatation	Drugs (antihypertensive)
	Sepsis
Reduced cardiac output	Coarctation (thoracic or abdominal)
	Myocardial dysfunction (congenital heart disease, valvular disease, cardiomyopathy)
	Pericardial tamponade, cardiogenic shock
Renal	
Renal vascular disorders	Vasculitis, malignant hypertension
	Hemolytic-uremic syndrome, disseminated intravascular coagulation
	Mechanical renal artery occlusion (surgery, emboli), renal vein thrombosis
Glomerulonephritis, specific diseases	Postinfectious, mesangiocapillary
	Rapidly progressive
Tubular necrosis, cortical necrosis	Renal ischemia (prolonged prerenal causes)
	Nephrotoxins (aminoglycosides)
	Pigmenturia (myoglobinuria, hemoglobinuria)
Interstitial nephritis	Drugs: penicillin, rifampicin, thiazides, furosemide (frusemide), allopurinol
	Infections
	Infiltration (leukemia, lymphoma), connective tissue disease
Postrenal	
Intrarenal obstruction	Crystal deposition (uric acid, methotrexate, acyclovir, triamterene, sulfonamides)
	Protein deposition (myoglobin, hemoglobin)
Extrarenal obstruction	Ureteric, pelvic:
	(Intrinsic obstruction (tumor, stone, clot, pus, fungal ball, papilla)
	(Extrinsic obstruction (retroperitoneal and pelvic malignancy, fibrosis, ligation)
	Bladder (stones, clots, ureteroceles, tumor, neurogenic)
	Urethral (valves, stricture, phimosis)

There are causes other than renal failure that may produce a rise in urea: increased protein load (catabolic states with fever, sepsis, gut hemorrhage), and increased resorption by the renal tubules (volume depletion, heart failure, obstructive uropathy). In contrast, creatinine, is a reliable index of glomerular function as it is released at a constant rate from skeletal muscle and excreted mainly by glomerular filtration.

Although oliguria or anuria is a common sign of ARF, beware of nonoliguric forms. Anuria always demands prompt attention as this is commonly due to obstructive uropathy, acute tubular necrosis or cessation of renal blood flow.

In critically ill patients, ARF is often multifactorial in origin and sepsis is commonly the precipitating factor. In contrast, acquired ARF in the community has usually a single identifiable cause.

EVALUATION

A careful history and examination may give clues to the etiology. A history of vomiting, diarrhea, diuretic use, blood loss, dehydration and symptoms compatible with heart failure suggest a prerenal cause, whereas fever, rash, vascular disease, musculoskeletal symptoms and hematuria may suggest renal parenchymal disease. Poor urinary stream and palpable bladder point to obstruction, but in the very young this can be only excluded by thorough investigation.

Examine urine sediment. A normal urine sediment suggests a prerenal or postrenal cause of ARF, whereas abundant cells, casts or protein suggest a renal pathology. In particular, pigmented granular casts and renal epithelial cell casts suggests acute tubular necrosis. The presence of white cell casts or eosinophil casts suggests acute interstitial nephritis, whereas the presence of red blood cell casts and heavy proteinuria favors a glomerulonephritis or some forms of vasculitis. A dipstick test positive for blood in the absence of red cells in urine is suggestive of hemoglobin or myoglobin.

Urine electrolytes and osmolality are also helpful in differentiating causes of uremia (see 'oliguria' below). Calculate the fractional excretion of sodium (FE_{Na}): in general, a value above 2.5%–3.0% is seen in most cases with intrinsic renal failure, and a value below 1% in most cases of prerenal uremia. In prerenal uremia, FE_{Na} may be higher in the presence of glycosuria, bicarbonaturia or use of diuretics. These indices are also unreliable in neonates, in nonoliguric forms of ARF and in obstructive uropathy.

In children, obstructive uropathy can be diagnosed only with a high degree of suspicion. Posterior urethral valves may present initially in the neonatal period with severe sepsis or shock; renal ultrasound examination is therefore essential in a child with ARF, to exclude obstruction.

In the absence of straightforward diagnostic clues, a cautious therapeutic trial with extracellular fluid expansion, urinary tract drainage, discontinuation of nephrotoxins, and improvement of cardiac index may be considered. Think about isotope renal scans, angiography, immunology tests—e.g. antinuclear antibodies, antineutrophil cytosolic antibodies, antiglomerular basement membrane (anti-GBM) antibody—and a renal biopsy to establish diagnosis in difficult cases.

Although renal failure is classified as prerenal, renal or postrenal rather arbitrarily, the mechanisms that lead to renal insufficiency significantly overlap. For appropriate management of ARF, accurately assess the cause, minimize further renal damage, correct and prevent physiological disturbances and attempt reversal of the renal injury where possible and provide optimal conditions that will facilitate speedy spontaneous renal recovery. This includes removal of the agents that may increase renal damage, supply of adequate nutrition and maintenance of a good renal blood supply (Ch. 2.10).

Prerenal uremia

Prerenal uremia, if treated early, is readily reversible. If treatment is delayed, acute tubular necrosis may ensue. The causes are outlined in Table 3.5.1 and in Chapter 2.10. Consider stopping NSAID therapy, which can contribute to ARF by severe afferent arteriolar renal vasoconstriction, and ACE inhibitors which lower renal perfusion pressure. These drugs are particularly likely to be the offending agents in high renin–angiotensin states such as edematous disorders, volume depletion, hypotensive states, and bilateral renal artery stenosis.

Postrenal uremia

Pure postrenal ARF is commonly reversible and always treatable. It is usual to treat urethral obstruction (posterior urethral valves) by suprapubic catheterization initially. A nondilated system does not exclude an obstructive uropathy, hence in some cases retrograde pyelography may be needed. Ensure adequate drainage. Posterior urethral valves are often associated with renal dysplasia, hence relief of obstruction can lead only to a limited improvement. Extensive bladder tumors, retroperitoneal fibrosis, pelvic tumors, stones, pus, and clots are other causes that can cause ureteric obstruction in children. These cases need appropriate further investigations and specific treatment. Occlusion of distal tubules with crystals (uric acid, calcium oxalate, acyclovir, methotrexate, purines) or with proteinaceous material can also produce obstruction to urine flow. Acute urinary flow obstruction due to sludge (metabolic), crystals, stones, tumors, a prior transplant procedure or clots may cause ARF. Abdominal ultrasound imaging is often diagnostic. However, in anuric states urinary tract dilatation may not be visible on imaging, and retrograde ureteric catheterization may be both diagnostic and therapeutic.

Renal uremia

Disorders with primary vascular damage (reno-vascular disease, vasculitis, hemolytic–uremic syndrome, thrombotic thrombocytopenic purpura), glomerular damage (postinfectious glomerulo-nephritis, IgA nephropathy, anti-GBM disease, crescentic glomerulonephritis, systemic lupus ery-thematosis nephritis), interstitial nephritis and tubular damage (as a consequence of acute ischemia, hypotension, sepsis or toxins, e.g. am-inoglycosides) can lead to ARF.

Radiographic contrast agents in sick children may lead to renal failure and should be avoided if possible. If necessary, low-osmolar nonionic con-trast agents should be used and good renal perfu-sion and high urine flow should be maintained with saline infusion.

The pathophysiologic basis of pigment-induced ARF always involves a concomitant element of extracellular volume depletion and renal ischemia. Iron pigments derived from muscle and blood may also play a role in catalyzing the formation of free radicals, which can destroy the cell mem-branes. Therefore, from a clinical perspective, maintenance of adequate extracellular fluid vol-ume and renal perfusion, the administration of mannitol, and perhaps urinary alkalinization (which increases the solubility of hemoglobin and myoglobin, thereby reducing cast formation) may provide adequate protection against pigment-induced ARF in the predisposed.

If the cause of renal failure still remains obscure, a percutaneous renal biopsy should be consid-ered. This may reveal various forms of acute glomerulonephritis, vasculitis or interstitial nephritis that may need therapy with immune modulation, steroids and plasma exchange.

SPECIFIC CONDITIONS

Hemolytic–uremic syndrome

Hemolytic–uremic syndrome (HUS) is the most common cause of ARF in infants and young chil-dren in developed countries. It occurs predomi-nantly in the summer months, often in small epidemics. It is usually associated with a prodro-mal illness with bloody diarrhea (90% of cases) and affects children aged 1–7 years. This diarrhea-associated HUS (D+ HUS) is usually due to a vero-toxin-producing organism, often identifiable in stool as *Escherichia coli* 0157, although there are other pathogens and mechanisms that are now recognized to cause HUS. Thrombocytopenia, microangiopathic hemolytic anemia and microvascular thrombosis are common features. Extrarenal manifestations such as cerebral symp-toms, pancreatitis, cardiac failure and hemor-rhagic colitis, although uncommon, may occur especially in atypical forms of HUS (D–HUS). Despite modern therapy mortality is still high (about 5%) in HUS. Many children with diarrhea-associated HUS tend to begin recovery within the first 2 weeks of illness. The treatment is mainly supportive, but plasma exchange has a place in therapy of D–HUS and for the extrarenal manifes-tations of D+HUS.

Acute nephritis

The most common type of acute nephritis is post-streptococcal glomerulonephritis, and a signifi-cant proportion of patients need dialysis. Various other forms of nephritis associated with autoim-mune disorders may present in ARF including vasculitis (e.g. Henoch–Schönlein purpura, SLE nephritis, microscopic polyarteritis, Wegener's granulomatosis, anti-GBM disease) and infective endocarditis with shunts. In addition to the immunological investigations—antinuclear anti-bodies (ANA), anti-double-stranded DNA anti-bodies (anti-ds-DNA), autoantibodies, anti-GBM antibodies, and antineutrophil cytoplasmic autoantibodies (ANCA)—a renal biopsy is often necessary for accurate diagnosis. In the acute phase of management, steroids, cytotoxic agents and plasma exchange may be required in addition to supportive therapy.

Acute interstitial nephritis may present in ARF. Drugs such as furosemide (frusemide) and NSAIDs, immune-mediated diseases (IgA nephropathy, SLE), infections (bacterial, including *Yersinia*, viral, fungal, rickettsial) are recognized causes. Check urine for eosinophils, a useful dia-gnostic feature. The mainstay of treatment is sup-portive care and the prognosis is usually good. Steroids and cytotoxic agents may be necessary in the treatment of immune-mediated causes.

Sometimes ARF occurs in patients with nephrotic syndrome due to mesangiocapillary glomerulonephritis which may present with features similar to those of acute post-streptococcal proliferative glomerulonephritis.

Infections

Various infectious agents can produce nephritis similar to that of post-streptococcal glomerulonephritis (e.g. *Mycoplasma*, *Leptospira,* atypical mycobacteria, varicella, cytomegalovirus, Epstein-Barr virus, *Toxoplasma*, rickettsia, hepatitis virus B and C). Serological tests and a renal biopsy are often required for the diagnosis. Treatment is mainly supportive.

Acute tubular necrosis/papillary necrosis

Acute tubular necrosis (ATN) may result from any insult, for example prolonged renal ischemia or hypoxemia, exposure to nephrotoxins (exogenous and endogenous) or prolonged urine outflow obstruction. Endogenous toxins include free hemoglobin (acute intravascular hemolysis as in glucose 6-phosphate dehydrogenase deficiency), free myoglobin (severe rhabdomyolysis) and accumulating toxic metabolic substances of inborn errors of metabolism (maple syrup urine disease, methylmalonic acidemia). Exogenous toxins include cyclosporin, amphotericin B, β-lactam antibiotics, aminoglycoside antibiotics, and cisplatin. Indomethacin and captopril can produce renal failure mainly by affecting renal hemodynamics, changes that could be irreversible if prolonged.

Snake, insect, and arachnid envenomation may cause renal injury, particularly in tropical countries. Hemolysis, disseminated intravascular coagulation (DIC) and the venom itself may contribute.

Sickle cell hemoglobinopathy is a well-known cause of papillary necrosis due to sickling of the abnormal red cells. This often results in gross hematuria. Recurrent episodes of sickling can lead to a sickle cell nephropathy causing an irreversible urine concentration defect. Approximately 1 in 10 subjects in sickle cell crises have been found to be in ARF, and often sepsis and volume depletion are recognized as the precipitating cause.

In hypovolemia, the combined influence of a decrease in renal perfusion pressure and afferent arteriolar constriction reduces glomerular filtration (see Table 3.5.1, oliguria below, and Chapter 2.10 for more details). The increase in tubular hydrostatic pressure due to obstructive casts and debris shed from ischemic proximal tubular brush-border epithelium and back leakage of filtered fluid through leaky tubular epithelium further reduce GFR in the maintenance phase of acute ischemic ATN. Therefore current clinical therapy is directed towards maintenance of adequate renal perfusion pressure, administration of renal vasodilators to restore renal blood flow, and establishment of a solute diuresis to wash out intratubular debris. Also, following ischemia, an influx of calcium results in renal tubular cell calcium overload which may activate several enzymes, leading to membrane and organelle disruption and dysfunction. However, calcium channel blockers have not been useful in effectively preventing or attenuating the onset of post-ischemic ATN.

Thrombosis

Renal vein thrombosis is not uncommon in neonates. Birth asphyxia may be a precipitating cause but rarely thrombophilic states (e.g. protein S or protein C deficiency) may be responsible. These infants usually present with hematuria in the neonatal period, with enlarged, firm, palpable kidneys. Rarely these patients may need dialysis. The thrombosis in this condition commences within the kidney and spreads into the larger veins, hence clot removal is unlikely to play a part in its recovery. Some cases with thrombosis involving the inferior vena cava, however, have benefited from thrombolysis using tissue plasminogen activator. Natural recovery from this condition is slow, and is mainly due to the recovery of the associated acute tubular necrosis. In addition to supportive therapy and thrombolysis in selected cases, anticoagulation may be necessary to avoid progression of the thrombosis, especially if there was associated inferior vena cava thrombosis that might impose a risk of pulmonary embolism.

Renal arterial thrombosis, rarely occurs alone and is usually associated with umbilical artery catheterization. It may occur also in association with renal venous thrombosis. Thrombolysis as above and anticoagulation should be considered, especially in early stages of the disease.

Renovascular disease

Renovascular disease may present in renal failure with associated severe hypertension. Renal failure in this circumstance could be a consequence of the renovascular disease, the hypertension, or both. Adequate control of blood pressure, followed by specific investigations and treatment of the cause is necessary. Administration of ACE inhibitors can be a precipitating cause of acute renal failure in these subjects, especially with bilateral severe renal artery stenosis, and should be avoided.

Postcardiopulmonary bypass

Cardiopulmonary bypass is an important cause of oliguric renal failure and its onset post operatively is a recognized factor that influences clinical outcome. The risk of ARF increases with central venous hypertension and/or low cardiac output states. High doses of inotropes have also being identified as a risk factor, but not the preoperative renal function.

Postrenal transplantation

Renal failure following transplantation is not uncommon and is often reversible with prompt attention. Acute tubular necrosis is the most common cause of ARF early after transplantation. Ureteric obstruction, urinary infection, cyclosporin toxicity, arterial or venous thrombosis and acute rejection are other causes of ARF in these children. The use of acyclovir is a recognized contributory factor.

Acute renal failure occurring in children early after bone marrow transplantation is multifactorial in origin and when it occurs is associated with a high mortality rate. Similarly, ARF may occur after other organ transplantation.

Nonoliguric ARF

Some patients may experience sudden deterioration in renal function without oliguria. This form of nonoliguric renal failure is known to be associated with hypercalcemia, obstruction, aminoglycosides, sepsis and other nephrotoxins. The condition has a better prognosis than oliguric forms of renal failure. These subjects maintain urine output because of a reduction in the resorption capacity of the functioning nephrons.

Tumor lysis syndrome

Rapid breakdown of malignant cells on the introduction of chemotherapy can lead to rapid accumulation of metabolites, especially uric acid (leading to urate deposition and uric acid nephropathy), potassium, phosphate and urea. This can cause ARF and be life-threatening. Adequate hydration, pretreatment with allopurinol and early hemodialysis reduce the severity and mortality.

Nephrotic syndrome

'Minimal change' is the most common cause of nephrotic syndrome in children. Complications associated with nephrotic syndrome such as hypovolemia, sepsis (peritonitis), renal vein thrombosis and drug toxicity (ACE inhibitors) may precipitate ARF (histologically ATN in 60%). The renal failure is often reversible, but can have an unpredictable duration (few days to several months).

HIV nephropathy

Human immunodeficiency virus nephropathy may first present in ARF or nephrotic syndrome. The histological lesions associated vary from minimal change and mesangial hyperplasia to focal segmental glomerulosclerosis.

THERAPEUTIC PRINCIPLES
Prevention

Prevention of ARF is the goal in patients at high risk of this condition, e.g. children with sepsis, extensive trauma, pigmenturia (hemoglobinuria, myoglobinuria), crystalluria (uric acid, methotrexate, acyclovir), nephrotoxins (radiographic contrast media, cisplatin, amphotericin B), and major cardiac and vascular surgery. Vital signs, volume status, hydration and electrolyte status should be carefully monitored. Judicious volume expansion and solute diuresis and alkalinization (in pigmenturia) may be beneficial. Efforts should be made to maximize cardiac output and renal blood flow with inotropes. Once acute renal failure is established, attempts to increase renal blood flow neither improve GFR nor attenuate the course of ARF.

Nutritional considerations

Patients with ARF need energy supplementation. Elevated levels of cortisol, catecholamines, and glucagon promote gluconeogenesis. Insulin levels may be low and insulin resistance may occur which acts to inhibit protein synthesis. Impaired energy intake promotes catabolism and worsens metabolic derangements of ARF. The benefits of amino acid or protein supplements are still debatable in ARF. Whenever possible the enteral route should be used for nutritional supplements and high-energy feeds should be administered, e.g. 8.4 kJ/ml (2 kcal/ml). Aim for 630 kJ/ml (150 kcal/kg) per day.

Treatment of the cause

Treatment of sepsis using appropriate antibiotics and of immune complex-mediated renal injury using steroids, cytotoxic agents or plasma exchange should be considered at the earliest opportunity once the diagnosis is established.

Monitoring

Many subjects may need frequent biochemical investigations (see Ch 2.10 for details). Daily or twice-daily measurement of body weight, frequent blood pressure, oxygen saturation (SaO_2), continuous ECG, respiratory rate, pulse rate and hourly urine output is required.

Management of physiological disturbances

Water

Although fluid retention is normal in renal failure this may not be present if severe fluid depletion has been the cause, in which case fluid repletion may be necessary. Water requirement in a child in renal failure is determined not only by body size but also by the catabolic state, environmental temperature and humidity, body temperature, and the urine output and other losses (for details of management see below).

Electrolytes

Hyponatremia in renal failure is generally due to salt and water overload, but more water than sodium although uncommon can be a consequence of sodium depletion, especially if sodium depletion has contributed to the onset of renal failure. Treatment is by water restriction and occasionally dialysis. The details are discussed in the section on sodium and Chapter 2.10.

Hypernatremia is rarely seen in ARF, unless hypernatremic dehydration has contributed to its onset.

Hyperkalemia is a serious complication of ARF. Continued potassium intake from dietary sources, blood products and the catabolic state with continued release of potassium from body stores (hemolysis, tumor lysis) aggravate this situation rapidly leading to cardiac dysrhythmias. The ECG is a sensitive indicator of potassium's effect on the heart. Monitor the results of calcium infusion by measuring ionized calcium levels. In addition, increasing the pH of the acidotic patient may be useful, and the most rapid way of doing this in the ventilated patient is hyperventilation. Intravenous sodium bicarbonate may be more effective if the patient has a metabolic acidosis (see Ch. 2.10 for details). In nonanuric patients consider a loop diuretic, e.g. furosemide (frusemide) 1 mg/kg and dialysis may be indicated in some cases (see Ch. 2.10).

Hypokalemia and renal failure can coexist. Additional potassium should not usually be given. In patients receiving peritoneal dialysis, add 4 mmol/L of KCl to the dialysate. In hemofiltration, use replacement fluid with 4 mmol/L of potassium if plasma potassium concentration is below 3.5 mmol/L, otherwise 1.0 mmol/L (see Chapter 2.10 and below for other management issues).

Hyperphosphatemia occurs in renal failure owing to diminished urinary excretion of phosphate. Although this is usually modest, rapid increases can occur in the presence of hypercatabolism, diffuse tissue injury, tumor lysis, and rhabdomyolysis leading to tissue deposition of calcium phosphate. An associated hypocalcemia is also usually seen. Mild elevation of plasma phosphate concentration can be treated by administration of oral phosphate binders such as calcium carbonate or aluminum hydroxide but marked increases in phosphate especially if associated with symptomatic hypocalcemia should be treated with hemodialysis. The efficacy of peritoneal dialysis in removing phosphate is poor.

Hypocalcemia is common in ARF and is usually asymptomatic because ionized calcium is maintained at normal levels by the associated acidemia. However, aggressive correction of acidemia can precipitate tetany and other symptoms of hypocalcemia. In the presence of ARF, parathyroid hormone (although markedly increased) is unable to mobilize calcium from the bone as in normal circumstances owing to a tissue resistance. Usually lowering the serum phosphate concentration is the only treatment needed to improve serum calcium levels. If hypocalcemia is symptomatic, infusion of calcium gluconate may be considered.

Hypercalcemia rarely complicates the diuretic phase of ATN, perhaps because of mobilization of deposited calcium salts with normalization of 125 dihydroxy vitamin D_3 levels and loss of skeletal resistance to parathyroid hormone. Occasionally dialysis with calcium-free dialysate may be necessary to alleviate this problem see 'calcium' in Ch. 2.10).

Hypermagnesemia to a modest degree is usually seen in ARF. Therefore, avoid use of magnesium-containing compounds such as antacids as this may accentuate the problem. Usually no specific treatment is needed.

Acid–base balance

Acidosis in renal failure is mainly due to impaired excretion of nonvolatile acids and decreased renal tubular resorption and regeneration of bicarbonate. Therefore severe acidosis with respiratory compensation may be seen. Slow correction of acidosis may be necessary, by administration of alkali. With dialysis the acidosis often is self-correcting. Beware of other causes of acidosis that may present with renal failure (more details are given later in this chapter).

Hypertension

Hypertension is common in renal failure. Often this is a consequence of salt and water overload, which must be treated first, but in certain cases humoral factors such as renin may operate. Occasionally, patients have a hypertensive crisis at presentation (neurological features, increased intracranial pressure, damage to other target organs such as eyes, heart, kidney). Such patients need very careful treatment of blood pressure, with direct arterial pressure monitoring to avoid rapid reduction of blood pressure. Only one-third of the desired blood pressure reduction is recommended over the first 24–48 hours. Convulsions should be controlled by anticonvulsants (diazepam, phenytoin) and hypertension using intravenous sodium nitroprusside or labetalol. Oxygenation and perfusion of vital organs should be maintained. In intractable cases intermittent positive-pressure ventilation with muscular paralysis, continuous dialysis—continuous venovenous hemofiltration (CVVHF), continuous venovenous hemodiafiltration (CVVHDF)—and intracranial pressure monitoring may be necessary.

Hyperuricemia

Hyperuricemia in renal impairment is due to diminished renal excretion. It is probably not harmful unless there is tissue breakdown (tumor lysis) that may lead to acute uric acid nephropathy. Treatment consists of administering xanthine oxidase inhibitors and prehydration. If acute uric acid nephropathy is suspected (presence of uric acid crystals in urine and spot urine uric acid/creatinine ratio >1) this should be aggressively treated with dialysis.

Anemia

Anemia occurs in ARF and is multifactorial in origin. Deficiency of erythropoietin, dilution effects due to fluid overload, frequent venepuncture, gastrointestinal losses, marrow suppression, and hemolysis are contributory. Cautious blood transfusion (beware of fluid overload) and erythropoietin therapy (in chronic cases) may be required in addition to supplementation of iron and folic acid.

Bleeding

Clinically significant bleeding may complicate the course of 5–20% patients with ARF. Usually the coagulopathy is due to the associated diseases (HUS, DIC, liver disease) or treatments (transfusions, anticoagulation). Acute renal failure per se may impair platelet function. Several therapeutic maneuvers can improve coagulopathy (Table 3.5.2).

Infections

Infection-associated complications are the most common cause of death in ARF. Common sources of infection are operative sites, the urinary tract, and intravascular access lines. The usual symptoms and signs of infection such as leukocytosis and fever may be less pronounced. Strict aseptic techniques, close monitoring of lines, prompt culturing and selective use of antibiotics are of paramount importance.

Pulmonary complications

In addition to pulmonary edema due to fluid overload, aspiration, infection and acute respiratory distress syndrome are common respiratory problems seen in patients with ARF. In addition, several disease processes can cause simultaneous renal and respiratory failure, such as Goodpasture's syndrome, Wegener's granulomatosis, systemic lupus erythematosus, polyarteritis nodosa, cryoglobulinemia, and renal vein thrombosis with pulmonary emboli. Development of pulmonary complications is one of the most ominous prognostic factors in patients with ARF.

Gastrointestinal complications

Anorexia, nausea, and vomiting are symptoms commonly seen in patients with advanced renal failure. Gastrointestinal hemorrhage, stress gastritis or ulcers can also occur. The use of antacids or H_2-blockers may prevent or reduce these.

Jaundice of multifactorial origin and mild elevations of plasma amylase are frequently seen in critically ill patients with ARF. Careful clinical and laboratory assessment is needed to exclude acute pancreatitis.

Neurologic complications

Confusion, disorientation, somnolence, coma, myoclonus, and seizures can occur. There are several possible causes of neurological dysfunction which are often operative. Medication-induced encephalopathy, metabolic disturbances, primary neurological disorders, systemic disorders such as vasculitis, endocarditis, HUS, and malignant hypertension are other etiologic factors.

Medication-related complications

Many pharmacological agents are excreted via the kidneys. Therefore in the presence of renal failure such medication should be reduced or abandoned to avoid toxicity.

✔ KEY POINTS

➤ Look for treatable causes. Promptly ascertain and treat prerenal and postrenal causes of ARF as this improves the chances of reversibility
➤ Fluids:
  – ensure adequate circulating volume
  – maintain fluid restriction (give only insensible loss, approximately 400 ml/m² per day and any other losses)
  – reduce sodium load, minimize potassium
➤ Hypertension: correct salt and water overload — Antihypertensive therapy may be needed
➤ Present hyperkalemia by reducing potassium intake and reducing catabolism; if it is already present, treat urgently
➤ Correct acidosis gently with bicarbonate (but assess risk of salt load, hypertension and hypernatremia)

TABLE 3.5.2 **Bleeding diathesis in uremia; therapeutic strategies**		
Treatment	**Time for onset**	**Duration**
Desmopressin	1–4 h	8–12 h
Fresh frozen plasma, platelets	Immediate	12–24 h
Cryoprecipitate	1–4 h	12–24 h
Blood transfusion	Few hours	Several days

➤ Anemia—consider transfusion (beware of fluid status, may need transfusion concurrently with dialysis)

➤ Nutrition: do not forget that an adequate energy intake is essential to minimize catabolism

➤ Drugs: avoid nephrotoxins and renally excreted drugs (if needed, then reduce dosage and monitor levels)

➤ Anticipate complications. Never delay dialysis or hemofiltration until dangerous complications develop. Refer early

➤ Is it acute or chronic renal failure? Are there any features that may support this. Perhaps X ray evidence of osteodystrophy, growth failure, anemia, kidney size on ultrasound.

POTENTIAL PITFALLS

Urinary chemistry is not helpful in:

- nonoliguric renal failure (as is a result of few abnormally functioning nephrons)
- infants (urine chemistry needs to be interpreted cautiously as kidney function is immature even in health)
- in the presence of glycosuria, bicarbonaturia or after use of diuretics (as natural homeostatic mechanisms are interfered with)
- in obstructive uropathy

Secondary carnitine deficiency

Patients on hemodialysis treatment lose carnitine in the dialysis fluid and secondary carnitine deficiency may occur leading to muscular dysfunction. Therefore, carnitine supplementation may be necessary especially during long-term dialysis.

Recovery phase

Watch for polyuria in the recovery phase. There is also associated electrolyte loss, and both fluid and electrolytes may need supplementation in large amounts. Saline 0.45% with glucose 2.5% with added calcium and potassium, is a reasonable replacement fluid in this situation.

WATER AND ELECTROLYTE DISTURBANCES IN THE CRITICALLY ILL

WATER

Infants have a slightly higher proportion of body water than adults, up to 80% compared with 60%. This is mainly due to a higher extracellular fluid volume. Babies produce more urine because their food intake is liquid, and they need a higher energy input for growth and have a higher solute load. Because critically ill patients may be hypercatabolic (rather than anabolic), solute load excreted by the kidneys may be higher than in health.

Illness may compromise the ability to regulate water and electrolytes. Either patients cannot conserve water properly (kidneys excrete too much), as in diabetes insipidus, causing dehydration, or they cannot excrete enough, and tend to become water-overloaded, as in the syndrome of inappropriate antidiuretic hormone (SIADH). Hence the concept of 'maintenance water requirement' is not applicable to critical care practice. In health it is the kidneys, not the clinician, that maintain water homeostasis. The figures given in Chapter 2.10, formula 3, provide sufficient water in a healthy child with normal metabolic rate—approximately equivalent to 24 ml water for 100 kJ (100 ml water for 100 kcal) energy expenditure—to allow for insensible water losses and allow excretion of the normal solute load—approximately 2.4–9.6 mOsmol per 100 kJ (10–40 mOsmol/100 kcal) of energy expenditure—such that the urine osmolality is approximately equal to that of plasma, and in the middle of the kidneys' normal wide range of concentrating ability (urine osmolality 60–1200 mOsmol/kg). Normal kidneys can accommodate a wide range of water intake. The clinician must allow for possible errors in either direction, but should remember that it is easier to replenish water when depleted than to remove excess when overloaded. In anuria the clinician must reduce water input to insensible losses only, which are approximately 30% of the figures in formula 3 (Ch. 2.10). Adequate energy input, however, should be a priority in order to minimize catabolism, and where necessary water removal (by dialysis or filtration) may be required to achieve this.

Oliguria

Most oliguria in acutely ill children is not renal failure. Physiological oliguria, a normal response of the kidney, can be caused by hypovolemia, dehydration, or low cardiac output. This is sometimes called prerenal failure, even though initially there is no true renal failure present. Hyperosmolar urine with low urine sodium concentration (fractional sodium excretion <0.5%, see formula 1 in Ch. 2.10) and high urine creatinine concentration (> 4000 μmol/L) suggests that the kidneys are behaving appropriately to a prerenal threat. However, GFR can become reduced with a rising plasma creatinine level, yet with preservation of urine of high quality. If a high urine sodium (fractional sodium excretion > 3%) is demonstrated, established renal failure is likely to be the cause of the oliguria (see Table 2.10.2, Ch. 2.10).

Inappropriate ADH secretion can also cause oliguria, in which there is renal water retention despite existing water overload. This is caused by excessive release of ADH which would normally be suppressed in the presence of such high extracellular fluid volume. There is hyperosmolar urine with a high urine sodium concentration, and hemodilution with hyponatremia (see Table 2.10.2). The natriuresis is caused by natriuretic hormone stimulated by the hypervolemia. Loop diuretics can usually stimulate kidneys to increase urine output when the cause of the oliguria is acting prerenally and there is water retention, including in SIADH.

Replacement of circulating volume

Although there has been a long-standing debate over the relative merits of colloid and crystalloid, with inadequate scientific evidence to support either view, standard practice in many pediatric critical care units is to use colloid for the following reasons:

1. It makes sense to replace lost plasma with a plasma substitute.
2. Anecdotal experience is that circulating volume expansion is faster and more effective with colloid.
3. It is acknowledged that approximately three times more crystalloid than colloid is needed to restore hypovolemia to normal circulating volume. The extra volume enters the interstitial extracellular space causing edema, including pulmonary edema, which may not be desirable in the critically ill. This 'three times rule' is based on the fact that the extravascular extracellular fluid space (150–160 ml/kg) is twice the intravascular space (70–80 ml/kg).
4. There may already be interstitial edema, especially in any child with systemic inflammatory response syndrome in sepsis, trauma, burns or after abdominal surgery ('third space edema'), or in nephrotic syndrome; hence the advantage of treating the intravascular space only.

However, exogenous albumin may also leak into the interstitial space in capillary leak syndromes. It will drag water with it and thereby worsen edema, and will increase the protein load that will eventually have to be metabolized and excreted.

Another question is which colloid to use? Human albumin solution 4% or 5% is expensive, often in short supply and not totally without risks. It has a longer half-life after infusion than gelatine hydrolysates which cause slightly more allergic reactions (although still rare) and which may contain high calcium levels. Studies have shown inferior volume restitution in newborns with gelatin derivatives. Newer starch derivatives, e.g. hydroxyethyl starch, are becoming more popular and may prove superior to albumin. They may last even longer in the circulation and may have a superior oncotic effect of drawing water from the interstitium into the circulation, and may improve the coagulation profile.

Polyuria

In the presence of stable renal function, if urine output cannot be measured, polyuria (> 4ml/kg·h) is confirmed by a urine creatinine concentration below 1000 μmol/L in babies and below 2000 μmol/L in older children, based on their relatively constant urine creatinine output of 100–200 μmol/kg per day. Urine output may be very variable in polyuric states, and thus water overload or depletion may easily occur if strict attention is not paid every hour to the hydration state. The best approach is to replace the previous hour's urine output together with an allowance for insensible and other measured losses.

SODIUM

Total body sodium is 80–100 mmol/kg, of which only 30 mmol/kg is in extracellular fluid, the rest being slowly exchangeable in bone. Normal daily intake is 2–3 mmol/kg in healthy infants on breast milk or formula, and usually 1–2 mmol/kg in older children. Up to 1 mmol/kg is retained in growth. Inability of infants and children (under 2 years old) to excrete a sodium load efficiently, (the kidneys are geared to sodium retention), may in fact be a physiological adaptation for growth. Whereas infants turn over a quarter of their body water per day (older children a tenth), sodium turnover is only 1–2% on a normal diet. More than 99% of filtered sodium (200–400 mmol/kg per day) is resorbed by the renal tubules, so that, in health, urine sodium concentration is low, less than 20 mmol/L or fractional excretion below 1% (see formula 1 Ch. 2.10). A sodium load is therefore excreted slowly, but the kidneys have the capacity to excrete up to 10 mmol/kg per day or as little as 0.1 mmol/kg per day. This does not mean that an ill child can be safely given a large quantity, because sodium retention means extracellular fluid expansion which may be undesirable, for example in heart failure, renal failure, brain injury and lung injury. As with water it is easier to replenish sodium, as a volume challenge with 0.9% saline, Hartmann's or Ringer's solutions or plasma substitutes, than to remove excess.

There continues to be controversy concerning rapid correction of hyponatremia. Although de-myelination syndromes, including central pontine myelinolysis, have been described in adults with rapidly corrected severe hyponatremia, possibly caused by rapid osmolar disequilibrium, these syndromes have not been reported in sympto-matic children where the hyponatremia has devel-oped rapidly. The approach outlined in Chapter 2.10, including use of hypertonic saline, has so far been shown to be safe and may improve outcome in critically ill children with hyponatremia and cerebral edema.

A second use advocated for hypertonic saline is in the early management of severe traumatic brain injury, especially associated with multi-trauma and hemorrhagic shock. Although hypertonic saline improves brain compliance there is insufficient evidence yet to justify its use routinely.

Hyponatremia in acute brain injury poses a spe-cial problem because it is often multifactorial. Iatrogenic hyponatremia should be avoided by water restriction in the presence of oliguria caused by SIADH, and by avoiding the use of hypotonic fluids. Some children appear to have unexplained renal sodium wasting even in the absence of SIADH. This has been termed 'cerebral salt wast-ing'. Its mechanism remains unclear but inappro-priate secretion of natriuretic peptides may play a part. Treatment is according to the principles in Chapter 2.10 with water and sodium repletion, avoiding overhydration.

POTASSIUM

Total body potassium is approximately 50 mmol/kg, with more than 95% being intracellular. Intake in health is 1–3 mmol/kg per day, up to 1 mmol/kg is retained in growth. As with sodium and water the kidneys regulate excretion over a wide range to maintain homeostasis. Rapid changes in plasma concentration in critically ill children are likely to be related to changes in acid–base balance with an associated intracellular–extracellular shift. Renal failure causes slow potas-sium accumulation. β_2-adrenergic drugs such as salbutamol for asthma may cause hypokalemia, although this is rarely of clinical importance and is not associated with potassium depletion.

Hyperkalemia is more dangerous than hy-pokalemia, especially in the presence of acidosis and hypocalcemia, and is a medical emergency if the level exceeds 6.5 mmol/L.

CHLORIDE

Chloride turnover is high compared with sodium and potassium, and is of the order of 5–10% of the total body content of approximately 35 mmol/kg.

This is mostly in the extracellular fluid. Because chloride is generally administered with sodium, and chloride follows sodium in membrane ion fluxes, extracellular ion changes are usually considered in terms of sodium, chloride being often neglected. Chloride depletion may be associated with sodium depletion in dehydration states. It may be replaced by bicarbonate and it is known that chloride depletion without sodium depletion may cause chronic 'metabolic' alkalosis. Chloride depletion is rare in pediatric intensive care practice because chloride is administered in excess to the body's needs as sodium or potassium chloride. Potassium is often better given as phosphate as there are many situations where potassium and phosphate depletion coexist, such as diabetic ketoacidosis.

ACID–BASE DISTURBANCES

Disorders of acid–base physiology are common in acutely ill children. The time-honoured system of defining acid–base state by changes in P_{CO_2} (respiratory) and standard base excess (metabolic) according to the nomograms of Siggaard-Andersen (or their derivatives) remains the most familiar and practical way of analysing a disorder in any individual patient. The concept of base excess has been criticized by many because of its imprecision and because it assumes constant concentrations of plasma albumin and blood hemoglobin. Blood gas machines, however, continue to provide this information derived by computer rather than from the nomograms relied on decades ago. There is, however, another way of expressing the total buffer base in any body fluid, known as the 'strong ion difference' (SID). This is the concentration, or rather activity, of weak anions, principally bicarbonate, albumin and phosphate. It can be estimated from formula 1 (see box).

Formula 1

$$SID_{apparent} \text{ (mEq/L)} = [Na^+] + [K^+] + [Mg^{2+}] + [Ca^{2+}] - [Cl^-] \text{ (all in mmol/L)}$$

It can be more accurately derived from the plasma bicarbonate (as calculated from pH and P_{CO_2} by the blood gas machine), albumin (g/L) and phosphate (mmol/L) by the formula 2:

Formula 2

$$SID_{effective} \text{ (mEq/L)} = [HCO_3^-] + [albumin] \times (0.123 \times pH - 0.631) + [phosphate] \times (0.309 \times pH - 0.469)$$

Plasma albumin at 40–45 g/L is 0.6 mmol/L but contributes 11 mEq/L to the weak base at pH 7.4. Phosphate at 1.5 mmol/L contributes 2.7 meq/L. Hypoalbuminemia may cause a mild metabolic alkalosis if it is compensated for by bicarbonate retention.

The anion gap is essentially the strong ion difference less the bicarbonate, and is mostly albumin in healthy individuals. It is elevated if bicarbonate has been replaced by lactate or other normally unmeasured anions, but not if replaced by chloride. The difference between $SID_{apparent}$ and $SID_{effective}$ (the strong ion gap) is the quantity of anions of strong acids, not normally measured, including lactate, sulfate, keto acids, etc. Although the concept of strong ion difference may not replace that of in vivo base excess, it may help us to understand disorders of acid–base state in critically ill children in the future.

The decision whether or not to treat an acid–base disturbance is often harder than deciding how to treat it. Compensating mechanisms should generally not be treated, otherwise the primary disturbance is exacerbated. For example, respiratory acidosis caused by hypoventilation secondary to a primary metabolic alkalosis, such as in severe vomiting in pyloric stenosis, should not be treated with assisted ventilation, otherwise life-threatening alkalosis may occur. Similarly, a metabolic alkalosis (chronic renal bicarbonate retention) compensating for chronic respiratory failure, e.g. in an infant with chronic pulmonary insufficiency of prematurity, has developed to prevent chronic acidosis which might inhibit growth and development. It should not be treated unless the child has been ventilated for an acute exacerbation, e.g. an acute rise in P_{CO_2} from 8 kPa to 12 kPa (60 mmHg to 90 mmHg) but then the alkalosis prevents the infant from reestablishing adequate spontaneous breathing. The secret here is not to overventilate, but to use 'permissive hypercapnia', i.e. not to lower the P_{CO_2} below the chronic value, in this case 8 kPa (60 mmHg). It is generally best not to intervene to ventilate a child with hyperventilation who is compensating for severe metabolic acidosis, for example in diabetic ketoacidosis, because it may not be possible to achieve the degree of hypocapnia that the patient achieves spontaneously.

A common mistake is to attempt to restore pH to normal. Normal acid–base physiology depends on a system which maintains extracellular pH close to 7.4 most of the time, but which permits marked metabolic acidosis at times of extreme exertion with anerobic metabolism, without danger to the individual. Metabolic acidosis, caused physiologically by lactic acid release from cells, provides the following advantages:

- it protects cells against the effects of hypoxia
- it assists oxygen unloading from hemoglobin by shifting the oxygen–hemoglobin dissociation curve to the right.

Some of the alleged problems of acidosis, for example negative inotropy or failure of inotropes to work at a pH below 7.2, have little experimental support. Acidosis causes pulmonary vasoconstriction but only extreme acidosis causes arrhythmias and depresses level of consciousness.

Plasma pH has been measured as low as 7.0 in healthy athletes during extreme exercise, illustrating the ability of the system to cope with sudden metabolic acid loads, the pH change being modulated very rapidly by changes in ventilation, and long-term by renal compensation. Patients with severe metabolic acidosis usually recover completely, e.g. diabetic ketoacidosis with pH 6.8, suggesting that even pathological acidosis is not, in itself, harmful. The outcome is poor only when the underlying disease has a bad prognosis, e.g. Gram-negative septicemia or hypoxic-ischemic multiorgan failure. In sepsis and ARDS lactic acid is produced by the lungs, and actively taken up, even at low pH, by other tissues. The pathogenesis of lactic acidosis in these conditions remains poorly understood. For this reason attention should be paid to treating the underlying condition rather than metabolic acidosis itself. In modern practice it should be uncommon to use alkalizing agents in high anion gap acidosis, at least as boluses for rapid pH correction.

Sodium bicarbonate has many alleged adverse effects, especially when given rapidly:

- increased intracellular acidosis—this is a theoretical problem with little scientific support and probably only applies if a large quantity of bicarbonate, e.g. full correction, is given over a short time. For example, if a pure metabolic acidosis (pH 7.2, bicarbonate 15 mmol/L, base excess –12) is fully corrected over 1 hour with 4 mmol/kg of bicarbonate, only a small proportion of bicarbonate will be converted to carbon dioxide. This would approximate to 1 mmol/kg which is equivalent to only about 10 minutes of normal CO_2 production
- increased hemoglobin-oxygen affinity
- hypokalemia
- hypocalcemia (decreased plasma ionized calcium)
- sodium load
- osmolar load
- late metabolic alkalosis
- exacerbation of effects of hypophosphatemia.

Sodium bicarbonate is especially unlikely to be helpful in lactic acidosis, unless the patient is sodium depleted, because the patient will end up sodium overloaded with a metabolic alkalosis (high plasma bicarbonate). Lactic acid causes acidemia because it is a strong acid at physiological pH. It can only be removed by dialysis against a bicarbonate dialysate which reverses the process whereby lactate has replaced bicarbonate in the extracellular fluid or by promoting hepatic and splanchnic uptake and metabolism by optimizing the hepatic and splanchnic circulation.

Slow sodium bicarbonate treatment may have a role in the management of normal anion gap acidosis where excessive chloride therapy would exacerbate hyperchloremia. Half correction of the base deficit over several hours, followed by 2 mmol/kg per day is a suitable recipe. In diabetic ketoacidosis bicarbonate is not recommended, even in severe acidemia with pH less than 7.0, unless there is evidence that keto acids have been excreted by osmotic diuresis more than chloride. If the rise in anion gap is no more than the fall in bicarbonate level, then it may be helpful to include about a quarter of the sodium replacement as bicarbonate given just as slowly as the rest of the repair. This may avoid the patient ending up hyperchloremic and tachypneic after the metabolic disorder is corrected.

Tris(hydroxymethyl)aminomethane (THAM, trometamol, or tromethamine) is an alternative alkalizing agent, less often used in pediatric intensive care practice. It is a nonionic alkali, *MW* 121, available as a 0.3 molar solution. It has half the osmotic load of bicarbonate, but 3.3 times as much water is administered. When combined with hydrogen ions it is excreted as THAM-H^+Cl^- by the kidney which may eliminate the extra water by osmotic diuresis. The effect is therefore to regenerate bicarbonate (which replaces chloride) from CO_2, thereby reducing P_{CO_2} without any osmolar load. Sodium carbonate and dichloroacetate are other alkalizing agents which may prove efficacious in treating acidosis while reducing P_{CO_2}, with less of an osmolar and sodium load than bicarbonate.

CEREBRAL EDEMA IN DIABETIC KETOACIDOSIS

Cerebral edema is a rare complication of DKA, and is usually fatal if presenting with symptoms or signs of cerebral herniation. It usually occurs after several hours of metabolic repair when the patient appears to be improving clinically and biochemically. Asymptomatic brain swelling may occur even before treatment begins. Acute osmotic dysequilibrium between brain and plasma probably occurs, related to the existence of intracellular molecules such as inositol and glutamine ('idiogenic osmoles') which protect brain cells from shrinking during the dehydration state. Sudden extracellular fluid hypo-osmolality may be involved, for example if excessive hypotonic fluid is given rapidly, or intracellular movement of sodium and potassium after insulin treatment occurs. Newer regimens of slow rehydration and slow metabolic correction may not provide the whole answer to this problem.

CONTROVERSIES IN WATER AND ELECTROLYTE MANAGEMENT

Hypertonic saline is advocated by some for management of hyponatremic states, especially for initial treatment of severe, symptomatic hyponatremia, and as an osmotic agent in head injury. There is some evidence for the former but its place has yet to be defined in managing trauma.

Some advocate the use of bicarbonate to treat metabolic acidosis, only if there is continuing bicarbonate wasting or lactate production with sodium depletion.

The role of dopamine in increasing renal blood flow and urine output has never been defined in children. It is doubtful whether there is a significant effect, other than via its inotropy.

The role of hemofiltration as a means of eliminating inflammatory mediators in systemic inflammatory response syndrome has yet to be defined, although this is a promising new indication. Peritoneal dialysis may also be effective.

The use of THAM as an alkalizing agent has never been evaluated in children. It may have a place in the future in treating severe acidosis.

The harmful effects of alkalosis may often be underestimated. The role of acidification with hydrochloric acid has not yet been defined.

The strong ion gap (difference between $SID_{apparent}$ and $SID_{effective}$—see formulae 1 and 2) is a new concept which may replace anion gap and base deficit. It has not yet been evaluated in critically ill children.

✓ KEY POINTS

➤ Individualize treatment. Consider water, sodium, potassium and other electrolytes separately. Consider the needs of the individual child. There is no such thing as a 'maintenance fluid' that suits all situations

➤ Correct abnormalities of body water and electrolyte composition slowly. This applies especially to acidosis, hyponatremia, hypernatremia and dehydration

➤ Err on the side of giving too little water. It is easier to correct underhydration than overhydration, the latter being more harmful anyway

➤ Review frequently—at least twice daily, the requirements for water, electrolytes and volume

➤ Measure electrolytes and acid–base values frequently—at least 12-hourly—in acutely ill children

➤ Do not neglect magnesium and phosphate

➤ Do not overlook urine chemistry investigations, which provide much useful information in disorders of water and electrolytes

➤ A low fractional sodium excretion is very reassuring in the presence of oliguria or other suspicion of renal failure. Treat the cause and the kidneys can usually be made to excrete urine

➤ Do not forget trace elements: depletion of copper, zinc, manganese and selenium are all not uncommon in critically ill children

➤ The insensible fluid losses can be very high (100–150 ml/kg per day) in premature neonates and those exposed to an overhead heater. In general, 40–60 ml/kg per day is an appropriate figure for replacement of insensible losses. However, close attention should be paid to this and accurate weighing twice a day is recommended.

✗ COMMON ERRORS

➤ Failure to recognize hypovolemia, especially in hypoalbuminemic states

➤ Failure to correct hypovolemia

➤ Failure to act on a rapidly rising plasma potassium level over 6.0 mmol/L

➤ Overestimating the degree of dehydration

➤ Assuming that all hyponatremia means sodium depletion

➤ Assuming that all hyponatremia with oliguria is SIADH

➤ Correcting dehydration too fast

➤ Correction of acidosis without attention to hypocalcemia

➤ Blood transfusion without provision for fluid removal (diuresis)

➤ Rapid reduction in blood pressure in hypertensive encephalopathy

➤ Rapid reduction of urea by dialysis

➤ Prescribing ACE inhibitors in ARF

➤ Failure to stop NSAIDs and other nephrotoxic agents in ARF

ADVANCES IN TREATMENT

NITRIC OXIDE

Nitric oxide is a major counterbalancing vasodilator of the renal circulation. Its inhibition reduces GFR. The place of nitric oxide donation in ARF is yet to be established. In animal models L-arginine administration has been shown to prevent and reverse ARF.

PLASMAPHERESIS

The use of plasmapheresis is controversial, but it may be beneficial in special situations (e.g. HUS, immune-mediated disease, and empirically in multiorgan failure).

ANTIBODIES AGAINST CYTOKINES

The use of antibodies against cytokines is still experimental.

METABOLIC DISORDERS

Maple syrup urine disease

Branched-chain amino acid (BCAA) accumulation is usually treated by a BCAA-free high-energy diet and peritoneal dialysis with or without exchange transfusion. Peritoneal dialysis is not very efficient in removing BCAA. Treatment with CVVH or CVVHDF is effective .

Hyperammonemia

In hyperammonemia (inborn errors of urea synthesis) a similar situation applies with ammonia being poorly removed by peritoneal dialysis, hence the need to consider CVVH or CVVHDF.

DRUGS FOR PREVENTION OF ARF

In established renal failure there are no proven pharmacological agents that can reverse renal injury. Dopamine and diuretics may be beneficial in the early phase and experimentally calcium channel blockers and nitric oxide inhibitors have been shown to have some beneficial effect.

NEWER PLASMA SUBSTITUTES

See 'replacement of circulating volume' above.

FURTHER READING

1. Shusterman N, Strom BL, Murray TG et al. Risk factors and outcome of hospital acquired acute renal failure. Am J Med 1987; 83: 65
2. Davidman M, Olson P, Kohen J et al. Iatrogenic renal disease. Arch Intern Med 1991; 151: 1809
3. Badr KF, Ichikawa I. Prerenal failure: a deleterious shift from renal compensation to decompensation. N Engl J Med 1988; 317: 623
4. Stein JH. Acute renal failure: lessons from pathophysiology. West J. Med 1992; 156: 176
5. Anderson RJ, Schrier RW. Acute tubular necrosis. In: Schrier RW, Gottschalk CW, editors. Diseases of the kidney. 5th ed. Boston: Little, Brown, 1993: pp. 1287–1318
6. Groeneveld AB, Tran DD, van der Meulen J et al. Acute renal failure in the medical intensive care unit: predisposing, complicating factors and outcome. Nephron 1991; 59: 602
7. Siegler RL. The hemolytic uremic syndrome. (review). Pediatric Clini North Am 1995; 42: 1505–1529
8. Venuto RC. Pigment-associated acute renal failure: is the water clearer 50 years later? J Lab Clin Med 1992; 119: 452
9. Better OS, Stein JH. Early management of shock and prophylaxis of acute renal failure in traumatic rhabdomyolysis. N Engl J Med 1990; 322: 825
10. Siegel NJ, Van Why SK, Boydstun II, Devarajan P, Gaudio KM. Acute Renal Failure. In: Holliday MA, Barratt TM, Avner ED, editors. Pediatric nephrology, 3rd ed. Baltimore: Williams & Wilkins, 1994: pp. 1176–1203
11. Griffin KA, Bidani A. Guidelines for determining the cause of acute renal failure. J Crit Illness 1989; 4: 32
12. Mathew A, Berl T. Fractional excretion of sodium: use early to assess renal failure. J Crit Illness 1989; 4: 45
13. Miller PD, Krebs RA, Neal BJ, McIntyre DO. Polyuric prerenal failure. Arch Intern Med 1980; 140: 907
14. Finberg L, Kravath RE, Hellerstein S, editors. Water and electrolytes in pediatrics. Physiology, pathology and treatment. 2nd ed. Philadelphia: WB Saunders, 1993
15. Ichikawa I, Yoshioka T, editors. Pediatric textbook of fluids and electrolytes. Baltimore: Williams & Wilkins, 1990
16. Brem AS. Disorders of potassium homeostasis. Pediatr Clin North Am 1990; 37: 419–427
17. Rodriguez-Soriano J. Potassium homeostasis and its disturbances in children. Pediatr Nephrol 1995; 9: 364–374
18. Bunchman TE, Donckerwolcke RA. Continuous arterial-venous diahemofiltration and continuous veno-venous diahemofiltration in infants and children. Pediatr Nephrol 1994; 8: 96–102
19. McClure RJ, Prasad VK, Brocklebank JT. Treatment of hyperkalemia using intravenous and nebulised salbutamol. Arch Dis Child 1994; 70: 126–128
20. Arieff AI, Ayus JC. Treatment of symptomatic hyponatremia: neither haste nor waste [editorial]. Crit Care Med 1991; 19: 748–751
21. Kox WJ, Gamble J. Fluid resuscitation. Baillière's Clinical Anesthesiology 1988; 2: 443–776
22. Mackenzie A, Barnes G, Shann F. Clinical signs of dehydration in children. Lancet 1989; ii: 605–607
23. Bellomo R, Kellum JA, Pinsky MR. Transvisceral lactate fluxes during early endotoxemia. Chest 1996; 110: 198–204
24. Stewart PA. Modern quantitative acid–base chemistry. Can J Physiol Pharmacol 1983; 61: 1444–1461
25. Figge J, Mydosh T, Fencl V. Serum proteins and acid–base equilibria: a follow-up. J Lab Clin Med 1992; 120: 713–719
26. Feld LG. Hyponatremia in infants and children: a practical approach. J Nephrol 1996; 9: 5–9
27. Ganong CA, Kappy MS. Cerebral salt wasting in children. The need for recognition and treatment. Am J Dis Child 1993; 147: 167–169

3.6 Hematologic problems

Stephen Keeley

Hematologic abnormalities in critically ill children are usually secondary to an underlying severe illness.

ANEMIA

Anemia reduces the oxygen-carrying capacity of blood, reduces oxygen delivery to tissues and increases myocardial work. Normal erythropoiesis requires an adequate intake of iron, folate and vitamin B_{12}, adequate erythropoietin production and intact stem cell function. The normal hemoglobin concentration varies with age (Table 3.6.1).

CAUSES

Causes of anemia are:

- blood loss:
  - trauma
  - gastrointestinal hemorrhage
  - surgery
  - sampling
- impaired red blood cell (RBC) production:
  - marrow failure (e.g. shock, poisoning, chemotherapy, nutritional deficiency)
  - erythropoietin deficiency (e.g. renal failure)
  - disorders of DNA synthesis (e.g. Fanconi's anemia)

- disorders of hemoglobin synthesis (e.g. sickle cell disease)
- abnormal RBC maturation (e.g. parvovirus B19 infection)
- increased RBC destruction:
  - membrane defects (e.g. hereditary spherocytosis)
  - metabolic defects (e.g. glucose 6-phosphate deficiency)
  - immune-mediated (e.g. ABO, Rh, autoimmune)
  - mechanical (e.g. hemolytic–uremic syndrome, cardiopulmonary bypass)
  - toxins (e.g. snake venoms, drugs such as quinidine and penicillin)

In critically ill children, the most common cause of anemia is blood loss and the next most common is hemolysis—usually due to mechanical disruption of the RBC membrane in diseases such as hemolytic–uremic syndrome (HUS) or as a component of disseminated intravascular coagulation (DIC)—that outstrips the capacity of the marrow to compensate. *Haemophilus influenzae* type b (Hib) and other pathogens such as *Clostridium welchii*, *Streptococcus pneumoniae*, *Staphylococcus* and *Escherichia coli* sometimes cause hemolysis. The anemia of acute inflammation (due to sampling, bone marrow suppression, impaired erythropoietin responsiveness and reduced iron availability) often accompanies severe infections. Severe megaloblastic anemia may develop after a few days of any very severe illness, and may be associated with thrombocytopenia and leukopenia. Treatment with folate, 0.1–0.3 mg/kg (maximum 15 mg) i.v. daily, and cyanocobalamin, 20 µg/kg i.m. daily for 7 days then weekly, rapidly corrects this anemia.

In the absence of a dietary risk factor or blood loss, initial investigation of anemia should include examination of the blood film, reticulocyte count, mean corpuscular volume (MCV), stool for occult blood and urinalysis. The presence of reticulocytosis implies that the marrow is normal and that the erythropoietin response is intact. This suggests chronic

TABLE 3.6.1 **Change in hemoglobin concentration with age**		
Age	**Hemoglobin (g/dl)**	**Concentration (g/L)**
Newborn	13.5–19.5	135–195
3 months	9.5–13.5	95–135
1 year	10.5–13.5	105–135
5 years	11.5–13.5	115–135
10 years	11.5–15.5	115–155
15+ years: female	12–16	120–160
15+ years: male	13–16	130–160

blood loss or red cell destruction. A low reticulocyte count suggests abnormalities of bone marrow or stem cell or deficient erythropoietin production.

SICKLE CELL DISEASE

Sickle cell disease (SCD) is the most common of the hemoglobinopathies and is found predominantly in people from Africa or the Middle East.

A single amino acid substitution on the beta chain of hemoglobin causes deformation of the RBC into a sickle shape when exposed to cold, hypoxia or dehydration. Red cell rigidity leads to reduced tissue blood flow, intermittent vascular occlusion and hemolysis.

Vasoocclusion crises in the bones, lung, brain and spleen cause pain and permanent ischemic tissue damage. In homozygous children 90–100% of the Hb is HbS compared with 20–30% in the heterozygote (sickle cell trait), so the heterozygote is almost always asymptomatic. Sickle cell disease is diagnosed by Hb electrophoresis.

SEPSIS IN SICKLE CELL DISEASE

Infections occur suddenly, are often fatal and are the leading cause of death in children with SCD. Most SCD patients are functionally asplenic by the age of 12 months owing to repeated splenic infarction and hemorrhage. They are at risk of infection by encapsulated organisms such as Hib, *Streptococcus pneumoniae* and *Salmonella*. Pneumonia (due to *Streptococcus pneumoniae*, Hib, *Staphyloccus. aureus* or *Mycoplasma*) may be difficult to distinguish from pulmonary infarction. Blood cultures should be taken and cefotaxime given if there is any doubt about the diagnosis. Routine immunizations must be kept up to date. Homozygotes must be vaccinated against Hib and *Pneumococcus*, and given prophylactic penicillin V (phenoxymethylpenicillin) 12.5 mg/kg 12-hourly. Any febrile illness is a medical emergency. If the temperature is above 38.5°C, a blood culture is taken and cefotaxime (50 mg/kg i.v. 6-hourly) started. Supportive treatment of septic shock, including blood transfusion and inotropic drugs, may be required. In SCD, sickling causes several types of crisis which may require intensive care.

ACUTE CHEST SYNDROME

Signs

Clinical signs include:

- fever, cough, pleuritic pain and tachypnea
- pulmonary infiltrates and pleural effusion on chest radiography

Cause

- In most cases of acute chest syndrome no cause is found. Possible causes are:
- infection (*Streptococcus pneumoniae* or *Mycoplasma* sp.)
- rarely, fat embolism due to a vasoocclusive event in marrow

Management

Prevent hypoxia by the use of oxygen, analgesia and physiotherapy. Face mask CPAP may be required. Following blood culture give an antibiotic (cefotaxime 50 mg/kg i.v. 6-hourly). It is rarely possible to exclude pneumonia.

Correct any dehydration, then give maintenance fluids (Ch. 2.10). Pulmonary edema can occur. Exchange transfusion is indicated if Pa_{O_2} is below 9.3 kPa (<70 mmHg) despite face mask CPAP and F_{IO_2} is 0.6 or more.

STROKE

Stroke is usually due to thrombosis of a large vessel such as the middle cerebral or internal carotid artery. Partial occlusion of large arteries often causes silent watershed infarcts.

Signs

Stroke is uncommon before 1 year of age. Onset is:

- sudden, with seizures and hemiparesis
- rarely preceded by headache

Management

1. Control airway, breathing, and circulation.
2. Treat seizures.

3. Begin partial exchange transfusion (see below).

ACUTE SPLENIC SEQUESTRATION

Acute splenic sequestrian is uncommon, but fatal in 35% of cases. It is most common between 10 months and 30 months of age, and virtually never occurs after the age of 5 years. Signs include:

- shock (tachycardia, pallor and poor peripheral pulses)
- acute splenomegaly

Management

Urgent correction of hypovolemia is required, with boluses of 20 ml/kg 0.9% saline or colloid, repeated if necessary. Prompt blood transfusion (10–20 ml/kg) is given to release the trapped red cells.

Sequestration can recur.

TRANSFUSION IN SCD

Indications for transfusion:

- hematocrit below 0.2
- signs of decompensation due to anemia:
  - cardiac failure
  - mental state changes

Indications for partial exchange transfusion:

- any CNS event
- acute chest syndrome requiring IPPV
- severe infection
- acute priapism

A 2-volume exchange (i.e. 150 ml/kg) of reconstituted red cells (50% packed cells and 50% FFP) should reduce HbS to below 30%.

THROMBOSIS

Thrombosis occurs in 10% or more of PICU patients. It is usually associated with central venous catheters, and is frequently caused by catheter sepsis.

Spontaneous venous thrombosis is rare in children and pulmonary embolism is even more uncommon. In asphyxia, dehydration, septicemia and shock, altered blood flow, vessel injury and impaired endothelial function can trigger thrombosis.

Hypercoagulable states due to inherited deficiencies of protein C or S or antithrombin III rarely present in childhood. Developmental changes in the balance between procoagulants and inhibitors in newborns and early adolescents, however, leave these groups at particular risk of iatrogenic thrombosis.

VENOUS THROMBOSIS AND PULMONARY EMBOLISM

Signs include:

- swelling, discoloration and pain in the affected limb
- acute pulmonary embolus or stroke
- superior vena cava syndrome with cyanosis, chylothorax and edema of the upper chest and face usually indicates a central venous catheter-related thrombosis (due to infection, stasis and irritant drugs or fluids).

Doppler ultrasonography can demonstrate or exclude large vein thrombus in most cases. A venogram can be performed in the PICU when doubt remains.

MANAGEMENT

Heparin may prevent extension of the thrombus. Symptomatic thromboses require treatment:

- surgical thrombectomy
- infusion of fibrinolytics such as streptokinase, urokinase and tissue plasminogen activator (TPA)

Fibrinolytics are difficult to monitor and the risk of treatment-associated hemorrhage is up to 10% in a high-risk (e.g. neonatal) population. Their use is contraindicated in the presence of active bleeding or a significant risk of local bleeding; for 10 days after general surgery and 3 weeks after neurosurgery.

Local infusion directly into the thrombus (TPA 0.02–0.05 mg/kg·h or streptokinase 50 units/kg·h) can decrease the risk of hemorrhage by avoiding the need to deliver systemic doses of the agent (up to 1000 times the local dose). Success is most likely in thrombi less than 1 week of age, and where obstruction is incomplete and collateral flow poor. During local infusion, heparin (loading dose 50 units/kg then 10–30 units/kg·h) should be given, to keep the activated partial thromboplastin time 2–3 times normal.

If local infusion of streptokinase or TPA fails to lyse the clot, systemic doses can be used:

- streptokinase 4000 units/kg (maximum 250 000 units) over 10 minutes, then 2000 units/kg·h for 6 hours
- urokinase (4000 units/kg over 10 minutes, then 4000 units/kg·h for 6 hours) should be used instead of streptokinase if:
  - streptokinase has ever been used previously
  - infant < 3 months of age
  - patient is on hemodialysis
- TPA 0.5 mg/kg·h i.v. for 6 hours; infuse heparin 10 units/kg·h during TPA infusion

Monitoring thrombolytic therapy is difficult as there is no reliable laboratory predictor of bleeding. Maintain fibrinogen levels above 1.0 g/L. Thrombolytics should be stopped after 48–72 hours regardless of outcome and heparin therapy continued for 48 hours after the thrombus resolves, or changed to warfarin if thrombus persists.

Although pulmonary emboli are uncommon in children, there is a high risk of pulmonary embolus in any child with a proximal vein or atrial thrombus and anticoagulant therapy is indicated.

THROMBOCYTOPENIA

Platelets have a circulation time of approximately 10 days and the platelet count in a normal individual is usually stable over time. Paucity of functioning platelets leads to mucosal bleeding, petechiae and superficial bruising. A low platelet count is common in critical illness. Platelet clumping can cause apparent thrombocytopenia and is excluded by examination of the blood film.

CAUSES

Thrombocytopenia—a platelet count below 150×10^9/L—is usually due to accelerated destruction, a diminished marrow capacity to respond or resuscitation with platelet-poor fluids:

- destruction: platelet trapping within microvascular thrombi in DIC or HUS
- decreased production: ischemia, sepsis, marrow infiltration or chemotherapy
- increased consumption
  - immune (e.g. ITP)
  - nonimmune (e.g. DIC or heparin-induced thrombocytopenia)
- dilution (e.g. large-volume blood transfusion)
- sequestration (e.g. hypersplenism)

Malignancy and chemotherapy often cause thrombocytopenia (with associated granulocytopenia and anemia) but bleeding rarely requires PICU admission. Idiopathic thrombocytopenic purpura (ITP) is the immune cause of thrombocytopenia most likely to present with life-threatening hemorrhage. It presents with profound, isolated thrombocytopenia.

In some patients, weeks to months of easy bruising or mucosal bleeding may precede the catastrophic bleeding which leads to ICU admission. A drug history and a search for symptoms and signs of a connective tissue disease may be helpful (see below).

MANAGEMENT OF PLATELET-DEPENDENT BLEEDING

Management consists of platelet transfusion (Table 3.6.2) and aggressive treatment of any underlying disorder.

A high-risk patient is one in whom:

- bleeding has already occurred
- a known hemostatic abnormality coexists

Platelet transfusion may be indicated regardless of number if there is known platelet dysfunction. Transfused platelets should be ABO compatible, as ABO antigens are expressed on platelets and matching improves platelet survival. In infants and small children, units of transfused platelets may

TABLE 3.6.2 **When to give a platelet transfusion**

	High-risk patient (platelets ×10⁹/L)	Low-risk patient (platelets × 10⁹/L)
Prophylaxis	< 20	< 10
Surgery or active bleeding	< 75	< 50
CNS surgery or life-threatening bleeding	> 100	< 100

contain enough donor plasma containing anti-A or anti-B isoagglutinins to cause hemolysis of recipient red cells, so if ABO-compatible platelets are unavailable, platelets should be pooled and resuspended in reduced plasma volume.

One unit (70 ml) of platelets per 5 kg body weight should increase the platelet count by 50 × 10⁹/L. Platelet concentrate is viable for 5 days if stored at 22°C on an agitator but platelet numbers and function decline with time after collection. A leukocyte removal filter can be used with platelets.

IDIOPATHIC THROMBOCYTOPENIC PURPURA

Idiopathic thrombocytopenic purpura is a disorder of platelet number that responds readily to treatment directed at an immune-mediated process. Signs include:

- a characteristic pattern of bleeding: epistaxis, mucous membranes, pressure points, facial petechiae on coughing or crying
- no other detectable abnormalities on history and physical examination
- CNS hemorrhage in 0.5%
- isolated thrombocytopenia with normal to large platelets and normal red cell and white cell morphology
- antiplatelet antibodies may be detected

Treatment

Treatment is indicated if:

- the patient is actively bleeding
- there are florid petechiae and a platelet count below 10 × 10⁹/L

Intravenous immunoglobulin (1 g/kg over 8–12 hours daily for 2 days) increases the platelet count to more than 30 × 10⁹/L over 48 hours. Alternatively, give prednisolone 2 mg/kg per day for 2 weeks, then taper.

Severe life-threatening hemorrhage, especially intracranial hemorrhage, is most likely to occur in children with platelet count below 10 × 10⁹/L and the risk is unrelated to age, time course of the illness or responsiveness to therapy. In a child with intracranial hemorrhage due to ITP, a trial of platelet transfusion plus intravenous γ-globulin or steroid is warranted. If this fails to raise the platelet count within 24 hours, or if there is a history of refractoriness to treatment, progressive neurological deterioration or an initial Glasgow coma scale score of less than 10, an emergency splenectomy is performed which increases the platelet count within hours.

X COMMON ERRORS

➤ Reliance on platelet transfusions alone to treat life-threatening bleeding. These patients show a negligible increase in platelet number after transfusion
➤ Relying on steroids or immunoglobulin in a previously unresponsive patient
➤ Using desmopressin to enhance platelet function (function is normal in ITP)
➤ Belief that ITP is a benign condition

DISSEMINATED INTRAVASCULAR COAGULATION

Disseminated intravascular coagulation is commonly present in the critically ill. It may be mild and subclinical, or severe and life-threatening.

Insults such as sepsis, malignancy, ischemia or trauma trigger the coagulation system, generating thrombin and simultaneously activating fibrinolysis. Circulating thrombin cleaves fibrinogen to form fibrin monomers, which are polymerized in the circulation to form microvascular thrombi in which platelets are trapped. Simultaneously, plasmin (derived from plasminogen) actively cleaves fibrinogen, leading to the generation of breakdown products. These products are markers of fibrinolysis and inhibit polymerization of fibrin, thereby exacerbating the bleeding tendency created by the consumption of coagulant proteins and the incorporation of platelets into small vessel thrombi.

The effects of DIC are:

- microvascular thrombi, causing ischemic organ damage
- exacerbation of shock, acidosis and pulmonary dysfunction due to the primary insult
- consumption of platelets and clotting factors causing bleeding, which is rarely life-threatening

Signs

The signs of DIC may be difficult to separate from those of the primary disorder. Oozing may occur from puncture sites, surgical wounds and from the nose after nasal intubation. Bleeding often occurs at the same time as lactic acidosis and encephalopathy appear and kidney, liver and lung function deteriorate.

The outcome for DIC depends mainly on the underlying disease and to a lesser extent on the disruption in organ function caused by microvascular thrombi.

Management

Treat the underlying cause (e.g. infection). Supportive treatment is required for organ dysfunction:

- oxygen, IPPV/CPAP for respiratory failure (Ch. 2.1)
- plasma volume expansion and inotropic drugs for circulatory failure (Ch. 2.3)
- hemofiltration or dialysis for renal failure (Ch. 2.10)
- replacement of depleted clotting factors and platelets if necessary (Ch. 2.8)

- platelets: give 10 ml/kg, repeated if necessary if the platelet count is below 20×10^9/L in nonbleeding patients, or below 50×10^9/L in bleeding patients
- give cryoprecipitate (0.2 unit/kg) if the child is bleeding and fibrinogen level is below 1 g/L
- give fresh frozen plasma (20 ml/kg, repeated if necessary) if bleeding and if PT and APTT are prolonged
- heparin (10 units/kg·h after an i.v. bolus of 50 units/kg) is only used if vascular occlusion is a prominent aspect of the DIC (e.g. after an incompatible blood transfusion)

TRANSFUSION MEDICINE

The oxygen-carrying capacity of blood is determined by the hemoglobin concentration and its saturation. Oxygen delivery falls as Hb and hematocrit fall, but there is no critical level of Hb or hematocrit below which transfusion is essential. While optimum values for tissue oxygen delivery can be determined in the laboratory, clinical experience suggests that a wide range of Hb or hematocrit is tolerated, depending on age, organ function and the rate at which Hb decreases. Outside the context of acute blood loss, transfusion requires assessment of compensatory responses including heart rate, respiratory rate, breath sounds, activity level, ventilation or oxygen requirements and laboratory data such as pH and blood lactate. While too liberal a transfusion policy inhibits erythropoietin production and exposes the child to blood from multiple donors, a rigid policy based on a few measurable values such as hematocrit may lead to inadequate restoration of red cell mass and may delay recovery. Maintenance of a hematocrit of 0.3–0.35 seems sensible.

BLOOD PRODUCTS

Most cellular blood products should only be given to ABO-compatible recipients to avoid antibody-mediated hemolysis (Table 3.6.3). Red cells require additional crossmatching of recipient against donor to avoid other antibody/antigen-mediated

TABLE 3.6.3 ABO compatibility of transfused blood

Recipient blood group	RBC antigen	Natural antibodies	Compatible donor red cells
A	A	anti-B	A, O
B	B	anti-A	B, O
AB	A, B	–	A, B, AB, O
O	–	anti-A, anti-B	O

interactions. Crossmatching takes 10 minutes to an hour or more.

Whole blood

Whole blood is rarely available, is an inefficient use of blood and should not be used to treat anemia. One unit contains 450 ml of blood and 60 ml of anticoagulant. The hematocrit is 0.35–0.4, and 6 ml/kg whole blood increases Hb by 10 g/L.

Indications for the use of whole blood are:

- hypovolemic shock due to blood loss
- exchange transfusion

Packed red blood cells

Removal of plasma from whole blood and replacement with an adenine-saline solution results in a product with a volume of 350 ml and hematocrit of 0.5–0.65. Transfusion of 3 ml/kg packed red cells increases the Hb by 10 g/L or the hematocrit by 0.03. Indications for its use include:

- rapid or continuing blood loss
- symptomatic anemia

The use of blood products should be minimized by:

- avoiding or rapidly controlling blood loss
- maximizing oxygen delivery by volume repletion, vasoactive drugs and mechanical ventilation with oxygen (Ch. 2.1).
- minimizing oxygen consumption (by sedation, analgesia, temperature control or mechanical ventilation)
- stimulating hematopoiesis (administer iron, folate, vitamin B_{12}, erythropoietin)

HAZARDS OF BLOOD TRANSFUSION

The benefits of blood component therapy must be weighed against its risks in every case before the therapy is started (Table 3.6.4).

Acute hemolytic transfusion reactions

The incidence of acute reactions is 1 per 600 000 units of donor blood. The usual causes are:

- clerical mishap (incompatible transfusion)
- high-titer hemolysin in donor plasma
- transfusion of overheated, frozen, badly stored or outdated blood

Transmission of infectious disease

See below.

Bacterial contamination

Bacterial contamination is a rare cause of cardiovascular collapse soon after transfusion. One in 300 blood components has a positive culture: mostly skin flora. Organisms are Gram-positive bacteria (including *Staphylococcus aureus*); coliforms; and *Yersinia enterocolitica*. Sources may be:

- donor bacteremia from occult infection, tooth brushing, defecation, etc.
- inadequate preparation of donor skin
- leaking blood bags

Signs include tachycardia; tachypnea; hypotension; cyanosis; fever; rigors; vomiting; diarrhea; DIC; and renal failure.

The risks are greater with platelets (stored at 22°C), especially when stored longer than 5 days. The risks are less with FFP and cryoprecipitate.

Alloimmunization of the recipient

Exposure to multiple donors leads to antibodies against HLA antigens on leukocytes. The problem is minimized by transfusing leukocyte-depleted products.

Febrile reactions

Alloantibodies in the recipient react with cellular antigens on donor platelets or leukocytes.

TABLE 3.6.4 Complications of massive transfusion

- Fluid overload
- Impaired clotting
  - dilution
  - reduced production
  - DIC
- Hyperkalemia, then later hypokalemia
- Citrate toxicity[a] (increased by hypothermia or liver disease)
  - metabolic acidosis, then later alkalosis
  - low ionized calcium
- ARDS and multiple organ failure
  - microaggregates
  - damaged transfused cells
- Poor function of donor cells (RBCS, leukocytes, platelets)
- Hypothermia[b]

[a]Citrate toxicity can be prevented by infusion of 10 ml of 10% calcium gluconate for every liter of blood infused. Note—excess calcium will cause more problems than the citrate. The calcium infusion must be infused through a different venous line to the one being used for the blood.
[b]Storage of blood at 4°C can result in central cooling. Infusion through blood warming devices can reduce this complication. Note—blood warming requires proper, regulated devices to be safe.

Graft-versus-host disease

Transfused, viable T lymphocytes engraft, proliferate within the recipient and react against host tissues to cause graft-versus-host disease (GVHD). Signs include skin rashes, liver dysfunction, and diarrhea.

Any cellular blood component can cause GVHD, which can be prevented by irradiating the product before transfusion. Children who require irradiated blood include:

- all neonates
- children who have undergone bone marrow or stem cell transplantation
- all immunocompromised patients
- recipients at risk of immunocompromise (e.g. all patients with interrupted aortic arch, truncus arteriosus or tetralogy of Fallot, unless DiGeorge syndrome has been excluded)
- any child receiving a directed donation from a blood relative

TRANSMITTED INFECTIONS

Post-transfusion hepatitis and retroviral infections are the main infection risks of transfusion of whole blood, packed cells, platelets, FFP, cryoprecipitate and granulocytes. All blood components except recombinant factors VIII, IX and XIII carry a risk of transmitting infection. Heat-treated products such as albumin, Prothrombinex and human factor VIII carry less risk than single-donor components such as packed cells, FFP or platelets. Multidonor packs such as pooled immunoglobulin carry the greatest risk. Improved donor screening and testing have reduced the incidence of these infections, but some risk remains.

Hepatitis B

In 8–10% of asymptomatic hepatitis B virus (HBV) carriers, the usual serological markers are undetectable. Forty per cent of donors capable of transmitting HBV are undetected by HBV surface antigen screening. The risk of transmission in Australia is 1 in 66 000 to 1 in 200 000 units of blood.

Hepatitis C

Seroconversion takes approximately 70 days, during which time undetected transmission of hepatitis C virus in donated blood is possible. The current risk of transmission in Australia is 1 in 120 000 units of blood.

Human immunodeficiency virus

Testing for HIV relies on antibody production to the virus. Detectable seroconversion takes 2–3 weeks after exposure. Sensitive donor screening procedures and the low prevalence of the infection in the donor population have greatly reduced but not totally eliminated the risk, estimated to be 1 in 600 000–1 000 000 units of blood.

Cytomegalovirus

Approximately 50% of donors are positive for cytomegalovirus (CMV). Despite the presence of antibody, the virus can persist in leukocytes. Immunocompromised patients who are CMV-negative are at risk of pneumonitis, hepatitis and enteritis from acquired CMV infection. Blood products that may contain leukocytes (e.g. packed cells, platelets and granulocyte concentrates) should be obtained from a CMV-negative donor or leukocyte filtered. Acellular components do not transmit the virus.

BLOOD SUBSTITUTES

At present no oxygen-carrying blood substitutes including modified Hb solutions and perfluoro-carbon emulsions can replace red cells. Progress has been limited by toxicity of these solutions and biologic properties incompatible with use in the critically ill human.

TREATMENT OF TRANSFUSION REACTION

Fever is commonly due to leukocyte antibodies in multiple transfusions, preventable by leukocyte-poor red cell transfusion. Give:

- acetaminophen (paracetamol) 10–15 mg/kg orally every 4–6 hours
- diphenhydramine 1–2 mg/kg orally, every 6–9 hours (1–2 mg/kg i.v. for anaphylaxis)

Hemolysis due to incompatible blood constitutes an emergency. Symptoms include fever, dyspnea, shock, bleeding, rigors, discomfort at the infusion site, chest pain and loin pain.

Action:

- discontinue transfusion but maintain intravenous access/infusion using a new administration set and 0.9% saline or dextrose saline
- treat for shock if present (Ch 2.3)
- follow pulse, blood pressure, urine output, temperature
- contact the blood bank immediately; save and return the blood product
- send to the laboratory a 5 ml (clotted) blood sample from the child and the next urine passed

✓ **KEY POINTS**

➤ Any febrile illness is a medical emergency in SCD
➤ For any acute crisis in sickle disease: assess and correct airway, breathing and circulation, give oxygen, correct acidosis and start i.v. fluids
➤ Spontaneous venous thrombosis and pulmonary embolism are rare in children
➤ Thrombolytic therapy should be stopped after 48–72 hours regardless of outcome
➤ A child with thrombosis in the atria or venae cavae requires long-term anticoagulation
➤ 1 unit/5 kg of platelets increases the platelet count by 50×10^9/L (50 000/mm³)
➤ 3 ml/kg packed red cells increases the hemoglobin concentration by 10g/L

FURTHER READING

1. Lane PA. Sickle cell disease. Pediatr Clin North Am 1996; 43: 639–664
   – (*Overview of recent treatments for the various manifestations of SCD*)

2. Ferguson WS. Hematologic disorders. In: Todres ID, Fugate JH, editors. Critical care of infants and children. Boston: Little, Brown; 1996
   – (*Review of the hematologic problems seen in critically ill children and those that cause children to become critically ill. Uses treatment algorithms*)

3. David M, Andrew M. Venous thromboembolic complications in children. J Pediatr 1993; 123: 337–346
   – (*Authoritative literature review of presentation, causes, diagnosis, prevention and treatment of childhood thromboembolic disease*)

4. British Committee for Standards in Haematology Blood Transfusion Task Force. Guidelines for administration of blood products: transfusion of infants and neonates. Transfus Med 1994; 4: 63–69
   – (*Guidelines on donors, storage, testing, indications and hazards*)

5. Hall LM, Perry EH. Blood products and transfusion. In: Reisdorff EJ, Roberts MR, Wiegenstein JG, editors. Pediatric emergency medicine. Philadelphia: WB Saunders; 1993
   – (*Extensive information on various blood products*)

3.7 Immunological disease

Nigel Klein

Dramatic advances have been made in the diagnosis of immunological diseases. The molecular basis of all of the major X-linked immunodeficiencies has now been elucidated, and the causes of many autosomal defects determined. In addition, developments in bone marrow transplantation have led to an increase in the number of patients eligible for this form of therapy. In spite of these developments, children with immunological abnormalities still account for a considerable number of admissions to intensive care units and are still associated with a very high mortality rate of between 40% and 60%. Early recognition and appropriate management is therefore critical to the survival of immunodeficient individuals. This chapter addresses the three common scenarios in which children with immunological abnormalities are managed during critical illness:

- admission without prior recognition of an immunological defect
- admission of known immunodeficient children
- children with other diseases who develop immunological abnormalities while receiving intensive care

PATHOPHYSIOLOGY

At birth, babies possess the essential elements of all components of the immune system, including a range of both nonspecific and specific defenses against microorganisms. However, it is only after encountering a wide range of potential pathogens that these defenses will fully mature to provide adequate protection in later life. The importance of acquiring a fully competent host defense system in this way is illustrated clinically by the problems encountered in immunodeficient individuals. These patients suffer not only from severe and persistent infections due to common organisms, but are also vulnerable to a range of unusual or opportunistic pathogens. The role played by each component of the host defense system can be deduced from the nature of infections associated with specific immunological defects, many of which present in childhood (Table 3.7.1).

There have been major advances in the understanding and diagnosis of immunodeficiency. It is now apparent that defects exist in a wide range of genes that regulate leukocyte development and function. These include cell surface molecules such as cytokine receptors, protein kinases involved in signal transduction and cytokine production. The majority of these defects lead to a reduction in the total number of lymphocytes or a reduced or absent subset of lymphocytes. Table 3.7.2 summarizes some of the immunodeficiencies that may be encountered in critical illness.

PREVIOUSLY UNDIAGNOSED IMMUNODEFICIENCY

RECOGNITION

It is vital to recognize immunodeficiency as early as possible. Immunodeficient children usually present with persistent or severe infections. In severe disease, most children will present before 6 months

TABLE 3.7.1 **Defects in the various components of the immune system render an individual susceptible to specific types of infection**

Immune defect	Infectious susceptibility	
Antibody	Bacteria	Staphylococcus, Streptococcus Haemophilus influenzae, M. catteralis
	Viruses	Enteroviruses
Cellular immunity RSV	Bacteria	Mycobacteria, Listeria
	Viruses	CMV, herpes, measles,
	Fungi	Candida, Aspergillus
	Protozoa	Pneumocystis
Neutrophils	Bacteria	Gram-positive, Gram-negative
	Fungi	Aspergillus, Candida
Complement	Bacteria	Neisseria, Staphylococcus

TABLE 3.7.2 **Primary immunodeficiencies which may lead to ICU admission**

Immunodeficiency	Ig	B cells	T cells	N	Molecular defect	Inheritance
T–B+ SCID:						
X-linked	↓	→ or ↑	↓	→	IL-2 gamma chain	XL
AR	↓	→ or ↑	↓	→	JAK-3 kinase	AR
T–B– SCID	↓	↓	↓	→ or ↓	RAG, ADA and reticular dysgenesis	AR
Hyper-IgM syndrome	↓IgG ↓IgM	→	→	→ or ↓	CD40 ligand	XL or ?
Agammaglobulinemia	↓	↓	→	→	Btk mutations	XL
MHC class II deficiency	→	→	↓CD4	→	MHC II transcription	AR
ZAP-70 deficiency	→	→	↓CD8	→	Zap-70 kinase	AR
Leucocyte adhesion deficiency	→	→	→	↑	Beta-2 integrins	AR
Chronic granulomatous disease	→	→	→	→	NADPH oxidase	XL/AR

Ig, immunoglobulin; N, neutrophils; XL, X-linked; AR, autosomal recessive; SCID, severe combined immunodeficieny; ADA, adenosine deaminase deficiency; Btk, Bruton's tyrosine kinase

of age. The most common presentation is of lower respiratory tract infections (Figure 3.7.1) although infections at other sites may also be evident. In addition, failure to thrive is a frequent accompaniment of severe combined immunodeficiencies (SCID). All children presenting with severe or persistent infections should be considered to be immunodeficient until proved otherwise. This is because the range of potential pathogens differs from those encountered in infants with an intact immune system and may have a major bearing on both management and prognosis (Table 3.7.1). Children with an immunodeficiency may have a history of recurrent infections. These patients may also have evidence of an enteropathy and are frequently failing to thrive. Many of the immunodeficiencies are inherited as X-linked or autosomal recessive traits. Parental consanguinity and a family history of unexplained family deaths, particularly of boys, may therefore be of diagnostic significance. Associated features of syndromes associated with immunodeficiency, e.g. velocardiofacial syndrome, should also be looked for. A rash may be indicative of a rare form of SCID, Omenn's syndrome or maternal engraftment.

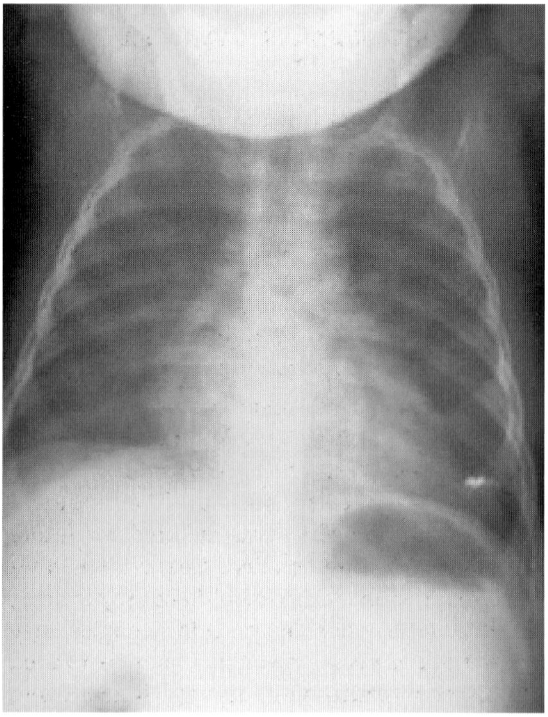

INVESTIGATION OF IMMUNOLOGICAL COMPETENCE

Children with suspected immunodeficiencies should be investigated to determine the exact nature of the underlying defect. Initial investigations should include a full blood count, which will demonstrate reduced lymphocytes in the majority of children with severe immunodeficiency. Serum immunoglobulins should also be determined as soon as possible. Maternal antibody and prior administration of blood products will influence the levels of IgG, but IgA and IgM determination can still be of diagnostic value. Further

Figure 3.7.1 Child with lower respiratory tract infection (*Pneumocystis carinii*)

Detection and management of immunodeficiency

- Suspect immunodeficiency
- Take a careful history and perform a careful examination
- Aggressive investigation for the identity of causative organisms
- Aggressive treatment of suspected organisms
- Early investigation of immune deficiency
- Plan discharge with immunologists to prevent future problems
- Save appropriate samples if patient dies before a diagnosis is made

---

tests should be directed towards the most likely cause, as assessed from the history and general examination. Currently available immunological investigations can not only quantify the essential elements of the immune system, but also provide a functional assessment of immunocompetence and in many cases identify the genetic basis for the immunological defect (Table 3.7.3). A DNA sample should also be stored for mutation analysis, and cells separated and stored for detection of specific proteins, e.g. Btk or JAK-3 kinase (see Table 3.7.2). Children infected with HIV may present with identical features and therefore a diagnosis of HIV should be sought after formal pretest counseling. In children less than 18 months old, maternally derived antibody may give rise to a false diagnosis of HIV. It is therefore important to obtain direct evidence of infection, usually by performing HIV polymerase chain reaction (PCR) analysis.

TREATMENT

Initial treatment should be directed at the acute cause of illness. As this is usually infective, identification of the causative organism or organisms should be aggressively sought. Nasopharyngeal aspirates, tracheal aspirates or bronchoalveolar lavage material should be examined for bacteria, *Pneumocystis carinii*, fungi and viruses—particularly respiratory syncytial virus (RSV) and cytomegalovirus (CMV). Blood cultures, buffy coat culture and PCR for CMV should also be performed if a pulmonary infection is suspected. Fluid from other sites of suspected infection, e.g. cerebrospinal fluid, should be examined.

Immunodeficient children may also harbor opportunistic infections in the gastrointestinal tract. Stools should be cultured for enteroviruses, CMV, and *Campylobacter,* and examined for *Cryptosporidium* and *Giardia lamblia*.

Empirical antimicrobial therapy should be started as soon as possible if the patient is critically ill. It is frequently necessary to treat pulmonary infections with high-dose trimethprim and sulfamethoxazole (co-trimoxazole), ganciclovir, broad-spectrum antibiotics and antifungal therapy. Methylprednisolone should be included if *Pneumocystis carinii* pneumonia (PCP) is detected, as this form of adjunctive therapy has dramatically improved the outcome of this infection (Fig. 3.7.2). Similarly, there are some data to support a trial of surfactant therapy if no improvement is seen with full PICU support and appropriate antimicrobial therapy. Intravenous immunoglobulin or fresh frozen plasma should be considered in patients with combined immunodeficiencies. *Blood products should be CMV-negative and irradiated* to prevent engraftment of donor lymphocytes.

INVESTIGATION OF CRITICALLY ILL CHILDREN

If a child is critically ill and survival is unlikely before immunological investigations have been performed, it is vital that appropriate samples are taken before or just following death. In addition to a full blood count, serum should be saved for immunoglobulin determination, an EDTA sample (5–10 ml) should be saved for gene mutation analysis, and cells (5–10 ml EDTA or heparinized) should be separated and stored for cell and protein analysis. Lymphocyte subset enumeration can be performed on an EDTA sample for up to 48 hours when maintained at room temperature. A skin biopsy can also be taken, stored at 4°C in tissue culture medium and fibroblasts cultured for future DNA studies. In some conditions, e.g. chronic granulomatous disease and Wiskott–Aldrich syndrome, simple investigations on parental samples may reveal a carrier phenotype. This can be performed at a future outpatient visit. As many immunodeficiencies are genetically determined, it is important to try and make a diagnosis as prenatal testing may be possible in future pregnancies.

TABLE 3.7.3 **A summary of investigations used to elucidate the nature of an immunodeficiency**

Test	Function
Lymphocytes	
Lymphocyte subsets	Determines the number of T cells, B cells and NK cells
Immunoglobulins	To measure the levels of IgG, IgM, IgA and IgE and IgG subclasses
Specific immunoglobulin responses to known antigens, e.g. vaccines	Tests the ability to mount an appropriate antibody response
T-cell proliferation in response to antigens and mitogens	A functional test of cell-mediated immunity
Neutrophils	
Nitroblue tetrazolium (NBT) test	Defective in chronic granulomatous disease
Surface adhesion molecules (CD18, CD15s)	Test for leukocyte adhesion deficiency
Complement	
Individual complement components	Reduced in complement deficiency states and other diseases
Total haemolytic complement	Functional test for complement
DNA	Mutation analysis, chromosomal breakage syndromes
Cell lysates	Protein analysis, e.g. for Bruton's tyrosine kinase and JAK-3 intracellular kinase
Engraftment studies	To test for maternal and blood product engraftment

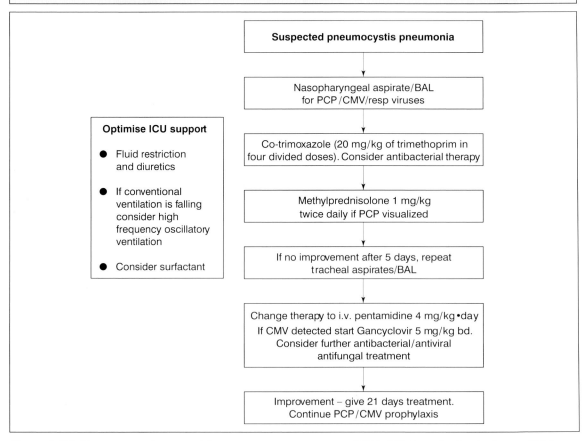

Figure 3.7.2 Management of suspected *Pneumocystis carinii* pneumonia (PCP). BAL, bronchoalveolar lavage; CMV, cytomegalovirus

CARE FOLLOWING DISCHARGE

The recent discovery of the genetic basis for many of the primary immunodeficiencies is likely to have a profound impact on future management. Gene therapy, in which a normally functioning gene is transfected into defective progenitor cells, has already been performed for adenosine deaminase deficiency. It is hoped that this form of therapy will soon be available for some of the other conditions outlined in Table 3.7.2. Until that time, however, management will continue to consist of:

- antimicrobial prophylaxis to prevent infection
- appropriate antimicrobial therapy to treat infection
- immunoglobulin replacement therapy for defects in antibody function or production and replacement of missing factors such as adenine deaminase or cytokines
- bone marrow transplants for severe immunodeficiencies

If the child is recovering from the acute illness, and the diagnosis of immunodeficiency is confirmed, future treatment should be planned. For some conditions, e.g. agammaglobulinemia or hyper-IgM syndrome, therapy with intravenous immunoglobulin replacement therapy and/or prophylactic trimethoprim with sulfamethoxazole (co-trimoxazole) may be sufficient. However, improvements in bone marrow transplantation have led to the increasing use of this treatment. Patients should be HLA-typed and potential bone marrow donors sought so that transplantation can proceed as quickly as possible. Further episodes of severe infection may be fatal.

KNOWN IMMUNODEFICIENCY

If a child is admitted with a known primary immunodeficiency, the principles of treatment described above should be applied. That is, the likely organisms responsible for the admission are diligently searched for and aggressively treated. It is important to note that immunodeficient patients treated with a bone marrow transplant are often receiving immunosuppressive therapy to prevent graft-versus-host disease and are therefore particu-

larly susceptible to infections owing to both the immaturity of their graft and immunosuppressive therapy. Infections contracted prior to transplantation may be particularly problematic. The prognosis for CMV and RSV infections in this context is poor. A lung biopsy should be performed early, as evidence of immune-mediated lung injury requires immunosuppressive therapy. The outcome for children admitted with an opportunistic infection despite treatment of the underlying immunodeficiency and prophylactic antimicrobial therapy is poor. It is important to discuss the prognosis with the patient's family and to consider the appropriateness of continuing therapy if the patient fails to improve or is slowly deteriorating.

CRITICAL ILLNESS AND IMMUNE FUNCTION

Patients with multiorgan failure may become hyporesponsive to endogenous mediators of inflammation. Antiinflammatory cytokines such as interleukin 10 (IL-10) may inhibit proinflammatory cytokine production (IL-1, IL-6, tumor necrosis factor) and render patients susceptible to opportunistic infections (Figure 3.7.3). In a small trial, patients with cytokine hyporesponsiveness were identified as having a reduced population of monocytes expressing MHC class II antigens. These patients appeared to benefit from treatment with interferon gamma.

In another study it was shown that infants receiving total parenteral nutrition as a sole source of nutrients acquired a neutrophil defect. These patients are particularly susceptible to coagulase-

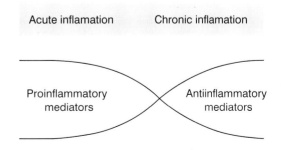

Acute inflamation	Chronic inflamation
Proinflammatory mediators	Antiinflammatory mediators

Figure 3.7.3 Chronic inflammation may be associated with immune hyporesponsiveness due to antiinflammatory cytokines

negative staphylococcal infections. Enteral nutrition appears to diminish the risk of this infection and should therefore be instituted as early as possible.

It is clear that patients requiring critical care can acquire immunological deficits. There is insufficient evidence to support the widespread use of interferon gamma therapy in patients with multiorgan failure. However, it is important to be aware that patients in the PICU may become relatively immunodeficient and are therefore at increased risk from infection, particularly from intravascular catheters, endotracheal tubes and peritoneal dialysis tubing. Vigilant attention to handwashing, nutrition and exposure to overt infection within the unit is essential.

✔ **KEY POINTS**

➤ Think of immunodeficiency in all infants admitted with a severe or unusual infection
➤ Vigilantly search for pathogens
➤ Aggressively treat presumed or identified infections
➤ Only administer irradiated, CMV-negative blood products
➤ Investigate immunodeficiency and save appropriate samples if the child dies before a diagnosis has been made

FURTHER READING

1. Steim, ER. Immunological disorders in infants and children, 4th ed. Philadelphia: W. B. Saunders; 1996
2. Klein N, Curtis N. Paediatric infectious diseases. In: Lissauer T, Clayden, G, editors. An illustrated textbook of paediatrics. 1996
3. Primary immunodeficiency diseases. Clin Exper Immunol 1997; 109(suppl.): 1–28
4. Dock WD, Randow F, Syrbe U et al. Monocyte deactivation in septic patients: restoration by IFN-gamma treatment. Nat Med 1997; 3: 678–681
5. Okada Y, Pierra A, Klein N. Neutrophil dysfunction: the cellular mechanism of impaired immunity during total parenteral nutrition in infancy. J Paediat Surg 1999; in press

3.8   Infectious disease

Vas Novelli, Mark J. Peters and Simon Dobson

Infections are the most common cause of acute illness in children. Life-threatening infections account for about 25% of children requiring admission for pediatric intensive care, and result in significant morbidity and mortality. Most infections are community-acquired; around one-third are nosocomial or hospital-acquired. Respiratory tract infections with associated respiratory failure, CNS infections, and sepsis syndromes constitute the bulk of critical infectious conditions. Increasingly, infections in the immunocompromised host (including children with HIV infection) are requiring intensive care. Optimal initial management and treatment of children critically ill with serious infections constitutes an important part of comprehensive pediatric care.

MENINGITIS

Despite advances in antibiotic therapy and increasing availability of pediatric intensive care, mortality and morbidity rates for bacterial meningitis remain substantial. The mortality rate is around 5–10% and up to a third of survivors of bacterial meningitis suffer permanent neurological sequelae. Bacterial meningitis is predominantly a disease of infants and young children with an incidence of around 5–7 per 100 000 persons. In developed countries, *Streptococcus pneumoniae* and *Neisseria meningitidis* have become the predominant causes of meningitis in children, owing to the near-eradication of invasive *Haemophilus influenzae* type b (Hib) infections following the introduction of Hib vaccine into the childhood immunization program. The increasing incidence of meningitis due to *Streptococcus pneumoniae*, resistant to conventional antibiotics, is however a cause for great concern worldwide. Table 3.8.1 shows the most common causative organisms responsible for bacterial meningitis in children.

PATHOPHYSIOLOGY

Although the CNS effects of bacterial meningitis were thought to be the direct result of the toxic effects of bacterial products it is now known that the host inflammatory response itself is chiefly responsible for the clinical findings and sequelae. Current research efforts are thus aimed at ways to modify this host inflammatory response. Following colonization of the upper respiratory tract of a susceptible individual, organisms subsequently invade the blood stream, and gain access to the subarachnoid space via the choroid plexus. Encapsulated organisms are particularly invasive because of their ability to evade host recognition and clearance. The bacteria replicate rapidly releasing bacterial products (endotoxin, lipotechoic acid) which stimulate macrophages and endothelial cells to produce cytokines (TNF, IL-1β, IL-6, PAF), which in turn potentiate the inflammatory response, causing endothelial cell injury. The result is increased capillary permeability leading to cerebral edema, raised intracranial pressure and decreased cerebral blood flow. Vasculitis and thrombosis can also contribute to brain ischemia. Irreversible focal or diffuse cerebral damage may then occur.

CLINICAL FEATURES

The onset of acute meningitis can present as a fulminant infection with rapidly progressive signs and symptoms (e.g. shock, purpura, DIC, coma); this presentation is more common in meningococcal meningitis. More commonly, presentation of acute bacterial meningitis is insidious, with a preceding nonspecific febrile illness often lasting several days, followed by the onset of signs and symptoms more characteristic of meningitis. Common initial manifestations include fever, vomiting, lethargy, poor feeding and irritability. These symptoms are followed by the appearance of the classical signs of meningitis: neck stiffness, bulging fontanelle, photophobia, positive Kernig's sign, impaired consciousness, seizures and focal neurological signs. These classic signs may be absent or difficult to elicit in very young children. Symptoms and signs in young children tend to be

TABLE 3.8.1 Bacterial meningitis: common causative organisms and antibiotic therapy

Age (months)	Common pathogen	Empiric antibiotic therapy[a]
0–1	Group B streptococcus Escherichia coli Klebsiella pneumoniae Listeria monocytogenes	Ampicillin + cefotaxime or Ampicillin + aminoglycoside
1–3	Group B streptococcus E. coli, K. pneumoniae Haemophilus influenzae Neisseria meningitidis Streptococcus pneumoniae	Ampicillin + third-generation cephalosporin
> 3	H. influenzae Streptococcus pneumoniae	Third-generation cephalosporin

[a]Vancomycin (60 mg/kg per day in four divided doses) should be added if highly resistant pneumococcal meningitis is suspected.

nonspecific and subtle (e.g. poor tone, lethargy, jaundice, less interest in feeding, respiratory distress, vomiting or diarrhoea). Hence the diagnosis may be delayed. Up to 20% of patients may develop seizures in the first few days of the illness.

INVESTIGATIONS

A lumbar puncture is necessary for a definitive diagnosis. Usually a Gram stain, cell count, CSF biochemistry and bacterial culture are performed on the cerebrospinal fluid obtained. Although generally safe, an LP is contraindicated in some circumstances, including those in which there is raised intracranial pressure (see below). In these circumstances, the LP is best deferred till the patient is stabilized. Empiric antibiotic therapy must nevertheless be commenced promptly. Computed Tomographic scanning of the head may be helpful in patients with focal neurology, signs of raised ICP and/or deteriorating neurologic state (increasing obtundation or seizures). There may be radiological evidence of a subdural empyema, abscess, infarction or hydrocephalus. A normal CT scan does not, however, entirely exclude raised ICP.

Contraindications to lumbar puncture

Contraindications include:

- raised intracranial pressure:
  - alteration in conscious level
  - papilledema
  - prolonged seizures

  - presence of focal neurologic signs
  - hypertension, bradycardia
  - fixed dilated or unequal pupils
  - absent doll's eye movements
  - decerebrate or decorticate posture
- cardiovascular and respiratory instability
- bleeding disorder
- localized infection at the site of LP

Note—Neither the absence of papilledema on physical examination nor a normal CT scan of the head can be relied on to rule out raised ICP.

Where immediate LP is not possible efforts should be made to identify the pathogen via other cultures. Blood cultures are of considerable value as 80–90% are positive in patients with bacterial meningitis. Throat swabs may be positive in those with Neisseria meningitidis infections. Gram staining and cultures of petechial lesions may lead to a specific diagnosis. Latex agglutination tests may detect relevant bacterial antigens in the CSF, blood or urine, even after antibiotic therapy has begun bacterial culture results are often negative. In some centers, PCR technology, which is able to detect small amounts of bacterial DNA from blood or CSF, is now available.

MANAGEMENT

It is essential that diagnosis and treatment of bacterial meningitis are not delayed. Prior to transfer to the PICU, children with suspected meningococcal disease or meningococcal meningitis should be given an immediate dose of a parenteral antibiotic, either penicillin (benzylpenicillin) 50 000 units/kg or a third-generation cephalosporin (e.g. cephotaxime (250–300 mg/kg). Ideally all patients with bacterial meningitis should be monitored on a PICU for the first 24–48 h. The following are the major problems to anticipate.

Early problems associated with bacterial meningitis include:

- cerebral edema, raised ICP, uncal herniation
- shock
- electrolyte disturbances, SIADH
- disseminated intravascular coagulation
- seizures

Give supplemental oxygen, obtain good vascular access and treat poor perfusion or any shock state with repeated intravenous boluses of fluids (crystalloid or colloid). Inotropic support may be required. Consideration should also be given to elective intubation (especially for severe meningococcal cases—see Ch. 6.2).

Treatment of raised intracranial pressure may require the following additional measures:

- elevation of the head of the bed (30°)
- fluid restriction—two-thirds maintenance. Fluids should not be restricted until hypovolemia/hypotension are corrected as maintenance of an adequate circulating volume is essential for cerebral perfusion, particularly in the presence of raised ICP.
- intubation and ventilation (initially to normocapnia 3.5–4.0 kPa)
- mannitol—boluses of 0.25 g/kg (not routinely necessary)

Coagulation disturbances are corrected with vitamin K and fresh frozen plasma. In mild cases of bacterial meningitis, any dehydration is first corrected over 24–48 hours and then followed by slight restriction of fluids.

Antimicrobial therapy

The choice of antibiotics depends on the likely infecting organism for the particular age group, pharmacokinetic properties of the drug (e.g. CSF penetration), and the prevalence and type of antibiotic resistance reported locally. Antibiotic therapy should be started immediately after lumbar puncture and not withheld pending initial results of the CSF examination. The most frequently used antibiotics (or combinations) are listed in Table 3.8.1. These are given intravenously until results of culture and sensitivity tests are known, when modification of therapy may be appropriate. Antibiotic levels in serum (peak and trough) must be obtained in the first 48 h if aminoglycoside or vancomycin therapy is instituted, in order to minimize the likelihood of otoxicity or nephrotoxicity.

Chemoprophylaxis

Patients with bacterial meningitis caused by *N. meningitidis* or *H. influenzae* type b are considered infectious for at least the first 24 h after the start of appropriate therapy, and hence should be kept in respiratory isolation. For meningococcal meningitis, the index patient, all household contacts (> 28 hours per week) and nursery contacts require chemoprophylaxis with rifampicin (10 mg/kg, max. 600 mg/dose, every 12 h for 2 days) to eradicate nasopharyngeal carriage of the organism. Patients receiving ceftriaxone do not require prophylaxis as this antibiotic is effective in clearing *N. meningitidis* from the nasopharynx. For *Haemophilus influenzae* type b meningitis, rifampicin (20 mg/kg per dose, max. 600 mg/dose, once daily for 4 days; 10 mg/kg for infants < 1 month) is recommended for the index patient and for all household contacts when there is an incompletely immunized child less than 48 months old in the household.

Controversial care

Steroids

Dexamethasone (0.15 mg/kg per dose every 6 h for 4 days), administered at the same time as the antibiotics or immediately before, has been shown in some trials to be beneficial in diminishing neurological damage and deafness associated with bacterial meningitis. The evidence is robust for *H. influenzae* type b meningitis, but is less clear for other forms of bacterial meningitis. According to the American Academy of Pediatrics (AAP) Red Book Committee recommendations, steroids should be considered as adjunctive therapy in bacterial meningitis, but the decision is left to the individual clinician.

ENCEPHALITIS

Acute encephalitis is an inflammation of the brain substance induced directly or indirectly by microbial agents.

Manifestations of encephalitis in children include headache, fever, photophobia, vomiting, focal seizures, alterations in conscious level and personality changes. Other manifestations such as hemiplegia, ataxia, choreoathetosis, cranial nerve palsies and bowel and bladder dysfunction may also be seen. The clinical course may be rapidly progressive in some patients. The incidence varies in different countries, but European data suggest an incidence of 8–10 per 100 000 children under 15 years old. Some patients may also have coexistent signs and symptoms of meningitis (meningoencephalitis).

PATHOGENESIS

Microbial agents (usually viruses) cause encephalitis by direct invasion or by production of an inflammatory reaction in the CNS leading to areas of demyelination. This latter condition is commonly referred to as a postinfectious encephalomyelitis or acute disseminated encephalomyelitis (ADEM), and is characterized by a biphasic illness, i.e. an initial nonspecific illness such as a URTI followed 2–3 weeks later by onset of neurological symptoms. The encephalitis that occurs following an acute exanthem (e.g. measles, rubella) also conforms to this pathogenesis. This is in contrast to the directly invasive form which results in encephalitic symptoms from he start of the illness. Table 3.8.2 shows the most common causes of encephalitis. Some agents cause a characteristic clinical picture, e.g. cerebellitis is often associated with varicella-zoster virus, while the development of fever, focal seizures and coma is more characteristic of herpes simplex virus encephalitis. It must be emphasized

that in the majority of cases of encephalitis (50–60%), an etiologic agent is never identified despite exhaustive tests.

Transmission routes of the various agents causing encephalitis are multiple and include the fecal–oral route (enteroviruses), the respiratory route via droplet spread (influenza A and B, Mycoplasma pneumoniae), direct contact (HSV-1 and -2), and tick-borne (Lyme disease, Rickettsiae) and insect-borne (arboviruses) spread.

INVESTIGATIONS

The following investigations should be obtained:

- MRI scan or CT scan of head
- EEG
- chest X-ray
- throat swab and stool for viral culture
- serum—acute and convalescent; for serology (neurotropic viruses, Lyme disease, Mycoplasma, etc.)
- CSF (if not contraindicated, e.g. by raised ICP) for cell counts, bacterial culture, TB culture, viral culture, PCR (HSV, CMV, toxoplasmosis, enteroviruses)

MANAGEMENT

Supportive therapy (see also section on meningitis) should include:

- ventilatory and hemodynamic support
- control of raised ICP (may need invasive monitoring)
- fluid balance and correction of biochemical disturbances
- control of seizures

General supportive therapy of all the systems compromised is indicated in the critically ill child,

TABLE 3.8.2 **Common infective causes of acute encephalitis/meningoencephalitis**	
• Viruses:	HSV-1 and -2, CMV, EBV, VZV, enteroviruses, mumps, measles, rubella, HIV, arboviruses, rabies
• Nonviral causes:	Mycoplasma pneumoniae, Lyme disease, Toxoplasma gondii, leptospirosis, Brucella, typhus, Rocky Mountain spotted fever, trypanosomiasis, TB
• Postinfectious causes (ADEM)	Measles, mumps, rubella, influenza, VZV, enteroviruses

with particular emphasis on neuroprotective techniques. This will maximize the likelihood of a good outcome.

Serial EEGs may be helpful to track the course of the disease.

Specific therapy

Therapeutic agents include:

- empiric antibiotics (e.g. cefotaxime) to cover the possibility of bacterial meningitis, until this is excluded
- acyclovir (500 mg/m^2 per dose, 3 times a day), the only antiviral agent with activity against some neurotropic viruses (HSV, VZV, RBV), should be commenced in all cases when etiology is unclear (await PCR results on CSF)
- erythromycin for treatment of *Mycoplasma pneumoniae* encephalitis, pending results of serology and/or PCR on CSF if available
- Corticosteroids for ADEM, if this is a possibility (characteristic lesions predominantly in white matter on MRI scan, representing areas of demyelination); not recommended in the child with encephalitis and cerebral edema

PREVENTION AND OUTCOME

The spectrum of illness severity with encephalitis is large. Good recovery is expected in the majority of children who suffer from a typical, mild form of acute encephalitis. In 10–20% there may be permanent neurological sequelae. Mortality is around 5%.

Advice should be given to those travelling to endemic areas on minimizing contact with ticks and other insects. A vaccine is available for prevention of Japanese B encephalitis in people travelling in rural areas of the Far East.

GROUP B STREPTOCOCCAL INFECTIONS IN INFANTS

Group B streptococcal infection always warrants special consideration in infants. Early and late forms of infection occur. In early onset disease

(usually occurs in the first 48 hours of life) there is a relationship to maternal risk factors. Presentation is commonly with fulminant sepsis, respiratory failure and pneumonia. Mortality rate is 50%. Late onset disease has little correlation with maternal risk factors. There is a lower risk of mortality and symptoms are more variable. A high percentage of these infants have meningitis.

EARLY ONSET DISEASE

The infant usually looks critically ill. Cardiovascular collapse is common and is frequently preceded by feeding difficulty followed by respiratory difficulty and then apnea. The majority of these infants require assisted ventilation and all need supplemental oxygen. Approximately one-third are hypotensive on presentation. Where thrombocytopenia and DIC develop, with clinical evidence of bleeding; platelets, and transfusion with fresh frozen plasma or cryoprecipitate are indicated. Seizures are common, particularly in those with meningitis. Hypoglycemia must be prevented, partly because of the essential nature of glucose as an energy substrate for the brain, but also because there is evidence that hypoglycemia superimposed on asphyxia, or associated with hypotension, greatly increases the risk of permanent neurological sequelae. Levels of asphyxia, hypoglycemia and hypotension, which alone would not cause brain damage, will do so in combination.

LATE ONSET DISEASE

Late onset disease occurs in the first 3 months of life, caused by secondary hospital or community acquired pathogens. It has an even higher incidence of meningitis (75% of the infected infants) but an overall mortality rate which is considerably lower (10–20%) than early onset disease. Meningitis can develop overtime or be the presenting feature of this illness. Pneumonia or empyema are common. Septic arthritis, osteomyelitis and cellulitis, particularly involving breast tissue may occur.

Most early signs and symptoms are nonspecific. Most laboratory tests do not help differentiate this infection from other causes of serious infection in neonates, with the exception of blood or CSF culture, and latex agglutination studies (performed on concentrated urine). Many infants present in shock with metabolic acidosis and a depressed level of conciousness, although there may be a brief prodrome of feeding difficulty and progressive respiratory symptoms. An important differential diagnosis in this age group is the coarctation syndrome, and femoral pulses should be specifically examined during initial assessment.

TREATMENT

Neonatal advanced life support strategies are often required to resuscitate and provide ongoing care. Appropriate antibiotic regimens are shown in Table 2.7.1 with dosages in the drug appendix. Give oxygen early. Have a low threshold for intubation and assisted ventilation. Give IV fluid volume expansion (10 cc/kg normal saline by bolus). Withhold feeds. Give fluids IV. Monitor acid base status and glucose concentration; check electrolytes.

BRONCHIOLITIS

Bronchiolitis (Ch. 3.1) is a clinical syndrome characterized by respiratory distress, hyperinflation of the chest, and a wheeze with fine inspiratory crackles heard on auscultation. It tends to occur during the winter months when epidemics are seen.

Bronchiolitis predominantly affects infants during the first year of life. The cause is usually viral, with respiratory syncytial virus being responsible for the majority of cases. Other viruses that may cause bronchiolitis include parainfluenza, adeno- and influenza viruses. *Chlamydia* may also cause a similar syndrome. Secondary bacterial infection is rare. Factors predisposing to the development of bronchiolitis include a family history of asthma, maternal cigarette smoking, premature delivery with significant neonatal respiratory problems (needing assisted ventilation), lower socioeconomic status and day-care attendance.

PATHOPHYSIOLOGY

Respiratory syncytial virus causes direct damage to the respiratory epithelium with resultant inflammation, mediated predominantly by neu-

trophils. This leads to small airways obstruction, which may be partial or complete, and results in areas of hyperinflation and atelectasis, with *V/Q* mismatch. Transmission of the virus is usually by direct contact with contaminated secretions via droplets or fomites. The illness generally commences with mild fever and coryza, and progresses over several days to cough, tachypnea and wheeze, indicating lower respiratory tract involvement. Feeding difficulties associated with increasing dyspnea are the usual indications for admission to hospital. Infection with RSV may also cause a pneumonia with very few signs in the young infant; apneic episodes may be the presenting problem, along with lethargy and poor feeding. Up to 1–2% of infants with RSV infection will require admission to hospital.

Conditions that increase the risk of severe RSV infection include:

- underlying lung disease (bronchopulmonary dysplasia)
- cardiac defects, especially those with pulmonary hypertension
- cystic fibrosis
- immunodeficiency disorders
- cancer chemotherapy
- premature birth

INVESTIGATIONS

The diagnosis is a clinical one, but a chest X-ray will usually show evidence of hyperinflation and patchy areas of atelectasis or pulmonary infiltrates. A diffuse pneumonitis or ARDS-like picture may also be seen. Immunofluorescence testing for the presence of viral antigens in nasopharyngeal aspirates may lead to a definitive diagnosis of RSV or other virus. Oxygen saturation monitoring and blood gas analysis are useful to assess the severity of the illness. It may be appropriate to also consider a sweat test and immunological investigations in some patients (recurrent episodes, severe or protracted illness).

Assessment of severity

Clinical indicators of severity of RSV infection include:

- moderate infection:
  - tachycardia
  - RR > 50/min
  - use of accessory muscles
  - sub-costal recession
  - inability to feed
- severe infection:
  - cyanosis/severe respiratory difficulty
  - physical exhaustion
  - toxicity
  - oxygen saturation < 90%
  - rising $P\text{CO}_2$

MANAGEMENT

The mainstay of treatment is good supportive care. This involves monitoring for the presence of hypoxia, apnea and exhaustion. Supplemental oxygen is given, along with intravenous fluids or feeds depending on the child's condition. Assisted ventilation is required in anticipation of respiratory failure and in those who become exhausted or encephalopathic. Nasal CPAP may be beneficial in some patients, thus avoiding the necessity of intubation. Antibiotics are only indicated for very sick intubated patients in whom a secondary bacterial infection is suspected. The important points of treatment are:

- monitoring—including frequent clinical assessment, pulse oximetry, apnea monitoring, and in the severely affected infant, frequent blood gas analysis
- oxygen therapy—give humidified oxygen via a head box or nasal cannula to maintain saturation levels > 90%
- intravenous fluids are required in children unable to take fluids owing to respiratory distress:
  - correct dehydration and then give two-thirds maintenance fluids
  - nasogastric tube feeding is best avoided (aspiration risk and reduced excursion of left leaf of diaphragm)
- antibiotics are not routinely recommended (secondary bacterial infection is rare)
- corticosteroids are not indicated
- bronchodilators rarely show benefit; however, some older infants may benefit from salbutamol or ipratropium bromide
- ribavirin (see below)

Controversial care

Ribavirin

Although initial studies suggested a benefit from ribavirin (aerosolized by a small particle generator, 18 h a day, for 3–7 days) given via an oxygen hood, tent or into ventilator tubing, more recent studies have cast doubt on this. The AAP Red Book Committee suggests that it is not yet possible to issue firm guidelines on the use of ribavirin because of the concerns about cost, benefit, safety, and variable clinical efficacy. PICU physicians should *consider* ribavirin aerosol therapy for those groups of infants at risk for severe RSV infection (see above), including infants less than 6 weeks old and severely ill patients with or without mechanical ventilation.

Other treatments

Inhaled nitric oxide and artificial surfactant therapy have all been used with some success in severe RSV disease, although no randomized controlled trials have been reported. Extracorporeal membrane oxygenation has been used as rescue therapy for very severe disease with excellent results. The use of respiratory syncytial virus – immunoglobulin – intravenous as adjunctive therapy has not been evaluated in formal trials, although some units use this product in children with SCID who have RSV infection.

SOFT TISSUE INFECTIONS

Soft tissue infections, such as erysipelas and cellulitis, are rarely life threatening, as infection is generally confined to relatively superficial tissues, and systemic manifestations are uncommon. However, systemic illness can occur in the presence of exotoxins. These toxins mediate disease far from the site of bacterial infection, causing severe fever, hypotension, and multiorgan dysfunction in toxic shock syndrome. Other, highly virulent *Streptococcal* species are also able to cause tissue infection with profound local destruction, in necrotizing fasciitis.

NECROTIZING FASCIITIS

Necrotizing fasciitis is a deep seated infection of the subcutaneous tissue, caused by toxin producing virulent bacteria (often *Streptococcus pyogenes*), characterized by widespread destruction of fascia and fat. There is often associated shock and multi-system organ failure, comparable to streptococcal toxic shock syndrome. Because of its dramatic clinical presentation, necrotizing fasciitis has generated considerable interest in recent years, with a significant increase in the recognition and reporting of this entity. Whether this increase represents increasing clinical detection, or emerging streptococcal virulence is not clear.

PATHOPHYSIOLOGY

Predisposing risk factors include varicella, penetrating and blunt trauma, minor cuts, burns, and surgical procedures. Although immunocopromise is a risk factor, necrotizing fasciitis is also seen in the immunocompetent host. It can occur both as a polymicrobial infection, involving anaerobes and other gram positive bacteria, or as a predominantly Group A Streptococcal infection. Depending on the clinical scenario, it can involve various anatomic sites, including the abdomen (usually following surgery), the extremities (usually following trauma), and the head and neck region, or the perineum.

The pathogen is thought to reach the subcutaneous space either via hematogenous spread, or via direct innoculation. Initially an area of cellulitis may be present, accompanied by local pain and fever, or diffuse swelling of a limb may be the first clinical sign. Importantly, significant changes in the overlying skin may be absent, and the level of discomfort is often disproportionate to the clinical findings. Within hours to days, spreading erythema develops followed by the formation of dusky blue blisters, representing progressive liquefactive necrosis. Involvement of nutrient arteries can lead to further ischemia.

Streptococcal exotoxins, which may act as superantigens, not only mediate direct tissue damage, but also generate a profound host response (responsible for the majority of tissue destruction) and systemic manifestations.

MANAGEMENT

Early diagnosis is crucial for appropriate management, and is aided by CT scan. Gas in the affected tissues suggests clostridial infection. Aggressive surgical debridement is essential, and may include limb amputation. Antibiotic therapy is partially guided by cultures obtained at surgery, but broad spectrum empiric treatment should include clindamycin, penicillin, and an aminoglycoside. Strep is usually exquisitely sensitive to penicillin, but clindamycin has a unique role in inhibiting toxin production.

Other therapies, such as hyperbaric oxygen therapy and IVIG remain controversial.

TOXIC SHOCK SYNDROME

Shock and organ failure, associated with the presence of streptococcus or staphylococcus, define TSS. Most often, *Streptococcal* TSS occurs as a complication of a localized strep *infection*, whereas *Staphyloccal* TSS occurs most often from a site of *colonization*. In the latter case, high clinical suspicion is necessary to consider this diagnosis in the absence of tissue manifestations. Whereas *Staphyloccal* TSS used to be associated with menstruation and the use of highly absorbent tampons, one third of *Staphyloccal* TSS cases now are 'non-menstrual' in origin, and cases are seen in prepubescent children.

Initial symptoms may include myalgia, nausea, malaise, chills, fever, nausea, vomiting, and diarrhea. An erythematous rash, with subsequent desquamation, is particularly characteristic of *Staphyloccal* TSS.

Lab studies are consistent with a significant host inflammatory response, with a profound leukocytosis and leftward shift, as well as thrombocytopenia, hypocalcemia, hypoalbuminemia, azotemia, and an elevated creatine kinase.

MANAGEMENT

A child critically ill with TSS will require multisystem support, with particular attention to maintaining circulating volume in the face of hypotension. Appropriate antibiotics must cover both *Streptococcus* and *Staphyloccus* when the infecting organism is unclear. Cloxacillin is the drug of choice for *Staphyloccus* TSS, unless MRSA is a concern, in which case vancomycin is appropriate.

Streptococcus TSS should include antibiotics as for *necrotizing fasciitis.*

TUBERCULOSIS

Tuberculosis is a mycobacterial infection spread by infected respiratory droplets. Worldwide, it is of enormous importance as a cause of morbidity and mortality, and in developed countries there has been a significant resurgence over the past 10 years. The majority of tuberculosis cases continue to occur in immigrants, and in blacks, Hispanics, aboriginal people, and in those dwelling in the inner city and in poverty.

The hallmarks of disease are cough, fever, and weight loss. However, the clinician must also suspect TB in more acute presentations, in order to diagnose miliary TB, and tuberculous meningitis. TB is an important differential diagnosis in the case of an unexplained pleural effusion, an atypical pulmonary infiltrate with or without respiratory failure, and with severe, atypical cervical lymphadenitis. TB in the HIV-infected child can be particularly devastating.

PEDIATRIC AIDS

The WHO estimated that by the end of 1997 there were 30 million people worldwide living with HIV, of whom more than 1 million were children under 15 years old. There were an estimated half million deaths amongst children in 1997. More than 90% of infected individuals live in the developing world, mainly in sub-Saharan Africa. By the year 2000, an estimated 40 million people will have been infected with HIV worldwide, including 10 million children, and 40 million children will have lost one or both parents to HIV. In the USA, as in the European region, around 7000 children have thus far been reported with AIDS. The route of transmission of HIV in these children is vertical, i.e. from mother to child, in 80–90% of cases. Other routes of transmission are by administration of infected blood or blood products and in some cases following sexual abuse. Vertical transmission can occur in utero, intrapartum or postnatally via breastfeeding. It is thought that in the majority of cases infection occurs in late pregnancy or during delivery. In developed countries the perinatal transmission rate is 15–25%; the major risk factors identified for vertical transmission include the HIV status of the mother (advanced clinical disease is more likely to transmit virus), vaginal delivery, prolonged rupture of membranes, presence of other sexually transmitted disease, and preterm delivery. The administration of zidovudine to the mother during the latter part of pregnancy and during delivery, as well as to the newborn child for the first 6 weeks of life, decreases the risk of vertical transmission to only 8% if breastfeeding is avoided.

PATHOPHYSIOLOGY

Human immunodeficiency virus infection is due to a human cytopathic RNA retrovirus (usually HIV-1), which is tropic for CD4+ T-helper lymphocytes. Other cells infected include macrophages and CNS glial cells. The major consequences of infection are a gradual CD4+ T-helper cell depletion which leads to a cell-mediated immunodeficiency state. With ongoing immunosuppression, major opportunistic infections and cancers (AIDS-defining illnesses) tend to occur, the diagnosis then being one of fullblown AIDS.

The natural history of perinatally acquired disease is that up to a quarter of infants will be rapid progressors and develop AIDS in the first year of life (this tends to be the group of most interest to the intensive care pediatrician). Table 3.8.3 shows the major AIDS indicator diseases and the percentages of total reported cases in children with vertically transmitted HIV disease. The remainder experience incubation periods of up to 10 years,

TABLE 3.8.3 **Most commonly reported AIDS indicator diseases in children with vertically acquired HIV infection**	
AIDS indicator disease	**Percentage**
● *Pneumocystis carinii* pneumonia	30–40
● Lymphocytic interstitial pneumonitis	25–30
● Recurrent bacterial infections	20–25
● HIV encephalopathy	15
● Failure to thrive, wasting	15
● *Candida* esophagitis	10
● CMV infection	5–10
● Atypical mycobacteria	5
● Neoplasms	< 5

during which they remain asymptomatic. They may then develop HIV-related symptoms which often include combinations of the following:

- generalized lymphadenopathy
- hepatosplenomegaly
- parotitis
- failure to thrive
- lymphocytic interstitial pneumonitis
- PCP as the initial presentation

Progressive immunosuppression inevitably occurs after this with resulting AIDS.

INVESTIGATIONS

Informed consent must be obtained from parents prior to testing a child with suspected HIV infection. The diagnosis should be made as soon as possible so that antiretroviral therapy can be considered along with other treatments the patient may be receiving. A positive HIV antibody test (ELISA) is diagnostic of HIV infection only in children over 18 months old. In these children, confirmatory tests are often carried out to make the diagnosis secure (e.g. western blot analysis). In younger infants, because placentally transmitted HIV antibody may persist for up to 18 months, diagnosis is dependent on the demonstration of virus or HIV viral DNA in the blood sample. Hence viral cultures or more commonly HIV PCR testing for DNA sequences of the virus are generally used to confirm infection status in young infants (at least two positive tests, 1 month apart, in a child at least 3 months of age). Other pertinent laboratory investigations may show low levels of CD4 cells (both absolute number and percentage of total lymphocyte count) and hypergammaglobulinemia. In the follow-up of HIV-infected patients, laboratory parameters that are measured regularly (at least every 3 months) include T cell subsets and HIV viral load.

CLINICAL SYNDROMES

Opportunistic infections

The most common AIDS-defining illness, occurring in up to 40% of infected children, is *Pneumocystis carinii* pneumonia (PCP). Presentation is usually in the first 6 months, and in the UK, PCP in an infant is often the first indication of HIV infection in the affected family. The clinical features tend to be nonspecific and include cough, dyspnea, tachypnea, and recession with few chest sounds. The chest X-ray usually shows an interstitial pattern of pneumonitis; diagnosis is by bronchoalveolar lavage which demonstrates typical protozoal cysts when material is stained with methenamine silver. Most infants with PCP will require ventilatory support. Unfortunately the outlook for ventilated infants with PCP is often not good; there is substantial mortality and morbidity in this group. Patients who survive go on to develop other AIDS-defining illnesses (especially HIV encephalopathy), although this may change in the future owing to the introduction of combination antiretroviral therapy.

Cytomegalovirus may cause disseminated disease in HIV-infected infants (colitis, hepatitis, pneumonitis and retinitis) as a result of congenital infection or perinatally acquired disease through breast milk. Often CMV is also found in the BAL in infants with PCP. Although this may represent asymptomatic shedding, invariably if the CMV is not treated, recovery tends to be prolonged and complicated. Other opportunistic infections such as toxoplasmosis and cryptococcal meningitis are extremely rare in children.

Bacterial infections

Children infected with HIV are prone to recurrent bacterial infections, often caused by the group of encapsulated bacteria responsible for ordinary childhood infections:

- *Streptococcus pneumoniae*
- *Haemophilus influenzae*
- *Salmonella* sp.
- *Staphylococcus* sp.

The most common presentations are pneumonia and/or bacteremia. A sepsis picture with shock and/or meningitis caused by either pneumococcus or *Haemophilus influenzae* is also well described. There may be underlying lymphocytic interstitial pneumonitis (LIP) in some patients who develop recurrent pneumonia. Response to intravenous antibiotics is often dramatic in these patients; however, some go on to develop bronchiectasis.

Other AIDS-defining illnesses

Other presentations include:

- failure to thrive—occurs more frequently in developing countries and has a multi-factorial etiology: poor oral intake, HIV enteropathy and gastrointestinal infections
- HIV encephalopathy can present with developmental delay, cognitive defects or a spastic diplegia
- HIV cardiomyopathy with resultant cardiomegaly and heart failure may be due to infection of myocytes with HIV
- HIV nephropathy presents with a nephrotic syndrome; a renal biopsy may show a focal glomerulosclerosis

MANAGEMENT

Treatment for HIV-infected children in the PICU includes the following:

- antiretroviral therapy
- treatment of the presenting infection/opportunistic infection
- general supportive care
- attending to the psychosocial needs of the child and family

The standard of care now consists of starting infected infants on combination antiretroviral therapy, often with two nucleoside reverse transcriptase inhibitors (NRTI) and one protease inhibitor (PI). A widely used combination in pediatrics consists of zidovudine plus lamivudine (3-TC) plus nelfinavir. Other drugs used in various combinations include didanosine, stavudine, nevirapine, indinavir, saquinavir and ritonavir. There is controversy about when to start therapy but all agree on the following criteria:

- all children with an AIDS-defining diagnosis
- all children with symptomatic HIV infection
- all children with rising HIV viral loads and falling CD4+ counts:
  - *young infants*—HIV viral loads persistently > 100 000 copies/ml; CD4 counts < 15–20% of total lymphocytes

- *older children*—HIV viral loads > 20 000–50 000 copies/ml; CD4 counts < 15–20% and/or CD4 < 300 × 10°/L

Specific therapy for PCP includes high-dose IV trimethoprim and sulfamethoxazole (15 mg/kg trimethoprim, 75 mg/kg sulfamethoxazole per day, 6 h doses), along with steroids for the first 10 days (prednisolone or equivalent, 2 mg/kg per day, 12 h doses), and then weaned over the next 7–10 days. Some intensive care physicians/pediatricians give several doses of endotracheal surfactant over 24–48 h, if there is a clinical deterioration despite maximum therapy.

Significant CMV infection is treated with ganciclovir (10 mg/kg per day, 12 h doses for 3 weeks). Long-term maintenance therapy with ganciclovir (5 mg/kg per day) is required for patients with CMV retinitis, usually via a central line.

The initiation of empiric antimicrobial therapy is appropriate for all HIV-infected children admitted with a potentially severe bacterial infection. Broad-spectrum antibiotics such a third-generation cephalosporin, in combination with an anti-staphylococcal agent if *Staphylococcus aureus* is suspected, should be commenced pending results obtained from blood cultures, sputum cultures and tracheal aspirates or BAL.

The social and psychological aspects of the disease must not be forgotten. Families need a tremendous amount of support to come to grips with an HIV diagnosis as well as a life-threatening complication in their child. This is best done in collaboration with members of a pediatric HIV multidisciplinary team which would include a specialist, psychologist, social worker and HIV counselor.

PROPHYLAXIS OF INFECTIONS

Daily or thrice-weekly trimethoprim and sulfamethoxazole (150 mg trimethoprim, 750 mg sulfamethoxazole, per square metre) is indicated in most patients for PCP prophylaxis. There is evidence that daily administration may be effective for prophylaxis against recurrent bacterial infections. Children with HIV should receive all regular immunizations (including live vaccine MMR unless their disease is very advanced) with the exception of BCG. Inactivated polio vaccine is given in preference to the oral vaccine. Children over 2 years old should also receive pneumococcal vaccine. Varicella-zoster immunoglobulin is recommended in immunosuppressed individuals who come into contact with varicella.

KAWASAKI DISEASE

Kawasaki disease is an acute febrile illness of unknown etiology, affecting predominantly infants and young children, in whom it is a leading cause of acquired heart disease. It is characterized by a prolonged remittent fever, mucositis, conjunctivitis, polymorphous rash, cervical adenopathy and edema of the hands and feet with subsequent desquamation. Cardiac involvement with coronary arteritis and aneurysm formation may occur with fatal consequences. The disease is most prevalent in Japan, where epidemics may occur every 3 years. In the UK the disease is underdiagnosed, but an estimated incidence of 1.49 per 100 000 children has been reported. About 80% of affected patients are less than 4 years old.

PATHOPHYSIOLOGY

Clinical features suggest an infectious cause, but no microbial agent has yet been conclusively implicated. Current evidence suggests the disease is the result of superantigen activity, i.e. a toxin with superantigen properties is able to cause widespread activation of the immune system, with massive cytokine release and the consequent initiation of generalized inflammatory changes and vasculitis. The pathological lesion in Kawasaki disease is thus a vasculitis affecting small to medium muscoloelastic arteries throughout the body, but with a predilection for the coronary vessels. Disruption of the tunica media and formation of coronary artery aneurysms are a major complication.

DIAGNOSIS

The diagnosis is based on the presence of five of six principal criteria without other explanation for the illness:

- fever of more than 5 days' duration
- changes in the mucous membranes or oropharynx

- conjunctivitis
- polymorphous rash
- cervical adenitis
- changes in the extremities:
  - swollen, erythematous hands and feet
  - desquamation of skin of hands and feet

Other abnormalities seen include diarrhea, arthritis, sterile pyuria, uveitis, and aseptic meningitis. The disease is divided into three phases: an acute phase lasting up to 14 days, until the fever resolves; a subacute phase from day 10–14 to day 28; and a convalescent phase from 6–10 weeks after onset of disease. The various clinical manifestations occur during different phases of the illness. During the acute phase, the major manifestations include fever, rash, conjunctivitis, edema of the hands and feet and changes in the oropharynx. Although fever and other acute signs have usually resolved during the subacute phase, thrombocytosis, desquamation of hands and feet and joint involvement are prominent. This phase lasts until all clinical features and thrombocytosis resolve. The convalescent phase lasts until the ESR is back to normal. Unfortunately, atypical cases of Kawasaki disease can occur, with fewer than the required number of diagnostic features.

Laboratory investigations

Diagnostic findings include:

- normocytic normochromic anemia
- elevated white cell count with predominance of neutrophils and band forms
- thrombocytosis, occasionally $> 1000 \times 10^9/L$ (subacute phase)
- raised ESR and CRP
- hypoalbuminemia
- ECG and echocardiography may show cardiac involvement (acute stage)

Differential diagnosis of Kawasaki disease

The following conditions must be excluded:

- scarlet fever
- staphylococcal toxin disease

- leptospirosis
- viral exanthemata
- rickettsial disease
- Stevens–Johnson syndrome
- drug reaction
- juvenile rheumatoid arthritis

MANAGEMENT

The goal of treatment is to reduce the vasculitic process and prevent or treat any subsequent cardiac complications that may develop. Cardiac involvement in Kawasaki disease may include the development of a myocarditis and/or pericarditis during the acute phase which can lead to the development of heart failure or arrhythmias. Coronary artery aneurysms (CAA) may develop during the subacute phase and are usually apparent by 3–4 weeks. Coronary artery thrombosis as a complication of CAA usually occurs during this period but may occur much later (years). Echocardiograms are generally obtained at diagnosis, 1–2 weeks into the illness and at 4 weeks.

Initial treatment

1. Assess cardiac status: clinical, CXR, ECG, echocardiogram, cardiac enzymes.
2. Treat any arrhythmias or cardiac failure.
3. Administer a single high dose of intravenous immunoglobulin (2 g/kg) over 10–12 h if child is not in cardiac failure. Consider an alternative regimen if patient in cardiac failure (IVIG 400 mg/kg per dose, daily for 4 days).
4. Commence high-dose aspirin therapy (80–100 mg/kg/24 h in four divided doses) until fever subsides.
5. Give low-dose Aspirin (3–5 mg/kg/ 24 h) once fever has subsided, and continue for up to 2 months (at least until the thrombocytosis has resolved).

The administration of IVIG within 10 days of the start of the illness leads to a decrease in the incidence of coronary artery abnormalities from 20% to below 5%. If CAA do develop, dipyridamole is often prescribed as an added 'antiplatelet agent'.

Coronary artery thrombosis is managed with appropriate analgesia and fibrinolytic therapy (streptokinase) followed by anticoagulation.

Controversial care

Persistent or recrudescent fever following treatment with IVIG may warrant a further course of IVIG (1–2 g/kg). Although data are scanty, retreatment with IVIG is nevertheless commonly given.

Because steroids are used in the treatment of most forms of vasculitis, some investigators have suggested their use in patients who do not respond to repeated doses of IVIG and have progression of coronary artery abnormalities (single daily doses of IV methylprednisolone, 30 mg/kg).

INFECTIONS IN THE IMMUNOCOMPROMISED CHILD

Children who are immunocompromised are predisposed to a variety of infectious complications. This may be the result of problems within one or more components of their host defense, either due to the presence of disease (congenital or acquired) or as a result of treatment (e.g. chemotherapy, bone marrow transplant). With the increasing availability of sophisticated medical technology and more prolonged survival of patients with immune deficiencies, infections in immunocompromised hosts are expected to become more common. Table 3.8.4 shows the pathogens most likely to cause infections according to the component of the immune system primarily affected.

Often, as well as more than one component of the immune system being affected, other factors exacerbate the susceptibility to infection (presence of indwelling lines, breaks in skin, disruption of mucosal barriers secondary to radiotherapy or chemotherapy) in the immunocompromised patient.

PATHOPHYSIOLOGY
Neutropenia

Neutropenia is the most frequent form of compromised immunity in children and is generally

TABLE 3.8.4 Pathogens causing infections in the immunocompromised host

Cell-mediated immunity	Humoral immunity	Phagocytes	Complement
Viruses	*Bacteria*	*Bacteria*	*Bacteria*
CMV	Haemophilus	Staphylococci	Neisseria
Measles virus	Pneumococcus	Gram-negative organisms	Pneumococcus
Herpes virus	Streptococcus	Salmonella	Haemophilus
RSV	Meningococcus		
Rotavirus	Staphylococcus	*Fungi*	
Enterovirus	Pseudomonas	Candida	
		Aspergillus	
Bacteria	*Protozoa*		
Mycobacterium	Giardia lamblia		
Listeria	Cryptosporidium		
Fungi	*Viruses*		
Candida	Echo virus		
Aspergillus	Polio virus		
Nocardia	Hepatitis B virus		
Cryptococcus			
	Other		
Protozoa	Ureaplasma		
Pneumocystis	Mycoplasma		
Cryptosporidium			

associated with cancer and its treatment. The risk of infection is related to the absolute neutrophil count. The frequency and severity of infection become greater as the neutrophil count drops below $1.0 \times 10^9/L$, and the risk rises dramatically as the count drops below $0.1 \times 10^9/L$ and approaches zero. Risk of infection is also greater when there is a rapid drop in neutrophil count compared with a slowly evolving neutropenia, and in cases of prolonged neutropenia. The portals of entry for organisms are usually the alimentary canal and the respiratory tract, with the most common organisms being Gram-negative bacilli (*Escherichia coli, Klebsiella pneumoniae, Pseudomonas aeruginosa*), Gram-positive cocci (*Staphylococcus aureus, Staphylococcus epidermidis*), and fungi (*Candida, Aspergillus*). In the 1960s and 1970s Gram-negative bacilli predominated, but now Gram-positive organisms including staphylococci (*Staphylococcus aureus, S. epidermidis*), α-hemolytic streptococci and enterococci are more common. The single most important association with the development of invasive mycosis is the duration of neutropenia after the initiation of empiric antibiotic therapy. It is now standard practice to start empiric broad-spectrum antibiotic therapy in children who have neutrophil counts of $0.5 \times 10^9/L$ or less and become febrile, and to add antifungal therapy if the fever continues beyond 4–5 days.

Cellular immune dysfunction

Defects in cell-mediated immunity can result from congenital disorders such as DiGeorge syndrome, SCID and Wiskott–Aldrich syndrome, or from acquired defects secondary to lymphomas, immunosuppressive drugs, HIV and other chronic illnesses. Patients are highly susceptible to infections with intracellular organisms such as *Salmonella, Listeria*, mycobacteria, herpesviruses (CMV, HSV, EBV), as well as fungi (*Histoplasma, Cryptococcus*) and protozoa (*Pneumocystis carinii, Toxoplasma*). Many of these infections (those caused by herpesviruses, fungi and *Pneumocystis carinii*) that occur in patients with congenital T cell deficiencies or HIV infection are primary infections, whereas in older children with secondary immunodeficiencies they tend to be reactivated disease.

Humoral immune dysfunction

Protection against the common encapsulated organisms such as *Haemophilus influenzae* and *Streptococcus pneumoniae* depends on the production of adequate amounts of immunoglobulins. Congenital defects include X-linked agammaglobulinemia and common variable immunodeficiency. Although patients with these conditions are mainly susceptible to pyogenic bacterial infection involving the upper and lower respiratory tract, progressive viral (echovirus) and protozoal (*Giardia*) infections may also occur. Patients with asplenia, whether congenital, surgical or functional (e.g. sickle cell disease) are prone to overwhelming sepsis with encapsulated organisms. These patients have abnormalities of their reticuloendothelial systems, and deficiencies of tuftsin and of opsonizing antibodies.

Complement deficiencies

Deficiencies of the complement system (C5–C9, late complement components) result in an increased risk of recurrent meningococcemia and gonococcemia. Fulminant meningococcemia is also associated with properdin deficiency (alternate complement pathway).

CLINICAL SYNDROMES AND TREATMENT

The clinical syndromes in immunocompromised patients that are pertinent to intensive care pediatricians include pulmonary infections, septic shock and CNS disease.

Pulmonary infiltrates

In patients with fever and neutropenia, a localized pulmonary infiltrate should be considered to be bacterial and be treated with broad-spectrum antibiotics (piptazobactam plus an aminoglycoside) to cover the usual childhood pathogens, Gram-negative bacilli and Gram-positive cocci, while awaiting more intensive evaluation such as results of a BAL. Some clinicians also add a macrolide to cover for the atypical pneumonias (*Mycoplasma, Legionella*). If there is a lack of response to the initial treatment, antifungal therapy needs to be added to cover for *Candida* and *Aspergillus,* and other causes should be considered (e.g. mycobacteria). Unfortunately, some patients with severe neutropenia, fever and respiratory symptoms suggesting a pulmonary infection may have a 'normal' chest X-ray, which only demonstrates an infiltrate later when the neutrophils return. It is imperative that these patients receive full antibacterial and antifungal cover and an aggressive diagnostic evaluation.

Interstitial infiltrates in immunocompromised patients, especially those with T cell defects or those on steroid or other immunosuppressive therapy, usually represent a nonbacterial process. *Pneumocystis carinii*, CMV and atypical pneumonias are the most likely causes. Initial empiric antimicrobial therapy should include antibacterial and antifungal agents effective against these pathogens, pending results of further investigations, e.g. immunofluorescence on nasopharyngeal aspirates, BAL, tracheal aspirates or lung biopsy. If PCP is diagnosed, the addition of steroids as adjunctive therapy is appropriate, and if there is no response over 5–7 days, switching from trimethoprim and sulfamethoxazole (co-trimoxazole) to intravenous pentamidine should be considered. The addition of surfactant to the regimen is controversial.

Septic shock

In febrile, neutropenic patients, the most common causes of septic shock are Gram-negative and Gram-positive bacilli, and fungi, especially *Candida* species. A standard approach is adopted for initial care of most critically ill children. Broad-spectrum antibiotics are commenced (piptazobactam plus an aminoglycoside), and vancomycin is added if there is concern about the presence of methicillin-resistant *Staphylococcus aureus* (MRSA) or *S. epidermidis.* If the septic shock is associated with perianal cellulitis, specific anerobic cover (metronidazole) should be added to the above regimen. Although often associated with a more benign bacteremia, central venous catheter-associated infections may clinically resemble septic shock.

CNS infections

The spectrum of CNS infections includes meningitis, meningoencephalitis, encephalitis and brain abscess. These may be caused by the pathogens commonly infecting immunocompetent children or opportunist organisms. Infections of the CNS are rare causes of fever in patients with neutropenia, but patients with cell-mediated immune defects seem to be particularly prone to CNS disease caused by intracellular organisms such as *Listeria,*

Cryptococcus and *Toxoplasma*. Table 3.8.5 shows the various causes of CNS infections in the different immunocompromised patient groups. A CT or MRI scan of the head may be helpful in making a diagnosis (e.g. multiple ring enhancing lesions in toxoplasmosis), as may a CSF examination (if LP is safe to perform), serology testing and a brain biopsy (if indicated). Specific treatment of CNS infections depends on identification of the causative organism.

PREVENTION OF INFECTION

Patients with immunodeficiency disorders must be nursed in high efficiency particulate airflow (HEPA)-filtered rooms to prevent nosocomial infections, including colonization with *Aspergillus* species. Prophylactic therapy with trimethoprim and sulfamethoxazole (co-trimoxazole) to prevent PCP, and with acyclovir to prevent HSV reactivation may also be appropriate, and Itraconazole or fluconazole can be administered for fungal prophlyaxis. Discussion with an infectious disease specialist is advisable.

NOSOCOMIAL INFECTIONS

Hospital-acquired infection is a major cause of morbidity and mortality in hospitalized children, especially those in intensive care. All hospitals should have an infection control committee, usually chaired by the hospital microbiologist or infectious diseases physician. It is the responsibility of this committee, having taken into account local epidemiologic factors, to establish procedures and policies to prevent nosocomial infections. Written guidelines should include advice on general hygienic practices applicable to all patients (standard precautions—

formerly universal precautions, and isolation procedures for infected patients (transmission-based precautions)). It must be emphasized that hand washing before and after each patient contact remains the most important routine practice in the control of nosocomial infections.

Pathogenesis

Nosocomial infections are those acquired as a result of a hospital stay and may present during the period of hospitalization or after discharge. Reported rates vary but are estimated to be 4–5 per 100 discharges in children's hospitals.

Respiratory tract infections, gastrointestinal infections and bacteremias are the most common pediatric nosocomial infections. Bacteria (Gram-positive and Gram-negative) tend to account for 60–70% of cases; viruses (e.g. RSV, rotavirus) account for around 25%, and tend to be more important etiologic agents in children than in adults. Nosocomial infections may occur as localized outbreaks (e.g. a rotavirus outbreak on an NICU), or as sporadic cases (e.g. an MRSA sternal wound infection on a surgical ward). These can be further subdivided according to whether they are exogenously or endogenously acquired (endogenously acquired pathogens are derived from the patient's own microbiological flora). The following simplified guidelines are based on recommendations issued by the Centers for Disease Control in 1996.

CONTROL OF NOSOCOMIAL INFECTIONS

Standard precautions

Standard precautions are designed to prevent the transmission of blood-borne pathogens (e.g. HIV,

---

TABLE 3.8.5 Pathogens causing CNS infections in immunocompromised patients

CNS infection	Neutropenia	T cell-mediated deficiency	Humoral immunity
Meningitis	*Staphylococcus epidermidis* *Candida* Gram-negative bacilli	*Cryptococcus* *Listeria*	*Streptococcus* *Haemophilus*
Encephalitis		Herpesviruses Adenovirus *Toxoplasma*	Enteroviruses
Brain abscess	*Bacillus cereus* *Aspergillus*	*Nocardia*	

hepatitis virus) from both recognized and unrecognized sources in hospitals. Standard precautions should be in use for all patients and apply to blood, all body fluids, secretions, nonintact skin, and mucous membranes. Techniques and equipment include:

- **handwashing** (before and after each patient contact)
- gloves
- masks, eye protection, face shields
- gowns
- mouthpieces, resuscitation bags (to avoid mouth-to-mouth resuscitation)
- proper handling of patient care equipment and linen (e.g. soiled with blood, secretions)

Transmission-based precautions

Transmission-based precautions are extra precautions instituted for patients known or suspected to be infected with pathogens that may be transmitted by the airborne route, by droplet spread or by direct contact.

Airborne transmission

Organisms are spread by airborne droplets or dust particles which are dispersed in the air and travel in air currents; this transmission is characteristic of varicella, TB and measles. Precautions include:

- single/isolation room
- negative air pressure ventilation with HEPA-filtered air
- masks
- respiratory protective devices for TB

Droplet transmission

Droplets are produced by coughing, sneezing, suctioning, etc., but do not remain suspended in air, and hence do not require specially ventilated rooms. Diseases spread in this way include *H. influenzae* type b infections, pertussis and influenza. Precautions include:

- private room (if possible)
- masks

Contact transmission

The most frequent route of transmission of nosocomial infections is by contact—either direct physical contact between susceptible host and infected patient (e.g. MRSA, rotavirus, RSV, Ebola virus), or indirect contact through a contaminated intermediate object, such as an unsterilized needle. Precautions include:

- single/isolation room (preferred; cohorting possible)
- gloves
- gowns

It may be necessary to combine airborne, droplet and contact precautions for organisms that may have more than one mode of transmission. Standard precautions should always be instituted for all patients in addition to any added precautions. Isolation rooms in the PICU setting are only necessary for infections caused by organisms spread by the airborne route. Older infection control precaution categories that may be still in operation include the following:

- strict isolation
- contact isolation
- respiratory isolation
- enteric isolation
- blood and body precautions
- protective isolation

Summary

The different transmission-based precaution requirements are summarized in Table 3.8.6 (see also Chapter 7.4 for accidental HIV exposure guidelines).

TABLE 3.8.6 **Transmission-based precautions for hospitalized patients (including standard precautions)**

Route	Single room	Masks	Gowns	Gloves
Airborne	Yes (HEPA)	Yes	No	No
Droplet	Yes (if available)	Yes	No	No
Contact	Yes (if available)	No	Yes	Yes

FURTHER READING

1. Abernathy R. Tuberculosis: An Update. Peds in Review 1997; 18: 50–58
2. American Academy of Pediatrics. Report of the Task Force on diagnosis and management of meningitis. Pediatrics 1986; 78(supplement): 959–982
 – (*Seminal paper on meningitis from the AAP, and a more recent update*)

3. American Academy of Pediatrics. Infection control for hospitalized children. In: Peter G, editor. 1997 Red Book: Report of the Committee on Infectious Diseases, 24th ed. Elk Grove Village: American Academy of Pediatrics; 1997; pp 100–107
4. Centers for Disease Control and Prevention. Guidelines for the use of antiretroviral agents in pediatric HIV infection. MMWR 1998; 47: (RR–4) 1–44
5. Chanock, SJ, Pizzo PA. Infectious complications of patients undergoing therapy for acute leukemia: current status and future prospects. Semin Oncol 1997; 24: 132–140

6. Davies EG, de Sousa C. How to investigate and manage the child with suspected acute encephalitis. Curr Paediatr 1993; 3: 106–113
7. Feigin RD, McCracken GH, Klein MD. Diagnosis and management of meningitis. Ped Inf Dis J 1992; 11: 785–814
 – (*An excellent overview*)
8. Landau L. Bronchiolitis. In: David TJ, editor. Recent Advances in Paediatrics, vol. 15. London: Churchill Livingstone; 1997; pp 1–10
 – (*A good, all-round up-to-date review*)

9. Rowley AH. Controversies in Kawasaki disease. Adv Ped Infect Dis 1998; 13: 127–141
 – (*An up-to-date review of the current problems in managing Kawasaki disease*)

10. Tunkel AR, Scheld MW. Acute bacterial meningitis. Lancet 1995; 346: 1675–1680
11. Textbook of Neonatal Resuscitation. Bloom RS, Cropley C (eds) American Academy of Pediatrics/American Heart Assoc 1994
 – (*Manual for the neonatal advanced life support (NALS) course; outlines all the resuscitation and support strategies appropriate for neonates and small infants*)

3.9 Diseases of early life

David Field

Although neonatal intensive care and pediatric intensive care have evolved from different origins they display considerable overlap from a technical and pharmacological perspective. Moreover in regard to mature infants and the range of conditions that can present in the first few weeks of life these two patient groups overlap.

Throughout most of the developed world there has been a move toward earlier discharge from hospital following delivery. This trend has caused an increased number of term newborns to present from home with conditions that in the past were considered to be part of neonatal practice. Once babies have left maternity services they are admitted as pediatric patients, so many infants who would previously have been dealt with by the neonatal service are now presenting as pediatric emergencies.

Most of the problems are considered in the organ-specific chapters of this book, but a number of issues merit special attention. These are considered in this chapter.

HISTORY

While it is essential in the assessment of any child to ask about problems relating to pregnancy and the perinatal period, these points assume greater importance when the child presents with serious medical problems in early life. The bulk of inherited disease presents at this stage. It is helpful to determine whether:

- the mother has a history of unexplained miscarriage (seen in some congenital and or genetic abnormalities)
- any other siblings are healthy (may be affected by the same inherited disorder)
- there is any family history of genetic disease
- the parents are blood relatives (this situation is common in some ethnic groups and is associated with a significantly increased risk of genetic disease in the offspring)

- there were any concerns regarding fetal development in pregnancy (e.g. oligohydramnios, seen in renal dysplasia; polyhydramnios, seen in conditions such as ileal atresia; low birthweight, seen in prematurity, intrauterine growth retardation, multiple pregnancy, and some genetic anomalies)
- there was any evidence of intrauterine infection

The particular importance of prematurity and the relevance of exposure to asphyxial insults are discussed below.

SYMPTOMS AND SIGNS

Babies are limited in the first weeks of life in their range of responses to serious illness. Note any specific features in the child's presentation (e.g. abdominal distention) but be alert to the possibility of this being part of a generalized disorder (e.g. abdominal distention may result from intestinal obstruction or be associated with paralytic ileus secondary to septicemia). Recurrent apnea or respiratory arrest are common modes of presentation in babies suffering from a variety of underlying disorders, particularly viral or bacterial infections. Often basic cardiorespiratory support has to precede attempts to reach a more specific diagnosis (particularly attention to airway patency and oxygen delivery).

INFANTS WHO HAVE RECEIVED NEONATAL INTENSIVE CARE

Between 5% and 10% of all newborns require admission to a neonatal unit. Approximately 1% of them need ventilatory support. These neonates have an increased chance of needing further hospitalization during the first year of life. Certain of them are at particular risk of developing medical problems after discharge from a neonatal unit.

Premature infants

Respiratory problems

The definition of a preterm baby is any infant delivered before 36 completed weeks of gestation. In practice it is those babies born before 31 weeks' gestation to whom the following remarks particularly apply. Many such infants are likely to have had significant lung disease secondary to their immaturity, and about half will have required assisted ventilation, and some develop chronic respiratory dysfunction in consequence.

The original description of the most extreme form of this condition led to the term 'bronchopulmonary dysplasia'. In current neonatal practice even with the advance of surfactant replacement therapy chronic lung disease still occurs, affecting perhaps a third of ventilated preterm infants; however, only a very small proportion have bronchopulmonary dysplasia. The remainder have lesser degrees of disruption to their normal pulmonary architecture at the level of the small airways and alveoli. None the less, all of these affected babies are more likely to develop acute pulmonary problems superimposed on their chronic dysfunction, for example:

- minor intercurrent infections (e.g. RSV bronchiolitis) may cause acute decompensation and respiratory failure of rapid onset
- they have an increased risk of 'asthma'
- there is an increased risk of apnea, e.g. in response to a simple upper respiratory infection, or elective general anesthesia

The most severely affected infants are oxygen-dependent at the time of neonatal discharge. These babies are also at risk for:

- acute failure of their oxygen supply
- chronic hypoxia from inadequate oxygen delivery over a prolonged period
- pulmonary hypertension and cor pulmonale—this may arise as a consequence of disruption to the normal pulmonary vasculature inherent in chronic lung disease, but is often compounded if chronic hypoxia coexists

When managing infants with a history of neonatal lung disease, even if it has apparently resolved, it is important to remember that the lungs are likely to be abnormal and that an increased vulnerability to sequelae can last well into early childhood. Radiological assessment of the child may be complicated by residual chest X-ray abnormalities.

Neurological damage

The combination of cardiovascular instability and the inherent fragility of immature cerebral vessels mean that sick preterm infants are particularly vulnerable to CNS insults in the form of hemorrhage or ischemia. Although hemorrhage is common, in most cases bleeding is limited, being confined to the ventricles, and of no long-term significance. However, where bleeding is more extensive there is an increased risk of posthemorrhagic hydrocephalus developing, and this condition often requires the insertion of a ventriculoperitoneal shunt. Shunt blockage at a later date may cause the child to present with vomiting, bulging fontanelle, drowsiness, irritability, apnea or fever (blockage typically arises secondary to infection). Where this diagnosis is suspected, urgent neurosurgical advice should be sought. Tapping or 'milking' shunts to obtain a CSF sample for diagnosis or temporarily relieve symptoms is often indicated but should only performed after expert advice.

Rarely hemorrhage will extend from the ventricular system into adjacent brain tissue (grade 4 hemorrhage). Ischemic lesions typically arise in vascular watershed areas (periventricular leukomalacia, PVL) in response to hypoxic ischemic insults either before or after delivery. In both these situations (where brain tissue is known to have been lost), there is a strong association with subsequent handicap. Infants affected in this way may show few specific signs in the first weeks of life, but can become difficult to manage, irritable and demanding children. This behavior increases their risk of nonaccidental injury. Fits may arise secondary to CNS damage, but positive diagnosis can be difficult as the manifestations are often subtle (yawning, grimacing, posturing). In addition it is often hard to differentiate clonic episodes from the normal tremulousness frequently seen in babies. In general, rapid movements and movements that can be abolished by holding an affected limb are not caused by convulsions.

Other problems

It is important to remember that premature babies may have been exposed to a wide variety of physiological and iatrogenic insults, many of which (e.g. necrotizing enterocolitis, steroid therapy, reduced immunoglobulin levels) may be significant in terms of their effects outside the immediate neonatal period; a history of prematurity should therefore always be evaluated in relation to any serious problem arising later in childhood.

Asphyxia in term infants

Intrapartum asphyxia can affect both term and preterm infants. In the latter group specific effects are sometimes difficult to separate from those of prematurity, but in mature babies clear clinical sequelae develop, often involving many organs. The effects on the brain are termed 'hypoxic ischemic encephalopathy' (HIE). The acute course of HIE may be turbulent, with abnormal CNS function (coma, seizures, altered tone). The presence of renal, hepatic, and/or cardiac impairment may all complicate the course. However, in the long term it is unusual for damage to persist outside the nervous system. Children who do suffer neurological impairment display great variation in their symptoms and signs (mild motor or developmental delay through to spastic quadriplegia with blindness). Presentation with critical illness is most likely to be as a result of:

- sepsis, pneumonia, infected (or blocked) shunt
- poor feeding (failure to thrive, aspiration)
- seizures
- nonaccidental injury (exacerbated by difficult behavior and constant crying)
- toxic sequelae of medication

History and examination should identify evidence of developmental delay, abnormal behavior, altered tone, and abnormal reflexes. Computed tomographic or MRI scan may demonstrate cerebral atrophy. If clear signs of permanent cerebral damage are evident, be sensitive to how this information is discussed or delivered, as parents may not be fully aware of or accept what is present.

ENVIRONMENT

The largest cohort of children with critical illness requiring intensive care are under 1 year of age. Where the child is only days old, the mother may still need medical care herself, breastfeeding may not be fully established, and the mother often requires extra help and support to maintain her milk supply through the child's illness. Conversely, when a breastfed infant dies suddenly it is important to arrange for the mother to receive advice re managing her milk supply artificially.

Where a child needing hospitalization is very young (particularly in the case of a newborn baby), parents may need additional emotional support to enable them to cope with the illness, to have the confidence to touch and provide basic care for their baby, and to enable normal bonding to take place.

TRANSPORT

A neonatal transport incubator can be used for moving babies weighing up to about 5 kg. An incubator is important since there is significant potential for infants to lose heat during the journey, because of their high surface area to body weight ratio. Observation and access are also easier. If such equipment is borrowed (e.g. for 'one-way' transport) it is vital to ensure that the accompanying disposables (endotracheal tubes, suction cannulas, etc.) are appropriate in size for the baby being transported rather than for a premature infant.

SUDDEN INFANT DEATH SYNDROME

Although recent years have seen a steady fall in the number of children dying of sudden infant death syndrome (SIDS), around 1 in 1000 children still dies in this way. The peak age is at 3 months. Many of these children present as emergencies, in which case full attempts at resuscitation should be offered until it is obvious that no response is going to occur. For the medical and nursing staff in attendance the death creates a number of obligations.

LEGAL

From the legal standpoint the approach to these deaths varies around the world. In the UK such deaths are considered to be potentially suspicious (caregiver inflicted) and must be reported to the coroner. The police are obliged to investigate the circumstances in which the death occurred. A postmortem is always ordered by the coroner.

THE CHILD

By definition deaths as a result of SIDS are unexplained. However, postmortem examination may reveal completely unsuspected disease (e.g. congenital heart disease), but other conditions will not be identified unless sought soon after death. Samples of blood and other body fluids should be taken to investigate for infection and metabolic derangement. Where an inherited disorder is suspected, skin biopsy (for fibroblast culture) and or blood sample (for DNA extraction) may permit confirmation of the diagnosis long after death. The exact approach to investigation varies according to local policy and must comply with the wishes of the local coroner.

THE FAMILY

The death of a child in these circumstances (i.e. with no warning) is obviously a terrible blow (Ch. 5.8). In the immediate aftermath the following should be clearly explained:

- that the child has died (be clear)
- no cause has been identified
- further tests (depending on local policy) may provide an answer at a later stage
- the police will be involved and/or a postmortem is mandatory (reflect local policy)
- there will be an opportunity to discuss all the results at a later stage; it is essential that a senior pediatrician is involved in counseling the family and that the family know who this person is and how to make contact.
- the death is not their fault (unless there is reason to suspect otherwise)

Once death has been confirmed, the parents will often welcome a chance to be with their child in private without interruption and without a time limit. The family doctor, health visitor and other professionals involved with the family must all be informed promptly.

APPARENT LIFE THREATENING EPISODES

Apparent life-threatening episodes (ALTEs) were, for many years, termed 'near-miss SIDS' but this description caused great alarm, was often misleading and diverted attention from underlying pathophysiology. The term 'ALTE' can be applied to a wide variety of different presentations (e.g. choking, altered consciousness, respiratory distress) with great variation in the severity of physiological disturbance (e.g. a choking episode may last a few seconds or lead to loss of consciousness).

When a child presents with an ALTE, initial resuscitation and management must first address the airway, breathing and circulation and be directed on a symptomatic basis (Chs 2.1, 2.2). Subsequently, a careful history of events up to the time of presentation and the actual mode of presentation will provide guidance with respect to investigation and probable diagnosis. The possible underlying causes are numerous and include:

- cardiovascular: undetected congenital heart disease, arrhythmia
- respiratory: infection (upper or lower respiratory; bacterial or viral), previously undetected congenital anomalies, abnormalities of respiratory control
- gastrointestinal: acute obstruction from volvulus, severe gastroenteritis
- renal: infection with secondary septicemia
- neurological: seizures of various etiology, altered consciousness (from whatever cause)
- metabolic disease: congenital adrenal hyperplasia causing an adrenal crisis
- nonaccidental injury: shaking injury, administration of toxic substances

This list indicates that there are important diagnoses to be excluded in all children presenting with an ALTE. In most cases this will require a period as an inpatient.

Even after the most exhaustive investigation, a group of children will remain who have had an ALTE but for whom there is no clear explanation of the 'attack'. These infants are at increased risk of going on to suffer SIDS, and as a result they merit close medical supervision, with psychological support for the parents. The role of monitoring devices at home is controversial (none fully protects against all underlying causes of sudden death). Many parents feel that an apnea alarm will reduce their anxiety about further episodes occurring, but many are quickly disillusioned (by the restrictions imposed by the devices and the stress of false alarms) and there is little evidence that monitoring of this type is effective. Markers of health such as good weight gain are more reliable indicators of wellbeing. It is good practice to ensure that parents of infants who suffer an ALTE are given training in basic life support and updated regarding changes in child care directives (e.g. not smoking at home, firm mattress in crib, placing infants on their backs to sleep).

NONACCIDENTAL INJURY

Nonaccidental injury (NAI) is common throughout the world. Presentation can take many forms (Ch. 4.3), and a number of affected children will come to medical attention as a result of an acute event. In relation to 'critical illness', one of three patterns can be observed:

- severe (sometimes multiple) injury (e.g. unexplained cerebral edema)
- a grave medical condition exacerbated by preceding neglect
- factitious (fabricated) illness or Munchausen syndrome by proxy

To diagnose NAI, always consider the possibility, particularly if there is something suspicious about a child's injuries:

1. Are the injuries compatible with the story? For example, a baby is very unlikely to suffer a fractured skull from rolling off a chair or sofa.
2. Is the site or distribution of injury unusual? For example, bruising to the inside of the thighs or abdomen is not compatible with an accidental cause.
3. Is there other evidence to support a diagnosis of NAI? Such evidence includes fractures through the epiphyseal plate of

long bones, gross wasting in the absence of organic disease, or other lesions characteristic of abuse.

In medical presentations (without overt trauma) clues may be more subtle and can include:

- the relationship between child and parents is unusual
- the child's clothing is inappropriate (e.g. in relation to the weather or state of cleanliness)
- the child's physical/and or emotional growth is abnormal
- the child's affect is bizarre (can be very 'flat' in children subjected to regular abuse)

In factitious presentations one parent, normally the mother, generates suspicion of illness in the child. Often this is achieved by manufactured signs, e.g. vomit containing blood put there by the mother. While this type of behavior may pose no immediate threat to the child, sometimes the infant can be at considerable risk (e.g. from repeated suffocation to mimic apnea or administration of strong sedatives to suggest 'blackouts').

PRESENTATION

Important acute modes of presentation of NAI include:

- unexplained acute cerebral edema (from shaking)
- unexplained loss of consciousness or other neurological disturbance (caused by drug administration or suffocation)
- unexplained painful limb—fracture found on X-ray
- obvious injury without explanation
- injury pathognomonic of abuse, e.g. bite or cigarette burn
- gross wasting in the absence of organic disease

Immediate care is governed by the nature of the child's presentation. However, if NAI seems a likely diagnosis, appropriate history and additional procedures are required at an early stage (i.e. once the child is stable) to ensure protection and investigation.

The full examination looks for evidence of abuse or neglect. Pay particular attention to:

- growth
- injury (this can be subtle, e.g. lacerations in the mouth, or show a peculiar distribution, e.g. cigarette burns)
- other signs of trauma (retinal hemorrhages from shaking)
- sexual abuse (anything other than cursory external examination should await support from an expert colleague, however, this type of injury is sometimes obvious)

In the case of factitious injury meticulous observation over time, sometimes with the aid of covert video surveillance, is necessary to make the diagnosis.

Investigations serve two purposes: (1) to aid the child's management and (2) to support or refute a diagnosis of NAI.

LEGAL ISSUES

Where a diagnosis of NAI remains a possibility the parents must be confronted and appropriate enquiries made. This stage *must* be carried out in conjunction with a senior pediatrician, social services and the appropriate authorities. The first legal step that is used in the UK (if parents will not cooperate voluntarily) is the emergency protection order (EPO). The order, which places the child or children under the care of the social services, lasts for up to 8 days. It can be challenged within 72 hours of issue. Only one extension is allowed, which is for a further 7 days. Applicants for an EPO are usually social service officers or the National Society for the Protection of Children (NSPCC). Where possible the child should remain at home, and the source of risk (e.g. an abusing parent) should be removed.

CONGENITAL AND INHERITED DISEASE

Earlier discharge of term infants from the maternity service contributes to the number of infants with metabolic and structural defects presenting as emergencies with the conditions described below.

TRACHEOESOPHAGEAL FISTULA AND ESOPHAGEAL ATRESIA

Tracheoesophageal fistula is almost invariably associated with esophageal atresia and hence presentation normally occurs soon after birth with copious frothy secretions (saliva) and choking. The diagnosis is made radiographically, with a nasogastric tube passed to the site of the obstruction. Stabilization is achieved by passing a Replogle (suction) tube. This permits all secretions in the upper pouch to be continuously aspirated. Intubation is a wise precaution where further choking episodes occur or transport for surgery is required.

GUT OBSTRUCTION

A variety of pathological problems can produce this picture (Ch. 3.12). Typically the child presents with bile-stained vomiting and abdominal distention. The degree of distention and speed of onset will vary with the site of obstruction. Significant fluid and electrolyte disturbance, shock or sepsis can coexist. Passage of meconium is often delayed, but where the obstruction is partial or 'high' some meconium may be passed. Immediate care involves:

- rehydration
- passage of a nasogastric tube, regular suction and nothing by mouth
- pain relief where required
- consideration of superadded sepsis
- surgical consultation

Upper and lower contrast studies (preferably performed by a specialist pediatric radiologist) are often helpful in making the diagnosis. Where volvulus secondary to malrotation is thought to be the diagnosis, surgery should proceed urgently in order to avoid ischemic damage to the bowel.

ANORECTAL ATRESIA

Although anorectal atresia should be readily apparent, diagnosis is sometimes delayed owing to a coexistent (vaginal) fistula which allows passage of meconium. Management follows the principles employed in other causes of gastrointestinal obstruction.

ABDOMINAL WALL DEFECTS

Gastroschisis

This is always apparent at birth since it is caused by an abnormality in the abdominal wall adjacent to the umbilicus. It is typically an isolated defect.

Exomphalos

Here too the defect is normally apparent at birth since gut is seen to extrude from the umbilical region, unlike gastroschisis, other congenital anomalies are frequently associated with this anomaly. In some cases of exomphalos the defect is minor. In this situation the bowel may be accidentally crushed when clamping the cord resulting in a late presentation with peritonitis or obstruction.

In both exomphalos and gastroschisis the immediate requirement is the prevention of fluid loss from the gut. The use of saline packs is not appropriate since this can cause massive heat loss from the bowel. Encasing the gut in a plastic bag or clingfilm is more satisfactory. Resuscitation with colloid and adequate fluid maintenance are essential prior to surgery.

In some cases of exomphalos the abdominal wall defect is small. In this situation the bowel may be accidentally crushed when clamping the cord. Sometimes a narrow defect must be enlarged emergently to relieve compression on the vascular supply to the prolapsed bowel. In both exomphalos and gastroschisis there is an increased risk of late obstruction secondary to adhesions. These infants can be seriously ill at presentation. Exomphalos can be associated with severe hypoglycemia—particularly when there is organomegaly and/or the infant is large for gestational age (> 90% for weight).

NEURAL TUBE DEFECTS

Recent years have seen a steady reduction in cases of neural tube defects (NTD) across the developed world as a result of folic acid supplementation and antenatal screening. Where the lesion is small and there is no evidence of neurological deficit, surgical repair and recovery are usually uncomplicated. Where the defect is large the following are assessed in planning further management:

- any neurological deficit in the legs
- evidence of bladder disturbance (i.e. constant dribbling of urine or no spontaneous voiding)
- evidence of lack of bowel control (patulous anus)

Where significant neurological damage or deficiency is present a conservative approach is adopted. Heroic surgery does not improve survival or reduce morbidity. Ninety per cent of cases have associated hydrocephalus. Typically this does not present until after the defect has closed either surgically or spontaneously. Neural tube defects are associated with a high incidence of urinary tract infection and the risk of renal damage.

RESPIRATORY DEFECTS

Most major defects involving lung parenchyma (e.g. diaphragmatic hernia, cystic deformity), present at birth with respiratory distress. Rarely presentation is delayed until days or weeks of age. In general late presentation indicates adequate underlying lung function and a good outcome can be anticipated.

Upper airway problems (e.g. choanal atresia or stenosis, micrognathia) can cause severe respiratory embarrassment in babies (particularly with superimposed infection).

CARDIAC DEFECTS

During the first few weeks of life pulmonary blood flow gradually increases as pulmonary vascular resistance falls. If the ductus arteriosus undergoes delayed closure, one or both of these factors can cause rapid decompensation of a major underlying cardiac anomaly which had previously been asymptomatic (Ch. 3.2).

CONGENITAL INFECTION

Many congenital infections present at or immediately after birth with features that are readily apparent, e.g. rash (rubella and CMV); hepatosplenomegaly (CMV and toxoplasmosis); choroidoretinitis (toxoplasmosis). However, these features may not be prominent and other features (e.g. hydrocephalus, developmental delay, prolonged jaundice, failure to thrive) may lead to a less acute presentation several days or months later.

Chickenpox (varicella) occurring early in pregnancy has a characteristic pattern of embryopathy with prominent neurological, skeletal and eye anomalies. However, where a mother contracts chickenpox late in pregnancy, the infant may be delivered incubating the virus but without the benefit of maternal antibody. Such infants may suffer overwhelming infection and require intensive care and treatment with acyclovir.

Human immunodeficiency virus infection in the newborn shows a variety of manifestations: neurological symptoms, profuse diarrhea and thrombocytopenia are typical. The diagnosis should always be considered where no explanation can be identified for a child's illness.

METABOLIC DISEASE

Metabolic disease is discussed in Chapters 2.9 and 3.11. The following points are relevant in relation to infants presenting in the first few days or weeks of life.

Making a diagnosis

At the time of presentation the full metabolic features of the condition are often evident, and it is possible to make a precise metabolic diagnosis. The appropriate samples (Ch. 3.11) should be obtained, even if they are simply stored in the first instance.

Many metabolic disorders present towards the end of the first week of life as a result of the increasing nutritional load, but this is not always the case. Congenital adrenal hyperplasia (21-hydroxylase deficiency) and medium-chain acyl-CoA dehydrogenase (MCAD) deficiency typically present outside the first week in response to some minor stress such as intercurrent infection. In the case of MCAD deficiency symptoms may not occur for some months.

Other causes of metabolic disturbance

Primary metabolic disease must be suspected and excluded in infants presenting with a marked biochemical disturbance. However, other conditions should be considered concurrently.

Acidosis

Both septicemia and cardiac lesions associated with reduced systemic blood supply (e.g. coarctation of the aorta) can produce severe metabolic acidosis.

Hypoglycemia

A range of inherited metabolic conditions and a number of hormonal abnormalities can result in hypoglycemia. However, in young infants glucose homeostasis is relatively precarious (stores are limited), and infants depend on regular feeds or provision of substrate. Physiological stress leading to hypoglycemia may complicate any serious illness, e.g. septicemia, inability to feed, hypothermia.

Electrolyte disturbance

Renal tubular abnormalities and disorders of adrenal hormone production will result in a disturbance of serum electrolytes. The changes observed are often not pathognomonic, and many conditions (e.g. gastroenteritis with inappropriate fluid replacement) may mimic the findings.

✔ KEY POINTS

➤ Be aware that the first few days of life are the most common time for congenital anomalies to present

➤ Where a presenting child has been born prematurely or received neonatal intensive care, send for the child's old notes urgently

➤ Infants who have chronic sequelae of neonatal lung disease may rapidly decompensate in the face of relatively mild respiratory infections

➤ Nonaccidental injury has many manifestations and should be considered where a child's condition cannot be adequately explained (including SIDS, near-drowning)

➤ Do not assume a diagnosis of NAI in a child with major bruising until a coagulopathy has been excluded

➤ Early discharge means that problems previously considered the province of the neonatal service (e.g. severe ABO incompatibility) are now presenting to pediatric services

✗ COMMON ERRORS

➤ Failure to explain the legal procedure to parents following the death of a child from sudden infant death syndrome

➤ Not informing the health visitor and family doctor after the sudden death of a child

➤ Assuming that a child with no murmurs and a normal heart size on X-ray has an anatomically normal heart

➤ Assuming that a child who has passed meconium cannot have an imperforate anus

FURTHER READING

1. Roberton NRC, editor. Textbook of neonatology, 2nd ed. Edinburgh: Churchilll Livingstone
2. Holbrook PR, editor. Textbook of paediatric critical care. Philadelphia: WB Saunders
– (*Comprehensive textbooks covering many aspects of both neonatal and pediatric intensive care*)

3. Alkalay AL, Pomerance JJ, Rimoin DL. Fetal varicella syndrome. J Pediatr 1987; 111: 320–323
– (*A review of 30 children with congenital anomalies associated with maternal varicella*)

3.10 Psychiatric emergencies and psychological effects of critical illness

Michael Fairley and Victoria Gilmore

A child or adolescent with emotional problems often makes us uncomfortable, particularly if their difficulties are similar to those we experienced at their age or currently experience with our own offspring. This section examines three behaviors that result in serious harm and discusses their immediate management and impact on staff. The second part of the chapter discusses the psychological effects of critical illness on the child and family.

SUICIDE AND PARASUICIDE

Together with traumatic injuries, suicide is the major cause of death in adolescents. Although girls make five times more attempts than boys, because of the violence of the means used, boys are five times more likely to die. At least a hundred attempts are made per fatality. Between 8% and 11% of 'normal' Australian secondary school students claim to have attempted suicide. Suicide is rare below the age of 11 years.

When asked why they tried to kill themselves, suicide survivors focus on the final precipitating event such as a loss, humiliation or disciplinary crisis. To an adult, the problem often seems transient or trivial. Of greater significance is the underlying mood, in particular, the presence of depression.

Some of the challenges faced in early adolescence include: physical growth and maturation; increased sexual drives; developing a sense of identity; testing of physical and academic ability and stronger peer relationships demanding independence from the family. Failure in these developmental tasks can result in depression. Other causes include preexisting psychiatric or developmental disorder, parental depression, chronic physical illness, family breakdown; and social adversity and migration.

RISK FACTORS

Risk factors for suicide include:

- depression
- drug and alcohol abuse
- access to means (firearms)
- being male, with a poor school record, unemployed, from a rural area
- a parent, friend or idol whose suicide provides a model
- a pattern of risk-taking or impulsive behavior
- isolation from supportive relationships

PARASUICIDE

Habitual repeat suicide attempters seek something other than death: tension release (after wrist cutting, the flow of blood is warm and comforting), respite from intolerable social circumstances (to obtain care) to manipulate relationships (prevent separation or to avoid punishment).

Harm arises from misadventure, such as underestimating the toxicity of acetaminophen (paracetamol) or the need to escalate the seriousness of the attempt to achieve the same effect.

ASSESSMENT

Signs and symptoms of depression must be sought. A high risk of further suicide attempts may be inferred from the persistence of suicidal ideation, threats and plans. More difficult to detect is the adolescent whose continued suicide intention is masked by a cheerful wish to get out of hospital. Exploration of the adolescent's fantasies about what would happen because of and after death may be helpful.

Research on the seriousness of intent, based on factors such as efforts to avoid detection, evidence of planning, lethality of means chosen, failure to give a warning, final acts and disappointment at failure, has not been very illuminating. A previous attempt is the best predictor of completed suicide. The risk of death increases with the number of attempts. Suicide may be tried again if the circumstances that led to the last attempt recur.

In parasuicides, signs of personality disorder (impulsiveness; intolerance of delay or frustration, inability to be alone) or drug and alcohol abuse should be sought.

MANAGEMENT

In overdoses, the possibility that multiple drugs, with or without alcohol, may have been ingested should be considered (Ch. 4.5). Specific serotonin reuptake inhibitors (SSRIs) have replaced tricyclic antidepressants as the treatment of choice for depression. Lower toxicity is a benefit, but in overdose—especially with other psychotropic drugs—a serotonin syndrome resembling neuroleptic malignant syndrome can emerge. Features include: agitation, vomiting, tremor, myoclonus, diarrhea, hypomania and confusion, hypothermia or hyperthermia, rhabdomyolysis, hypertension, cardiac arrhythmias and death. Treatment is to cease SSRI therapy and implement general supportive measures (Ch. 4.5). Medication is usually not helpful, the serotonin antagonist cyprohepta-cline has been used and dantrolene to control muscle rigidity and rhabdomyolysis.

All attempted suicide patients should have a psychiatric consultation before discharge. Severely depressed and suicidal patients should be transferred to an inpatient psychiatric unit unless effective community care is available. Involuntary treatment is necessary if the patient refuses treatment or seeks to leave against advice.

For lower-risk cases, outpatient follow-up is appropriate. The value of even a single interview should not be underestimated. The aims are acknowledgment of specific worries and reassurance that the adolescent is not unique in having such problems; that they can be understood and effectively helped. Strategies other than self-harm are examined. These should include access to timely and confidential help. Options for further assessment and treatment are also discussed at these interviews.

✗ COMMON ERRORS

➤ Not asking about suicide for fear of suggesting the idea

➤ Trying to persuade the patient of the many good reasons to keep living; this rarely proves convincing and is taken as proof of not understanding the young person's pain
➤ Showing anger with parasuicides by taunting them to do it properly next time
➤ Assessing mood or suicide potential while the adolescent is still affected by an overdose
➤ Accepting glib reassurance from the adolescent or parents that the attempt was an accident or aberration

DRUGS AND ALCOHOL ABUSE

Even where illicit drug use is common, alcohol intoxication or a combination of drugs and alcohol remains the most common reason for young adolescents to require acute hospitalization. Experimentation and peer pressure can lead to the consumption of large quantities of spirits by the naive drinker. Drug and alcohol use is heaviest in late adolescence. The pattern is usually weekend binges rather than the constant consumption frequently seen in adults.

Intoxication increases the risk of accidental injury, especially falls and pedestrians struck by cars. Ataxia produced by the sniffing of volatile substances makes these abusers particularly vulnerable to injury. It is important not to overlook the possibility that intoxication or withdrawal may be contributing to an altered state of consciousness in a victim of multiple trauma.

Drug-dependent parents tolerate frustration poorly and readily resort to pharmacological solutions, medicating their children to keep them quiet. Such children may present as cases of 'near-miss SIDS'.

ASSESSMENT

Delirium is established by the presence of a fluctuating level of consciousness, hallucinations (usually visual), misinterpretation (usually novel stimuli perceived as familiar) and agitation. This may be due to drugs (e.g. anticholinergic toxicity) or withdrawal. Marijuana, though usually producing somnolence and inertia, induces an acute paranoid psychosis in a small percentage of users. They will be hyperalert, frightened and suspicious.

The pattern of drug and alcohol use should be established. Is intoxication a regular feature of weekend parties? Are substances used to seek oblivion when the child is unhappy? Are stimulants or depressants preferred or are mixtures used? In younger children affected by drugs, family assessment is indicated as there may be a culture of drug abuse. The behavior may be encouraged by adults.

Evaluation of the child's mental state should be deferred until the psychoactive substance has cleared. Delirium can easily be confused with psychosis. Sedative or excitatory effects confound the assessment of depression.

MANAGEMENT

In a hospital environment where most patients are seriously ill, the appearance of self-inflicted injury (intoxication or suicide attempt) arouses ambivalent staff attitudes. Some wish to rescue the child while others think firm discipline is required. Punitive or judgmental attitudes should be avoided.

The drug and alcohol abuser wakes up feeling irritable or even aggressive. This is a product of disorientation, fear and the disinhibiting effect of the substances. Disturbed behavior in acute care areas is frequently managed by medication. In these cases, however, nonpharmaceutical measures are preferred because the agitation is usually transient and sedative medication only complicates the problem. The reassurance provided by a parent or familiar person is paramount. Limit the number of staff making contact, and talk quietly and slowly. A patient who is medically stable should be moved to a quiet room. Agitated, ambulant patients may be safer pacing about in an enclosed courtyard than confined to bed. If restraint is required, wait until sufficient people are available.

Only delirium or psychosis requires treatment with antipsychotic medication. Haloperidol (0.01 mg/kg up to 0.5 mg) can be used alone or in combination with diazepam (0.2 mg/kg). Beware of akathisia in which restlessness, pacing and an inability to sit still simulates agitation. Acute dystonia requires an anticholinergic agent, such as benztropine, but this may aggravate the delirium. Drug or alcohol withdrawal is rare in adolescents. Its management is summarized in table 3.10.1. If withdrawal is present, diazepam (0.2 mg/kg) is the sedative most commonly used; neuroleptics should be avoided.

A single episode sufficiently serious to require hospital treatment warrants psychosocial assessment. The young addict should be recognized and referred for appropriate follow-up, preferably by a specialist youth drug and alcohol

TABLE 3.10.1 **Diagnosis and treatment of withdrawal syndromes**		
	Clinical features	**Treatment**
Alcohol	Restlessness, anxiety, nightmares, depression, tremors, vomiting, sweating, diarrhea, seizures, confusion, hallucinations	Quiet surroundings, no alcohol, observe for seizures, hypoventilation, airway obstruction Assess concurrent illness (liver, pneumonia, head injury, fractures) Thiamin, multivitamins Treat dehydration; monitor serum K and Mg Diazepam 0.1 mg/kg; titrate against agitation; avoid oversedation
Benzodiazepines	Anxiety, confusion, insomnia, psychosis, seizures, anorexia, nausea, vomiting, tremor, sweating	Reintroduce diazepam and gradually taper the dose to zero over 1–2 weeks
Opiates	Irritability, confusion, hyperactivity, sweating, lacrimation, rhinorrhea, stuffy nose, pruritus, piloerection, vomiting, abdominal pain, diarrhea	Consider the possibility of sepsis Symptomatic treatment of withdrawal Clonidine partly relieves symptoms; titrate doses against symptoms and blood pressure

service. Contact can be made by the social worker or liaison psychiatrist.

Lack of supervision and inappropriate access to drugs and alcohol indicate neglect. To give a child substances to promote entertaining behavior or facilitate sexual activity is child abuse. Child protection authorities should be notified in these cases.

CHILD ABUSE

Trauma sufficient to warrant intensive care occurs in shaken babies, sexual assault with multiple injuries and some cases of physical abuse. Factitious Disorders (Munchausen syndrome by proxy) may involve serious metabolic disturbance or infection (Ch. 4.3). In most cases, government or local authority child protection services are already involved or are notified immediately. Staff of these bodies will make decisions regarding the child's safety. Difficulties arise when the parent is the perpetrator. If the parent is excluded, a substitute carer must be found to accompany and comfort the child. If contact with the parents is allowed, staff's abhorrence of their action can lead to the parent's needs for emotional support being ignored (including their grief as perpetrators and grief for their child's condition). Parents with a personality disorder, particularly if impulsive and aggressive, react belligerently to being blamed. Those troubled by guilt and poor esteem as parents stay away, surrendering the child's care to the hospital. Their absence confirms their unsuitability to care for the child, in the eyes of the staff. A similar process occurs with drug-addicted parents who are frequently neglectful. Return of the child to the parent's care, in such circumstances, is difficult for all. To prevent alienation of the parent-perpetrator, staff should treat the parents as normally as possible: encouraging the parents' efforts to be involved with the child, keeping them informed of developments, providing emotional support and avoiding the expression of judgmental attitudes.

The usual delay between initial presentation and the diagnosis of a Factitious Disorder is almost a year. During this period, abuse may be suspected but there is insufficient evidence to establish a case. When such a child presents, staff will have dual roles: forging a treatment alliance with the parent and investigating. The suspected perpetrator is allowed continued access to the child and not warned that he or she is being scrutinized for interference. This leads to concern by staff about exposing the child to unnecessary risk and entrapment of the parent by providing a situation that encourages continued abuse. Staff who regard this approach as deceitful, press for the suspected abuse to be discussed with the parent. Unfortunately, this period of observation is necessary to obtain the required evidence to present to court. The alternative—precipitate confrontation of the suspected perpetrator—results in indignant denial, withdrawal of the child from care, further interference to 'prove' that the illness is 'real' and increased artifice in deception. The Children's Court, when presented with suspicions and coincidences but no proof and seeing an attentive parent, usually with many character witnesses, has no alternative but to return the child to the parent's care. The rationale for this approach, as well as doubts and dissenting opinions, should be discussed at regular multidisciplinary staff meetings. A split may develop between those who believe abuse is occurring and those who believe the parent to be incapable of such an action. This must be addressed promptly to prevent damage to morale.

The emotional consequence of abuse for the child is a disruption of the child's sense of safety which leads to hypervigilance and lack of trust in adults. Insecure attachment to the caretaker is evident by 1 year of age, with anxious, avoidant or disorganized responses in the infant following separation. Attachment difficulties persist with a lack of mutual pleasure and an excess of negative responses, such as fear, placation and withdrawal, in childhood. The child also feels to blame for the parent's anger or neglect, resulting in low self-esteem. Difficulty with the regulation of emotional arousal results in angry outbursts. By school age, the delayed development of social skills can lead to poor peer relations, with even friendly approaches being met with aggression or withdrawal.

PSYCHOLOGICAL EFFECTS OF CRITICAL ILLNESS

The physical and emotional development of children is often adversely affected by critical illness or injury. Hospitalization is an exceptionally stressful event. A PICU stay, however short, further increases the level of stress for all concerned. The ability to decrease these emotional and psychological effects is a vital skill for health professionals working with critically ill children. The following section describes:

- behavioral traits displayed by children admitted to a PICU
- factors that affect the ability of children and their families to cope with this stressful life event
- strategies to help reduce the effect of critical illness or injury on the child and family

ICU SYNDROME

The ICU syndrome refers to the effects of admission to an intensive care unit and is best reported in the adult literature. Its manifestations include fear, anxiety, depression, hallucinations and delirium. Children, too, demonstrate physical and psychological effects from their PICU admissions. The responses of children to critical illness are affected by many factors including age, developmental stage and family support. Table 3.10.2 lists factors that contribute to a child's psychological and emotional state during or after admission and treatment for critical illness.

Despite the best efforts of experienced staff and devoted parents, such children during convalescence can demonstrate signs of emotional withdrawal. Some become passive and nonresponsive to painful procedures, while others may have extreme responses to recurrent and nonpainful procedures. Children may become distraught during simple procedures such as temperature measurement per axilla. They may physically retreat from any hospital staff who approach. Negativity with familiar events can appear and children may refuse anything and everything. Developmental regression is common in younger children and

---

TABLE 3.10.2 Factors affecting a child's psychological response to severe illness

- Age
- Developmental stage
- Personality type
- Loss of ability to control self and environment
- Sleep deprivation
- Pain
- Anxiety
- Previous experiences with illness or hospitalization
- Length of critical illness and duration of PICU admission
- Complications associated with the critical illness
- Drugs and other treatments administered
- Invasive and painful procedures
- Preexisting psychiatric disorders
- Family and social background including the coping skills of the child and family
- Parental involvement during the child's stay in the PICU
- Parental understanding of child's illness and treatments
- Staff responses to the child and the family

---

those who had previously been toilet-trained may revert to bed-wetting. Children recovering from severe illness or injury are often very demanding (especially of parents) and refuse to allow parents to leave them. They may actually demonstrate physical signs of terror such as trembling, tachycardia, hypertension and sweating.

We now recognize many ways of orienting care to help children and their families cope better and to decrease the severity of the psychological effects of their experience.

Empathetic staff

Nurses and doctors experienced in dealing with critical situations spend large amounts of time with children and families and are able to assess the coping skills of the child and family. They can respond to the 'whole' individual's needs effectively and avoid concentrating exclusively on physiological parameters or the technology of care.

The presence of a sympathetic nurse can reduce the anxiety and stress. A calm and sympathetic interaction between the nurse and the child, and provision of information about the illness and its expected course, help reduce the stress that parents are feeling. This improves their ability to cope with the child's illness, to act as parents and to respond more effectively to their child's needs. Development of a truly multidisciplinary team is a key element in providing child and family-oriented care (Ch. 5.5).

DEVELOPMENTAL NEEDS

Provision of a child-oriented environment includes understanding the developmental needs of a child, comprehensive communication and responding appropriately to their physical and emotional needs during admission. Ready access to family and familiar objects is essential.

Infants

Infants respond positively to the presence of their parents, a reassuring human voice and to basic comfort measures such as touch, positioning, swaddling, pacifiers, full stomachs, adequate sleep, and gentle, comforting caregivers. It is important to minimize the number of painful procedures and to optimize the way in which procedures are performed (e.g. by the use of topical or local anesthetic agents) and by providing comfort after necessary procedures.

Preschool children

Preschoolers are more complex and the emotional, psychological and developmental setbacks can be severe if care is not taken. Again, the presence of their parents is very important but there is no easy guide to how much parents should remain with their child. Every child and family is different, and staff can do no more than help parents to decide what is reasonable. Calm, age-appropriate explanation must always be given before procedures or changes in treatment. Careful use of simple, clear language can minimize misunderstandings. For example, if anesthesia is described as 'going to sleep', some children may become very fearful of bedtime if they wake in pain after an operation or recall having a black mask placed over their face at the start of anesthesia. Preschoolers need to be reassured that they have not become sick because they were naughty or bad.

Children in this age group are becoming independent in their bodily functions and daily living habits (e.g. feeding themselves and toilet-training).

Loss of control in these areas can distress children who are unable to use adult rationalization to explain the change in their circumstances.

Providing an alternate focus (parents reading, child blowing bubbles) gives the child choice and an area to maintain control during procedures. Health professionals should keep parents informed of the ways in which children normally react to serious illness and hospital admission, and of the temporary regressive responses that may occur.

Case example

S. was a 3-year-old boy with 40% flame burns and an inhalation injury admitted to an Australian PICU from a Pacific island. His French-speaking mother accompanied him, while his father and sister remained on the island. His treatment course followed the usual pattern with debridement, skin grafts and daily dressings. S. was still a very distressed boy on day 3 of admission despite a concerted pharmacological approach to management of his pain and anxiety.

S. is an extreme example of a preschooler admitted to PICU following a traumatic injury. He was separated from at least two very important people in his life (father and sister). He was distanced from most staff by language and culture, and mother although receiving all information through regular, formally translated sessions (including a telephone interpreter when it was considered necessary) remained very anxious.

S. had no control over his injured body. He had tubes in most orifices and invasive monitoring lines. His skin was swathed in bandages and he was undergoing painful procedures every day. In response hospital staff assessed his pain and anxiety state more frequently to better respond to his individual requirements. They also ensured that his mother was not only fully informed but had a real understanding of what was occurring. Nurses encouraged her to explain in simple clear language to S. what was happening and where his other family members were. Children's tapes in the French language were obtained.

Schoolchildren

School-aged children also benefit from the presence of their parents. Children in this age range require comprehensive age-appropriate explanation, discussion and reassurance about what is happening to them. They have vivid imaginations, can feel very anxious about inadequately explained impending events and need their questions answered in honest, direct terms. Be truthful and encourage questions when preparing school-aged children for procedures such as intravenous line insertion, physiotherapy or tracheal suction and for surgical wounds. Also maintaining their privacy is essential.

Adolescents

Adolescents are another particularly vulnerable group. Critical illness or injury for an adolescent already in a body-image crisis can be psychologically devastating. Separation from peers and their activities can lead to grief and anger, affecting how they deal with their situation. Returning young people to a dependent state just as they are starting to test their independence can have a profound psychological impact.

Honest explanations and scrupulous maintenance of privacy are essential. Adolescents and their parents must be involved in all decision-making. Whether peers are allowed to visit depends on the adolescent: some want to avoid being seen when they are ill, while others may demand peer contact. Listen to the adolescent and respond appropriately. Allowing their own music (preferably with earphones!), clothing and visual entertainment helps young people feel comfortable.

COMMUNICATION

The stress on parents can be reduced by arranging regular opportunities for communication. Nurses are usually able to discuss management issues informally with parents (and with the child when possible and appropriate). Information already provided can be repeated, expanded or confirmed.

Medical information can be discussed with parents at the child's bedside or in a sit-down session away from the bedside. Care should be taken that information provided at the bedside is appropriate for the child to hear. Assume that *all* children can hear what is being said at all times but may not understand. Misunderstood or partly understood bedside conversations can be as terrifying for an aware child as being told nothing at all about what is happening.

ANALGESIA AND SEDATION

The pain of wounds and unpleasant procedures such as catheter placement, physiotherapy and tracheal suction, and anxiety about all the strange and unpleasant aspects of critical illness and hospitalization are stressful and demoralizing for the child. Anxiety augments the child's perception of pain and the persistence or recurrence of inadequately relieved pain prevents the child from adequately processing all the information, thoughts and ideas which present themselves. Unrelieved pain also prevents the child from interacting normally with parents, siblings, friends and staff. The anxiety this causes in others, in turn amplifies the child's distress. Too heavy sedation, on the other hand, interferes with sleep–wake cycles and with the processing of sensory information, leading to disorientation and confusion. Thoughtful and meticulous use of non-drug methods of pain relief (e.g. posture, comfort, warmth, parents and food), frequent assessment of the appropriate level of comfort and sedation for *each child* by nursing and medical staff, and selection of appropriate drugs and doses, are much more effective than a standardized regimen for provision of analgesic and sedative drugs (Ch. 5.2).

The dose of narcotic and sedative drugs should be reduced slowly after prolonged exposure. Withdrawal symptoms can impair children's psychological (and physical) ability to cope with their situation. Although the child may be entering a convalescent phase, parents are often worried and distressed by signs of drug withdrawal.

PARENTS

It is recognized increasingly that families and even individual parents differ considerably in their needs, preferences and reactions regarding their child's care. Skilled care givers explore such things as how much parents want to be directly involved with care or in decision making, and what methods of communication work best.

By supporting the presence of parents, staff can promote the child's psychological and emotional wellbeing. Parents treated with consideration and fully informed rarely have a negative effect on their child. Keeping parents away from their child for the sake of staff ('controlled visiting') is a dangerous policy because many children become anxious and withdrawn ('well-behaved') in the parents' absence, and only act out their true emotions ('badly behaved') when the parents are finally allowed to visit.

Staying with a critically ill and often noninteractive child can be very difficult for parents. The physical and emotional exhaustion that goes hand-in-hand with a child's critical illness affects parents' ability to concentrate and to cope with what is happening to their child. Many parents have unspoken fears, including that staff many be less than fully motivated in their care when children are not their usual 'cute' selves following trauma, surgery or when paralyzed for ventilation. Encouraging parents to express their fears has value. Photographs of the child when well provide a useful cue for initiating such conversations.

ENVIRONMENT

Areas where children are treated should be designed to meet the needs of children and their families. Big, open units meet the needs of staff but provide a distressingly busy, noisy and brightly lit environment for critically ill children. Lighting and noise should be reduced whenever possible, especially at night. Observation remains important, but selective lighting and bed screens can be used to highlight particular children, for example those undergoing procedures or whose condition is deteriorating, while allowing other children to rest or sleep undisturbed.

Providing familiar toys, books and music makes the environment friendlier for children. Other measures such as murals and mobiles soften the landscape in the unit and show that the focus of the unit is on the children and their needs.

✓ KEY POINTS

➤ Have an open and flexible visiting policy and encourage parents to visit as often as possible
➤ Tailor pain relief and sedation to the needs of each child
➤ Keep the parents and the child fully informed

➤ Always assume that a child can hear what is said at the bedside
➤ Provide a quiet, private and child-friendly environment
➤ Allow for the needs of children of different developmental stages

✗ COMMON ERRORS

➤ 'Controlled visiting'
➤ A bright, noisy, 'busy' PICU
➤ Fixed sedation and analgesia regimens
➤ Inadequate explanations to child and parents
➤ Careless bedside conversations

FURTHER READING

1. Khan AU. Psychiatric emergencies in pediatrics. Chicago: Year Book; 1979
   – (*Good sections on chronic illness, nonorganic disease, the dying child, irate parents and psychiatric assessment*)

2. Walsh TL, Scully R. Psychiatric aspects of critical care. In: Holbrook PR, editor. Textbook of pediatric critical care. Philadelphia: WB Saunders; 1993
   – (*More extensive coverage including delirium, pain and dying*)

3. Smith JB, Browne AM. Critical illness and intensive care during infancy and childhood. In: Curley MAQ, Smith JB, Moloney-Harmon PA, editors. Critical care nursing of infants and children. Philadelphia: WB Saunders; 1996
   – (*Thorough review of developmental aspects of the psychological stresses imposed on the child by critical illness*)

4. Curley MAQ, Meyer EC. The impact of the critical care experience on the family. In: Curley MAQ, Smith JB, Moloney-Harmon PA, editors. Critical care nursing of infants and children. Philadelphia: WB Saunders; 1996
   – (*Review of stresses on the family, and the role of nurses in the management of stress*)

5. Todres ID, Earle M, Jellinek MS. Enhancing communication: the physician and family in the pediatric intensive care unit. Pediatr Clin North Am 1994; 41: 1395–1404
   – (*Coping mechanisms, communication and counseling from a medical viewpoint*)

6. Delbanco TL. Enriching the doctor/patient relationship by inviting the patient's perspective Ann Int Med 1992; 116(5): 414–418
   – (*An excellent review of processes that constructively enhance traditional values and practices via realistic modern methodologies*)

3.11   Genetic metabolic disorders

John Christodoulou

Genetic metabolic disorders are inherited diseases that interfere with normal metabolic function. When one of these conditions is detected clinically and by screening tests, specific biochemical investigations to establish the exact nature of the abnormality must be performed urgently if appropriate therapy is to be instituted early enough to prevent death or permanent damage.

Over 500 biochemically distinct inborn errors have been identified, but despite their diversity, most of these disorders manifest themselves in one of four clinical presentations (Table 3.11.1). Almost all inborn errors are autosomal recessive in inheritance, although there are a few exceptions.

Genetic clues to an inborn error of metabolism include:

- history of a similarly affected sibling or other affected relative
- parental consanguinity
- ethnicity (some disorders are more common in certain ethnic groups)
- parents come from the same small town or village
- parental isonomy (same last name)

DISEASES OF SMALL MOLECULES

PHYSIOLOGY

For most disorders of small molecules the clinical and biochemical consequences are due to either an accumulation of toxic metabolites, or a deficiency of essential products (Fig. 3.11.1).

Accumulation of toxic metabolites

Important points to remember include:

- most small molecule diseases affect enzymes in catabolic pathways
- catabolic processes such as infections or major surgery will overload already compromised enzyme function

---

TABLE 3.11.1 Classes of genetic metabolic disorders based on clinical presentation

ENCEPHALOPATHY

Acute

Disease of small diffusible molecules
- Amino acid disorders
- Organic acid disorders
- Fatty acid oxidation defects
- Hyperammonemias
- Primary lactic acidoses
- Encephalopathy with seizures

Chronic

Diseases of small diffusible molecules (see above)
Disease of organelles
- Mitochondrial disorders (defects in pyruvate and electron transport bioenergetics)
  - defects of pyruvate metabolism
  - defects of the tricarboxylic acid (Krebs) cycle
  - electron transport chain defects
- Lysosomal storage disorders
  - mucopolysaccharidoses
  - glycoproteinoses
  - gangliosidoses
  - other sphingolipidoses
  - leukodystrophies
- Peroxisomal disorders
  - defects of peroxisomal biogenesis
  - defects of several peroxisomal proteins
  - defects of single peroxisomal enzymes

DIFFUSE HEPATOCELLULAR DISEASE
(acute or chronic)
- Defects of carbohydrate metabolism
- Defects of amino acid metabolism
- Defects of metal transport
- Defects of protease inhibitors

MYOPATHY

Skeletal myopathy
- Acute rhabdomyolysis
- Chronic myopathy

Cardiomyopathy
- Lysosomal storage disorders
- Disorders of fatty acid metabolism

RENAL DISEASE

Glomerular and tubular disease
- Lysosomal storage disorder
- Enzyme defect

Transport defects
- Defective transport of individual or groups of similar molecules

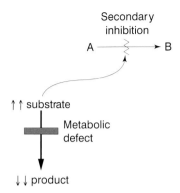

Figure 3.11.1 Biochemical pathology of inborn errors of metabolism. Inborn errors may cause the accumulation of a toxic substrate or deficiency of an essential product or may inhibit other important metabolic pathways

- noxious molecules that accumulate include:
  - amino acids
  - organic acids
  - fatty acids and their esters
  - ammonium
- hepatomegaly and signs of generalized hepatic dysfunction are often found

Brain involvement in the disease process reflects its vulnerability to metabolic disturbance, rather than greater enzymatic activity in the brain.

Product deficiency

Product deficiency disorders includes those that impair energy production, resulting in intracellular depletion of ATP:

- defects of gluconeogenesis
- defects of pyruvate metabolism
- Krebs cycle defects
- mitochondrial respiratory chain defects

Because the newborn period is a time of substantial catabolism, the breakdown of protein and fat results in increased delivery of metabolites to the pathway which is blocked by the genetic defect, and consequent elevations of the metabolite levels. Infants who have slightly more residual enzyme activity, with a less severe metabolic block, may escape presentation in the newborn period, only to develop symptoms later in infancy,

or even later in life, when they are exposed to catabolic stresses such as increased protein or fat intake (for example by a switch from breast milk to a cow's milk formula), or breakdown of body protein or fat due to infection, starvation, or trauma (including surgery). Many of the encephalopathic metabolic crises that intermittently affect even well-treated patients are also precipitated by catabolic stress. The recognition of subtle signs of impending metabolic decompensation, such as the development of ataxia or changes in behavior, permits the early institution of emergency therapy to prevent progression of the episode to acute encephalopathy.

ACUTE ENCEPHALOPATHY

Encephalopathy is the most common clinical presentation of genetic metabolic disorders. It can be acute, intermittent, chronic, or even nonprogressive. Patients with a severe enzyme defect often present in the newborn period or early infancy, but small molecule diseases may cause acute encephalopathy at any age, and must be excluded even in adults with unexplained acute encephalopathy. This category of inborn errors includes:

- aminoacidopathies (e.g. maple syrup urine disease)
- organic acidopathies (e.g. methylmalonic acidemia)
- fatty acid oxidation defects (e.g. medium-chain acyl-CoA dehydrogenase deficiency)
- urea cycle defects (e.g. ornithine transcarbamylase deficiency)
- primary lactic acidosis disorders (including defects of gluconeogenesis, Krebs cycle, pyruvate metabolism and the mitochondrial respiratory chain)

ACUTE ENCEPHALOPATHY IN THE NEWBORN

Remember the following points:

- it takes time for the offending metabolite to accumulate to toxic levels
- the infant is usually well for several days to a week after birth

- symptoms are usually nonspecific and include:
  - poor feeding
  - vomiting
  - lethargy
  - hypotonia
  - irritability
  - tachypnea and hyperpnea (if metabolic acidosis or hyperammonemia is also present)
  - seizures (usually a late feature, and imply a poor prognosis)
- cerebral edema occurs frequently with signs of raised intracranial pressure
  - progressive obtundation
  - bulging fontanelle
- failure to thrive is almost always present
- hepatomegaly is often present

The most common alternative diagnoses in an infant with acute encephalopathy are:

- sepsis
- perinatal hypoxia
- congenital malformation of the heart or gut
- intracerebral hemorrhage

The possibility of an inborn error is often considered only after these have been ruled out, but unless screening investigations for inborn errors are performed in parallel with testing for these more common diseases and appropriate aggressive treatment given, severe neurological damage or death may ensue. Screening tests that should be performed in any newborn or infant with acute encephalopathy are summarized in Chapter 2.9, Table 2.9.3.

AMINOACIDOPATHIES

Amino acids are essential for endogenous protein synthesis, but once anabolic needs are met, the surplus is degraded and used for energy. In the aminoacidopathies these degradative pathways are disrupted. Catabolism and excess amino acid intake lead to accumulation of the toxic metabolite.

Maple syrup urine disease

Maple syrup urine disease (Fig. 3.11.2) is an example of an aminoacidopathy:

- enzyme defect: branched-chain α-ketoacid dehydrogenase
- provoking substances: the branched-chain amino acids leucine, isoleucine and valine
- accumulating substances: α-ketoacids amino acids
- abnormal screening tests:
  - characteristic odor in body fluids
  - urine amino acid screen
- definitive test: plasma amino acid quantitation
- acute treatment: see Chapter 2.9
- long-term-treatment: see Chapter 2.9

ORGANIC ACIDOSES

Organic acidopathies should be considered in any patient with unexplained metabolic acidosis. Accumulation of organic acids, products of the later steps of the breakdown of the carbon chain of the amino acids, causes a more severe metabolic acidosis than that seen in the aminoacidopathies, with a compensatory hyperpnea. The catabolic pathways of the various amino acids result in the formation of many different organic acid intermediates, which for a particular disorder results in a characteristic biochemical signature, detectable by gas chromatography/mass spectrometry of urine or plasma.

Methylmalonic aciduria

Methylmalonic aciduria (Fig. 3.11.2) is an example of an organic acidosis:

- enzyme defect: L-methylmalonyl-CoA mutase (most common)
- provoking substances: isoleucine, valine, threonine and methionine, odd-chain fatty acids, and the side chain of cholesterol
- accumulating substances: propionic and methylmalonic acids
- abnormal screening tests: metabolic acidosis, increased anion gap
- definitive test: urine organic acid screen
- acute treatment: see Chapter 2.9
- long-term treatment: see Chapter 2.9

A clue to the presence of an organic acid accumulation is an increase in the anion gap (Ch. 2.10). Organic acidopathies must be excluded if the

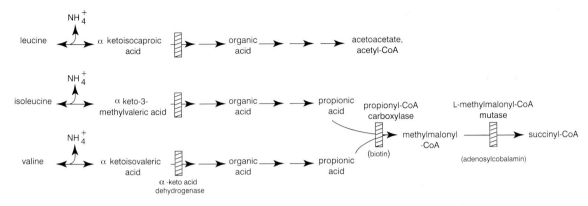

Figure 3.11.2 Defects of amino and organic acid metabolism. Excess amino acids undergo a series of catabolic reactions, producing organic acids which are then converted to simpler molecules. These examples are the catabolic pathways for the three branched-chain amino acids, leucine, isoleucine and valine. Many enzymes require vitamin cofactors: e.g. biotin is a cofactor for propionyl-CoA carboxylase, and adenosylcobalamin (a vitamin B_{12} derivative) for methylmalonyl-CoA mutase

anion gap is greater than 20 mEq/L, although most patients with an increased anion gap do not have an inborn error of metabolism, but an acquired acidosis either from lactic acidemia secondary to tissue hypoxia, or from ketone body accumulation (ketoacidosis), for example in diabetes mellitus. A normal anion gap does not exclude significant lactic acidemia, as it may remain normal until blood lactate level exceeds 6 mmol/L.

FATTY ACID OXIDATION DEFECTS

Following prolonged fasting in normal children, hepatic glycogen stores become depleted, causing the brain and muscle to use fatty acids liberated by lipolysis as the major energy source. These fatty acids undergo β-oxidation, generating ketone bodies, which can be directly utilized by muscle and brain (Fig. 3.11.3). The decrease in ketone body production in children with fatty acid β-oxidation defects results in hypoketotic hypoglycemia. These disorders are therefore usually exposed by fasting. Consequently, *an inherited disorder of fatty acid β-oxidation should be suspected in any child with*:

- fasting coma
- lethargy and vomiting, particularly if associated with hepatomegaly
- fasting hypoglycemia
- skeletal myopathy or cardiomyopathy

- acute life-threatening episodes
- family history of sudden infant death syndrome (SIDS)

Medium-chain acyl-CoA dehydrogenase deficency

Medium-chain acyl-CoA dehydrogenase deficiency (Fig. 3.11.3) is an example of a fatty acid oxidation defect:

- enzyme defect: medium-chain acyl-CoA dehydrogenase
- provoking situations: prolonged fasting, catabolic state
- accumulating substances: fatty acyl-CoAs and their esters
- abnormal screening tests: hypoglycemia, hypoketonuria, low plasma carnitine
- definitive tests
  - urine organic acid screen
  - fibroblast enzyme and mutation studies
- acute treatment: see Chapter 2.9
- long-term treatment: see Chapter 2.9

HYPERAMMONEMIA

Because ammonium is a potent neurotoxin, hyperammonemia needs urgent investigation for a possible inborn error of metabolism. Hyperammonemia, sometimes severe, is often

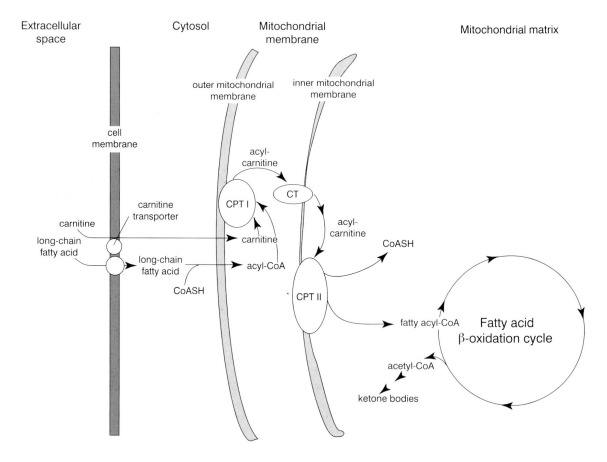

Figure 3.11.3 Fatty acid metabolism. The process of fatty acid oxidation removes one acetyl moiety with each cycle, generating ketone bodies which can be used by skeletal and heart muscle and brain, particularly during fasting. These enzymes (which form the β-oxidation cycle) are found within the mitochondrial matrix. Whilst medium- and short-chain fatty acids can freely traverse the mitochondrial membranes, long-chain fatty acids cannot, and must be first ligated to carnitine before being translocated across the membranes. This acylcarnitine is then converted back to its acyl-CoA form, where it can then undergo β-oxidation. Three enzymes are necessary for this process; carnitine palmitoyltransferase I (CPT I), carnitine-acylcarnitine translocase (CT) and CPT II. There are multiple isoforms of the β-oxidation enzymes, which show chain length specificity. The four enzymes of the cycle are the acyl-CoA dehydrogenases (very long chain, long-chain, medium-chain, and short-chain; 3-hydroxyacyl-CoA dehydrogenases (long-chain, and short-chain); the enoyl hydratases; and the ketothiolases

seen in the organic acidopathies and fatty acid oxidation defects, reflecting a secondary inhibition of the urea cycle by the accumulating metabolites of those disorders. Primary hyperammonemia caused by urea cycle defects usually presents in the first week of life (Fig. 3.11.4).

Ornithine transcarbamylase deficiency

Ornithine transcarbamylase deficiency (Fig. 3.11.4) is an example of a primary hyperammonemia:

- enzyme defect: ornithine transcarbamylase
- provoking situations: excessive protein intake, catabolic state
- accumulating substances: ammonium
- abnormal screening tests: hyper-ammonemia, respiratory alkalosis
- definitive tests:
  - urine and plasma amino acids
  - urine orotic acid
- acute treatment: see Chapter 2.9
- long-term treatment: see Chapter 2.9

Neurological impairment is seen in almost all late-diagnosed survivors, and these infants are at risk of further encephalopathic episodes following excessive protein intake or during catabolic periods.

Transient hyperammonemia of the newborn

Transient hyperammonemia of the newborn (THAN) is an acquired disorder of unknown cause found predominantly in low birthweight newborns. Major clues to the diagnosis are the early onset of the hyperammonemia, usually within 24 hours of birth, and the frequent association of lung disease. Hyperammonemia is often severe (up to 2500 μmol/L), and there are no specific biochemical markers. The condition must be treated in the short term like a urea cycle defect.

PRIMARY LACTIC ACIDOSIS

In a child with lactic acidosis, if poor tissue perfusion due to cardiac disease, hypovolemia, severe sepsis or some other cause of shock has been excluded, the possibility of an inherited defect of pyruvate metabolism, the citric acid (Krebs) cycle, gluconeogenesis, or of the mitochondrial respiratory chain should be suspected. Organs that are heavily energy-dependent, particularly the brain, heart, kidney, skeletal muscle and retina, are most often affected, causing a wide range of clinical signs (Table 3.11.2). Table 3.11.3 summarizes some of the important clinical and biochemical features which can help in distinguishing the groups of disorders causing a primary lactic acidosis.

These disorders are usually associated with raised blood and/or CSF lactate concentration, and may result in a metabolic acidosis with an increased

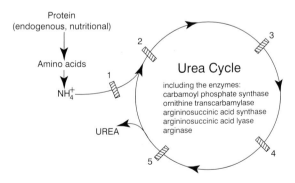

Figure 3.11.4 The urea cycle. Ammonium is a byproduct of amino acid catabolism and a potent neurotoxin, which must be rapidly removed from the circulation by the urea cycle. Defects in the urea cycle can cause life-threatening hyperammonemic coma during catabolic illnesses or excessive protein intake. Arginase deficiency is more often associated with a progressive cerebral palsy-like illness

---

TABLE 3.11.2 Clinical features of the mitochondrial respiratory chain disorders

General
- Small stature
- Anorexia

Central nervous system
- Neonatal acute encephalomyopathy, with severe lactic acidosis
- Leigh disease (subacute necrotizing encephalomyelopathy)
- Developmental delay
- Dementia
- Myoclonic seizures
- Ataxia
- Stroke-like episodes (often reversible)
- Dysphagia
- Progressive external ophthalmoplegia
- Sensorineural hearing loss
- Retinal degeneration
- Optic atrophy
- Peripheral neuropathy

Skeletal muscle
- Hypotonia
- Weakness
- Exercise intolerance
- Rhabdomyolysis

Gastrointestinal
- Malabsorption
- Diarrhea

Hematologic
- Sideroblastic anemia
- Neutropenia

Cardiac muscle
- Cardiomyopathy
- Cardiac conduction defects

Kidney
- Renal Fanconi syndrome

Liver
- Progressive hepatic failure

Endocrine
- Diabetes mellitus
- Diabetes insipidus

TABLE 3.11.3 **Differential diagnosis of inherited causes of primary lactic acidosis**

	Pyruvate metabolism	Defects of gluconeogenesis	Krebs cycle defects	Defects of the respiratory chain
Hypoglycemia	−	++[a]	−	− → +
Ketosis	−	− → +[b]	+	+
Lactic acidemia relative to feeding	Postprandial	Fasting	Postprandial	Postprandial
Ratio of BOB to acetoacetate in plasma (N < 1.5)	Normal	Variable	Normal	↑
Ratio of lactate to pyruvate in blood (N < 10)	Normal	↑	↑	↑
Neurological impairment	Usually severe	Depends on hypoglycemia	Moderate − severe	Nil → severe
Other clinical features	CNS malformations; dementia	Hepatomegaly during acute episodes	CNS malformations; dementia	May have multisystem disease incl. dementia
Example	Pyruvate dehydrogenase deficiency	Pyruvate carboxylase deficiency	Fumarase deficiency	Cytochrome *c* oxidase deficiency

[a]*Some cases of pyruvate carboxylase deficiency do not have hypoglycemia.* [b]*Not in glycogen storage disease type I.* BOB, β-hydroxybutyrate; CNS, central nervous system; N, normal.

anion gap, although in some cases the acidosis may be mild and the anion gap normal. In Krebs cycle disorders, urine organic acid analysis can help identify the accumulating organic acid, but for these and the other primary lactic acidoses, enzymatic assay in biopsied liver and muscle is required to confirm the specific enzyme defect. Structural abnormalities of the mitochondria are commonly found in the respiratory chain disorders including 'ragged red fibers', which contain peripherally situated clumps of mitochondria that stain red with the modified Gomori trichrome stain used for light microscopy.

The majority of the respiratory chain proteins are autosomal recessive or X-linked in inheritance. Defects in mitochondrial DNA (mtDNA), in contrast, are either maternally inherited, or sporadic, and screening for the more 'common' mtDNA mutations should be part of the diagnostic investigation for respiratory chain defects.

ENCEPHALOPATHY WITH PREDOMINATING SEIZURES

In the disorders described above seizures are a late feature, but there are four disorders in which early seizures are the predominant feature:

- nonketotic hyperglycinemia
- pyridoxine-dependent epilepsy
- sulfite oxidase deficiency
- molybdenum cofactor deficiency

The clinical presentation of all of these can be suggestive of perinatal asphyxia, but without a supportive history.

Nonketotic hyperglycinemia

Nonketotic hyperglycinemia (NKH) has a rapidly progressive course in the neonate with profound hypotonia, progressive obtundation, seizures, hiccoughs and apnea. Survivors usually have poorly controlled seizures and profound intellectual handicap:

- enzyme defect: glycine cleavage system
- provoking situations: none
- accumulating substances: glycine
- abnormal screening tests: hyperglycinorrhachia, hyperglycinemia, hyperglycinuria
- definitive tests:
  - raised CSF to plasma glycine ratio
  - liver or lymphoblast enzyme assays

- acute treatment: benzoate, NMDA receptor antagonists
- long-term treatment: none is effective

Pyridoxine-dependent epilepsy

Pyridoxine-dependent (vitamin B_6-dependent) epilepsy begins in the first weeks of life (or even in utero), and should be excluded in any infant or child with an unexplained seizure disorder. Traditional anticonvulsants do not control the seizures:

- enzyme defect: unknown
- provoking situations: fever sometimes worsens seizures
- accumulating substances: none
- abnormal screening tests: none
- definitive test: clinical response to pyridoxine, with EEG normalization
- acute treatment: pyridoxine (100 mg given over 10 minutes—be prepared for transient apnea)
- long-term treatment: pyridoxine (50–200 mg per day)

Other children with pyridoxine-dependent epilepsy may have a later onset (as late as 18 months of age), may be initially or partially responsive to other anticonvulsants, or may have seizure-free periods on no medications.

The outcome is variable. Some patients have good seizure control and normal development, but many others are intellectually impaired, although this may reflect late diagnosis.

Sulfite oxidase deficiency

Sulfite oxidase deficiency, a defect of cysteine catabolism, or a defect in the biosynthesis of its molybdenum cofactor, produces a remarkably similar phenotype, which usually has its onset in the neonatal period. Typical clinical features in the first week or two of life include feeding difficulties, intractable generalized seizures, and truncal hypotonia with peripheral hypertonia. Those who survive beyond the neonatal period develop progressive destructive brain changes with severe calcification, choreoathetoid movements and lens dislocation. Milder variants have also been described, with less severe neurological and somatic abnormalities and a later onset of symptoms. Features of the disease are:

- enzyme defect: sulfite oxidase or its molybdenum cofactor
- provoking situations: none
- accumulating substances: sulfite, S-sulfocysteine
- abnormal screening tests: increased urine sulfite, S-sulfocysteine, thiosulfate, low serum uric acid in molybdenum cofactor deficiency
- definitive test: liver or fibroblast enzyme assay
- acute treatment: none is effective
- long-term treatment: none is effective

ACUTE ENCEPHALOPATHY BEYOND THE NEWBORN PERIOD

A child or adult with a small molecule disease may have good health for years or decades, and may then present unexpectedly with an acute encephalopathy. In these patients there is sufficient residual enzyme activity to catabolize the substrate when they are in good health, but the added stress of a catabolic episode causes excessive substrate accumulation. In the intermittent variant of maple syrup urine disease, for example, the child is biochemically normal except when challenged by the catabolism of intercurrent illness or excessive protein intake. Ataxia and decreased conciousness then develop, due to accumulation of the branched-chain α-keto acids.

Occasionally a patient with a disease of this type may not present until adult life. The initial presentation of ornithine transcarbamylase deficiency in female carriers may be during the catabolic phase after childbirth. Older patients with small molecule diseases may present with loss of consciousness, ataxia, disorientation or frank psychosis.

The intermittent or late-onset forms of the small molecule inborn errors are commonly misdiagnosed as Reye's syndrome because of the presence of encephalopathy, cerebral edema, and mild liver dysfunction (increases in aspartate transaminase with fatty infiltration of the liver, hypoglycemia and hyperammonemia). Thus, the diagnosis of Reye's syndrome should only be made after the exclusion of small molecule inborn errors.

MANAGEMENT OF INHERITED SMALL MOLECULE DISORDERS

Acute resuscitative therapy

In patients suspected of having an inborn error of metabolism, it is important to implement immediate resuscitative treatment while the diagnostic investigations are in progress, treatment should include elements addressed in Chapters 2.9 and 2.10 to correct the metabolic disturbance:

- provision of fluid, electrolytes, and glucose
- correction of the metabolic acidosis
- hemodialysis or hemofiltration
- specific therapy according to the disease

and in chapters 2.4 and 2.6 to manage the encephalopathy:

- support circulation (avoid hypotension)
- ensure adequate oxygenation (avoid hypoxia)
- maintain cerebral perfusion (avoid cerebral ischemia)

Specific therapies include *nutritional modification,* such as appropriate energy supplements (e.g. intravenous lipid and amino acid supplements free of the offending precursor amino acids in MSUD). *Cofactor administration* will sometimes improve the function of a genetically defective metabolic pathway (e.g. vitamin B_{12} in some cases of methylmalonic aciduria, since adenosylcobalamin is a cofactor for L-methylmalonyl-CoA mutase).

Use of *alternate metabolic pathways* is another possibility: for example, administration of sodium benzoate in hyperammonemia diverts a toxic substrate to a benign, excretable form.

Long-term therapy of small molecule diseases

For many small molecule disorders, dietary modifications are used to maintain low levels of the toxic metabolites. For example, for MSUD patients, enough leucine, isoleucine, and valine are provided to allow normal growth by giving very small amounts of normal protein-containing foods

but avoiding excess of these amino acids which would be catabolized to form the toxic keto acids. An artificial formula including the other essential amino acids, vitamins, minerals and other trace nutrients is provided. Regular blood monitoring of amino acids is necessary. Normal or near-normal neurological outcome is possible for the well-managed patient, depending on the degree and duration of the initial encephalopathic episode, the severity of subsequent metabolic crises, and the quality of the long-term metabolic control.

ACUTE HEPATOCELLULAR DISEASE

ACUTE LIVER DISEASE IN THE NEWBORN

A few inborn errors may present with acute hepatic failure (Table 3.11.4). Galactosemia, hereditary fructose intolerance, and tyrosinemia type I generally first present in the newborn period or infancy, but symptoms may not appear until later. Hepatomegaly, jaundice (direct and indirect hyperbilirubinemia), abnormal coagulation (re-flecting severe impairment of hepatic synthetic functions), increased liver enzymes (reflecting hepatocellular damage), and hypoglycemia are often found. The renal Fanconi syndrome is a feature of these disorders as well as of Wilson disease, and is characterized by the impaired proximal renal tubular transport of glucose, phosphate, amino acids, protein, bicarbonate, electrolytes, and other solutes. Accurate diagnosis of these four diseases is important because they are treatable and because the child's family will need genetic counseling. Defects of the mitochondrial respiratory chain, fatty acid β-oxidation, and Niemann–Pick disease may also present with neonatal hepatic dysfunction.

Galactosemia

Galactosemic neonates often present with jaundice, hemolysis and/or Gram-negative sepsis, well before the metabolic diagnosis is suspected. Delayed treatment will result in intellectual disability:

- enzyme defect: galactose-1-phosphate uridyltransferase
- provoking substances: galactose-containing foods

TABLE 3.11.4 Genetic metabolic disorders causing hepatocellular disease

Disease	Defect	Onset of liver disease	Renal Fanconi syndrome	Other features	Specific laboratory tests
Galactosemia	Galactose-1-phosphate uridyl transferase (GALPUT) deficiency	Neonate only	Frequent	E. coli sepsis and hemolysis in newborns; cataracts; intellectual disability; ovarian failure	RBC screening test and enzyme assay
Fructose intolerance	Fructose-1,6-diphosphate aldolase deficiency	After fructose ingestion	Frequent	Vomiting; hypoglycemia; history of fructose ingestion must be actively sought	Enzyme assay in liver; mutation analysis
Tyrosinemia type I	Fumaryl acetoacetate hydrolase (FAH) deficiency	Any age, but esp. in neonates and infants	Frequent	Rickets	Succinylacetone in urine; elevation of α-fetoprotein
Alpha-1-antitrypsin [(α_1-AT)] deficiency	α_1-AT	Neonate only	None	Adult-onset emphysema	Pi typing of serum α_1-AT
Wilson disease	Liver-specific copper transporter protein	After about 6 years of age	Variable	Kayser–Fleischer ring; hemolytic anemia; extra-pyramidal disease in adolescence	Low plasma ceruloplasmin; elevated urine and liver copper

- accumulating substances: galactose, galactose 1-phosphate, galactitol
- abnormal screening tests: positive urine reducing substances (negative on specific urinary testing for glucose), newborn screening for RBC galactose metabolites, abnormal liver enzymes, coagulopathy
- definitive test: RBC enzyme assay
- acute treatment: supportive management and remove galactose from diet
- long-term treatment: exclusion of galactose from diet

Despite early diagnosis and good dietary compliance, subtle defects in intellectual function are often present, and primary or secondary ovarian failure occurs in more than 80% of affected females.

Hereditary fructose intolerance

Vomiting is the common presenting sign of fructose intolerance, and in the infant or small child is associated with hypoglycemia, gastrointestinal discomfort, failure to thrive, and rickets. It is important to take a careful dietary history, as ingestion of only small amounts of fructose or sucrose provokes symptoms in a young child. Older children develop an aversion to sweet foods:

- enzyme defect: fructaldolase B
- provoking substances: fructose-containing foods
- accumulating substances: fructose, fructose 1-phosphate
- abnormal screening tests: hypoglycemia, hyperuricemia, hypophosphatemia, abnormal liver enzymes, coagulopathy
- definitive tests: liver assay or mutation analysis
- acute treatment: supportive management and remove fructose from diet
- long-term treatment: exclusion of fructose from diet

Tyrosinemia

Patients with tyrosinemia type I may present with acute liver disease in the first month or later (even after 1 year), with chronic liver disease and rickets. Because the defect is in the tyrosine catabolic pathway, dietary phenylalanine and tyrosine restriction is needed, which improves the hepatic dysfunction in the short term:

- enzyme defect: fumarylacetoacetate hydrolase
- provoking substances: phenylalanine, tyrosine
- accumulating substances: succinylacetone
- abnormal screening tests: liver enzymes, coagulopathy, raised blood α-fetoprotein
- definitive tests: liver assay
- acute treatment:
  - supportive management
  - remove tyrosine and phenylalanine from diet
- long-term treatment
  - restriction of dietary phenylalanine and tyrosine
  - NTBC
  - liver transplantation

Liver transplantation offers the only cure at present. The drug 2-(2-nitro-4-trifluoromethylbenzoyl)-1,3-cyclohexanedione (NTBC) has been found to be very effective in improving renal tubular and hepatic function, and can be used in conjunction with dietary therapy to normalize blood tyrosine levels until liver transplantation is possible.

Alpha-1-antitrypsin deficiency

Alpha-1-antitrypsin is a major protease inhibitor and in the most common variant of this disease, a mutant polypeptide accumulates in the hepatocyte:

- enzyme defect: α1-antitrypsin
- provoking substances: none
- accumulating substances: α1-antitrypsin as inclusions within hepatocytes
- abnormal screening tests: liver enzymes, cholestatic jaundice, coagulopathy
- definitive tests: blood α1-antitrypsin Pi typing
- acute treatment: supportive management
- long-term treatment:
  - liver transplantation for cirrhosis
  - avoidance of cigarette smoke

  - α1-antitrypsin infusions for the pulmonary disease

Low plasma levels of functional α1-antitrypsin result in the unimpeded activity of neutrophil elastase in the lung, progressively destroying the alveoli, resulting in premature emphysema in adults. This disorder is often associated with cholestatic jaundice, and in most patients the liver disease improves without treatment, although about 5% progress to cirrhosis. Apart from hepatic transplantation, there is no treatment for the liver disease.

ACUTE LIVER DISEASE BEYOND THE NEWBORN PERIOD

Like tyrosinemia, hereditary fructose intolerance, Niemann–Pick disease, and α1-antitrypsin deficiency, Wilson's disease can present as either early acute or later chronic hepatopathy, but in contrast to them, it is rarely apparent before the age of 6 years, and neurologic disease may be the presenting problem:

- enzyme defect: liver-specific intracellular copper transporter protein
- provoking substances: copper
- accumulating substances: copper (within the liver)
- abnormal screening tests: liver enzymes, coagulopathy, hemolysis
- definitive tests: low blood ceruloplasmin, high urine copper excretion, increased hepatic copper, mutation analysis
- acute treatment:
  - supportive management
  - tetrathiomolybdate?
- long-term treatment:
  - penicillamine, zinc
  - liver transplantation for cirrhosis

Patients may present with acute disease in childhood with fulminant liver failure and hemolytic anemia, or more insidiously in the second or later decades with cirrhosis. Older individuals may initially have only extrapyramidal (rarely seen before the age of 12 years) or neuropsychiatric signs. The Kayser–Fleischer ring, a dull copper-coloured granular deposit at the limbus of the cornea, is seen in most but not all adults, but may be absent in up to a third of children presenting with acute liver disease.

CONCLUSION

With early and prompt diagnosis, specific and effective treatment for inborn errors that present with acute metabolic failure is often possible, with very gratifying short-term and long-term results. Families with affected children can be alerted to the risk of recurrence, through genetic counseling. In many instances, presymptomatic treatment of affected relatives, carrier testing, and prenatal diagnosis can be offered.

✔ KEY POINTS

➤ In newborn encephalopathy, to prevent death or permanent brain damage, perform screening tests and start appropriate treatment for a metabolic disorder while waiting for alternative diagnoses (e.g. sepsis) to be excluded

➤ The anion gap may remain normal until blood lactate concentration exceeds 6 mmol/L

➤ Suspect a metabolic disorder if a child has lactic acidosis without heart failure, shock or sepsis

➤ Immediate resuscitation includes securing the airway, breathing and circulation, providing fluid, electrolytes and glucose; correcting metabolic acidosis; and considering hemofiltration or dialysis and disease-specific therapy

➤ Management of the encephalopathy is largely supportive, with close attention to the maintenance of adequate cerebral perfusion pressure

FURTHER READING

1. Christodoulou J, McInnes RR. A clinical approach to inborn errors of metabolism. In: Rudolph AM, Kamei R, editors. Rudolph's fundamentals of pediatrics (2nd ed.). Stamford: Appleton & Lange; 1994; pp. 181–208
   − (*Practical approach to diagnosis and management*)

2. Saudubray JM, Ogier H, Charpentier C. Clinical approach to inherited metabolic diseases. In: Fernandes J, Saudubray JM, Van den Berghe G. (eds). Inborn metabolic diseases: diagnosis and treatment, 2nd ed. Berlin: Springer; 1994; pp. 3–39
   − (*Approach to differential diagnosis of clinical syndromes*)

3. Fernandes J, Saudubray JM. Diagnostic procedures: function tests and postmortem protocol. In: Fernandes J, Saudubray JM, Van den Berghe G. (eds). Inborn metabolic diseases: diagnosis and treatment, 2nd ed. Berlin: Springer; 1994; pp. 41–46
   − (*Very practical discussion of common biochemical tests, sampling procedures and interpretation used in diagnosis of metabolic disorders*)

4. Ogier de Baulny H, Saudubray JM. Emergency treatments. In: Fernandes J, Saudubray JM, Van den Berghe G. (eds). Inborn metabolic diseases: diagnosis and treatment, 2nd ed. Berlin: Springer; 1994; pp. 47–55
   − (*Brief review of emergency treatment: dietary, supportive and toxin removal*)

5. Saudubray JM, Charpentier C. Clinical phenotypes: diagnosis/algorithms. In: Scriver CR, Beaudet AL, Sly WS, Valle D, (eds). The metabolic and molecular bases of inherited disease, 7th ed. McGraw-Hill; 1995; pp. 327–400
   − (*Comprehensive discussion of the diagnosis of inborn errors according to their clinical and biochemical mode of presentation*)

6. Surtees RAH, Leonard JV. Metabolic encephalopathy in inborn errors of metabolism. In: Eyre JA. (ed) Coma. Clinical Paediatrics International practice and research. London: Baillière Tindall 1994; 2(1) 65–80
   − (*A practical review and outline of the two major elements of therapy, correction of the metabolic disturbance and management of the encephalopathy*)

7. Volpe JJ. Hyperammonemia and other disorders of amino acid metabolism (chapter 14) and: Disorders of organic acid metabolism (chapter 15). In: Volpe JJ. (ed) Neurology of the Newborn. 3rd ed. Philadelphia: W.B. Saunders. 1995 515–541 and 542–564
   − (*Detailed reviews from the stand point of the infant presenting in early life with data on metabolic consequences, neuropathology and clinical features plus acute therapy*)

3.12 Gastrointestinal illness

Andrew J. Macnab

ACUTE ABDOMEN

Severe abdominal pain, present for more than 6 hours, constitutes an 'acute abdomen'. In the newborn, acute abdominal pain, distention and vomiting frequently follow as a result of congenital abnormalities within the gastrointestinal tract or sepsis. In children, the most common lesion requiring surgery is acute appendicitis which must be differentiated from mesenteric adenitis.

The nature of the pain can be helpful. Intestinal distention produces colic which is intermittent. In contrast, pain due to infection tends to be continuous and made worse by movement, deep breathing, loud crying or palpation. Because of its embryological origin, the intestine generates pain that is felt in the midline initially, although localization often occurs as the process develops.

Pain of sudden onset suggests torsion or perforation. Pain from pancreatitis is often lessened when the child is sitting. Renal colic frequently radiates anteriorly and inferiorly to involve the scrotum and groin. In contrast, testicular pain is often referred to the umbilical area. Pain from inflammation of the lower surface of the diaphragm can radiate to the shoulder. Children with an organic cause (and the likelihood of needing surgery) are more inclined to keep their eyes open during abdominal palpation than those with an inorganic cause.

Absolute constipation (absence of stool or flatus) follows bowel obstruction and all peritonitis.

LABORATORY INVESTIGATIONS

Blood

Blood counts commonly show an elevated level of white blood cells (12–18×10^9/L, $12\,000$–$18\,000$/mm^3). A normal white cell count does not exclude appendicitis, although an elevated count with a predominance of polymorphs is usual.

Electrolytes, glucose, blood urea nitrogen (BUN) and creatinine, AST, ALT, alkaline phos-

phatase, amylase, and calcium should all be measured. Establishing the presence of acidosis or alkalosis and the electrolyte status, particularly of potassium, is important.

Urine

Urine samples should be sent for microscopy, culture and analysis.

Stools

A stool specimen is required for culture, and for occult blood testing.

Radiography

An abdominal X-ray series is required (supine and upright) and a chest film, to assess the gas pattern and exclude perforation, and because of the frequency of pneumonia as primary or secondary pathology.

Consider investigation of the urinary tract (e.g. intravenous pyelogram or ultrasound).

Other

Consider sickle cell testing where appropriate.

MANAGEMENT

Consider early discussion with surgical colleagues. An outline for the management of a child with an acute abdomen is shown in Table 3.12.1.

CAUSES OF ABDOMINAL PAIN

Appendicitis

Paraumbilical pain often begins suddenly and vomiting follows. Over a few hours the pain becomes localized in the right iliac fossa (one in four children only have pain in this location). Mild fever is common (39°C), stools may be normal, loose or con-

TABLE 3.12.1 **Management of the child with an acute abdomen**

Address ABC
Initiate care
- Vital signs
- Obtain i.v. access
- Give fluid bolus (crystalloid 10 ml/kg)
- Assess for signs of shock (treat or monitor for evolving signs)
- Pass nasogastric tube, keep child nil by mouth

Secondary survey
- Additional history
- Full physical examination (hydration, pain, associated symptoms or diseases, genitalia, rectal examination)
- Initial laboratory studies, plain X-rays

History of trauma (establish whether blunt or penetrating)
- Maintain circulation
- Discuss with surgeon (prior to giving analgesia)
- Consider CT scan (with contrast—see abdominal trauma)
- Unstable blunt or penetrating trauma—probably requires surgery, reassess for hypovolemia, crossmatch blood

Stable patient
- Maintain good i.v. access
- Serial vital signs
- Monitor physical status
- Consider other studies, therapy

Signs of peritonitis
- Discuss with surgeon
- Consider additional i.v. fluid bolus
- Consider antibiotic to cover gut flora (ampicillin, gentamicin, clindamycin)
- Repeat plain X-rays (after 6–8 hours)
- Measure serial abdominal girths

All patients
- Provide supportive care
- Monitor clinical and laboratory progress
- Treat underlying cause (surgical or medical)
- Consult appropriately
- Perform additional studies and laboratory tests (ultrasound scans, pregnancy tests, chest X-ray, as indicated)

stipated. Diarrhea or urinary symptoms and tenderness predominantly on deep palpation suggests an appendix that is retrocecal or pelvic in location (urine microscopy shows no pus cells). Children have a thin appendix wall and less developed omentum. Consequently, perforation produces generalized peritonitis, indicated by a rising pulse rate and white cell count above $12 \times 10^9/L$ (12 000/mm³).

Ileus

Ileus is a loss of effective persistalsis in the absence of physical obstruction. Abdominal distention is caused where intraluminal fluid and air accumulate, vomiting and decreased or absent bowel sounds can follow. Trauma, sepsis, surgery or hypokalemia are common causes.

Intussusception

Intussusception is characterized by sudden, initially brief episodes of pain occurring with relative regularity (child often screams out and pulls up legs). Between pains, the child appears comfortable. This pain usually begins before vomiting occurs. Normal or slightly loose stools may precede the characteristic 'redcurrant jelly' stools (for 6–12 hours after pains begin). The abdomen is rigid and tender only during attacks. Between episodes of pain a right upper quadrant mass (in the outline of a sausage) is often felt associated with a relative emptiness of the right upper quadrant. The rectum feels empty. Blood is usually present (although occasionally children have no bleeding). This condition is most common in infants (less than 2 years old). Ultrasonography is diagnostic, as are lower gastrointestinal contrast studies which can also accomplish hydrostatic reduction.

Volvulus

Volvulus occurs with twists or kinks of the bowel which compromise the vasculature of the mesentery. In older children, pain is often generated by activity or excitement (e.g. while watching a sports event or riding on a train). Initially, pain can be intermittent but once continuous is dull and associated with vomiting (bilious) and signs of obstruction. In both conditions, fluid shifts and bleeding can lead to presentation with severe hypovolemia, necrotic bowel can be present and also superimposed sepsis (antibiotics should include coverage for anaerobic pathogens).

Urinary tract infections

Urinary tract infections are a common cause of abdominal pain, vomiting, fever, abdominal distention, diarrhea and septicemia. Frequency of micturition is often noted. In infants, poor feeding and vomiting may lead to dehydration and infrequent passage of urine. Older children do sometimes report dysuria but it is less frequent than in adults. Children with appendicitis often have a phase of urinary frequency in the evolution of their disease and microscopic hematuria is common.

Trauma

If the acute abdomen follows trauma, establish whether there is blunt or penetrating injury (Ch. 4.4).

VOMITING

Vomiting is a common symptom in children as it is a manifestation of a variety of infectious conditions both inside and outside the gastrointestinal tract including gastroenteritis, urinary tract infection, otitis media and meningitis. Moreover, vomiting may be the principal symptom for some of the rare inherited disorders of intermediate metabolism, or it may be a sign of increased intracranial pressure from hydrocephalus or a brain tumor.

The common causes of vomiting are shown in Table 3.12.2. It is important to distinguish whether the vomiting is bilious or nonbilious. The former is of greater concern as it suggests obstruction in the small bowel distal to the second stage of the duodenum. The higher the level of obstruction, the more likely vomiting is to occur with the onset of obstruction. In upper small bowel obstruction, as with other causes of obstruction proximal to the ampulla of Vater, hypochloremic alkalosis results (often with hypokalemia). With obstruction below the ampulla of Vater, vomiting of alkaline secretions results in acidosis and hypokalemia. Where the lower bowel is obstructed, although abdominal distention may appear over a matter of hours, vomiting may not develop for several days. The presence of fecal material in vomit suggests 'low' colonic obstruction.

In pyloric stenosis, vomiting is nonbilious, forceful, projectile and occurs abruptly during or immediately following a feed. The condition usually presents in infants at 2 months of age. Visible gastric peristalsis (the appearance of a golf ball moving under the skin over the stomach area) often precedes vomiting. A 'pyloric tumor' is most easily felt with the left hand by an examiner on the left side of an infant who is actively feeding. Ultrasound studies confirm the diagnosis. The treatment is surgical pyloromyotomy.

TABLE 3.12.2 **Causes of vomiting**

Acute		Chronic
Gastrointestinal	**Nongastrointestinal**	**Gastrointestinal**
Congenital anomalies:	CNS:	Gastroesophageal reflux
• atresia	• raised ICP	
• tracheoesophageal fistula	• drugs	Chronic mechanical obstruction
• malrotation and volvulus	• intoxicants	
• pyloric stenosis		Motility disorders
	Urinary infections	
Meconium ileus		Intestinal inflammation:
	Systemic infections	• celiac disease
Intussusception	Pneumonia (lobar)	• Crohn's disease
	Diabetic ketosis	• infections
Infection:		• duodenal ulcer
• gastroenteritis		• gastritis
• peritonitis		• gastric ulcer
• appendicitis		
• hepatitis		Other:
• necrotizing enterocolitis		• anorexia, bulimia
		• cyclic vomiting
		• fecal impaction

DIARRHEA

The normal stools of a breastfed infant are unformed, can be passed as frequently as hourly and may be green in colour. Once lactation has become established (third to fifth day) relatively short gut transit times and frequent stools are common. By the end of the first month of age stool frequency has decreased (once every 1–3 days) and stools are of a pasty consistency. Diarrhea is defined as an increase in the stool volume and frequency from the individual's normal baseline. Gastroenteritis is rare in the exclusively breastfed child but any infant may have loose stools at the start of an acute infection (e.g. urinary, respiratory or ear infection). Loose stools are also common during antibiotic therapy owing to disturbance of the normal flora.

The majority of children with acute diarrhea will have an infectious (usually viral) cause and their illness will be self-limiting. An acute diarrhea may last for 2 weeks. Diarrhea for longer than 2 weeks is defined as chronic. Table 3.12.3 lists the causes of acute and chronic diarrhea.

The priorities in assessment are recognition of severe degrees of dehydration, electrolyte disturbance or other life-threatening complications. The smaller the child, the lower its ability to tolerate fluid loss. The nature of the stools should be checked by the clinician. Taking the temperature rectally or performing a rectal examination often stimulates the evacuation of a fresh stool. *Note—* profusely watery stools may be mistaken for urine, particularly by parents.

It is important to determine whether the diarrhea is grossly bloody. Bloody diarrhea suggests a colitis which may have an infectious, allergic or vasculitic etiology. The infectious causes include *Shigella, Salmonella, Yersinia, Campylobacter* or *Escherichia coli.* Rotaviral gastroenteritis never results in bloody diarrhea. Other conditions to consider include Henoch–Schönlein purpura and hemolytic–uremic syndrome.

Cryptosporidium infection is most common in healthy infants and children from daycare. *Campylobacter* and *Giardia* can be acquired from pets. *Clostridium difficile* infection usually follows antibiotic therapy a few weeks earlier. Food-borne toxins and pathogens (*Staphylococcus aureus,*

TABLE 3.12.3 Causes of diarrhea

Acute diarrhea
- Ischemia
  - anoxia
  - infarction
- Local infections (noninvasive)
  - rotavirus
  - adenovirus
  - *Giardia lamblia*
  - *Cryptosporidium*
  - *Escherichia coli*
- Systemic infections (invasive or toxigenic)
  - *Campylobacter*
  - *Salmonella*
  - *Shigella*
  - *Yersinia*
  - *E. coli*
  - *Clostridium difficile*

Chronic diarrhea and failure to thrive
- Mucosal
  - postinfectious enteritis
  - cow's protein allergy
  - celiac disease
  - immunodeficiency
  - acrodermatitis enteropathica
  - congenital villous atrophy
  - microvillus inclusion disease
  - abetalipoproteinemia
- Intraluminal
  - pancreatic insufficiency
  - bile salt deficiency
  - CHO enzyme deficiencies
- Secretory
  - infectious toxins
  - neuroblastoma
  - carcinoids
  - Zollinger–Ellison syndrome
  - laxative abuse
  - congenital chloride losing diarrhea
  - endocrinopathies

Clostridium perfringens) commonly cause symptoms on the day of ingestion; *Staphylococcus* gives violent vomiting 1–6 hours after ingestion, *Clostridium* colicky abdominal pain and watery diarrhea 12–18 hours after ingestion. Some fish (e.g. tuna, mackerel) contain a material (scombroid) which causes gastrointestinal tract disturbance with superimposed signs of histamine toxicity (urticaria, angioedema, bronchospasm, flushing and sometimes blisters on the oral mucosa).

Rashes (macular, papular) can occur in viral gastroenteritis, and *Shigella* and *Salmonella* infection.

Typhoid has a typical (rose spot) rash. Joint pains may occur with *Campylobacter, Shigella* and *Yersinia.* Seizures may be the presenting feature of illness due to *Shigella* (secondary to a neurotoxin). Pain (similar to that of mesenteric adenitis) often complicates *yersinia* infection (secondary to ileitis).

Physical examination requires airway, breathing and circulation to be addressed, and the issues of potential hypovolemia and hydration status (Table 3.12.4) need particularly careful assessment (including vital signs, weight, state of the mucous membranes, fontanelle, skin turgor, capillary refill and presence or absence of tears). Within the secondary survey, the full physical examination addresses pain, associated symptoms or diseases, and includes examination of the genitalia and rectum. Assess the severity of the child's overall condition. Severe dehydration, the presence of shock, peritonitis, gross elevation of body temperature, associated respiratory difficulty or signs of trauma make the nature of the child's condition potentially more critical.

MANAGEMENT

The management of infants with mild dehydration includes fluid replacement with oral rehydration solutions and rapid reintroduction of starchy foods. Breastfed infants with mild diarrhea should continue to breastfeed. Infants with moderate to severe dehydration should receive intravenous rehydration over 4–6 hours and feeding should then resume. In most infants and children with bacterial enteritis the disease has a self-limited course and does not require antibiotic therapy. In more severe cases, treatment with the therapeutic agents listed in Table 3.12.5 may be required.

INGESTION OF FOREIGN BODIES

The majority of ingested foreign bodies are swallowed and go through the gastrointestinal tract without difficulty. Sometimes, however, they will lodge at a point of narrowing within the esophagus. Some objects require removal and occasionally complications such as perforation occur. The three areas of functional narrowing in the esophagus are:

- inferior to the cricopharyngeal muscle
- at the aortic arch
- just proximal to the diaphragm

Simultaneous aspiration of material into the upper airway can occur and a choking spell frequently precedes presentation. Foreign bodies in the esophagus or the airway can cause secondary dysfunction in the other structure from swelling or the overflow of secretions. Hot-dog segments are one of the most common foreign bodies to cause problems, particularly if they are superheated in a microwave. A local burn with edema and narrowing can develop, and even when the foreign body is in the esophagus, the thermal trauma that results in the upper airway can produce signs indistinguishable from epiglottitis.

Coins in the esophagus require endoscopic removal before localized pressure necrosis develops (a fistula can result). On PA X-ray the flat surface is seen (whereas in the airway the edge of the coin is seen). Small alkaline batteries can cause pressure necrosis or a burn. These batteries are particularly dangerous in the esophagus and require urgent removal. Clues usually come from the history, but in a smaller, symptomatic child where an object has to be identified, radiological studies can be helpful. Coins appear flat and have a sharp edge. In contrast, the PA view of a battery suggests concentric double densities, and on lateral view rounded edges are seen with a step-off evident where the cathode and anode join.

Foreign bodies that pass into the stomach generally pass through the gastrointestinal tract without problem.

The signs and symptoms listed below suggest that a foreign body remains in the esophagus:

- gagging
- reluctance or refusal to feed
- increased salivation
- drooling
- retching
- fear or discomfort associated with swallowing
- complaints of feeling 'something stuck' (in older children)
- retrosternal pain radiating through to the back

TABLE 3.12.4 Signs and symptoms of dehydration according to severity

Signs or symptoms	Mild		Moderate		Severe	
	Infants	Children	Infants	Children	Infants	Children
Fluid deficit (ml/kg)	50	50	100	60	150	90
Body weight loss (%)	5	3	10	6	15	9
Skin:						
turgor	Poor		Doughy		Tenting	
color	Pale		Gray		Mottled	
temperature	Cool		Cool		Cold	
Mucous membranes	Dry		Very dry, no tears		Parched	
Urine:						
output	May be ↓		Oliguric		Anuric/oliguric	
specific gravity	May be ↑		↑		↑↑	
Laboratory studies:						
BUN	WNL		↑		↑↑	
Na⁺	WNL		↑		↑↑	

pH	WNL		Acidosis		Extreme acidosis	
Vital signs:						
HR	May be ↑		↑		↑↑	
BP	WNL		↓		↓↓	
General appearance	Sleepy eyes slightly sunken		Sunken fontanelles, sunken eyes, lethargic		Sunken fontanelles, obtunded, shocky	

WNL, within normal limits
From: Brown PA, Blayney F, Brown CA, Gregg-Evans K, editors. Pediatric intensive care nursing. Aspen; Rockville: 1989

TABLE 3.12.5 Therapeutic agents for bacterial gastroenteritis

Infective organism	Drug
Campylobacter	Erythromycin 10 mg/kg per dose every 6 hours (use aminoglycosides i.v. in critical illness)
Clostridium	Vancomycin 5–10 mg/kg per dose orally 6-hourly OR metronidazole 7–10 mg/kg per dose orally 8-hourly
E. coli (pathogenic)	Trimethoprim-sulfamethaxozole (co-trimoxazole) 5 mg/kg per dose i.v. or orally 12-hourly Ampicillin is an alternative for sensitive pathogens
Giardia	Metronidazole 5 mg/kg per day orally 8-hourly OR quinacrine (mepacrine) 2 mg/kg per dose orally 8-hourly
Salmonella[a]	Ampicillin 50–75 mg/kg per dose 6-hourly i.v. or i.m. Trimethoprim-sulfamethoxazole (co-trimoxazole) orally as an alternative Cefotaxime 25 mg/kg per dose i.v. 6-hourly may be required for critical illness *Note*—neonates, children with meningitis or osteomyelitis are special cases where different dosage or prolonged treatment may be required
Shigella	Trimethoprim-sulfamethoxazole (co-trimoxazole) 5 mg/kg per dose orally or i.v. 12-hourly (ampicillin is an alternative)

[a]Not all children with Salmonella infection require treatment. The group at risk are those likely to develop invasive disease, e.g. small infants less than 3 months of age, children with immune compromise, malignancies, splenic dysfunction, or hemoglobinopathies, those with congenital heart disease at risk for endocarditis, and those likely to have enteric fever.

MANAGEMENT

Coexisting airway compromise will require immediate intervention to secure the airway. In general, it is preferable to examine such children under anesthesia, in the operating room wherever possible. In less urgent cases, radiology will often identify the site of lodgment.

Keep children 'nil by mouth' pending radiological studies (PA view of the neck, chest, abdomen and base of skull). Consider endoscopy for the items described above and pointed objects capable of causing perforation. Such children should have endoscopy while intubated in the operating room.

STRESS ULCERS

Stress ulceration occurs in association with major underlying illness—severe burns, sepsis, shock, major trauma (particularly head injury), prolonged surgery or serious illness in neonates. Drug therapy (e.g. aspirin, NSAIDs and high-dose corticosteroids) can also cause erosive gastritis. Stress ulceration is seen in all age groups; it can present with severe hemorrhage or perforation. There is no association with *Helicobacter pylori*. The diagnosis needs to be considered in any child with hematemesis or blood in the gastric aspirate associated with major illness. Lesions can occur anywhere in the gastrointestinal tract, the duodenum being more commonly affected than the stomach. The pattern of involvement varies from superficial erosive lesions to deep ulceration. The mechanism is unclear but increased acidity in the stomach and compromise of normal protective mechanisms probably contribute.

MANAGEMENT

1. Acute management—provide oxygen, obtain intravenous access, restore the circulation and consider replacing blood lost.
2. Give antacids (aluminum hydroxide/ magnesium hydroxide) 0.5 ml/kg per dose (to a maximum of 30 ml per dose) every 2–4 hours via a nasogastric tube, or ranitidine 3 mg/kg per dose i.v. every 8 hours.

Prophylactic treatment should be provided for the following group of patients to prevent secondary gastric hemorrhage from stress ulceration adding to the morbidity of the underlying condition:

- patients with:
  - burns
  - sepsis
  - shock
  - major head trauma
- critically ill neonates
- postoperative patients after major surgery
- children receiving high-dose steroids, NSAIDs or large doses of aspirin
- any critically ill or injured child

GASTROINTESTINAL HEMORRHAGE

> Gastrointestinal hemorrhage is a common and potentially life-threatening emergency

Definitions:

- hematemesis: vomiting of blood (bright red or 'coffee grounds')
- hematochezia: passage of bright red blood in stool
- Melena: passage of (altered) dark red or black blood in stool, or normal-looking stools that test positive for blood (guaiac test)
- 'redcurrant jelly' gelatinous cherry-red material in stool

SITE OF BLEEDING

Most children (50%) bleed from the colon and/or rectum, 33% from the small intestine and 10% from a lesion proximal to the ligament of Treitz. Blood shortens gut transit time (potent cathartic). Bleeding causing melena and hematemesis usually originates above the ligament of Treitz, but if transit time is delayed small bowel bleeds can cause melena. Hematochezia usually signifies bleeding distal to the terminal ileum. 'Redcurrant jelly' stools occur with intussusception or Meckel's diverticulum.

Stools will also test positive if they contain swallowed blood, e.g. after nasopharyngeal trauma, epistaxis, or in a newborn who has swallowed maternal blood (intrapartum or from a cracked nipple).

Following anoxic damage to the bowel mucosa (e.g. in near-drowning), occult positive stools are often passed that are loose, blue-gray in color, foul-smelling and may contain sloughed tissue.

Not all stool coloration is pathological. Stools that test negative for blood but are red or black in color can follow ingestion of beets, tomatoes, food coloring or wax crayons, or blueberries, prunes, iron, charcoal, licorice or bismuth, respectively.

EVALUATION OF A CHILD WITH GASTROINTESTINAL HEMORRHAGE

Determine the site, cause (Table 3.12.6) and extent of bleeding, and whether it is ongoing at the time of the evaluation. Check the adequacy of respiration and for cardiovascular compromise. Give immediate fluid resuscitation if necessary. Crossmatch blood, check coagulation status and hemoglobin level. When the patient is stabilized, pass a nasogastric tube and determine the site of bleeding. In patients with small amounts of bleeding or with occult positive stools, proceed as follows:

- history:
  - pattern of bleeding, color, character
  - frequency
  - acute or chronic
  - associated pain
  - syncope, dizziness, tachycardia
  - other systemic diseases
  - family history/history of bleeding disorder
  - medication history
  - social history
- physical examination:
  - vital signs
  - pallor
  - abdominal pain or mass
  - hepatosplenomegaly
  - rectal examination
  - cutaneous signs
- laboratory studies
  - complete blood count with platelets
  - reticulocyte count
  - electrolytes
  - hepatic and renal function tests
  - coagulation profile
  - sample to blood bank (for group and crossmatch)
  - consider blood gas and urine analysis
- special studies:
  - nasogastric tube (blood in aspirate—bleeding proximal to ligament of Treitz)
  - barium studies of the upper or lower bowel
  - upper or lower endoscopy (nuclear medicine)
  - Meckel's scan *Note*—false negative with absence of gastric mucosal tissue
  - arteriography
  - exploratory laparotomy

TABLE 3.12.6 Causes of major bleeding

Upper gastrointestinal tract	Lower gastrointestinal tract

- Lesions in pharynx
- Esophageal varices
- Esophagitis
- Gastritis
- Ulcers (gastric, duodenal)
- Mallory–Weiss tear
- Vascular lesion
- Foreign body, mass
	- Infections (*Campylobacter, Salmonella, Shigella, E. coli, Yersinia*)
	- Meckel's diverticulum
	- Colitis (ulcerative, Crohn's, infections, ischemic, chemical, cow's milk or soya protein)
	- Vascular lesion (hemangioma)
	- Mass (polyps, duplication, tumors, foreign body)
	- Intussusception, volvulus
	- Trauma:
	   – hemolytic-uremic syndrome, Hirschsprung's disease (colitis)
	   – vitamin K deficiency
	   – anoxia

TREATMENT

Specific therapeutic measures include:

- secure airway if necessary
- elevate the (autotransfusion) legs
- replace intravascular volume with crystalloid (two i.v. lines)
- type and crossmatch for packed cells or whole blood
- Consider:
  - CVP line
  - urinary catheter
  - gastric lavage to monitor ongoing hemorrhage
  - H$_2$-blockers
  - vitamin K (5–10 mg i.v. or i.m.)
  - endoscopic coagulation
  - Sengstaken–Blakemore tube
  - intravenous vasopressin
  - intraarterial embolization
  - surgery

MANAGEMENT OF MASSIVE BLEEDING

> Massive gastrointestinal hemorrhage is a life-threatening emergency: emergency treatment must precede diagnostic evaluation

Priorities for management of bleeding:

- brief history (extent and nature of bleeding, previous episodes, bleeding disorder)
- vital signs
- vascular access and replacement of vascular volume
- laboratory studies (complete blood count, liver function tests, coagulation studies, crossmatch)
- nasogastric tube
- full history and physical examination
- transfusion and intravascular support
- determination of probable cause

Specific interventions

Peptic disease:

- endoscopy

- antacids (0.5 ml/kg per dose, hourly); keep gastric pH above 4 in acute bleeds
- H$_2$-blockers
- sulcrafate (not during acute bleeding)
- if bleeding is unremitting consider:
  - endoscopic coagulation or injection
  - surgical repair or resection

Varices:

- octreotide
- vasopressin
  - initial dose 20–40 μg per 1.73 m^2 over 20 min i.v., diluted in 5% dextrose
  - infusion (to follow) 0.1 μg per /1.73 m^2 per min
  - side-effects include increased BP, arrhythmia, oliguria, tissue necrosis
- endoscopic sclerotherapy or band ligation
- Sengstaken–Blakemore tube (tamponade)
- if bleeding is unremitting, consider:
  - emergency portosystemic shunt
  - esophageal devascularization

Mallory–Weiss tear:

- vascular anomaly
- endoscopic ablation

Surgical intervention

Indications for surgery in gastrointestinal hemorrhage are:

- Meckel's diverticulum
- necrotic bowel
- intussusception (failed hydrostatic reduction in children > 2 years)
- duplication cyst
- bowel neoplasm
- arteriovenous malformation
- massive life-threatening bleed

In absence of a diagnosis consider the intraoperative bowel washout (via appendectomy) with colonoscopy to locate lower bowel bleeding site.

CONTROVERSIES IN CARE

Nasogastric lavage (with 0.9% saline) to control bleeding is controversial. Theoretically, iced fluid reduces gastric blood flow but can rapidly lower a small child's core temperature and may compromise platelet aggregation. A nasogastric tube can be passed when there are esophageal varices and is valuable to determine the extent and site of upper gastrointestinal bleeding, monitor pH and administer antacids. *Note*—constipation follows the use of aluminum-based products, diarrhea follows magnesium-based products.

FURTHER READING

1. Gray DWR, Dixon JM, Collin J. The closed eyes sign! An aid to diagnosing non-specific abdominal pain. Brit Med J 1988; 297: 837

2. Reynolds SL. Missed appendicitis in a pediatric emergency department. Ped Emerg Care 1993; 9(1): 1–3

3. Stevenson RJ, Ziegler MM. Abdominal pain unrelated to trauma. Pediatr Rev 1993; 14(8): 302–311

4. Cochran EB, Phelps SJ, Tolley EA, Stidham EL. Prevalence and risk factors for upper gastro-intestinal tract bleeding in critically ill pediatrics patients. Crit Care Med 1992; 20: 1519–1523

–   (*Four papers addressing specific aspects of gastrointestinal disease in children*)

5. Roy CC, Silverman A, Alagille D. Pediatric clinical gastroenterology, 4th ed. St. Louis: Mosby; 1995

–   (*A comprehensive text for in-depth topic review*)

Environmental emergencies

4

4.1 Burns

Russell Taylor

Extensive burn injuries (greater than 40% body surface area) in children occur infrequently in Western countries. Different mechanisms of injury are characteristic of different ages:

- toddlers sustain scald injuries from incidents in the home: especially from the spilling of hot fluids on the face, neck, chest and arms, and from accidental or nonaccidental immersion in bathrooms and laundries
- older children and adolescents burn themselves in many ways, usually involving the careless use of matches and petroleum products, and occasionally the mixing of chemicals to produce unstable explosives

Although most burns are accidental, it is important (particularly in younger children) to consider the possibility of nonaccidental injury. Factors that may suggest this include:

- delay in presentation
- an account of the incident that changes or is incompatible with the clinical pattern of injury

In these circumstances, medical social workers should be involved early, for further social assessment.

Irrespective of the mechanism of injury, the severity of the burn is determined by the percentage of body surface area burned, the depth, and the anatomical site of injury. Survival in children is expected in burns of up to 80% of body surface area, but the complications of management and the likelihood of long-term physical and psychological sequelae increase with increasing burn surface area and according to the anatomic distribution and depth of the burn.

Fluid, electrolytes and protein are lost from the circulation at the site of the burn, and elsewhere in the body. There is also increased evaporative loss as a result of skin damage. Losses at the burn site are the result of increased capillary permeability, due both to direct injury and to production and release of mediators such as histamine, thromboxane and cytokines by the burn wound. The hypothalamic stress response is activated by afferent nerve stimulation: ACTH is released from the anterior pituitary gland, increasing glucocorticoid and aldosterone production, and increased amounts of antidiuretic hormone are released from the posterior pituitary. The effect of these hormones is to retain salt and water within the intravascular space and to maintain the circulating blood volume.

HYPERMETABOLIC RESPONSE

Burn injury and the resulting pain stimulate the sympathetic nervous system to release catecholamines from the adrenal medulla, which in turn stimulates hepatic glycogenolysis and gluconeogenesis. Glucocorticoid released by ACTH stimulation also causes the breakdown of skeletal muscle protein to amino acids, which become the precursors in the gluconeogenic pathway. Catecholamines also stimulate lipolysis in adipose tissue, increasing the plasma concentration of free fatty acids.

Nutritional support of the hypermetabolic state is essential to ensure efficient wound healing in these patients. Protein catabolism cannot be reversed by increasing amino acid availability alone. It can be reversed by anabolic agents, such as growth hormone and insulin-like growth factor 1 (IGF-1). Hormone treatment significantly improves wound healing in severely burned children. Supplementation with amino acid and vitamins, specifically arginine and vitamins A, B and C, provides optimal nutritional support for the healing burn wound.

FIRST AID

The child's clothing must be removed immediately, the flames smothered and cold water (*never* ice or ice slurry) applied to the burned area by compress or by immersion in a bowl for 10–20 minutes. This dramatically reduces the pain of a burn.

ASSESSMENT

HISTORY

It is important to document:

- the *time of injury*, because the time elapsed since the patient was burned will affect the rate of intravenous fluid resuscitation
- the *causative agent*, e.g. scald, flame, contact or chemical
- the *circumstances* of the burn:
  - in flame burns in particular, it is important to record whether the injury occurred in an open or enclosed space, e.g. car or home, and whether there is a significant risk of smoke or toxic fume inhalation (Ch. 4.2)
  - in scald injury, it is important to detemine, if possible, the water temperature and the duration of exposure (Fig. 4.1.1)
- *First aid:* if you are the first point of contact, it is important to determine what first aid has occurred, e.g.
  - for how long was cold water used?
  - was ice inadvertently used, with the possibility of cold injury?
- *previous medical treatment:*
  - what fluids have been administered since the injury, and in what volumes?
  - what drugs, including analgesics, have been given: what doses, and by what route?
  - past medical history, current medication and immunization record

EXAMINATION

The child with major burns should be examined in a warm room and the whole body exposed. The child's airway, breathing and circulation are assessed and rapidly resuscitated. A general assessment of the patient should be made for evidence of hypovolemia and shock, i.e. pallor, sweating, cool mottled extremities or disorientation. In general terms, the younger the child, the more likely shock is to occur for a given extent of burn. The respiratory system (including inhalation burn injury, Ch. 4.2) and conscious state are assessed. The child is examined rapidly but carefully for signs of other injuries, as children may suffer falls or be struck by debris during fires. Vital signs including heart rate, blood pressure, respiratory rate, mucosal color (or Hb saturation), rectal temperature, conscious state (e.g. Glasgow coma scale score), and pupil size and reaction are recorded on arrival and half-hourly.

Estimation of burn surface area

The adult formula (the 'rule of nines') is not applicable to children, because the proportions con-

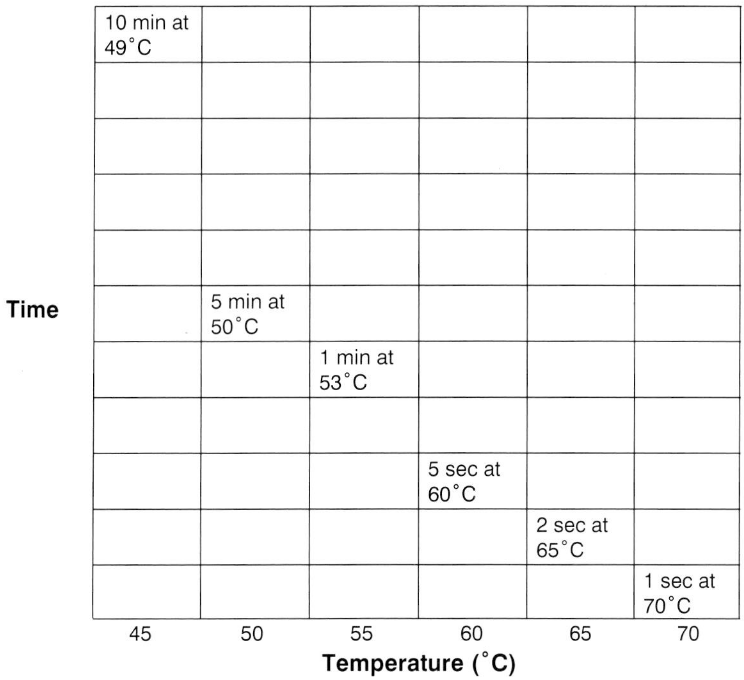

Figure 4.1.1 Duration of exposure to hot water needed to cause full-thickness burns

tributed by the head and limbs vary at different ages. The burn area should be recorded accurately on a body chart, and the area calculated with aid of the Lund–Browder chart (Fig. 4.1.2). In practice, the extent of the burn is rarely underestimated, but overestimation is common and frequently leads to excessive fluid resuscitation.

Assessment of burn depth

Burn depth can be very difficult to assess particularly in a scald injury, as the depth tends to vary within the injured area.

Epidermal burns

Epidermal burns are superficial and painful: they may just be areas of erythema or minor blistering.

Dermal burns

The distinction between superficial dermal burns and deep dermal burns can only be made definitely after 10–14 days. Deeper burns are usually less painful and do not blanch with pressure. A superficial dermal burn is usually erythematous, moist, blanches to pressure and, if sensation is tested (this is not routinely done), will be very sensitive.

Full-thickness burns

Full-thickness burns usually occur with flame and contact burn injury, although a severe and prolonged scald injury can also result in complete skin loss down to the subcutaneous fat, and sometimes fascia, muscle and bone. Muscle and bone involvement is more commonly seen with electrical burn injury.

BURNS OF SPECIFIC BODY AREAS

FACIAL BURNS

In a child with severe burns to the face, it is important to consider whether there has been any airway burn and if an artificial airway should be established before swelling makes tracheal intubation or tracheostomy impossible (Ch. 4.2).

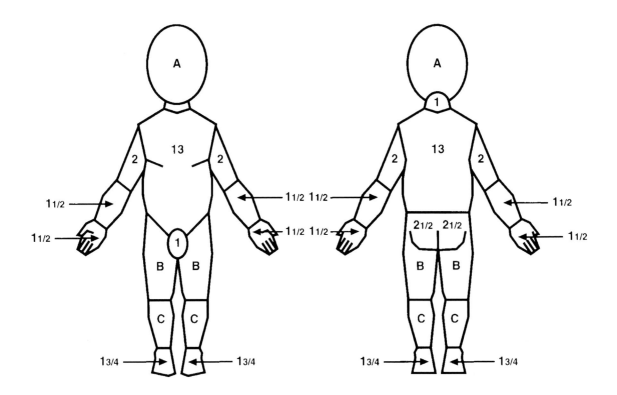

Areas affected by growth: % body surface area

Age in years	0	1	5	10	15
A 1/2 of head	91/2	81/2	61/2	51/2	41/2
B 1/2 of one thigh	23/4	31/4	4	41/4	41/2
C 1/2 of one leg	21/2	21/2	23/4	3	31/4

Figure 4.1.2 Lund–Browder calculation of burn surface area

CIRCUMFERENTIAL BURNS

For circumferential limb and trunk burns, escharotomy should be considered if the peripheral circulation to the limb is jeopardized, or if the respiratory excursion is impeded. Although these procedures are usually performed at a specialist burn center, delays in transfer or long transfer times may necessitate early escharotomy at the initial receiving institution. Escharotomy is only required for full-thickness burns, so no anesthesia is needed as the tissue is without sensation. The incision should be made in the midaxillary line (for chest burns) from the proximal to the distal end of the constricting eschar. For limb burns, the incision is made in the medial and lateral line of the limb and of the digits, including across joints. The incision is made down to living tissue: usually this means only down to subcutaneous fat, deep enough to allow the edges of the wound to gape. It is not necessary to incise the deep fascia unless a compartment syndrome has developed or the burn is very deep (e.g. an electrical burn).

PERINEAL BURNS

For severe perineal burns, early urinary catheterization is essential. It provides accurate estimation of urinary output and is much easier to perform before perineal swelling occurs. A fine balloon catheter of Silastic material should be used. If no Silastic catheter is available and the transfer time is long (several hours), other types of catheter may have to be used, with the risk of later urethral stricture.

EYES

In the presence of a facial burn, it is important to document whether any damage has occurred to the eye before the eyelid swells, making examination impossible. The examination should be performed by an ophthalmologist if available and includes staining the conjunctiva with fluorescein and using ultraviolet light to exclude corneal ulcers. If mucosal injury to the cornea is found, antibiotic ointment should be instilled. It is important to reassure the family and the patient that the edema will subside in the ensuing 2–3 days, and that it is very rare to have any significant residual eye injury.

AIRWAY OR RESPIRATORY BURN AND SMOKE INHALATION

The presence of an airway burn (Ch. 4.2) should be assumed in a child who was burned in a closed space such as a room or a motor vehicle, or if there is singed nasal hair, intraoral or circumoral burns, or an obvious voice-change. If there is any doubt, oxygen (8 L/min) should be given by mask, before and during transfer.

TRANSFER OF A BURNED PATIENT

The transfer critera for a patient should be discussed directly with a pediatric burn surgeon, or with the physician in charge of the pediatric emergency transfer service (Ch. 1.5). It is usually recommended that any child with greater than 5% partial or full-thickness burn should be transferred to a tertiary facility.

During transfer, most burns can be covered with a foam transport dressing (if available) or with a clean sheet. The child should be wrapped in a space blanket to prevent heat loss during the transfer.

The longer the transport time, the more extensive the resuscitation measures needed before departure. All children should have intravenous or intraosseous access established prior to transfer and fluid resuscitation commenced (see below). Morphine by repeated small i.v. bolus may be titrated against the child's pain. Doses of morphine 0.025 mg/kg i.v. are repeated as necessary to a maximum of 0.15 mg/kg 4-hourly, although in severely distressed children this maximum dose may be exceeded.

A nasogastric tube is only required when the child's conscious state is impaired. A urinary catheter should only be inserted if this can be done under aseptic conditions. All observation sheets, fluid balance charts and drug charts should be sent with the patient.

HOSPITAL MANAGEMENT

RESUSCITATION

Intravenous access

A peripheral venous catheter should be inserted when the burned area is greater than 10% of body surface area. It should be located in unburned skin, but in children with extensive burns this is not always possible. A cannula placed through burned skin should be secured with a suture. In shocked infants and children, intravenous access may sometimes be very difficult, and an intraosseous needle can be used during the early stages of resuscitation (Ch. 6.1), but an intravenous cannula should always be inserted and secured before long transfers once the veins are filled by the initial resuscitation, as intraosseous cannulas can be less reliable during transport.

Fluid regimens

There are many different formulae available to calculate the resuscitation volumes required. The following regimen (Fig. 4.1.3) is a reliable guide to a child's requirements. The volume of fluid in ml (50% isotonic serum albumin and 50% Hartmann's solution) for the first 24 hours is determined by formula 1 (see box).

Formula I Estimation of 24-hour fluid volume.
fluid (ml) = 3 × body weight (kg) × body surface area burned (%)

Half of that volume should be given in the first 8 hours from the time of injury and the other half over the next 16 hours. This formula is only intended as a guide. The amount may have to be altered according to the urine output and the warmth and color of unburned skin, since over- or underestimation of the area or depth of burn will cause over or underestimation of the resuscitation fluid requirements. In addition to this fluid, the child's maintenance fluid requirements (Ch. 2.10) are given as 0.45% saline in 5% dextrose. Urine output should be measured to assess the response to fluid resuscitation. In children, the target is 0.75–1.0 ml of urine per kg body weight per hour.

Name _____   Date of birth _____

% of BSA burned _____   Time of burn (24 hour) clock _____

Weight in kg _____   Time IV commenced _____

Date _____

Burn resuscitation 3 x kg x % = _____ ml*	1st 24 hours after the burn	1st 8 hours after the burn	2nd 8 hours after the burn	3rd 8 hours after the burn
Type of fluid: a. 50% as 5% albumin b. 50% as Hartmanns or normal saline. Both fluids given concurrently	_____ ml _____ ml	1/2 of 24 hour volume _____ ml _____ ml	1/4 of 24 hour volume _____ ml _____ ml	1/4 of 24 hour volume _____ ml _____ ml
B. Maintenance fluid N/2 saline in 5% dextrose	_____ ml	1/3 of 24 hour volume _____ ml	1/3 of 24 hour volume _____ ml	1/3 of 24 hour volume _____ ml
Total: A + B Resuscitation + Maintenance fluid	_____ ml	_____ ml	_____ ml	_____ ml

Urine output expected: 0.75 ml/kg/hour = _____ ml
* In less severe burns, 2 ml/kg per % BSA burned is sufficient

Figure 4.1.3 Fluid resuscitation of a burned child during the first 24 hours following injury (BSA, body surface area)

Maintenance fluid

Oral fluid

Most children with burn injuries tolerate oral fluids. Initially, all children may be offered small amounts of milk and, if tolerated, the quantity can be increased hourly. Usually, after a few hours, the patient is receiving most maintenance fluid by mouth, except for those with very severe burns.

Intravenous fluid

If oral fluids are not tolerated, maintenance fluid is given intravenously.

After the first 24 hours, the fluid requirement is very hard to predict. In general, the capillary leak decreases progressively and the volume of intravenous fluid resuscitation is reduced accordingly. The volume of resuscitation fluid used in the second 24 hours is approximately half of that in the first 24 hours. A large urinary output in the first 24–48 hours usually implies overresuscitation, and fluid administration should be reduced. The type of fluid used (red cells, albumin, sodium content) depends on the urine output, serum electrolytes and hemoglobin concentration. Maintenance fluid requirements are unchanged.

MANAGEMENT OF HYPERMETABOLISM

Early continuous enteral feeding through a nasogastric or nasojejunal tube (Table 4.1.1) is the mainstay of current management (Ch. 5.3). Administration of energy and protein minimizes the breakdown of body protein, especially in muscle and lymphoid tissue, and promotes wound healing. Enteral feeding also maintains the integrity of gut mucosa and thus may prevent bacterial translocation across the gut wall, reducing the load of bacteria and bacterial endotoxin reaching the Kupffer cells of the liver and seeding distant organs. In the early phase of care, a wholeprotein feed based on cow's milk (4.2–6.3 kJ/ml, 1–1.5 kcal/ml) is used. The energy requirement used is the recommended daily intake for age and weight of the child plus 63 kJ (15 kcal) per 1% body surface area burned. Up to 15% of the energy

> **TABLE 4.1.1 Indications for insertion of a nasogastric or nasojejunal tube**
>
> - Age > 10 years and burns > 20% BSA
> - Age < 10 years and burns > 15% BSA
> - Facial burn preventing feeding by mouth
> - Tracheal intubation
> - Unable to take 65% of estimated energy needs orally by day 2
> - Unable to take 80% of estimated energy needs orally by day 3
>
> BSA, body surface area

requirement is derived from protein (up to 3–5 g/kg of protein per day). Half of the energy is supplied by carbohydrate and the remainder by fat. The onset of diarrhea sometimes requires a temporary reduction in the amount of energy per ml of feed.

WOUND CARE

In children with extensive deep burns, the burn wound is washed and dressed daily. The burned area should be washed with saline or antiseptic solution, and dressed with topical silver sulfadiazine cream and a nonadherent dressing. Superficial dermal burns require only tulle gras dressing, covered with gauze and a crepe bandage, changed after 5 days.

TIMING OF SURGERY

Excision of burned tissue and skin grafting begins 3–4 days after injury, once the child is hemodynamically, metabolically and hematologically stable. This is preferable to commencing very early (a day or two after the burn injury), or delaying intervention until the burned tissue separates from the body. Each session is limited to approximately 10% of the burned area and to about 2 hours of operating room time. The hypermetabolism of burn injury does not cease until the whole burned area is covered. Excision of burned tissue is essential to prevent, or at least reduce in frequency, the episodes of septicemia. All burned tissue should be excised within 3 weeks. In very large burns, the amount of skin available for grafting is limited. Covering this area with cadaveric skin is preferable to the porcine substitute.

BURNS PREVENTION

Strategies or prevention of burns (Ch. 1.4) include:

- the reduction of domestic hot-water temperature to 50–55°C
- exclusion of small children from kitchens, by temporary physical barriers in passageways, while cooking is in progress
- the use of heat-resistant fireguards, which completely surround open fires and other hazardous heaters at a suitable distance, to reduce the possibility of contact burns
- removal of matches and cigarette lighters from the reach of children. Only childproof cigarette lighters should be allowed to be sold
- the use of nonspill cups for hot drinks; disposable cups used for hot drinks should always have a broad base and be fitted with a lid
- a continuing publicity campaign run by government or local authority to warn of the dangers of 'fooling with fuel'
- community-based programs to encourage child safety

✔ KEY POINTS

➤ First aid: completely undress the child
➤ First aid: apply cold water (never ice or ice slush) for 10–20 minutes
➤ Transfer any child with a burn exceeding 5% body surface area to a tertiary center
➤ Secure venous or intraosseous access and start fluid resuscitation before transfer
➤ Prevent hypothermia
➤ Consider the possibility of inhalation injury: give oxygen
➤ Reduce the resuscitation fluids if urine output remains above 1 ml/kg•h
➤ Consider the need for escharotomy if the burns are circumferential
➤ Commence enteral feeds early

✗ COMMON ERRORS

➤ Delay in securing the compromised airway
➤ Inadequate first aid measures (insufficient application of cold water)
➤ Accidental induction of hypothermia by:
  – prolonged application of cold sheets, water-soaked towels or ice as first aid measures
  – exposing and treating the patient in an unwarmed room
  – not wrapping patient in space blanket during transfer
➤ Overresuscitation with intravenous fluids because of:
  – overestimation of the burn surface area
  – overestimation of burn depth
  – inadequate weight assessment
  – failure to reduce intravenous fluid resuscitation in the face of sustained high urine output.

CONTROVERSIES IN CARE

USE OF ANTIBIOTICS

Antibiotics should not be used routinely, but only when there is a suspicion of systemic infection: a sick, febrile patient (temperature above 39°C), with leukopenia and thrombocytopenia. Cultures of blood and burn wound must be taken before antibiotics are given to identify the causal organism and its antibiotic sensitivity. The organisms commonly involved in burns sepsis are *Staphylococcus aureus* and a wide range of Gram-negative organisms, especially *Pseudomonas* species. If there is evidence of systemic sepsis, broad-spectrum cover with an aminoglycoside (e.g. gentamicin) and an anti-staphylococcal agent (e.g. flucloxacillin) is started before the results of cultures are available.

A single dose of these antibiotics is also given at the time of surgery, to prevent the bacteremia which always accompanies the excision of colonized burned tissue.

MANIPULATION OF THE STRESS RESPONSE

Adrenergic β_1-receptor blockade, β_2 stimulation and the administration of human growth hormone and insulin-like growth factor, may improve the outcome after severe burns. Growth hormone accelerates wound healing at the skin-graft donor site by 25%. Massively burned children can then be taken to the operating room for further skin grafting about 2 days earlier, reducing by 30–40 days the time taken to achieve total wound closure.

FURTHER READING

1. Herndon DN. The 1994 Presidential address. Accepting the challenge. J Burn Care Rehabil 1994; 15: 463–469
   – *(Excellent summary of pathophysiology and management)*

2. Monafo WW. Initial management of burns. N Engl J Med 1996; 335: 1581–1586
   – *(Reviews fluid resuscitation and management of the burn wound)*

3. Rose JK, Herndon DN. Advances in the treatment of burn patients. Burns 1997; 23: S19–S26
   – *(Review of recent improvements in burn care)*

4.2   Smoke inhalation

Robert Henning

Respiratory failure is the most common cause of death in the first hour after burn injury. Three per cent of burned children suffer an inhalation injury, most commonly when the victim is burned in an enclosed space such as a burning building or motor vehicle. These children are 20% more likely to die than those without an inhalation injury.

PHYSIOLOGY

HEAT

Airway injury due to flame or dry heat is limited to the mucosa of the mouth, pharynx, larynx and subglottic area, while inhalation of steam, which has a high specific heat, causes severe injury to the whole trachea, to the bronchi and sometimes to the lung parenchyma. Inhalation of hot gases causes erythema, edema, hemorrhage and ulceration of the mucosa. The mucosal edema and the consequent airway obstruction increase over 48–72 hours. Swelling of the tongue occurs later, and the tongue may become fixed because of swelling of the tissue planes of the neck. Scald injuries to the upper airway in toddlers who attempt to drink hot coffee usually cause only mild stridor which resolves spontaneously, or after inhalation of nebulized epinephrine (adrenaline), but may cause severe swelling of the supraglottic structures with eschar formation, requiring tracheal intubation.

CHEMICAL INJURY

Smoke consists of carbon particles suspended in a mixture of gases. The particles are coated with toxic substances such as hydrochloric acid, ammonia, ketones and organic acids. Most smoke particles are large and are deposited in the nasopharynx, larynx or trachea where they contribute to the obstruction of large airways or cause damage because of their heat content or the toxins on their surface. Small particles and gases cause injury to small airways and alveoli.

Strong acids and alkalis in smoke such as HCl and NH_3 cause mucosal cell necrosis and severe edema of the larynx, large and small airways and alveoli. Water-soluble gases such as acrolein, NH_3 and HCl cause intense upper airway irritation, coughing and increased ventilation which increases the exposure of the lower airway and lung parenchyma to other toxins including carbon monoxide and hydrogen cyanide. With more prolonged smoke exposure, central nervous system depression by hypoxia, CO_2, CO and HCN causes hypoventilation. Lipophilic hydrocarbons and phenols cause pulmonary vascular injury and toxicity to distant organs.

Mucus production is increased, and slough formed by soot, mucus, edema fluid and dead epithelium lines and obstructs the large and small airways and alveoli. Ciliary activity and surfactant production are suppressed, predisposing to atelectasis, secondary bacterial infection of the airways, pneumonia and in some cases, septicemia. Work of breathing is greatly increased by atelectasis, pneumonia and alveolar edema combined with skin burns of the chest, and the increase in airways resistance caused by slough and mucosal edema.

ASPHYXIA

Oxygen concentrations may be very low (2–10%) for a distance of several meters around fires in enclosed spaces. Hypoxic injury to the brain and heart (seen when the inspired oxygen concentration is less than 8%) combines with carbon monoxide and cyanide poisoning to cause collapse, unconsciousness and death or severe residual brain injury in some victims.

CARBON MONOXIDE

Carbon monoxide is bound by hemoglobin 250 times as strongly as oxygen. It reduces the amount of hemoglobin available for carriage of oxygen and reduces its ability to release oxygen to the tissues. Carbon monoxide also binds to brain cytochromes, injuring neurons by interrupting aerobic metabolism. The acute effects of CO poisoning are similar to those of a global hypoxic–ischemic insult, affecting especially the brain, heart, kidneys, liver and bowel. Myocardial depression due to carbon monoxide adds an ischemic insult to that caused by the low oxygen content of blood. The onset of neuropsychiatric effects of CO poisoning, including apathy, coma, dementia, seizures, and choreoathetosis may be delayed from day 1 to up to 240 days after injury. These effects may be seen despite an initial carboxyhemoglobin concentration of less than 30% (even as low as 7%).

CYANIDE

Cyanide binds to cytochrome aa_3 (the terminal enzyme in the respiratory chain), blocking oxidative phosphorylation and oxygen utilization. A cyanide concentration of 110–135 p.p.m. causes death after 30–60 minutes and 180 p.p.m. causes death in 10 minutes. Many organs are injured, but those with the highest metabolic rate (the brain and heart) are the most sensitive. Myocardial depression reduces cardiac output and blood pressure, while brain cell injury causes hypoventilation, coma and death. A metabolic acidosis is seen in cases of significant cyanide intoxication, due to lactate accumulation from anaerobic metabolism.

MANAGEMENT

PREHOSPITAL

Unconscious children and those with upper airway obstruction or respiratory difficulty at the fire scene should ideally be intubated immediately if there are personnel available with the necessary experience in difficult intubation in children. Otherwise, the child should be given high-flow oxygen by mask (10 L/min) and transferred urgently to hospital.

The stomach should be decompressed with a wide-bore nasogastric tube draining freely into a bag, as acute gastric dilatation and consequent regurgitation-aspiration, impairment of venous return and restriction of diaphragmatic movement are very common in children with burn inhalation injury.

Positioning on the side, jaw thrust and jaw support, and the use of a Guedel airway may be needed to maintain an adequate airway in an unconscious child.

Some burned children may have suffered a head injury (e.g. in vehicles burning after a collision or from falling in a burning building), and if this appears likely, it should be treated appropriately (Ch. 2.6).

EMERGENCY ROOM

Inhalation burn injury is more likely to be present in children with facial burns, conjunctivitis or rhinorrhea and in those trapped in a closed space (e.g. a burning vehicle).

Stridor, wheezing, dyspnea, cough and a hoarse voice are rarely present on arrival at the hospital. Signs of supraglottic injury and impending airway obstruction include low-pitched stridor which may be inspiratory, expiratory or both. Swallowing may be difficult and the child may drool and prefer sitting to lying down. A hoarse voice implies a laryngeal injury. When airway obstruction is marked, there may be tracheal tug and sternal and intercostal retraction.

INTENSIVE CARE

If significant airway obstruction appears in the first few hours after injury, the trachea should be intubated to protect the airway, as the swelling and obstruction are likely to increase in severity over the next 2–3 days. Stridor and signs of upper airway obstruction are often absent when the child first arrives at the hospital, but increase in severity over the next 4–6 hours. In general, it is safer to intubate the trachea early rather than later, when swelling of the mucosa, tongue and neck tissues will make it much more difficult to see the larynx, identify landmarks and enter the trachea. Inhalational anesthesia is used for tracheal intubation, as for any patient with upper airway obstruction (Ch. 6.3).

Endotracheal tube fixation and patency are critically important in these patients, as reinsertion of a dislodged or blocked endotracheal tube may become impossible when edema is at its maximum, and emergency tracheostomy may be difficult and dangerous in the presence of neck burns. Nasotracheal tubes are more readily secured than orotracheal tubes, provided that there is no contraindication to their use, such as basal skull fracture or a severe coagulopathy. In the presence of a facial burn, endotracheal tubes may be secured by cotton tapes tied around the neck or attached firmly by four-point fixation to a skull cap. Sedation and splinting of the child's arms may be needed to prevent displacement of the precious endotracheal tube.

Adequate humidification, frequent tracheal suction and close nursing observation are essential to the safe management of a child with an inhalation injury of the airway. A child who is suspected of suffering from an inhalation injury, but in whom airway obstruction is still only mild, should be observed closely in a well-lit ward. There is no evidence of a therapeutic benefit from mist tents or steroids in these circumstances. Although nebulized epinephrine (adrenaline) may reduce the severity of large and small airways obstruction caused by edema, its use may not benefit the patient if it merely allows the postponement of tracheal intubation to a time when intubation becomes difficult or dangerous.

If tracheal intubation is impossible or the laryngeal inlet cannot be seen, the safest options are:

- passage of an orotracheal tube over a fiberoptic laryngoscope
- in a child 12 years or over – needle or surgical cricothyroidotomy
- in a child under 12 years – needle cricothyroid-otomy.

Rigid bronchoscopy or fiberoptic bronchoscopy via an endotracheal tube may be needed to assess and remove slough and debris when airway obstruction persists after tracheal intubation. In the first 48 hours after injury, fiberoptic laryngoscopy under local anesthesia and light sedation may be used in children in the emergency room and the intensive care unit to assess the severity and progression of laryngeal and supraglottic edema and (in conjunction with physical signs) to judge the need for tracheal intubation. Hypoxemia and the alveolo-arterial oxygen difference ($AaDO_2$) increase in severity over the first 72 hours after injury. Cyanosis may be difficult to assess in the presence of skin burns, especially facial and mouth burns. Pulse oximetry does not reliably estimate hemoglobin saturation when CO is bound to hemoglobin (saturation reads high), when the skin perfusion is poor due to hypovolemia, or when the limb is very edematous. A shallow tachypnea implies parenchymal lung disease, while hyperventilation is caused by metabolic acidosis due to shock or cyanide or carbon monoxide poisoning.

Blood gases should be measured at presentation and every 2–6 hours for the next 2 days and whenever the child's condition deteriorates. Metabolic acidosis in a burned child may be caused by hypovolemia, by hypoxemia, or by CO or cyanide toxicity. Hypercarbia may be caused by severe upper airway or lower airway obstruction or by smoke injury to the alveoli. Depression of the respiratory center by cyanide or CO, by opiate drugs, cerebral hypoxia, or by an associated blunt head injury may also contribute, while splinting of the chest wall by pain, edema or a circumferential eschar may cause hypoventilation. Any factor that causes hypercarbia also causes hypoxemia, which may also be caused by intrapulmonary right-to-left shunt and by ventilation–perfusion inequality due to destruction of small airways or alveolar injury.

If the PaO_2 falls below 8 kPa (60 mmHg) despite the administration of 10 L/min of oxygen by mask, the trachea should be intubated and continuous positive airway pressure (CPAP) 5–15 cmH$_2$O or intermittent positive-pressure ventilation (IPPV) with positive end-expiratory pressure (PEEP) 5–15 cmH$_2$O applied (Ch. 6.4). In severe inhalation injury, the early institution of IPPV/PEEP before the appearance of hypoxemia results in better short-term survival than the commencement of IPPV/PEEP later when hypoxemia appears. In general, the management of impaired gas exchange in inhalation injury is that of acute respiratory distress syndrome (Ch. 3.1). Twelve hours after injury, any beneficial effect of a high FIO_2 on carbon monoxide elimination is outweighed by the risk of pulmonary oxygen toxicity, and the FIO_2 should be kept below 0.5 as far as possible. To minimize iatrogenic lung injury, tidal volumes and peak airway pressures should be restricted at this stage to the minimum levels needed to achieve a PaO_2 of 7 kPa (50 mmHg) or more and an arterial pH of at least 7.15—this usually means a $PaCO_2$ no higher than 10.5 kPa (80 mmHg).

A sudden increase in respiratory distress, especially with signs of large airway obstruction such as stridor, cyanosis or widely transmitted wheeze (which can be unilateral), may represent life-threatening obstruction of a large airway due to movement of a cast, or separation of a piece of sloughed mucosa requiring urgent bronchoscopy for its removal. Sudden dyspnea may also be caused by a tension pneumothorax. Signs of mediastinal shift including displacement of the trachea in the sternal notch or of the apex beat may not be detectable when there are burns of the neck and chest. If these signs appear, urgent chest X-ray is indicated, while if the situation is extremely urgent, needle thoracentesis of the hemithorax that has the poorer air entry is needed. Escharotomy of the chest wall may reduce the hypoventilation and the restrictive lung defect caused by circumferential chest burns (Ch. 4.1).

Wheezing may appear after a few hours, caused by edema, mucus production and separation of sloughed mucosa in large and small airways. Gas trapping with chest hyperinflation and pulsus paradoxus may increase in severity over the next 96 hours. Areas of reduced air entry, wheezes and crackles may be audible despite the difficulty of chest auscultation when there are extensive skin burns of the trunk. Bronchodilator drugs such as salbutamol (albuterol) have little effect when wheezing is due to narrowing of large airways or the presence of large casts or mucous plugs, but a trial of salbutamol may improve gas exchange and mobilize secretions in some cases. The use of corticosteroids for wheezing is only justified in known asthmatic patients or in children dependent on exogenous steroids. When a wheeze is widely transmitted, bronchoscopy may be needed to exclude or relieve large airway obstruction by casts or mucous plugs.

Carbon monoxide or cyanide poisoning is likely to occur in fires in closed spaces and when the victim was unconscious at the scene. Hypotension, pulmonary edema, confusion, hallucinations, convulsions or headache should lead to a suspicion of CO or cyanide poisoning. Cherry-red coloration of mucous membranes is far less common than cyanosis in patients with carbon monoxide poisoning. A child with cyanide poisoning may be stuporose or comatose, hypotensive and tachycardic with flushed skin and slow, gasping respiration. Venous blood may be bright red because of poor oxygen utilization in a child with cyanide intoxication.

If smoke inhalation is suspected, blood is taken immediately for measurement of carboxyhemoglobin (COHb) and plasma cyanide levels. If cyanide levels cannot be obtained quickly in a child with a history of smoke exposure, a metabolic acidosis and the physical signs of cyanide toxicity, the sodium nitrite/sodium thiosulfate antidote should be administered without waiting for assay results. The COHb concentration depends on the time elapsed since exposure and on the oxygen concentration inhaled in the meantime, as well as on the COHb concentration at the scene, so that the history of exposure and the child's conscious state may be the best guides to treatment of CO toxicity when the COHb level is low.

Any child who has suffered smoke exposure in an enclosed space should receive high-flow oxygen by mask. A child who has been unconscious at the scene of the fire or since should be intubated to permit the administration of 100% normobaric oxygen, especially if the child is to be transported to another hospital by air. If the COHb concentration on arrival at hospital is 30% or greater, hyperbaric oxygen therapy should be considered if it can be achieved with minimal risk to the child (i.e. the child's airway, breathing and circulation are stable and can be kept stable in the conditions of the hyperbaric chamber). Two or three hyperbaric treatments of 2.5 atmospheres lasting 90 minutes are given in 24 hours.

Any child with heavy smoke exposure (especially closed space fires or loss of consciousness) and a metabolic acidosis or a high carboxyhemoglobin concentration should be given cyanide antidote treatment. This consists of sodium nitrite, 10 mg/kg given i.v. to a maximum of 300 mg plus sodium thiosulfate 400 mg/kg to a maximum of 12.5 g given i.v. over 20 minutes and repeated after 30–60 minutes if necessary. Methemoglobin concentration is monitored during treatment and should remain below 10%. Amyl nitrite may be inhaled if i.v. access is delayed.

In the first hours after a burn inhalation injury, a plain AP chest X-ray usually shows little more than mild hyperinflation. Later, signs of atelectasis, secondary bacterial pneumonia or ARDS (Ch. 3.1) may appear. If the child's gas exchange deteriorates, and dyspnea and the respiratory rate increase, a plain AP chest radiograph may reveal a pneumothorax, a collapsed lung or lobe, a pleural effusion, pulmonary edema, an endotracheal tube displaced downwards into a bronchus or consolidation consistent with the onset of secondary bronchopneumonia

TRANSPORT CARE

Interhospital transport often occurs when upper airway edema is increasing rapidly and gas exchange is deteriorating. If there are early signs of stridor, wheezing or arterial desaturation, it is safer to intubate the child before transfer to protect the airway and to permit the use of CPAP or positive pressure ventilation if necessary during the retrieval. At the receiving hospital, the situation can be reviewed carefully, and the child extubated if appropriate. When significant carbon monoxide exposure seems possible (see above), it is safer to intubate the child before transfer in order to administer 100% oxygen, as mask oxygen therapy can only achieve a maximum FIO_2 of 0.5–0.6. Humidification and tracheal toilet are critically important, and sufficient suction catheters of the appropriate size must be carried. Examine the chest X-ray to exclude a pneumothorax before departure. Carry adequate analgesia, sedation, muscle relaxant drugs, cyanide antidote and resuscitation fluids when retrieving burned children. Consider performing bilateral chest escharotomies (after consultation with the receiving surgeon) before departure if ventilator inflation pressures are high owing to circumferential chest burns.

CONTINUING CARE

The main continuing problems are airway management, ventilatory support, fluid and nutritional therapy and care of associated skin burns (Ch. 4.1), and the monitoring and treatment of sepsis. Secondary bronchopneumonia causes 6% of deaths in the first week after respiratory burn injury and 42% after the third week. Routine bacteriologic surveillance reveals only colonizing organisms, so culture specimens of blood and tracheal aspirate should be taken only when there is a clinical suspicion of pneumonia (e.g. new fever, rising white cell count with a left shift, deteriorating gas exchange and the appearance of new alveolar opacities on chest X-ray). The antibiotics chosen should cover the pathogens found by culture. If antibiotics are given before culture results are available because of a clinical suspicion of pneumonia, they should cover the pathogens most commonly found in this situation: *Staphylococcus aureus* and Gram-negative bacilli including *Pseudomonas*. Flucloxacillin plus an aminoglycoside is an appropriate combination. The use of prophylactic antibiotics has not been shown to affect mortality or morbidity in controlled trials in patients with respiratory burn injury, but is known to predispose to the development of antibiotic-resistant bacteria. Their use is not recommended.

CONTROVERSIES IN CARE

PROPHYLACTIC STEROIDS

Prophylactic steroids treble the mortality from sepsis in patients with respiratory burn injury. Their use is not recommended.

SURFACTANTS

Surfactant administration has not been shown to reduce pulmonary edema or the surface tension of alveolar fluid in animal models of burn inhalation injury.

HYPERBARIC OXYGEN THERAPY

There is evidence that hyperbaric therapy improves survival and neurological outcome in patients with high COHb levels at presentation and in those found unconscious at the fire scene.

CARE FOLLOWING DISCHARGE

Complete healing takes up to 4 weeks in moderately severe smoke inhalation injury. Tracheal scarring and stenosis, bronchiectasis and bronchiolitis obliterans are sometimes found. Regular follow-up should be arranged to monitor the progress of these problems. Three years after the injury, about a third of children have normal lung mechanics, a third have some obstructive defect, a fifth have a restrictive defect and the remainder have a combined restrictive and obstructive defect.

✓ KEY POINTS

➤ High-flow oxygen (maximally humidified) for all nonintubated patients

➤ Intubate to protect the airway before stridor becomes severe, especially before transport. Intubation may become very difficult or impossible later

➤ Careful tracheal toilet to remove mucosal slough and large soot particles

➤ Consider hyperbaric oxygen treatment in all children found unconscious at the scene and in all those with a high carboxyhemoglobin level (> 15%) at presentation

➤ Give cyanide antidote to any child with heavy smoke exposure, metabolic acidosis or a high carboxyhemoglobin level

➤ In ventilated children, adopt a policy of permissive hypercapnia to avoid iatrogenic lung injury

✗ COMMON ERRORS

➤ Postponement of intubation until swelling in and around the pharynx is severe

➤ Inadequate fixation, humidification and suction of the endotracheal tube

➤ Failure to protect the airway and ensure adequate oxygenation before transport

➤ Underestimation and undertreatment of significant carbon monoxide exposure, especially in children found unconscious at the fire scene

➤ Failure to realize that oximetry is an unreliable measure of oxygenation when CO is bound to Hb

➤ Administration of steroids and prophylactic antibiotics

➤ Use of excessive ventilator pressures and tidal volumes in an attempt to achieve normal blood gas levels

FURTHER READING

1. Crapo RO. Causes of respiratory injury. In: Haponik EF, Munster AM, editors. Respiratory injury: smoke inhalation and burns. New York: McGraw-Hill, 1990
   – *(Review of the pathophysiology of lung injury)*

2. Pruitt BA, Cioffi WG, Shimazu T, Ikeuchi H, Mason AD. Evaluation and management of patients with inhalational injury. J Trauma 1990; 30: S63–S68
   – *(Review of assessment and management: mostly in adults)*

3. Davies JWL. Toxic chemicals versus lung tissue—and aspect of inhalation injury revisited. J Burn Care Rehabil 1986; 7: 213–222
   – *(Careful investigation of the pathogenesis of lung injury)*

4. Sharar SR, Heimbach DM, Hudson LD. Management of inhalation injury in patients with and without burns. In: Haponik EF, Munster AM, editors. Respiratory injury: smoke inhalation and burns. New York: McGraw-Hill, 1990
   – *(Good discussion of management: mostly adult focus)*

5. Vreman HJ, Mahoney JJ, Stevenson DK. Carbon monoxide and carboxyhemoglobin. Adv Pediatr 1995; 42: 303–334
   – *(Review of carbon monoxide poisoning in childhood)*

6. Tibbles PM, Perrotta PL. Treatment of carbon monoxide poisoning: a critical review of human outcome studies comparing normobaric oxygen with hyperbaric oxygen. Ann Emerg Med 1994; 24: 269–276
   – *(Useful review of the evidence for and against the use of hyperbaric oxygen therapy in carbon monoxide poisoning)*

4.3 Trauma: nonaccidental injury

Arthur F. Cogswell

Child maltreatment has become so prevalent and the violence directed toward children so severe that it has warranted description in the USA as a public health crisis. The world literature suggests that the situation is likely to be little different in most developed countries.

The obligation to report the suspicion of nonaccidental injury (NAI) and being prepared to make the diagnosis enables us to prevent further injury. This section deals with identification of possible abuse scenarios, and management of the patient and the situation to achieve the best possible outcome; it does not address the complex question of why this abuse occurs.

DEFINITION

Child maltreatment is classified as *abuse* or *neglect*. The distinction is made on the basis of whether there are acts of commission or omission. In turn, abuse may be physical, sexual or emotional, and neglect may be physical, emotional, educational, or nutritional. These subdivisions are by no means exclusive, and any patient may well have been exposed to multiple forms of abuse and neglect. Children presenting to a PICU because of NAI usually represent the severe end of the spectrum and there is little doubt regarding diagnosis. However, the astute physician must always look for more subtle history and signs of maltreatment in cases where a diagnosis is obscure. These signs may indicate previous, less severe injury which can be an indicator of future risk. In this situation physicians must adopt a preventive approach, as appropriate management may be life-saving for the index case, and for existing and potential siblings.

EPIDEMIOLOGY

It appears that the incidence of child abuse worldwide has increased substantially since the 1970s, even allowing for increased detection and report-

ing. The number of children seriously injured through abuse has at least quadrupled in the decade since 1988. Males and females are maltreated equally overall, although females probably suffer more sexual abuse and males are more frequently physically abused. While physical abuse of younger children is no more frequent than in older age groups, the effects are more dramatic and mortality and morbidity are disproportionately high in infants. Those least able to defend themselves certainly suffer most.

Child maltreatment has no boundaries in terms of race, religion, sex, educational status, socioeconomic group, urban or rural setting, but there is a significantly increased incidence of all forms of abuse and neglect in low-income and large families. Children of single parents are at greater risk than those living with both parents. The perpetrator is typically a parent or parent equivalent, and most commonly will be young and poorly equipped to cope with the stresses of raising young children. The perpetrator may well have suffered abuse as a child. While both sexes abuse young children, men injure them fatally more often than women. The children involved are often 'different' in physical, behavioral or developmental terms.

Conservative data from the USA suggest that NAI kills at least 5 out of every 100 000 children aged 4 years and under. That translates to 2000 deaths per year or 5 per day, exceeding by far the contribution of the automobile, home fires, drownings and falls, making child abuse the *leading* cause of trauma death at age 1–4 years.

While the mortality rate is shocking, it is dwarfed by the morbidity seen in survivors. For those 2000 deaths per year in the USA there will probably be about a million substantiated cases of abuse out of 3 million reports. Serious permanent disabilities will cripple an estimated 18 000 children each year. The lifelong cost of emotional trauma pursuant to childhood neglect, physical and sexual abuse is incalculable. The need for preventive intervention from all quarters is clear.

CLINICAL MANIFESTATIONS

GENERAL

The possibility of NAI must be considered in all cases of serious trauma and in all situations where a child has developed a serious illness without clear cause. The key to detection is a broad experience of the range of what constitutes 'normal' in pediatrics (e.g. developmental progress, the natural history of medical illnesses, and the common forms of accidental trauma that are part of the day-to-day hazards of growing up). When something out of the ordinary occurs, when the history and physical findings are discordant, then the index of suspicion must rise.

Classical warning signs that child maltreatment may be an issue are listed in Table 4.3.1. Child abuse often occurs in a setting where a high-risk parent or carer and a high-risk child experience a crisis which triggers an abusive outburst. Inexperience, poverty, isolation and unemployment in the caregiver are major risk factors. Most often the cardinal finding is that the history offered to explain the injury is discordant with the type or degree of injury observed in the setting of the age and developmental status of the child. Delay in seeking medical attention is common and may negatively influence the outcome (e.g. in severe head or abdominal trauma, and burns) by superadding a secondary injury (e.g. due to hypoxia or ischemia).

The history should establish the child's developmental status prior to illness or injury, to determine the child's physical abilities with reference to the mode of injury. This may be important in determining the plausibility of the account of the injury and may be helpful in determining the appropriateness of the parent's expectations. Unfortunately, in many cases, the entire history may be a fabrication and has to be discounted as an explanation for the child's illness. Significant variations in the history detail when related to different interviewers, or at different times to the same interviewer, must be carefully documented, verbatim if possible. This is another hallmark of NAI.

Physical examination must be detailed and thorough, both clinically and on the written record for

---

TABLE 4.3.1 Warning signs for child maltreatment

History
- Parent or carer
  - poverty, unemployment
  - isolation
  - youth, inexperience
  - marital instability
  - inappropriate expectations
  - abused as a child
  - previously abused other children
  - cannot be located or leaves early
  - substance abuse
- Triggering situation
  - family crisis in finances, housing, health, etc.
- Injury:
  - delay in presentation
  - history vague or inconsistent
  - history does not explain findings of examination and investigation
- Child:
  - unwanted pregnancy
  - multiple pregnancy
  - in utero abuse or neglect
  - prematurity, low birthweight
  - abnormal or difficult child

Examination and investigation
- General
  - failure to thrive, malnutrition
  - child emotionally detached from parents or vice versa
  - multiple cutaneous lesions, varying ages
  - bruises or burns in shape of weapon
  - bites
  - bruises or burns in unusual location (see text)
- Head, CNS:
  - serious intracranial injury, < 12 months of age
  - serious intracranial injury, following reported trivial incident
  - skull fracture complex, diastolic, multiple
  - retinal haemorrhages
  - lateral face injuries, especially ear
  - lip or frenulum injuries
  - shaken infant complex (see Figure 4.3.1)
  - subdural haemorrhages of varying ages
  - unexplained coma or life-threatening event
- Skeletal:
  - metaphyseal and epiphyseal fractures
  - multiple rib fractures, varying ages
  - multiple limb fractures
  - avulsion of clavicle or acromion
  - any fracture at age < 12 months
- Abdomen
  - acute pancreatitis in childhood
  - severe viscus injury with reported trivial

medicolegal purposes. The patient's overall growth and nutritional status may be indicative of neglect preceding abuse. Significant malnutrition or failure to thrive in the absence of chronic medical illness should be regarded as suspicious. Evidence of old, previous abuse may be present in bruises and scars in various stages of healing. Bites, in particular, are strong evidence of abuse. All cutaneous lesions should be documented accurately by pattern, shape, color, measured size and location. Bruises should be described by color (Table 4.3.2). Estimation of age by color is only approximate. Good-quality photographs are an invaluable aid.

Toddlers typically suffer multiple minor falls as part of their normal development and have the bruises to match, usually on the anterior face, elbows and shins. Major injury or bruises to the genitalia, buttocks, back, abdomen, lateral body or lateral face should be considered suspicious. Bruises in the shape of an object may indicate a specific mode of abuse such as lash or whip marks, handprint bruises, belt buckle bruises, etc. Similarly, burn scars may indicate a specific weapon such as a cigarette, clothes iron or hot plate. The face may bear the brunt of abuse and careful examination of the ears and oral cavity is essential.

The genitalia must be carefully and compassionately examined, bearing in mind that sexual abuse may coexist with physical abuse. This examination demands special investigation procedures and the right environment (child chaperoned, discreet location). A knowledge of the range of a normal anatomy, especially in girls, is essential. Pregnancy must be considered a possibility in age-appropriate patients.

SKELETAL INJURIES

A skeletal injury is seen in up to one-third of physically abused children. The shafts of the long bones are the most common site. The injuries may be single and clinically obvious, but many children have multiple occult injuries detectable only by skeletal survey. The latter should be ordered in any infant less than 12 months of age with evidence of neglect or deprivation, all children less than 2 years of age with external evidence of abuse, any child with clinical evidence of a skeletal injury, and all unexplained deaths. The films should be reported by a radiologist with pediatric experience, as some of the findings are subtle and easily missed, and a medicolegal opinion may be required on the age of any fractures and the differential diagnosis. Whole-body 'babygrams' are not acceptable, and the survey should include specific separate films of skull, chest, limbs and vertebral column.

While no radiological lesion is absolutely diagnostic, some are highly specific for NAI. Most accidental fractures occur in children of school age, result from falls and are rarely associated with other serious injury. Most nonaccidental fractures occur in children less than 3 years old, presentation to medical attention is delayed, and other, older, occult fractures may be evident. Any fractures in infants less than 1 year old are highly suspicious of child abuse, as are metaphyseal and rib fractures in children of any age.

Metaphyseal–epiphyseal fractures are the classically described injuries of child abuse and include corner fractures, bucket-handle fractures and metaphyseal lucency. They are usually seen in the knee, wrist, elbow and ankle. They are all forms of the same injury, are virtually pathognomonic for abuse, and indicate severe shearing forces in the bone adjacent to the growth plate usually due to violent shaking.

Rib fractures are usually occult and not often accompanied by injury to the underlying lung. They are less frequent than limb fractures but more specific for child abuse, more frequent in infants, and often multiple, bilateral and posterior. They are caused by thoracic compression with the

TABLE 4.3.2 **Estimation of age of bruise or contusion**													
Day	1	2	3	4	5	6	7	8	9	10	13	21	28
	Red-blue		Blue-purple			Green		Yellow-brown			Resolved		

Adapted from Wilson EF: Estimation of the age of cutaneous contusions in child abuse. Reproduced with permission from Pediatrics 1997; 60: 750–752 (Copied from Pediatr Clin North Am 1990; 37(4))

violent forces exerted in shaking, and are very unlikely to be caused by CPR. Lateral fractures are less common, are seen in older children and often result from direct blows. Rib fractures are best seen radiologically 10–14 days after injury when callus formation enhances visualization.

Long-bone shaft fractures are seen in the tibia, fibula, radius and humerus and may result from indirect, nonaccidental trauma such as swinging, where a strong torsional force causes a spiral or oblique fracture. Transverse fractures usually result from direct trauma. When such fractures are seen in children less than 2 years of age, child abuse should be suspected, simply because of the forces involved. New periosteal bone formation will also be seen. This is the radiological picture of a maturing subperiosteal hematoma which usually results from forceful traction and torsion of a limb.

Vertebral column injuries may also be seen in infants in association with shaking, with a violent hyperflexion-extension injury causing compression fractures of the vertebral bodies in the lower thoracic or upper lumbar spine. These are seen radiologically as lucency of the anterosuperior edges of the vertebral bodies. Associated disk herniation may be seen as a narrowed disk space. These findings indicate the need for thorough neurological evaluation and possibly MRI scan for underlying spinal cord injury.

HEAD INJURY

Head injuries are by far the most common cause of mortality and long-term physical morbidity from NAI. The majority are closed head injuries. These may be externally obvious with clear signs of an impact injury, or they may be occult, as in the classic 'shaken infant' syndrome. Often the history given is of a minor traumatic incident around the home, while some children present in unexplained coma or respiratory arrest and the head injury is discovered only through investigation. Nonspecific symptomatology such as apnea, lethargy, irritability, seizures and vomiting are all common. The medical literature on this subject is extensive and clearly indicates that serious intracranial injuries found in infants less than 12 months of age should be regarded as nonaccidental in origin until proved otherwise. Minor household trauma is highly unlikely to result in significant intracranial pathology.

A significant number of cases of abusive head trauma are misdiagnosed. One study shows that up to 30% of children with nonaccidental injury are initially misdiagnosed and that 50% of these children were subsequently injured again before the true diagnosis was recognized.

History

A detailed history is essential and must include the developmental status and motor abilities of the child in order to determine the child's potential for accidental injury. An infant who is not yet mobile by crawling or rolling is unlikely to fall down stairs, and a child who is not yet standing is unlikely to climb out of a crib. In situations where a history of a fall or other incident is offered as an explanation for a head injury, detail the estimated height of the fall, surfaces involved, corroborating witnesses and associated injury. Changes in the child's conscious level from the time of the incident and the time line of associated complications such as seizure activity, irregular respiratory effort, cyanosis or pallor may indicate the possibility of secondary injury due to hypoxia or ischemia. Document significant delays between symptom development and presentation to medical help. If shaking is admitted, obtain a detailed description of the nature of the shaking and duration.

Examination

Examination should be directed at detecting signs of impact injury to the head, the associated injuries seen in shaken infants and evidence of previous unrelated trauma. Seventy per cent of children with significant head injury have associated skeletal injuries, many of which may be occult. The head injury itself may be occult (as in many shaken infants) and the absence of external signs of impact does not preclude life-threatening brain injury. The classical 'shaken infant' syndrome presents a complex of findings (Figure 4.3.1) without obvious external signs of trauma: there has been controversy as to whether impact may also be necessary to produce the injuries seen in such cases.

Scalp	bruising
Skull	fractures
Brain	hematoma, contusion, hemorrhage and edema
Skeleton	fractures of ribs, vertebral column and limbs
Trunk	bruising where held
Eyes	retinal hemorrhages

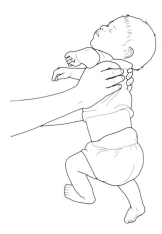

Figure 4.3.1 The shaken infant

The entire scalp should be examined for signs of soft tissue swelling or bruising, which must be documented and dated if possible. Impact injuries may be due to a blunt object blow or may be produced when the infant is thrown or swung against a surface. Skull fractures are empirical evidence of a serious force impact, although the pliable infant skull may sustain significant injury without developing a fracture. The eyes should be examined for signs of trauma, and ophthalmoscopy for retinal hemorrhages is essential. The latter are virtually pathognomic for nonaccidental injury. The oral cavity and ears are common sites of abusive injury which may accompany head injury. Full neurological examination will document focal signs of damage. The search for associated injury should include examination of the trunk and extremities for 'grip' bruises.

Investigations

Investigations should include a plain skull X-ray, followed by a CT scan of the head and, in selected cases, MRI of the brain and spinal cord, cervical spine X-rays and skeletal survey. If retinal hemorrhages are seen, a specialist ophthalmologist con-

sultation is worthwhile for medicolegal reasons, and for subsequent follow-up regarding long-term visual disability.

Skull fractures are seen in about half of the children with fatal abusive head injury. Accidental skull fractures are generally small, linear and parietal and are *not* associated with significant brain injury. Fractures that are diastatic, depressed, nonparietal, multiple, complex, bilateral or crossing the midline, and associated with significant intracranial injury, should be suspected of being nonaccidental in origin.

Subdural hematomas are the single most common finding in abusive head injury and half will also have skull fracture. While only 20% of patients dying from accidental head injuries have subdural hematomas, 90% or more of fatally abused head injury cases have subdural hemorrhage. These lesions are caused by rupture of the bridging veins between the brain and dura and indicate either a direct blow or violent shaking. They are seen most frequently in the interhemispheric fissure and may extend bilaterally over the cerebrum. Multiple subdural hematomas of varying ages indicate repeated violent head injury and are indicative of abuse. Magnetic resonance imaging is particularly useful for dating subdural hematomas and differentiating associated cerebral atrophy from communicating hydrocephalus.

Epidural hemorrhages are less common and usually associated with a fracture. Even in the absence of a fracture they indicate a violent force of injury.

Subarachnoid hemorrhage is often seen in association with subdural hemorrhage but may also be seen in association with cerebral edema alone, where it is strongly suggestive of abuse.

Intracerebral hemorrhage is usually seen in the white matter adjacent to the gray-white junction, and indicates direct trauma or violent shaking. Cerebral contusions are not frequently seen in infants but when they occur they are usually associated with an overlying fracture.

Cerebral edema may be focal or general and may take some days to develop following the injury before reaching its maximum and causing a mass effect with obliteration of the ventricles and loss of gray-white differentiation. The 'reversal sign' (the white matter having a higher attenuation than the gray) is occasionally seen and reflects severe cerebral edema. Diffuse cerebral edema may be the only abnormality found in some children following severe shaking, it may follow other forms of injury (such as asphyxiation) or be due to significant secondary injury from hypoxia or ischemia where presentation is delayed.

While all these findings in themselves reflect severe head injury, they rarely occur in isolation and frequently form part of a well-recognized pattern, which may be pathognomonic of child abuse. The American Society of Pediatric Neurosurgeons has stated clearly that new or healing extremity and/or rib fractures in infants presenting with new onset seizures, in association with retinal hemorrhages and intradural surface hemorrhages, should be regarded as nonaccidental injury.

ABDOMINAL INJURIES

Visceral injury due to blunt abdominal trauma is the second most common cause of death in child abuse and is typically seen in the older toddler. While accidental abdominal trauma results in mortality rates of only 4–12%, nonaccidental injury mortality rates of up to 50% have been reported, due primarily to the typically late presentation. Multiple visceral injuries are more commonly due to abuse rather than accident.

History

The history in most cases is vague or blames a trivial play incident for severe injury. Delay in presentation, with the child often in a moribund state, is by no means unusual.

Examination

Examination may show external signs of trauma such as abdominal wall bruising from kicking or punching, but life-threatening internal injuries may be present with few external indicators. More than 50% of children will have other, older injuries from other nonaccidental injuries.

Midline blunt injuries result in compression of viscera against the vertebral column and may result in acute pancreatitis or pseudocyst formation, and upper small bowel injury. Intramural hematoma of the duodenum or proximal jejunum may cause obstruction, becoming symptomatic over several days, or may rupture retroperitoneally. Hepatic contusion or hemorrhage is by no means rare, but the spleen and kidneys are rarely involved. Plain abdominal X-ray may show free gas in a viscus rupture, but ultrasound and/or CT scans will be required for complete assessment of liver, pancreatic or small bowel injury.

THERMAL INJURY

Burns and scalds may be the result of neglect or deliberate injury, and in the latter case are often inflicted with a punitive intent. They are a common manifestation of maltreatment, occurring in 10% of abused children. A significant proportion (up to 10% in some series) of hospitalized burns in children may be a manifestation of child abuse. While the peak age for accidental burns is in the exploring second year of life, deliberate burns are seen most frequently a little later. Most studies show that male children are at a higher risk and that children less than 12 months old are rarely abused by burning. Abusive burns may be emotionally and psychologically devastating for the victim and require long-term management.

Dry contact burns caused by cigarettes and hot implements are the most common abusive burns seen, although scalds and flame burns are more common in severe, hospitalized burn cases.

History

The history should identify the date and time of burn, its nature, where it occurred and circumstances leading to the event. Immediate treatment provided by caretakers should be recorded and any delays in seeking medical treatment should be documented. Previous history of other burns or 'accidents' should be sought. In the older child capable of communication, a history should be sought in the absence of the parents or caretakers.

Examination

Examination must document the nature, depth and extent of the burns and photographs may be particularly useful. Burn depth depends on temperature and duration of exposure, and the pattern of the burn may clearly indicate abuse or be in conflict with the history. An expert opinion from a plastic surgeon experienced in the care of burns may be required to determine whether the burn is consistent with the history provided. It may be useful to attempt a recreation of events using a doll or models and it may be necessary to have an expert examine the scene of the burn.

Some contact burns leave distinctive patterns, such as those inflicted by cigarettes or hot irons. Scalds may be in a pattern showing immersion, splash, pour or contact injuries. Accidental scalds typically affect the anterior lower side of the face, neck, shoulder, anterior chest and trunk, with a downward 'V' pattern reflecting liquid cooling with descent. In contrast, some burn patterns are typical of abuse. Pour or splash scalds inflicted from behind, 'glove and stocking' distribution full-thickness burns of a limb, or clearly demarcated forced immersion lines with flexural sparing, are all indicative of deliberately inflicted burns. Where the diagnosis is suspected, a skeletal survey should be considered and general examination made for signs of other abuse or neglect.

ASPHYXIATION

Nonaccidental asphyxiation may be due to suffocation or drowning. Suffocation may be caused by smothering or strangulation and may be clinically indistinguishable from near-miss sudden infant death syndrome, seizures, apneic episodes in the premature infant, symptomatic gastroesophageal reflux, or symptomatic RSV or pertussis infection. Any infant or child presenting following resuscitation from a life-threatening event or unexplained episode of loss of consciousness should be considered at risk unless a clear cause can be identified. Specific signs such as bruising or petechial hemorrhage over the face or neck, front and back, or inside the mouth, should be sought but will often be absent. Warning signs for nonaccidental injury include a past history of recurrent similar episodes which have not been investigated or clearly diagnosed, unexplained death in siblings, and a child who is outside the normal presenting age for SIDS or congenital metabolic disorders. A significant proportion of deaths attributed to SIDS are now believed to be caused by NAI.

Homicidal drowning usually occurs at home and may be difficult to distinguish from an 'accident'. True accidents usually happen in the bath in a setting where a parent has been distracted and an infant has been left unattended or with other siblings; the usual age is 9–15 months. Nonaccidental drowning should be suspected where the infant is older (15–30 months), and the bath is being taken at an unusual time, in the absence of siblings in the home. There may be obvious injuries to the face, neck or limbs where the child has been forcibly submerged and struggled and postmortem examination may reveal foreign matter in the lungs.

POISONING

Accidental intoxications are common in the exploring toddler (aged 2 years or more) and neglect may be an important factor. The substances involved are those the child can reach while exploring under the kitchen sink, in low, unlocked medicine cabinets, or in a container inadvertently left accessible (e.g. a purse or handbag).

Deliberate poisoning is usually seen in the slightly younger child (less than 2 years) and may present either with unexplained symptomatology or with exposure acknowledged but claimed to be accidental. Recurrent surreptitious poisoning is being increasingly reported as a manifestation of Munchausen syndrome by proxy. Where toxin exposure is unknown, diagnosis will be dependent on the astute physician detecting signs and symptoms of a specific toxidrome, or toxicological screening of blood and urine. Where toxin exposure has been acknowledged but claimed to be 'accidental', the history detailing the circumstances of exposure, in the light of the child's developmental capabilities, will be important.

The range of substances reported in nonaccidental poisoning is staggering. Suffice to say that whatever is available to the adult, either legally or otherwise, may be used to poison a child. Access to a poison information center or similar listing source for toxidromes may be important in translating a list of signs and symptoms into a diagnosis.

MUNCHAUSEN SYNDROME BY PROXY

This bizarre form of child abuse is being recognized with increasing frequency and detection requires a high index of suspicion. The background setting has been well described: the dedicated mother who refuses to leave the side of her ailing child; the father who is distant and rarely seen; the patient who has an illness that cannot be explained or defies adequate therapy, who undergoes multiple tests and procedures. Such a child may present with a simulated illness where the mother has been 'salting' specimens of the patient's body fluids, or with an illness actually produced by the mother using drugs, or trauma, to produce symptoms in her otherwise well child. Presenting symptoms include changes in conscious level, apnea or cyanosis, blood appearing in various body fluids or excretions, unexplained diarrhea or vomiting, unexplained rashes or fevers.

SEXUAL ABUSE

Sexual abuse may be suspected where a child shows physical evidence of sexual activity such as pregnancy, sexually transmitted disease, or perineal or anal trauma, or where the history clearly suggests the problem. The age, emotional status and other injuries in the patient will determine when and where the examination should be performed and whether anesthesia or sedation is required. Parents should be excluded if their presence is obviously distressing the child or if they are suspected to be the perpetrators. Where obvious trauma is involved, general anesthesia may be required for adequate gynecological and or general surgery examination and repair. Most pediatric centers have staff available who are specifically trained to perform medicolegally acceptable examinations and specimen collections. A 'rape kit' including the containers required for specimens of blood, semen, local swabs and fingernail scrapings should be available.

Physical examination should be performed within 72 hours of an assault, if possible, and must be thorough. Attention should be focused on the mouth, breasts, genitalia and anus for evidence of trauma. Photographs may be appropriate. Any material obviously foreign to the patient such as adult pubic hair, semen, etc. should be collected. Detailed examination of the genitalia is required and age-inappropriate changes should be sought. This assumes the knowledge of age-appropriate normal ranges. Evidence of anal or vaginal penetration may necessitate endoscopic or speculum examination and specimen collection.

MANAGEMENT OF THE SUSPECTED CHILD ABUSE CASE

Diagnosis of child abuse is dependent not only on detecting historical inconsistencies and demonstrating examination and investigation findings consistent with abuse, but also in establishing and excluding a reasonable differential diagnosis list. While the patient does not have to be subjected to a myriad of investigations to exclude every 'fine print' condition, the diagnostic process must withstand medicolegal scrutiny. For example, in a case of isolated intracranial hemorrhage where a shaking injury is suspected, physical examination should be directed to, and exclude, signs of a generalized bleeding diathesis and investigations must include a coagulation profile. An expert opinion from a physician experienced and skilled in the area of child abuse is invaluable, in order to ensure sufficient documentation and investigation to support the diagnosis of child maltreatment. Most tertiary pediatric centers now have a 'child protection team' or equivalent to provide that service, and they should be notified when the diagnosis of child abuse or neglect is being considered. Additional supportive expert consultations from radiology, ophthalmology, surgery, orthopedics, etc. may be invaluable for court proceedings. Where it is agreed that the diagnosis is possible, then notification of the case to the appropriate statutory authority, whether that be social services, police or both, must then follow. Most Western countries now have legislation mandating report of suspected child maltreatment. The physician who refuses to notify must accept responsibility for the potential return presentations of the same child or a sibling with an escalation of violence and also faces the prospect of litigation.

The notifying physician, as patient advocate, has a responsibility to provide a place of safety for the patient, and consideration of the same for any siblings, but does not have any responsibility in either establishing legal proof of abuse or the identity of the perpetrator. The temptation to play detective should be resisted, as should the temptation to assign blame to or assume the guilt of a particular party. Once notification has taken place, the attending physician and other staff should maintain a neutral role, avoid antagonizing the parents, and focus attention on the comprehensive medical management required by the patient. Make a point of explaining to the parents that the staff have a responsibility to care for the child, which means caring for the parents also, and that this will be done without reference to who may be responsible for the child's injuries. The parents will often require counseling and this should be provided by an appropriately trained professional. The complexities involved in many of the families will be challenging for the child protection team and the experienced counselors, and there is no place for well-meaning amateurs.

One of the most common clinical scenarios of possible NAI is the isolated intracranial injury in an infant with a plausible—if unlikely—history, and parents who strenuously deny any possibility of child maltreatment. This is a difficult area and the reader is well advised to consult the report by Wilkins (8 in the Further Reading list). Differentiation of maltreatment and accident will at times be challenging, and in such a situation a physician needs to consult expert opinions. In such a context, notification remains entirely appropriate, in order to permit a full investigation of the social and home setting. If, at the end of the day, sufficient doubt exists, then it is quite reasonable to leave the diagnosis open.

COURT APPEARANCES

Physicians will often be required to appear in court regarding cases of child abuse. A number of reviews are available giving advice regarding testimony and the reader is well advised to consult them (see Further Reading list—(1) is particularly good for practitioners in Commonwealth countries, while (2) is more relevant to American courts). See Ch. 5.12.

OUTCOME

The current outcome from child abuse and neglect is far from satisfactory. Many children are dying and many more are being maimed. Worst of all, a significant proportion of them or their siblings will have suffered a minor abusive injury previously that either went unrecognized or was recognized but not acted upon. Trauma due to maltreatment is one of the small group of disease entities that potentially can be entirely prevented. We all have a responsibility to review our own practice in terms of our recognition and reporting, and to encourage our statutory authorities to be vigorous in the follow-up of problem situations.

✔ KEY POINTS

➤ Child maltreatment is the leading cause of trauma death in children 4 years and under, and the major source of serious morbidity in survivors

➤ Missing the diagnosis and/or failing to report suspected cases places the index case and siblings at risk of further injury

➤ The diagnosis will be missed unless it is considered in *all* cases of serious trauma or severe illness without clear cause

➤ In evaluating such cases ask yourself, 'how did this happen?'. If the answer provided by the history leaves you uneasy, then review your history and repeat your examination, looking for warning signs (Table 4.3.1).

➤ Alarm bells:
  – age-inappropriate multiple bruises of varying ages
  – weapon outline bruises
  – any fracture in an infant, and metaphyseal and rib fractures in children of any age
  – intracranial injuries with a history of 'household accident'
  – protracted or repeated serious illness which is unexplained despite multiple investigations and defies all attempts at treatment

➤ Initiating a report of child maltreatment does not demand that the physician become a detective

➤ Case management should be based on comprehensive medical management in a place of safety for the patient and excluding reasonable alternative diagnoses

➤ The investigation of the family for issues relating to child maltreatment should be managed by a multidisciplinary team separate from the team respon-sible for management of the child's medical care

➤ Giving an expert opinion on whether an injury or illness constitutes child maltreatment demands a comprehensive and current knowledge of the literature and should not be undertaken lightly

✗ COMMON ERRORS

➤ Failure to admit any child 'at risk' to a place of safety (e.g. hospital) pending investigation

➤ Failure to consider the diagnosis in cases of trauma or severe illness

➤ Avoiding the diagnosis through a misplaced sense of compassion for apparently plausible parents

➤ The history taken is inadequate for medicolegal purposes

➤ Documentation of examination findings inadequate

➤ Medical management overly focused on a primary injury (e.g. unexplained cerebral edema), missing associated signs that provide a diagnosis (e.g. multiple rib fractures, retinal hemorrhages and metaphyseal fractures)

➤ Investigations to confirm the diagnosis or exclude the differential diagnosis list are incomplete or inadequate through ignorance of requirements

➤ Failure to report the suspicion of NAI

➤ Failure to consult other expert or specialist help

CHECKLIST FOR CASES OF SUSPECTED CHILD MALTREATMENT

NOTIFICATION

If you have reasonable suspicion that maltreatment has occurred you should notify the appropriate statutory authority in your area. Remember that you are not obliged to prove maltreatment, you are simply reporting your suspicions. It is the responsibility of the statutory authority to prove or disapprove the case.

If you are unsure, get help. It does no harm to consult. Consider expert consultation from clinicians experienced in dealing with child maltreatment cases, and from specialists in ophthalmology, radiology or other areas as required.

DOCUMENTATION

Record the following:

- detailed history as given by child's caregiver and as recorded by each person who interviewed the caregiver
  - are there inconsistencies?
  - does the history adequately explain all the findings?
  - is the past or family history significant (previous injury, illness, deaths)?
- detailed examination thoroughly documented
- Important negatives noted, e.g. no signs of a bleeding diathesis

INVESTIGATION

Check whether you need:

- examination of the crime scene by somebody who knows what to look for
- photographs of the scene
- photographs of the patient (medicolegal standard)
- X-rays:
  - skull, multiple views
  - formal skeletal survey
  - CT scan
  - MRI
- blood tests:
  - CBC, coagulation profile
  - calcium, magnesium, phosphorus, serum alkaline phosphatase
  - renal function
  - liver function, amylase
  - metabolic disease tests
  - toxicology
  - titer for sexually transmitted diseases
- urine tests:
  - toxicology screen
  - metabolic disease screen
  - pregnancy test
- other tests:
  - 'rape kit' samples
  - testing of parents for substance exposure
  - video monitoring of patient and/or carer

– do the siblings need to be examined?
– psychiatric assessment of child and/or carer
– developmental assessment
– growth chart
– full postmortem examination by an experienced pediatric pathologist

SPECIALIST CONSULTATION

Consider:

- child protection
- ophthalmology
- neurosurgery
- plastic surgery
- coroner
- radiology
- neurology
- metabolic diseases

MANAGEMENT

Essential questions are:

- is the patient safe? (if in doubt admit to hospital)
- are the siblings safe?
- are your notes adequate for medicolegal purposes?
- Ensure comprehensive management of the medical issues and leave further investigation of the maltreatment issue to the appropriate team.

FURTHER READING

1. Meadow R, editor. ABC of child abuse. London: Br Med J 1989
   – (*An excellent general review with good photographs and diagrams*)

2. Reece R, editor. Pediatr Clin North Am, 1990; 37, (4)
   – (*Entire edition dedicated to child abuse, chapters on imaging and court testimony particularly useful*)

3. US Advisory Board on Child Abuse and Neglect. A nation's shame: fatal child abuse and neglect in the United States. Washington: US Government Printing Office; 1995
   – (*The report makes devastating reading. Appendix contents a very useful detailed literature review listing*)

4. Monteleone JA, Brodeur AE. Child maltreatment, a clinical guide and reference. St Louis: GW Medical Publishing 1998

5. Ludwig S, Kornberg AE, editors. Child abuse, a medical reference. 2nd ed. Edinburgh: Churchill Livingstone
   – (*Two excellent, detailed reviews*)

6. Wilson EF. Estimation of age of cutaneous contusions in child abuse. Pediatrics 1977; 60: 750–752

7. Sedlak AJ, Broadhurst DD. Executive summary of the Third National Incidence Study of Child Abuse and Neglect. Washington: US: Department of Health and Human Services; 1996
   – (*Frightening statistics for those readers who think we live in a civilized world*)

8. Wilkins B. Head injury – abuse or accident? Arch Dis Child 1997; 76: 393–395

9. Sunderland R. Commentary on preceding review. Arch Dis Child 1997; 76: 396–397
   – (*A very useful summary of the complexities involved in assessing head injuries in children. Essential reading for anyone working in this field*)

4.4 Trauma of individual systems

Andrew J. Macnab

Traumatic injuries remain the leading killer of pre-school and school-aged children, adolescents and young adults. A significant proportion are predictable and preventable, and various management strategies have been shown to be effective in reducing mortality and morbidity.

Primary injuries occur with the exchange of energy between the environment and the body. These result in surface contusions and lacerations, fractures, and laceration or disruption of internal organs with associated damage to cell units and vasculature. Injuries are caused by 'impulsive loading', in which the body is set in motion but not struck, and from 'impact loading' where the body is hit directly or is suddenly stopped when in motion. In cases of impact loading, local injury occurs at the point of impact, shearing strains are exerted and contusion of the tissues opposite the point of impact can occur. Primary injuries are essentially irreversible, functional recovery depends upon the potential for healing, repair and regeneration of the individual tissue or organ.

Secondary injury can be influenced by treatment. Avoiding inappropriate management is often more important than intervening with specific therapy. Secondary brain injuries mainly result from inadequate oxygen delivery to areas of the brain temporarily compromised by the injury. Prevention of factors that can cause or aggravate secondary injuries is the major objective for physicians managing children following trauma, in particular provision of adequate oxygenation and perfusion, recognition of the extent of injury, protection of the cervical spine and anticipation of and intervention for potential complications.

There are important differences in the mechanisms involved in injury between children and adults. Children have a large head relative to the size of their bodies which makes them more vulnerable to accelerative injury and associated injury to the cervical spine. Young children are also more prone to injury because their brains are less myelinated than adults and their cranial

bones are thinner. Copious bleeding from scalp lacerations can lead to presentation in hemorrhagic shock and cerebral edema commonly follows severe injury.

The smaller the child, the smaller the airway and, therefore, the greater the risk of airway occlusion. The most common causes of preventable death following trauma are errors in management of the airway, breathing and circulation and the failure to recognize that multisystem injury is common in children. A child's exploratory nature and inexperience increase the risk of injury, and young children are vulnerable to child abuse or the effects of neglect by a parent or caregiver.

Children's physiology enables them to compensate for hypoperfusion more effectively than most adults initially. However, decompensation is abrupt; hence the need to anticipate progression to shock, minimize oxygen debt and support the circulation *before* overt signs of hypotension (which indicates significant shock) develop.

MANAGEMENT

PREHOSPITAL CARE

Management of the injured child begins at the scene of the incident. In all cases an overall assessment of the extent of the injuries is essential, with provision of the basic life support measures required. However, every unnecessary delay must be avoided in cases of severe injury, as successful resuscitation and survival without major neurologic handicap are related to the time elapsed between the injury occurring and the child's arrival at hospital.

Mismanagement or neglect while performing the 'ABC's are major causes of preventable complications. Pediatric airway skills are particularly important because of the high incidence of respiratory compromise associated with injury in this age group.

HOSPITAL MANAGEMENT

Hospital management always begins with a primary survey and measurement of vital signs to detect any problems with the airway, breathing, circulation or the cervical spine. The primary survey can usually be completed in approximately 30 seconds, but its importance cannot be overstated when determining the need for basic life support measures.

In conjunction with initiating supportive treatment the full extent of the child's injuries must be determined by physical examination. Although the secondary survey (Ch. 2.6) is intended to identify other associated injuries, as more history becomes available specific areas may require additional examination or investigations not ordered initially.

HEAD AND NECK

A sequence for examination of the head, face and neck, is given below (see also Ch. 2.6).

SCALP

Palpate the scalp, checking for laceration, swelling and depression. Palpate for fractures at the base of all lacerations. Control scalp hemorrhage.

SKULL

Look for signs along the base of the skull (the line connecting the mastoid process and the orbit). Basal skull fractures may produce signs along this line. Hemorrhage is often evident behind the eardrum. When CSF otorrhea is present, the fluid is invariably mixed with blood. Under these circumstances, clotting is delayed and a double-ring pattern forms where this fluid drops onto a sheet. When frank otorrhea is evident, avoid otoscopic examination because instrumentation can contribute to infection (which can spread to involve the meninges). Bruising over the mastoid process (Battle's sign) indicates a basal skull fracture.

Basal skull fracture

Basal fractures throught the floor of the skull are usually linear. They should be suspected on clinical grounds (difficult to recognize on X-ray). Clues to diagnosis are:

- bleeding from nose, eyes, or ears
- discoloration in the mastoid area (bruising behind the ear or Battle's sign) and/or 'raccoon eyes'
- blood and CSF behind the eardrum (causes a bulging tympanic membrane), otorrhea when the tympanic membrane is ruptured
- CSF rhinorrhea (75–90% of normal children have nasal secretions that give a positive glucose oxidase reaction)
- cranial nerve lesions (I, III, and VIII)
- air in the cranium

EYES

Examine the eyes early, as orbital swelling is likely to increase with time and may render the examination impossible. Look for bilateral periorbital hematomas (raccoon eyes), subhyoid hemorrhages and scleral hemorrhages without a posterior margin. Check for foreign bodies under the lids and signs of penetration injury. Visual acuity can be tested by having the child read, if old enough. Test the pupillary reflex to light and the corneal reflex to touch if the patient is unconscious. Use fundoscopic examination to look for retinal hemorrhage or papilledema. Proptosis can occur with crush injuries.

FACE

Palpate the face symmetrically, looking for tenderness or deformity. Children's teeth are often loose and may be displaced with a head injury. Check for stability among those that remain, and take care to avoid displacing teeth into the airway. Instability of upper incisors can indicate maxillary fracture, commonly associated with basal skull fracture. Rarely, displaced facial fractures can compromise the airway and, under these circumstances, pull the fractures segments forward to provide emergency clearing of the airway.

NECK

Examine the neck, bearing in mind the high frequency of associated cervical spine injury in pediatric trauma. Ensure that the head is held firmly while the cervical collar is removed. Look first for deformity, bruising or laceration. Palpate each of the spinous processes, feeling for tenderness in the conscious patient and for obvious deformity. Muscle spasm can indicate ligamentous injury. Neck lacerations may need to be explored surgically.

Replace the cervical collar prior to radiologic studies. These should show all seven of the upper vertebrae. If concerns persist, maintain protection with the cervical collar. Excessively large collars can make breathing difficult for small children.

If the patient is conscious, check for sensation in each of the extremities. Ask the child to move his or her fingers and toes to confirm motor function, and to squeeze your fingers to confirm upper limb strength. Lower limb strength can be checked by hip flexion. Any focal injury or deficit should be documented.

Repeat examination to confirm the adequacy of the airway, breathing and circulation is an ongoing part of management and assessment of progress, as is recalculation and recording of the Glasgow coma scale score (Ch. 2.6).

ABDOMINAL TRAUMA

Abdominal trauma includes all injuries (both blunt and penetrating) to the intraabdominal structures. Trauma to the lower six ribs in a child, whether blunt or penetrating, may result in serious injury to the underlying organs. Generally blunt trauma accounts for the majority of abdominal injuries. These are most commonly the result of motor vehicle trauma (as a pedestrian, cyclist, or occupant) where multiple injuries tend to be the rule rather than the exception. Falls from a height or against hard objects (including bicycle handlebars), and physical abuse account for the majority of other blunt injuries. Penetrating trauma is seen less frequently except in hospitals serving city populations where trauma secondary to knife and handgun injury occurs.

Blunt trauma

Blunt trauma is more difficult to evaluate than penetrating wounds. Physical findings are often minimal in spite of there being serious underlying injuries. Mechanisms of injury are:

- organ compression against the spine
- direct transfer of energy to an organ
- rapid deceleration causing tearing
- sudden increase in intraabdominal pressure causing rupture.

The solid organs are injured most frequently. Laceration of the spleen is the most common injury in children. Other vulnerable structures are the liver, pancreas, small bowel mesentery, duodenum and proximal jejunum. Associated injury to the kidney, ureter and bladder are dealt with under renal trauma.

PENETRATING TRAUMA

Penetrating trauma may produce laceration of solid organs and perforation of hollow viscera. Blood vessels, including the major structures, can be lacerated. Because hollow viscus injury is very common, secondary peritonitis often will develop. The onset may be immediate if bowel contents leak into the peritoneal cavity, but can also be delayed if peritoneal contamination is minimal or located in the retroperitoneum.

Major vascular injury can be life-threatening after penetrating trauma. Generally gunshot wounds inflict more serious injury and have a higher mortality rate than knife wounds. Surgical exploration of a gunshot wound of the abdomen is generally urgent because of the high likelihood of visceral and vascular injuries. Conversely, stab wounds require a selective approach. In one-third of injuries the peritoneal lining remains intact, and even in cases where the peritoneum is penetrated, only 50% of children have visceral injuries that require repair.

Evisceration of the abdominal contents can follow penetrating wounds. The exposed organs should be covered with moist, clean and sterile dressings. Replacement into the abdomen should not be attempted and care must be taken not to twist or kink the organs or their associated blood vessels or mesentery while awaiting surgical repair.

PHYSICAL EXAMINATION

Assessment for signs of hypotension and impending or actual shock is a priority following assessment of the adequacy of respiration. A secondary survey should look for associated injuries in other systems. For blunt trauma, note the following:

- bruises and contusion (these can indicate the location of underlying visceral damage)
- abdominal tenderness, guarding, rigidity or distention (this can indicate bleeding into the peritoneal cavity, perforation of the bowel or the onset of peritonitis)
- bowel sounds (these may be altered in nature or absent)
- referred pain (splenic, hepatic or diaphragmatic injury causes pain radiating to the shoulder; renal and ureteric trauma can cause pain referred to the groin)
- signs of spinal injury (these can be associated with abdominal distention and ileus)
- discoloration of the abdominal wall (seen in pancreatic injury)
- rectal examination (frank blood may be present and the location and tenderness of the prostate may point to genitourinary trauma)

The breathing pattern in children can change after abdominal trauma. Small children usually breathe with prominent abdominal movement. When peritoneal irritation occurs (either with blood or visceral contents) this can change to a pattern where chest breathing predominates. Such children also avoid deep inspiration (and to a lesser extent full expiration) because such movements aggravate pain. A similar sign is that a conscious child will lie still and avoid crying loudly (whimpering may still occur). These two signs are very reliable as markers for peritonitis.

Palpation of the abdomen can be complicated by voluntary guarding or an increase in abdominal muscle tone when the child becomes distressed. Light palpation is often most informative as a means of detecting increased muscle tone and discomfort. Deep palpation, particularly to elicit rebound tenderness, tends to precipitate crying and the risk of losing the cooperation and trust of the child. With an acute abdomen, rebound tenderness can be reliably detected by percussion or gentle shaking, and another technique is to ask the child to cough during palpation, rather than rapidly releasing manual pressure.

Rectal examination should include evaluation of the tone of the anal sphincter and the position of the prostate and integrity of the pelvis. The presence of blood strongly suggests rectal or colonic perforation. The important findings on rectal examination and the injuries associated with them are listed in Table 4.4.1.

The prostate is not always palpable in boys 5 years old or younger. A high-riding prostate or boggy mass palpable anteriorly suggests rupture of the membranous urethra. Signs of perianal trauma should be looked for, in addition to checking anal tone (anal tone can be decreased after sedative overdose—particularly with large doses of benzodiazepines—and the anus may be seen to gape, but sphincter tone is rarely totally absent).

Remember to examine the back ('log roll' the child if there is any possibility of spinal injury). Significant pain or crepitus with pressure over the symphysis pubis or anterior superior iliac spine suggests bony damage to the pelvis. A lack of dullness over the liver on percussion suggests perforation (pneumoperitoneum).

HEPATIC AND SPLENIC LACERATION

Hepatic and splenic lacerations are best diagnosed by CT scan of the abdomen. These lesions usually tamponade spontaneously, making surgical repair or resection rarely necessary. The child must be carefully assessed for signs of shock and regularly reassessed.

Nonoperative care requires close observation for signs of:

- hypovolemia, poor perfusion and deteriorating perfusion

TABLE 4.4.1 **Findings on rectal examination**	
Physical findings	**Injury**
Sphincter tone absent	Traumatic spinal cord injury
Prostate 'floating'	Rupture of the urethra
Disruption of bowel wall	Rectal perforation
Disruption of pelvic wall	Fractured pelvis
Presence of blood	Colonic or rectal injury
Sensation of fullness	Hemorrhage (retroperitoneal)

- hypotension
- a progressive decrease in hematocrit
- deteriorating signs on repeat physical examination

Surgical care is required when there is:

- ongoing requirement for significant blood transfusion (> 40 ml/kg) implies active bleeding
- shock not responding to vigorous medical therapy
- severe associated trauma necessitating surgical stabilization of the abdominal pathology

Where hepatic or splenic lacerations occur, the history should be reviewed to exclude a lap seat-belt injury as the cause. These seat-belts commonly cause a triad of injuries in young children. In addition to hepatic or splenic injury, visceral trauma occurs (contusion, perforation or avulsion from the mesentery) with fracture dislocation of the lumbar and/or sacral spine. Under such circumstances keep the child immobile and supine on a firm surface until spinal injury can be excluded. Associated injuries include pancreatic and blood vessel trauma. In the absence of positive history, this triad of injury should be suspected where there is a central bruise at or above the umbilicus and symmetrical soft tissue trauma over or above the anterior superior iliac spines. The fracture dislocation of the spine may result in paraplegia (Chance fracture).

INVESTIGATION

The number and types of studies will be dictated by the child's clinical state, the nature of the injuries and consultation with surgical and radiological colleagues. The primary investigations required in abdominal trauma are listed below:

Monitoring

Monitoring of physical signs and regular repeat physical examinations are required

Hematology

Investigations should include:

- complete blood count
  - a WCC of 20–30 × 10^9/L (20 000–30 000 mm^3) suggests splenic rupture
  - hemoglobin and hematocrit will probably be normal initially, even where significant hypovolemia from blood loss has occurred
- blood type and crossmatch
- amylase (consider liver enzymes)
  - amylase concentration is often normal initially, even in the presence of pancreatic trauma
  - liver enzymes can be elevated acutely in hepatic injury
- blood glucose, electrolytes, BUN and creatinine measurement
- blood gas analysis
- coagulation profile

Urine

Urine studies, routine and microscopic urinalysis (the presence of hematuria requires investigation for renal or urinary tract injury).

Radiography

| No child should be sent for X-ray until an assessment for signs of hypovolemia has been made and vital signs have been stabilized |

1. Chest X-ray: exclude pneumothorax, pleural effusion, rib fractures and loss of diaphragm integrity—herniation of bowel into chest.
2. Abdominal X-rays—upright, supine, left lateral decubitus views. Look for distention of bowel loops, and areas of increased density suggesting blood and air under the diaphragm suggesting perforation. (*Note*—80% of perforations are not evident on X-ray.) Look for disruption of normal vertebral alignment; check position of nasogastric tube.
3. Consider an intravenous pyelogram (cystogram, urethrogram) to assess injury to the renal tract.

4. Consider an abdominal CT scan (hepatic and splenic lacerations are best diagnosed by this study). *Note*—discuss with the radiologist giving 100 ml of water-soluble contrast medium (e.g. gastrographin) down the nasogastric tube 20 minutes prior to CT scan to detect leakage from a ruptured bowel.
5. Ultrasound studies are useful for major solid organ damage and can detect blood in the peritoneum.
6. Consider an upper gastrointestinal series, radionucleotide scans or angiography (discuss with surgeon/radiologist.

CONTROVERSIES IN CARE

Peritoneal lavage

Peritoneal lavage has a recognized place in the management of adult trauma victims, but its use in childhood is controversial.

The procedure should be performed by a surgeon under direct vision. An incision is made in the midline subumbilically (following local anesthesia). The lavage solution is 0.9% saline or Ringer-lactate solution (sterile, warmed and in a dose of 10 ml/kg). The presence of blood is generally not regarded as an indication in itself for laparotomy. However, the presence of white cells (> 500/ml), obvious vegetable fibers or an elevated amylase concentration are regarded as significant. The presence of bile usually indicates hepato-biliary trauma.

The controversy over peritoneal lavage in children arises from the fact that positive findings are not always present in children who subsequently require surgical exploration. Consider peritoneal lavage:

- as a diagnostic measure where the source of blood loss is obscure in a shocked child following trauma
- to determine the need for transport of a child to a tertiary care facility (under these circumstances the need for a lavage should be discussed with the surgeon at the receiving hospital, and if it is done, samples of the lavage returns should accompany the child)

MANAGEMENT

Successful management of the child with abdominal trauma depends on full resuscitation of the airway, breathing and circulation, serial monitoring of vital signs, repeated examination and correct interpretation of the diagnostic studies selected. The immediate priority should not be to make a specific diagnosis but to determine whether or not surgery is required and how urgent this intervention is. An outline of an approach to management is shown in Figure 4.1.1.

If an acute surgical emergency exists, the initial presentation, or serial reexamination of the child and the ensuing clinical course will identify it. Children can be divided into two groups: (1) those requiring immediate operative intervention, and (2) those who can receive conservative or nonoperative care. Conditions requiring immediate or urgent surgery are listed below. These children must be promptly resuscitated and minimal (if any) diagnostic tests are performed. The following abdominal injuries require immediate laparotomy:

- massive or continued hemorrhage which cannot be stabilized by transfusion (often associated with deterioration of vital signs)
- penetrating abdominal trauma (stab wounds with peritonitis: gunshot wounds to lower chest or abdomen)
- gastrointestinal perforation (pneumoperitoneum)
- rupture of the diaphragm
- bladder perforation, urethral rupture or renal vascular injury
- biliary tract rupture
- evisceration
- unclear diagnosis with suspicion of serious or potentially fatal injury (e.g. duodenal rupture or avulsion)

Children in the conservative group can still have significant or even potentially fatal traumatic injuries, but the nature of the injuries is such that hours or days may elapse before they are sufficiently evident for surgery to be indicated. Generally this group is sufficiently stable following resuscitation to undergo the investigations described above.

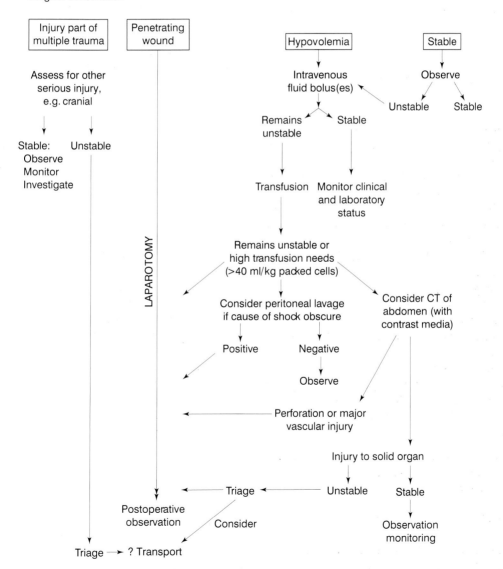

Figure 4.4.1 Management of abdominal trauma

Prehospital care

Prehospital care priorities are:

- give oxygen
- address ABC as effectively as possible
- apply local pressure to tamponade overt bleeding

Airway management and recognition and treatment of respiratory failure take precedence over abdominal injuries. Do not delay transfer to establish i.v. access, but endeavor to initiate this on route if required. Consider the intraosseous route to expedite access in the unconscious child. Nasogastric drainage is beneficial. The possibility of associated injuries (spine and head) should be considered.

Hospital care

Hospital care begins with reassessment of the ABC, starting dual intravenous access, passing a nasogastric tube (orogastric if basal skull fracture suspected), and vigorously addressing hypovolemia. After appropriate assessment insert a Foley catheter to monitor urine output and to assess hematuria. Cover penetrating wounds with sterile dressings, examine prolapsed viscera and ensure unrestricted blood flow (keep dressings moist). **No analgesics**: do not give narcotics to children until they have been assessed by or discussed with a surgeon. Regrettably, key symptoms can be masked by overzealous provision of analgesia. Carefully assess all penetrating wounds (ingress and egress). Monitor vital signs (blood pressure, pulse rate, respiratory rate and CVP). Consider broad-spectrum antibiotics and tetanus prophylaxis.

SPECIFIC INJURIES

Hepatic injury

The signs of extensive occult bleeding associated with right upper quadrant pain suggest this diagnosis. Most hepatic trauma does not require operative intervention. However, massive hemorrhage and shock can occur, hence the need to contact a surgeon and the operating room immediately. If this diagnosis appears probable, and if the child is deemed stable, a CT scan confirms the diagnosis.

Splenic injury

Left upper quadrant pain and referred pain to the shoulder tip (particularly following trauma over the lower ribs on the left side) suggests this injury. Most cases can be managed nonoperatively with careful, conservative monitoring and diagnosis by CT scan or nuclear scan.

Bowel perforation

Clinical and radiological assessment is notoriously difficult in acute injury. Observe for signs of progressive peritoneal irritation.

Penetrating trauma

Stabilize for shock. Do not remove objects impaled in the abdomen. Laparotomy is required for exploratory diagnosis and repair.

Rectal trauma

Rectal injury is suggested by blood on rectal examination (often with signs of pelvic fracture). Surgical intervention usually involves colostomy. Osteomyelitis can complicate combined injuries.

Duodenal trauma

Duodenal trauma is common after lap belt injury. Initial symptoms are often minimal, other than local pain. This is followed by severe vomiting 6–18 hours after the injury with clinical signs of small bowel obstruction. If the damage is limited to a hematoma, nonoperative therapy (nasogastric suction and i.v. fluids) is sufficient, but more extensive damage requires laparotomy. An associated pancreatitis is common.

Pancreatic trauma

Symptoms are epigastric or paraumbilical pain with vomiting, classically after a forward fall onto the abdomen (as in a bicycle handlebar injury). The amylase level may be normal or raised. Nonsurgical treatment (nasogastric suction and i.v. fluid) is usually effective.

Hemorrhage (retroperitoneal)

Severe back or pelvic injuries precede the appearance of hypovolemic shock accompanied by paralytic ileus. Initial resuscitation must be aggressive with oxygen, i.v. fluids, transfusion and nasogastric suction. If the condition is not self-limiting, angiographic embolization may be required.

Paralytic ileus

Paralytic ileus may follow minor or major injury. Gastric distention occurs (increased by air swallowing). Signs are nonspecific with abdominal pain and vomiting. Treatment is nonsurgical using nasogastric tube drainage and intravenous fluids, and is generally effective in approximately 12 hours. More severe gastric injury is suggested by fresh blood in the nasogastric tube aspirate, or free air seen on X-ray. Surgical repair is required.

Trauma to the biliary tree

This injury is uncommon but should be suspected where low-grade, persistent peritonitis occurs following trauma.

THE PREGNANT TEENAGER

Trauma occurs in 6–8% of pregnancies. Fetal loss from minor trauma is rare and is most common as a result of maternal death. Significant prevention is afforded by lap and shoulder seat-belt use in motor vehicles (a 50% reduction in maternal death or serious injury and no increase in the incidence of fetal death).

Pathophysiology of teen pregnancy

Cardiovascular changes

Cardiac output increases by 40% by the 10th week of gestation. During the last trimester a 25% reduction occurs (due to aortocaval compression). Blood pressure falls and pulse pressure widens during the first 6 months of pregnancy. Blood pressure returns to normal values near term (pregnant patients are never normally hypertensive). Circulating blood volume is increased by 50% by 34 weeks of gestation and the CVP is one third of normal at term when the resting heart rate is 80–90 beats/min.

Blood flows through the uterus at a rate equivalent to the entire maternal cardiac output every 8–10 minutes. Maternal hematocrit is 0.32–0.34 (32–34%) at 34 weeks of gestation and there is a physiological leukocytosis (18×10^9/L). Coagulation factors rise towards term and a normal fibrinogen level can exist even in the presence of disseminated intravascular coagulation (DIC). The gravid uterus elevates the diaphragm, but overall there is an increase in tidal volume, P_{CO_2} values are 4–4.5 kPa (30–34 mmHg) by term, with bicarbonate values of 19.5 mmol/L (V_{O_2} increases by 20%).

Practice points

Acute maternal bleeding or hypoxia result in uterine artery constriction and secondary uterine hypoperfusion. Fetal compromise can result in the absence of maternal clinical signs.

Placental abruption is common following severe blunt abdominal maternal trauma. Pre-mature labor is frequent, particularly following abruption. The wellbeing of a fetus should be checked by:

1. Fetal heart rate variability (baseline, beat-to-beat and long-term) and the presence of decelerations (decelerations and accelerations are less sensitive than beat-to-beat variability for fetal distress).
2. Late decelerations (type II) suggest fetal hypoxia. Type I (early) are usually innocent. Tococardiography is the optimal method for detecting abruption; ultrasonography is the best method of checking for the presence of a fetal heart.

If chest tube insertion is required the point of insertion should be one or two interspaces higher than usual.

Pregnant teenagers with an altered level of consciousness (especially with seizures) should be assessed for eclampsia

Management

Pre-hospital care:

- transport the patient to triage
- position the patients on their left side tilted 15° down (to avoid the uterus compressing the vena cava)
- give oxygen

Hospital care:

- anticipate occult maternal hemorrhage of 10–20% of blood volume
- after primary and secondary survey consider nasogastric tube and Foley catheter placement, monitor fetal heart rate at least every 10 minutes (*Note*—lowered fetal heart rate equals abruption until proved otherwise)
- laboratory studies:
  - conventional investigations for trauma
  - fibrinogen, FDP and Kleihauer–Betke test (for fetal maternal hemorrhage)
- treatment:
  - carefully maintain oxygenation and support circulating volume to avoid fetal hypoxia/ischemia. Position mother on left side to avoid vena caval compression and compromised cardiac return
  - consider blood transfusion early to prevent maternal anemia
  - tetanus prophylaxis may be given for the usual indications (there is no evidence of teratogenicity)

INTENSIVE CARE

Intensive care following abdominal trauma is comparable to that required by the multiple trauma victim and necessitates meticulous attention to monitoring respiratory and cardiovascular function, following clinical and laboratory parameters for signs of change, intervening to treat abnormalities and initiating additional investigation or surgical management as required.

Careful triage is important in this group of patients. All children with abdominal trauma require admission and any evidence of intra-abdominal bleeding, even if seemingly minor in a stable child, demands ongoing intensive care monitoring and discussion regarding the possible need for surgery and/or transport.

TRANSPORT

The process of interfacility transfer can aggravate and accelerate bleeding. Pain can be increased con-

siderably by movement. In addition to optimizing oxygenation, two secure sites for intravenous access are required. The child's condition should be carefully documented prior to analgesia being given to provide pain relief for the journey. Gastric drainage (with a large-bore tube to avoid blockage) makes the child more comfortable, as well as providing treatment for paralytic ileus and reducing the risk of vomiting and secondary as-piration. Assessment of the urinary tract should be sufficiently comprehensive for a Foley catheter to be passed prior to transfer unless the journey is less than 1 hour in duration.

RENAL TRAUMA

Renal trauma should be suspected where there are the following physical signs:

- pelvic fracture
- inability to void
- genital swelling
- blood at the urinary meatus
- hematuria
- high-riding prostate on rectal examination
- fractures of the lower ribs
- lower abdominal mass or tenderness
- a mass in the flank, a contusion or an obvious wound

Renal trauma is relatively rare. Approximately 5% of childhood trauma involves the kidney, and in 10% of these cases an underlying renal anomaly makes the kidney more vulnerable to trauma (hydronephrosis or horseshoe kidney).

MANAGEMENT

Priorities will depend on the overall condition of the child; 80–90% of children will have hematuria after renal injury. Try to determine the type, location and extent of injury and make an assessment of the status of the uninjured kidney. Generally minor contusions and lacerations can be managed conservatively, but these decisions should be made jointly with the pediatric nephrologist or surgeon. *Note*—the extent of the hematuria does not correlate with the severity of the injury. Similarly, the absence of hematuria does not rule out significant renal trauma.

Catheterization of the urethra should not be attempted until the integrity of the urethra is confirmed by a urethrogram. The optimal form of radiological study should be discussed with a radiologist; computerized tomography is often preferable to conventional intravenous pyelograms as trauma elsewhere in the abdomen can be detected in addition to lesions within the urinary tract.

Other associated injuries (such as a ruptured liver or intracranial injury) may be life-threatening and require immediate intervention, which can result in a delay in diagnosis of renal injuries. Children rarely exsanguinate from renal injuries. Those who present in profound shock usually have associated injuries. Paralytic ileus can accompany renal injuries if intraperitoneal damage has also occurred. An algorithm for the management of renal trauma is shown in Figure 4.4.2.

RESPIRATORY TRACT INJURY

LARYNGOTRACHEAL TRAUMA

Laryngotracheal injuries are relatively rare. These structures are predominantly cartilaginous and major trauma is required to cause significant injury. In addition the surrounding structures are mobile and the thoracic cage is intrinsically elastic. Laryngeal fractures are more common in older children and young adults. Hanging and choking injuries (both deliberate and accidental) can produce a variety of symptoms which include changes in the pattern of respiration and ability to phonate. There may also be difficulty with swallowing, hoarseness, stridor, hemoptysis, subcutaneous emphysema and signs of asphyxia. Physical signs can include local bruising, petechiae, edema, lacerations and crepitus from subcutaneous emphysema. After hanging, or strangulation from neck entrapment, localized injury or laceration may be evident.

Mild lesions are the most common. They are seen in younger children and clinical signs include edema, lacerations and hematoma.

Blunt or penetrating trauma can cause injury to the trachea and lower respiratory tract through shearing forces, by direct compression and distention against a closed glottis. Right-sided injury near the carina is the most common site of tracheal injury.

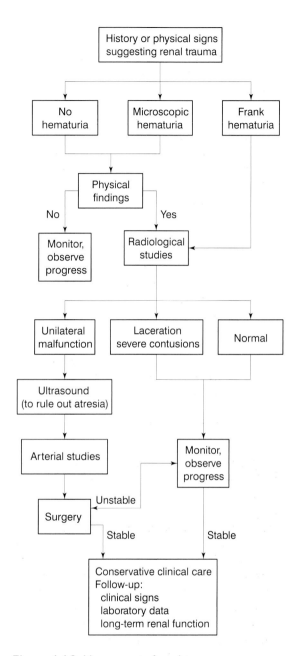

Figure 4.4.2 Management of renal trauma

Tracheal rupture follows major chest trauma, particularly injuries related to motor vehicle crashes, falls from a significant height, and the application of acute force to a localized area of the airway (e.g. neck entrapment in an automatic garage door). Findings include active bleeding with hemoptysis (usually where bronchial artery damage is associated), respiratory difficulty, progressive subcutaneous or mediastinal emphysema, tension pneumothorax, massive atelectasis or airway obstruction.

In children with injuries secondary to hanging or neck entrapment, there is a high risk of associated damage to the cervical spine which requires immobilization and maintenance of stabilization during investigation.

Traumatic tracheoesophageal fistula can develop 3–5 days after compression injuries that trap the trachea and esophagus between the sternum and the vertebrae. This type of injury leads to ischemic damage which is followed by necrosis and fistula formation. Another bizarre injury follows ingestion of superheated food into the esophagus (e.g. a piece of a microwaved snack). This creates a local burn in the esophagus and secondary thermal injury to the airway anteriorly with edema causing alteration of respiration and phonation, problems with secretions and the risk of airway obstruction. This is effectively a traumatic form of epiglottitis and should be managed similarly to epiglottitis from an infectious cause. See Chapter 3.1 for airway foreign body aspirations.

Resuscitative measures depend on the severity of the symptoms (Ch. 2.6). For mild cases, inhalation of a cool mist may be helpful. All children with signs or symptoms of airway involvement following trauma require admission and observation. Moderate cases may require urgent laryngoscopy and/or racemic epinephrine (adrenaline) to maintain airway patency. For severe symptoms bag-and-mask ventilation and/or endotracheal intubation must be attempted. If edema is present a smaller tube will be required. Hemorrhage and secretions can obstruct the field of view and localized swelling or discontinuity of part of the airway can result in unfamiliar anatomy. Intubation can be made easier by using a flexible light wand (lighted stylet) particularly in the prehospital or emergency room setting. The device gives more light and better visualization than a laryngoscope alone and blind intubation is aided by transillumination of the soft tissues of the neck. The optimal method of diagnosing the location and extent of a tracheobronchial lesion is bronchoscopy. Surgical repair is required for traumatic disruption. Tracheostomy or thoracotomy may be necessary.

LUNG CONTUSION

Lung contusion can occur in the absence of rib fractures or overt injury and can present either acutely or over a number of hours following trauma. Contusion to the lung tissue results in edema and progressive desaturation secondary to arterial venous shunting which can progress to frank hypoxia.

Diagnosis

The diagnosis is made by a combination of clinical examination and X-rays. Clinically, the child has respiratory difficulty with dyspnea and elevation of respiratory rate, and crepitations develop within the area of contusion. Active bleeding may occur (hemoptysis, blood in the endotracheal tube or with suctioning). Severe cases will be markedly hypoxemic, cyanosed and in great respiratory difficulty.

Immediately after contusion the chest X-ray may be normal but as symptoms develop patchy infiltrates or consolidation are usually evident. Computed tomographic studies identify contusion well.

Management

Management includes provision of oxygen and support of the airway and respiration. Intubation and mechanical ventilation may be required and either positive end-expiratory pressure or an element of continuous positive airway pressure is frequently beneficial. After the initial resuscitation of any coexisting hypovolemia due to other elements of trauma, fluid restriction is employed to limit the evolution of pulmonary edema. Symptoms can progress during the first day following injury and resolution is usually complete in 2–3 days.

VASCULAR INJURY

Major intrathoracic vascular injury is extremely rare in children and usually follows severe trauma such as an unrestrained injury in a motor vehicle or a long fall. The majority of children do not survive to reach hospital, dying from the combined effects of hypovolemia and associated injury (particularly head injury and loss of respiratory drive, and protective airway and respiratory responses). Of those who do survive most are unconscious, and have signs of shock, localized absence of pulses or obliteration of breath sounds, in addition, abdominal distention or signs of hemoperitoneum can occur. In the conscious child chest and limb pain accompany progressive signs of shock. If chest X-ray is possible, the classic signs are of widening of the mediastinum, apical capping of the lung, first or second rib fracture and deviation of the trachea away from the site of injury. Computed tomographic images show high-density collections within the pleural cavity, and can be used to identify intrathoracic vascular injury in the absence of signs of bony trauma. Angiography usually remains the definitive study.

MANAGEMENT

Management requires all facets of resuscitation to be applied with consummate speed, plus surgical consultation and possibly arteriography prior to emergency surgery. Most vascular injuries in childhood follow penetrating trauma. With peripheral vascular injury, initial management includes attempts to limit blood loss by tamponade of the bleeding site through manual compression. In hospital, surgical exploration to locate the site of injury and determine treatment options should be a priority. With extremity fractures where arterial laceration (or compression) is possible, urgent orthopedic consultation is necessary before fracture reduction so that the bony and vascular components of the injury can be addressed appropriately.

The incidence of vascular compromise compounding fractures in children is rare (< 0.5%). The vessels most prone to injury are those in proximity to supracondylar fractures. Ischemia for longer than 3 hours will have serious sequelae.

A controversial element of care is the use of systemic heparinization as a means of preventing thrombosis. If it has a place in management, it is for injuries that are isolated and not associated with a rapidly progressive hematoma.

The most reliable sign of vascular integrity is the return of peripheral pulses following fracture reduction. Doppler examination is valuable where distal pulses are either weak or impalpable. Serial examinations (preferably by the same observer) are essential.

With penetrating trauma arteriography is usually not indicated prior to surgery. Exploration of the wound is usually sufficient to locate the site of vascular injury. Arteriography is most relevant in the child who is not in shock and has questionable damage to an intraabdominal vessel (evidenced by abdominal tenderness and/or a mass) and those with cervicomediastinal trauma (e.g. with loss of carotid or arm pulsation, hemothorax, widening mediastinum, subpleural hematoma). In addition to confirming the diagnosis arteriography can delineate the optimal operative approach.

Doppler studies enable distinction between spasm and occlusion. Most vessels in spasm have some distal flow which increases with correction of hypovolemia. However, appropriate intensive care includes surgical consultation in such cases, rather than waiting and assuming that spasm will resolve over a number of hours. If the diagnosis made is incorrect irreversible ischemia and thrombosis can occur within this period.

Carotid artery injury can follow blunt or penetrating trauma to the neck. Clinical signs include the loss of carotid pulsation and/or expanding hematoma or persistent bleeding. Subcutaneous emphysema should be suspected as an associated complication where there is visible (bubbling) or audible (hissing) escape of air from the wound. Under these circumstances the airway must be secured and tracheal and esophageal exploration will need to accompany the vascular repair.

The first aid measures are the obvious ones of maintaining airway patency and oxygenation while applying direct compression to the bleeding site, obtaining vascular access, restoring circulating volume and mobilizing the appropriate surgical team.

ELECTRICAL INJURIES

Electrical injuries are a potent cause of death, serious injury and permanent disability. The main mechanisms of injury are:

- electrical
- thermal
- mechanical

Electrical current is either alternating (which causes repeated fibrillating stimuli to the myocardium) or direct (which causes a single countershock). There is electrical disruption of central nervous system integrity directly and through associated injury (vascular injury, coagulation and disruption of the respiratory center). Apnea tends to be more prolonged than cardiac dysfunction and anoxic secondary injury is a common sequela.

Thermal injury can be extreme. Superficial burns may occur due to combustion of clothing; deeper injury occurs where metal melts in contact with the skin (e.g. belt buckles or jewelry). Dry skin tends to deflect electricity over the body surface, but high-energy discharge or contact with a wet surface can result in thermal transmission through the body, evidenced by entry and exit wounds. Skin marking with electrical burns is often described as having a 'feathered' or 'tree-like' pattern.

Mechanical trauma is usually blunt, secondary to pressure waves or being thrown off balance, and is particularly common with lightning injury. Any organ system may be affected.

The severity of injury depends on multiple factors. Burns to the head carry a poor prognosis as do extensive muscle involvement or widespread damage to nerves or blood vessels. Delays in initiating cardiopulmonary resuscitation contribute to death. Failure to provide adequate respiratory support during the period of apnea is a major error.

LIGHTNING INJURIES

Lightning injuries may be due to a direct strike or a proximity strike involving another person or static object. The combination of massive electrical and thermal energy is highly disruptive and frequently causes death or permanent neurological disability. However, approximately 60% of victims survive if prompt CPR and ongoing respiratory support are provided. The most common effects of lightning strike are:

- central nervous system:
    - disruption of respiratory drive
    - loss of consciousness

- cerebral edema
    - convulsions
    - paralyses
    - intracranial bleeding
    - amnesia (retrograde)
    - aphasia
    - vertigo
    - psychological disturbance
- respiratory system:
    - apnea
    - lung contusion
- cardiovascular system:
    - asystole
    - myocardial damage
    - atrial or ventricular fibrillation
    - premature ventricular contractions
    - raised BP or shock
    - heart failure
- renal:
    - myoglobinuria
- auditory:
    - hearing loss (sensorineural, tympanic rupture)
- skeletal:
    - fractures
    - cervical-spine injury
- skin:
    - burns
    - rashes ('tree-like' pattern)
- other:
    - stress ulcers
    - SIADH
    - compartment syndrome
    - vascular spasm

Renal failure develops secondary to impaired perfusion or blunt trauma (myoglobin release can be a factor but is less common in lightning injury than other electrical trauma). Vascular injury may be temporary where spasm is involved, but permanent problems with circulation occur and compartment syndrome can develop.

TREATMENT AT THE SCENE

Resuscitation must be deferred, pending safe rescue of the victim who may still be in contact with the electrical source when found. This poses risks for the rescuers. Disconnecting the power supply is safer than attempts to isolate the victim using a nonconducting material (e.g. a wooden object). The priorities of the ABCs should be followed and respiratory support should be continued pending restoration of cardiac rhythm. Those victims not in asystole or apneic are likely to survive. Care with the cervical spine at the scene of injury should occur.

HOSPITAL CARE

Continue CPR with particular attention to respiratory support and review of circulatory adequacy. A history of clinical signs of mechanical trauma necessitates evaluation of the cervical spine. Electrocardiographic studies may show nonspecific ST segment changes or there may be evidence of myocardial infarction. Biochemical studies include measurement of lactate dehydrogenase (LDH). These isoenzymes are preferable to creatine phosphokinase (CPK) enzyme assay as electrical trauma to muscle tissue can release cardiac fractions of the CPK enzyme. Fluid management should be used aggressively to correct hypovolemia and maintain urine output. The principles are similar to those for other burns but larger volumes may be required to compensate for internal elements of electrical burn injury. Urine analysis for myoglobin is important. If myoglobin is present, clearance can be aided by promoting urine flow (2 ml/kg·h) until frank myoglobinuria ceases, then maintain flows of 0.5–1 ml/kg·h. Pigment deposition in the tubes may be reduced by therapy with mannitol and/or alkalinization of the urine. A CT scan can be valuable to detect blunt injury to internal organs or CNS-related injury.

Triage

These patients require admission for appropriate burn care, cardiac monitoring, respiratory support and fluid management. The presence of neurological deficit and the risk of cerebral edema make neurological consultation appropriate.

CRUSH INJURIES

Traumatic asphyxia is a syndrome that follows acute high-pressure compression of the chest. The most common cause is motor vehicle trauma where the child is physically run over by the vehicle. Automatic garage doors can cause similar injuries and children trampled on by crowds can present with crush injuries as a component of multiple trauma. Because the injury occurs when the child is conscious the chest compression occurs against a closed glottis (as the child cries out). There is a marked elevation of intrathoracic pressure which is transmitted peripherally through the venous system. The integrity of the valves within the veins is overcome with the result that the raised venous pressure communicates with the intracranial structures.

On examination there are petechiae and areas of suffusion with edema caudally from the point of crush injury, so that the head, neck and upper chest are usually involved. Frequently there is overt swelling of the eyelids, and conjunctival hemorrhages, fundal hemorrhages and proptosis are described. The flexibility of the child's skeleton means that rib fractures do not always occur. The child usually complains of chest pain, headache, breathing difficulty and sometimes disordered vision (secondary to CNS sequelae or retinal injury). The marks of the tire tread are often visible across the chest, and examination of the child below the point of contact usually reveals nothing abnormal. However, lung contusion is commonly associated and vascular injuries can occur. Seizures and airway compromise are also found.

Management involves appropriate support and monitoring of respiratory and cardiovascular function; and in addition evaluation of myocardial function, the central nervous system, a complete eye examination and an evaluation for abdominal injury are important.

COMPARTMENT SYNDROME

Compartment syndrome can be defined as an elevation of pressure within one or more tissue compartments in an extremity, which results in disturbance of circulation of blood to the muscles and nerves within that anatomical region. A high index of suspicion is required for this condition, which can follow a variety of blunt or fracture-related injuries. The mechanisms involved are complex and multifactorial and include external pressure, tissue swelling, hemorrhage within a confined space and the effects of progressive ischemia. Decreased arterial blood flow results and irreversible ischemic damage and necrosis will occur over a 4–6-hour period if surgical relief of the pressure within the affected compartments does not occur.

The diagnosis is made on the basis of careful and repeated neurovascular examination, looking particularly for changes in sensation initially (hyperesthesia and parasthesia) and pain in the muscles, particularly with movements that involve stretching, as the muscle fibers become ischemic. In an unconscious child these signs cannot be elicited, and the presence of a distal pulse does not exclude that a compartment syndrome exists or is evolving following trauma. Surgical intervention has to be based on the nature of the injuries and exploratory findings; often it is required prophylactically (as in the case of burns).

Surgical fasciotomy is most often required in the periphery (lower leg, hands and forearms).

Controversial elements of care include direct measurements of pressure within compartments which many feel are inaccurate and inappropriately time-consuming.

The ultimate diagnosis and management of compartment syndrome is surgical. However, having the suspicion and initiating surgical enquiry is a prime responsibility of any physician caring for a critically injured child.

SOFT TISSUE INJURIES

Clean soft tissue wounds that result from trauma are often minor; however, those that are extensive, complicated or result in avulsion of body parts require special care.

CLASSIFICATION

Wounds can be divided into those that are open or closed. Open wounds occur where the skin is broken and it is important to determine the age of the wound and the degree of contamination. The risk of contamination depends in large part on the nature of the object causing trauma, the time since injury and the extent of the tissue injured. The

dirtiness of the object or the degree of contamination with bacteria (e.g. human or animal teeth), the passage of 6 hours or more since injury, and large areas of crushed or devitalized tissue all increase the risk. The presence of foreign bodies, the location of the child at the time of trauma and the site of injury on the body are also relevant. Penetrating wounds contaminated by gut contents or those received in an environment where there is a high level of bacterial contamination (e.g. agricultural injuries) are particularly dangerous.

MANAGEMENT

The priorities for care are to arrest hemorrhage, establish if there are underlying fractures or communication with deeper structures, and minimize the risk of further contamination or extension of injury. Irrigation of the tissues involved with copious amounts of fluid is generally a sound principle, as is removal of foreign bodies and any devitalized tissue by debriding (the latter is particularly important for animal bites). Saline solution (0.9%) can be used to irrigate the majority of wounds. Fluid should be directed as deeply as possible into the tissue. Generally nothing is added to the irrigation solution as most antibacterial agents and surfactants are toxic to tissues or cell function. If the wound is to be closed, the surrounding skin surface should be cleansed prior to suturing (e.g. with iodine).

Delayed closure is used for open wounds where there is extensive soft tissue injury, where the site where the injury occurred was heavily contaminated (e.g. agricultural injuries), wounds that are over 24 hours old, most bites where there are deep areas of puncture or extensive tissue trauma, and wounds in poorly vascularized areas (e.g. the shin or elbow). Delayed closure involves appropriate irrigation, debriding and dressing with a review for potential closure at 72 hours.

Wound infection is reduced by irrigation and debriding and foreign body removal. If surgery is required for penetrating wounds preoperative intravenous medication is usually recommended (e.g. with penicillin).

Many animal bites require antibiotic prophylaxis. Human, camel and cat bites do, as do bites to the hand or the face or where there are deep punctures or delay in closure beyond 6 hours after the bite. The child receiving cancer chemotherapy or otherwise immunocompromised also benefits from prophylaxis. Options include penicillin G (benzyl penicillin) (200 000 units/kg per day), penicillin plus gentamicin (5 mg/kg per day) or ticarcillin plus clavulanic acid (200 mg/kg per day).

Children who are actually or effectively asplenic can also develop overwhelming infection following wound contamination with relatively benign organisms. The most common contaminating flora are *Staphylococcus aureus* and group A streptococci; *Pasteurella multocida* is common in cat and dog bites.

Many foreign bodies are evident radiologically. Two views are beneficial and identification is easiest when a radio-opaque marker is placed on the skin. Metal is readily visualized. Glass is usually detectable. The visibility of plastic fragments and wood fibers depends partly on their size.

Avulsed or amputated tissue (e.g. ears, fingers) should be saved in the hope of surgical reimplantation. Tissues should be handled gently, cleansed (preferably in Ringer-lactate solution) and protected by moistened gauze and a plastic bag. Tissue should be kept cool (in close proximity to, but not directly in contact with, ice chips). Avulsed secondary teeth should be transported in Ringer-lactate solution or milk en route to hospital. Gentle washing in Ringer's solution should precede reinsertion. Reinsertion optimally occurs less than 12 hours following trauma.

Additional investigations (e.g. CT scan) are indicated where penetrating soft tissue wounds may communicate with deeper structures, such as in abdominal wounds or dog bites to the head in a smaller child.

TETANUS PROPHYLAXIS

Tetanus prophylaxis is integral to the comprehensive care of trauma victims. The regimen used depends upon the immunization status and the age of the individual. A table of recommendations can be found in Chapter 7.3, page 559.

✔ KEY POINTS

TRAUMA

➤ Repeat examination to confirm the adequacy of the airway, breathing and circulation is an ongoing part of management and assessment of progress, as is recalculation and recording of the Glasgow coma scale score

➤ Always perform a detailed examination of the head and neck, and exclude other associated injuries. As more history becomes available, specific areas may require additional examination or investigation

➤ Prevention of factors that can cause or aggravate secondary injuries is the major objective for physicians managing children following traumatic injury

➤ Talk to the child: if the child is able to reply and give logical answers, the airway is patent and the child is being adequately oxygenated (a normal cry confirms the patency of the airway in an infant)

➤ With impairment of consciousness the tongue commonly obstructs the airway, and the relatively large size of a child's head can lead to airway compromise from excessive neck flexion: use the chin lift maneuver to open the airway.

➤ Monitor perfusion and blood pressure, bearing in mind that hypotension only occurs late in the evolution of shock (adequate circulation is suggested by a palpable *peripheral* pulse)

ABDOMINAL TRAUMA

➤ abdominal trauma in children is frequently part of the clinical presentation of multiple trauma

➤ hepatic and splenic injury is the most common form of serious abdominal trauma in children

➤ the absence of free air on abdominal films does not exclude bowel perforation

➤ hemoperitoneum and liver injury can progress rapidly to shock and urgent surgical exploration may be required

AIRWAY TRAUMA

➤ A variety of traumatic injuries can involve the upper and lower airway; even minor degrees of swelling produce disproportionally severe obstruction in the small airway of the child

➤ Clinical signs of respiratory distress should prompt early, elective intubation and support of ventilation; do not delay for blood gas analysis or chest X-rays

➤ Tension pneumothorax should be suspected where respiratory failure follows trauma or acute chest pain. Be prepared to do a needle aspiration for diagnosis or relief of symptoms. Do not wait for a chest X-ray in the severely distressed child

➤ Lung contusions can be asymptomatic initially. Close monitoring and a high index of suspicion are required for early intervention

➤ The frequency, depth and pattern of respiration help to determine if breathing is adequate. Administer oxygen if any doubt exists

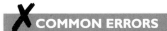

COMMON ERRORS

TRAUMA

➤ Mismanagement or neglect while performing the ABCs or initial management of trauma are major causes of preventable complications. Pediatric airway skills are particularly valuable because of the high incidence of respiratory compromise during injury in this age group

➤ Failing to prevent significant movement of the neck before the cervical spine has been protected or confirmed to be intact radiologically: keep a rigid cervical collar in place or stabilize the cervical spine manually during neck examination)

➤ Not maintaining circulating volume and blood pressure sufficiently to ensure cerebral perfusion and oxygen delivery.

ABDOMINAL TRAUMA

➤ Failure to provide gastric drainage with an adequately large nasogastric tube

➤ Failing to diagnose hypovolemia or impending shock (the hemoglobin or hematocrit may be normal initially, as may blood pressure)

➤ Sending a child for radiological studies prior to stabilization of the vital signs

➤ Failure to examine all six elements of the abdomen—anterior, posterior (including the back), both flanks, the pelvic floor and the diaphragm

➤ Failing to consider the possibility of spinal injury and moving the child with abdominal trauma

FURTHER READING

1. APLS. The pediatric emergency medicine course. 2nd ed. Elk Grove/Dallas: American Academy of Pediatrics/American College of Emergency Physicians; 1993
   – *(Thorough overview of trauma management priorities and explanation of related procedures)*

2. Lloyd-Thomas AR. ABC of major trauma: pediatric trauma. Primary survey and resuscitation 1. Br Med J 1990; 301: 334

3. Lloyd-Thomas AR. ABC of major trauma: pediatric trauma. Survey and resuscitation 2. Br Med J 1990; 301: 380
   – *(Two papers summarizing the priorities of the pediatric primary and secondary survey)*

4. Hung OR, Stewart RD. Lightwand intubation I. A new light wand device. Can J Anaesth 1995; 42(9): 820–825, 1995
   – *(A description of the technique for using a flexible lighted stylet to assist intubation)*

5. Ciarallo L, Fleisher G. Femoral fractures: are children at risk for significant blood loss? Ped Emerg Care 1996; 12(5): 343–346
   – *(A retrospective study indicating that multiple trauma victims, older children and those with a hematocrit below 30% often need blood transfusion, while those with isolated femoral fractures rarely lose sufficient blood to necessitate transfusion)*

6. Esposito TJ. Trauma during pregnancy. Emerg Med Clin North Am 1994;12(1): 167–199
   – *(The special circumstances of trauma in the pregnant patient)*

7. Jaffe KM, Massagli TL, Martin KM et al. Pediatric traumatic brain injury: acute and rehabilitation costs. Arch Phys Med Rehabil 1993; 74: 681–686
   – *(The economic costs of mild, moderate and severe brain injury—obvious cost benefit implications of minimizing severity and preventing secondary brain injury)*

8. Swischuk LE. Emergency imaging of the acutely ill or injured child. 3rd ed. Williams & Wilkins, Baltimore, 1994.
   – *(The subject material of this excellent book is 'bread and butter' radiology presented in a form that is practical and clinically useful. This book is particularly valuable for physicians who do not have ready access to radiologists with extensive familiarity with pediatric imaging.)*

4.5 Toxicology and poisoning

Tom Grattan-Smith

Clinicians who care for acutely ill children must be able to recognize that poisoning has or is likely to have occurred, assess its severity, initiate resuscitation, stabilize the patient and gain access to appropriate information. Information about the pharmacology and likely toxicity of individual compounds or combinations of compounds and the range of treatments available is readily accessible from poison information centers and from textbooks. Such information usually relates to adults and one should be cautious about extrapolating it to children.

EPIDEMIOLOGY

In the USA in 1992 there were 950 human exposures to poisons per 100,000 population (probably an underestimate). Most reported poison exposures occur in young children: 59% involve children less than 6 years old, with the highest incidence in those aged 1–2 years (37%).

In children younger than 6 years the vast majority of poisonings are unintentional. Disruption of the normal home environment by moving house, absence of one parent, pregnancy, diverts the attention of parents and predisposes to poisoning. Intentional poisoning (child abuse or Munchausen syndrome by proxy) occurs infrequently but should be considered in repeatedly poisoned children less than 3 years of age. Intentional self-poisoning is more common in older children and adolescents, and may be associated with a major disturbance such as depression and physical and sexual abuse.

PREVENTION

Preventive strategies (especially legislative) have greatly reduced mortality rates for child poisoning. Packaging legislation in many countries has made it more difficult for young children to gain access to toxins. Other methods include education of families about the toxicity of common household products and their safe usage and storage. A completely 'childproof' environment will never be achieved, so appropriate supervision of young children remains essential. Well-advertised telephone numbers for poison information centers provide rapid access to information for parents and hospital staff.

DIAGNOSIS

An approach to establishing the diagnosis of poisoning is shown in Table 4.5.1.

HISTORY

> Recognize the possibility of poisoning

Children often present with a clear history of known or possible exposure to a specific toxin. In other cases it is not clear that poisoning has occurred, and one must seek information from witnesses such as ambulance personnel, friends, relatives or other bystanders. The key to recognition is a high index of suspicion of poisoning, especially in any young child who presents with an acute unexplained illness. An altered level of consciousness, unusual behavior, unexplained trauma, unexplained metabolic acidosis or unexplained dysrhythmias should alert the clinician to the possibility of poisoning.

PHYSICAL EXAMINATION

The first priority is to recognize and treat actual or impending compromise of the airway, breathing or circulation. During the first examination, baseline observations of conscious state and vital signs are made and the child should be examined for the effects of the suspected compound and evidence of trauma. This examination should include:

- temperature
- heart rate and rhythm

- blood pressure
- respiratory rate and pattern
- level of consciousness
- pupil size and reaction
- presence or absence of sweating
- presence or absence of bowel sounds

These clinical signs, the ECG and pulse oximetry should be monitored closely.

If serious poisoning is suspected, investigations should include:

- urea and electrolytes
- plasma glucose
- liver function tests
- osmolar and anion gaps
- urinalysis
- X-rays looking for evidence of trauma, aspiration and opaque tablets in the esophagus, stomach or bowel
- timed measurements of blood levels of drugs such as acetaminophen (paracetamol),

theophylline or cyclic antidepressants may be used to guide treatment

MANAGEMENT

EMERGENCY DEPARTMENT MANAGEMENT

Treat the patient not the poison.

Minimize the patient's exposure to the toxin. For inhaled poisons the first priority is to remove the patient from the contaminated atmosphere. For skin exposure the skin should be thoroughly washed with water and soap. Remove contaminated clothing. For chemical eye injury, the eye is rapidly and thoroughly irrigated with water or saline for at least half an hour and until all contamination has been removed. Alkalis may require irrigation for many hours. Gut decontamination (see below) should be considered for ingested poisons.

TABLE 4.5.1 **Approach to a possible poisoning**

Consider the possibility of poisoning
- History:
  - missing tablets or compound
  - observed exposure
  - acute unexplained illness
  - **high index of suspicion**
- Physical examination
  - baseline observations of conscious state and vital signs
  - effects of the suspected compound
  - evidence of trauma.
- Investigations—**should not delay urgent treatment:**
  - specific effects: establish a baseline to detect later change
  - will drug levels be useful?
  - complications, e.g. aspiration, trauma

Management
- Supportive therapy
  - minimize the patient's exposure to the toxin
  - **ensure safety of staff**
  - ensure adequacy of the ABCs
  - treatment of complications, e.g. seizures, cardiac dysrhythmias
  - ICU support of organ systems
- gut decontamination
  - is the ingestion recent and serious enough to warrant decontamination?
  - does the compound bind to charcoal?
  - will repeated doses decrease absorption or enhance elimination? If not, proceed to whole bowel lavage
- Is further intervention indicated?
- Balance the risks and benefits – **treat the patient not the poison**
- enhancement of elimination (? dialysis, hemofiltration/perfusion)
- specific antidotes

Supportive therapy

Most patients who ingest a poison will survive intact if there is:

- appropriate support of the airway, breathing and circulation
- timely and effective gut decontamination
- treatment of complications such as seizures and cardiac dysrhythmias

Gut decontamination

Induced vomiting

Induced vomiting using syrup of ipecac 6% (1–2 ml/kg, maximum 30 ml) is rarely useful. Its efficacy is uncertain; it delays more useful treatment such as activated charcoal and may put the airway at risk. Contraindications include ingestion of corrosive compounds, hydrocarbons and compounds that may produce significant bradycardia or a rapid decrease in the level of consciousness.

Gastric lavage

Gastric lavage has a small role in gut decontamination. Its efficacy is also uncertain, but it may remove some of the ingested toxin and allow the gastric contents to be examined without delaying the administration of activated charcoal or whole bowel lavage. Because it is unpleasant and not clearly effective, gastric lavage is rarely indicated in a conscious patient.

Gastric lavage is most likely to be useful in the patient who presents early (less than 1 hour after ingestion, or later if the compound delays gastric emptying) with a potentially life-threatening ingestion and who is obtunded or comatose (in which case the patient will need to be intubated to protect the airway). Ingestion of corrosives or the presence of significant esophageal disease are absolute contraindications to its use.

Having ensured that the airway is protected, lie the patient on the left side and insert a large-bore (at least 32 FG even for small tablets), double lumen orogastric lavage tube. The stomach contents are then aspirated and an aliquot of 1–2 ml/kg of 0.9% saline is flushed in and then aspirated. This cycle is repeated until the aspirate is free of gross contamination by the ingested compound. A perfectly clear gastric aspirate need not be achieved so the process usually takes only a few minutes. Activated charcoal or whole bowel lavage solution can then be given via the gastric tube before it is removed.

Activated charcoal

Activated charcoal, given as a single dose of 1 g/kg or as repeated doses of 0.25 g/kg hourly, is the mainstay of gut decontamination. Repeated doses increase the charcoal to toxin ratio in the bowel and maintain the availability of binding sites. Charcoal administration interrupts the enterohepatic circulation of some toxins. Compounds that have already been absorbed may be removed from the blood by 'gastrointestinal dialysis'. Some compounds are not adsorbed to charcoal, including iron, lead, mercury, lithium, arsenic, cyanide, methanol and ethanol, ethylene glycol, strong acids and alkalis, organic solvents and hydrocarbons.

The use of laxatives such as sorbitol or magnesium sulfate with charcoal does not increase the clearance of drugs compared with charcoal alone and is not recommended. Children are usually reluctant to drink repeated doses of charcoal. Milk and flavorings reduce charcoal's adsorptive efficacy, so unmodified charcoal is given through a nasogastric tube (whose position has been checked by pH testing) in significant ingestions.

Charcoal should not be given in the absence of bowel sounds or in unintubated patients who are not conscious enough to protect their airway, as it can cause severe aspiration pneumonia.

Cathartics

Cathartic agents include saline, monosaccharides and whole bowel lavage (WBL) solutions. Osmotic cathartics such as magnesium citrate or mannitol may cause severe fluid and electrolyte shifts, whereas WBL solutions using polyethylene glycol cause no net fluid shift. Whole bowel lavage empties the gut by flushing, and enhances drug elimination by gastrointestinal dialysis and by interrupting enterohepatic circulation. It is the preferred cathartic technique in children of all ages. Indications for its use include:

- toxins that are poorly adsorbed by charcoal
- delayed-release drugs such as theophylline and verapamil
- iron tablets or watch batteries lying beyond the pylorus

The dose required for WBL is 15 ml/kg·h, increasing to 30 ml/kg·h (maximum of 2 L/h) if tolerated. Few patients will drink this volume and a gastric tube is usually required. Vomiting may require reduction of the administration rate or an antiemetic such as metoclopramide. The WBL solution is infused until the rectal effluent is clear, usually within a few hours.

INTENSIVE CARE MANAGEMENT

Intensive care management consists of supportive treatment for failure of organ systems (e.g. hypotension or cardiac dysrhythmias, respiratory failure, renal or hepatic failure, fits or encephalopathy). Enhancement of drug elimination should also be considered, and an antidote administered in the few cases when one is available.

Enhanced elimination

Indications for techniques to enhance elimination include:

- the patient is seriously ill or likely to become so
- the poison ingested can be removed in clinically significant quantities by the technique
- the likely benefit of the increased elimination outweighs the risks

The most commonly used methods are repeated doses of activated charcoal or whole bowel lavage (see above). The benefits of other methods such as forced acid or alkaline diuresis and extracorporeal techniques such as hemodialysis and charcoal hemoperfusion rarely outweigh their risks.

Forced acid or alkaline diuresis

The excretion of weak acids (e.g. salicylates) is enhanced by alkaline urine and that of weak alka-

lis (e.g. amphetamines) by acid urine. Promotion of a diuresis using mannitol or furosemide (frusemide) may also increase renal clearance. For most poisonings, the benefits of diuresis and pH manipulation do not warrant the risks of unwanted plasma electrolyte, pH and volume changes.

Dialysis

Hemodialysis and hemofiltration are only useful for elimination of massive overdoses of compounds which have a low molecular weight (< 500), a small volume of distribution (< 1 L/kg), are highly water-soluble and have low protein binding (< 90%). Such compounds include lithium, salicylates, ethanol and methanol. Peritoneal dialysis is less efficient than hemodialysis but may be more readily available and causes less cardiovascular instability in critically ill children. Dialysis techniques are described in Chapter 2.10.

Hemoperfusion

Compounds may be cleared from the blood by adsorption to activated charcoal or polystyrene resins contained in a hemoperfusion cartridge. Blood is pumped from a large vein through the cartridge and returned to the vein. Hemoperfusion is not useful for removal of fat-soluble drugs such as tricyclic antidepressants which have a large volume of distribution, because too little of the total toxin load in the body passes through the cartridge. Hemoperfusion has a small role in massive overdoses of drugs that:

- are water-soluble
- are adsorbed by activated charcoal
- have low fat and protein binding
- have low endogenous clearance (< 4 ml/kg·min)

The risks of extracorporeal toxin removal (by hemodialysis, hemofiltration or hemoperfusion) include complications of vessel cannulation, infection and bleeding complicated by heparinization and/or thrombocytopenia. Other problems include hemodilution, hypothermia, hypoglycemia and major electrolyte disturbances.

Antidotes and specific therapies

For a few toxins there is a specific therapy or antidote (Table 4.5.2). While these specific therapies—e.g. deferoxamine (desferrioxamine) for iron poisoning—and antidotes—e.g. *N*-acetylcysteine for acetaminophen (paracetamol)—may be effective, they all carry risks and should be used judiciously. The vast majority of patients who ingest toxins are successfully managed by gut decontamination and supportive therapy alone.

The toxidromes of cholinergics, anticholinergics, sympathomimetics, sympatholytics, and opiate, alcohol and sedative agents are shown in Table 4.5.3.

SPECIFIC POISONINGS

ACETAMINOPHEN (PARACETAMOL)

Acetaminophen is rapidly absorbed after oral ingestion and peak levels occur within 1–2 hours. Its volume of distribution is 0.9 L/kg.

Most acetaminophen is conjugated with sulfate and glucuronide in the liver, forming nontoxic metabolites. In toxic doses, the conjugation pathway is overwhelmed and depletion of liver glutathione stores allows a toxic metabolite to disrupt the liver cell membrane and inactivate intracellular proteins. Hepatotoxicity is the major feature of acetaminophen poisoning but the kidneys, heart

TABLE 4.5.2 **Common poisons and their antidotes**		
Poison	**Antidote**	**Route and dose duration**
Acetaminophen (paracetamol)	*N*-Acetylcysteine	See text
Beta-blockers	Glucagon	See text
Calcium channel blocker	Calcium	See text
Tricyclic antidepressants	Bicarbonate	1–2 mmol/kg i.v. for cardiac conduction delay or ventricular arrythmia. Titrate to effect and pH
Iron	Deferoxamine (desferrioxamine)	See text
Lead	EDTA	30–40 mg/kg per dose i.m. or slow i.v. (over 1 hour) 12-hourly for 5 days[a]
Mercury	Dimercaprol (BAL)	3 mg/kg per dose (max. 150 mg) i.m. 4-hourly for 2 days, then 6-hourly for 1 day and then 12-hourly for 10 days[a]
	Penicillamine	5–7.5 mg/kg per dose 6-hourly (max. 2 g per day) oral[a]
Arsenic	Dimercaprol (BAL) Penicillamine	As for mercury
Methanol	Ethanol	See text
Ethylene glycol	Ethanol	See text
Organophosphate insecticides	Atropine	0.05 mg/kg i.v., then 0.02–0.05 mg/kg per dose every 15–60 min until atropinized 12–24 h)[a]
(continue	Pralidoxime	25–50 mg/kg (max. 2 g) over 30 min, then up to 10 mg/kg·h (max. 12 g per day)[a]
Anticholinergics	Physostigmine	0.02 mg/kg (max. 1 mg) i.v. every 5 min till response (max. 0.1 mg/kg) then 0.5 – 2.0 μg/kg·min[a]
Narcotics	Naloxone	0.1 mg/kg i.v. stat (max 2 mg) then then 0.01 mg/kg·h[a]
Digoxin	Digoxin immune Fab	See text
Benzodiazepines	Flumazenil	5 μg/kg stat i.v. repeat every 60 s to max total of 40 μg/kg (max. 2 mg), then 2–10 μg/kg·h i.v.[a] (contraindications coingestion of tricyclic antidepressants or benzodiazepine therapy for seizure prevention)

[a] *Shann F. Drug doses, 9th ed. Collective Pty Ltd. 1996.*

TABLE 4.5.3 Toxidromes

Cholinergic (e.g. organophosphate insecticides)
- Central effects:
  agitation, confusion, seizures, coma
- Muscarinic effects:
  - **S**alivation, **L**acrimation, **U**rination, **D**efecation, **G**astrointestinal disturbances, **E**mesis/Eye disturbance (miosis, blurred vision) (**SLUDGE** mnemonic)
  - plus bradycardia and heart block, bronchorrhea and wheezing
- Nicotinic effects:
  muscle fasciculations, weakness, paralysis, tachycardia and hypertension

Anticholinergic (e.g. atropine, antihistamines)
(*'mad as a hatter, blind as a bat, red as a beet, hot as a hare and dry as a bone'*)
- Central effects:
  tremor, agitation, confusion, hallucinations, psychosis, seizures, coma, myoclonus
- Peripheral effects:
  fever, flushing, dry skin, dry mouth, dry eyes, mydriasis, ileus, urinary retention, tachycardia

Sympathomimetic (e.g. cocaine, amphetamines, theophylline)
- Central effects:
  agitation, hyperreflexia, confusion, delusions, paranoia, seizures, coma
- Sympathetic system effects:
  fever, flushing, sweating, mydriasis
- CVS effects:
  tachycardia, hypertension, dysrhythmias, myocardial infarction, cerebral hemorrhage

Sympatholytic (e.g. β blockers)
- Mixed central and peripheral effects:
  bradycardia, hypotension, miosis, reduced sweating and peristalsis, CNS and respiratory depression

Opiate, ethanol, sedative
- Classical opiate effects:
  coma, respiratory depression and pinpoint pupils
- Other effects:
  MILD TOXICITY: mood changes, impaired judgment, dysarthria and ataxia
  GREATER TOXICITY: lethargy, coma, respiratory depression, miosis (mydriasis with some sedatives), ileus, hypothermia, hyporeflexia

---

and pancreas are also injured. Severe acetaminophen poisoning is relatively uncommon (though occasionally seen) in children under 6 years of age.

In the first few hours after ingestion there are usually few symptoms or signs. Nausea and vomiting may be present but soon settle. After 36 hours, the prothrombin time becomes prolonged and levels of transaminases and bilirubin increase. By day 3 or 4, clinical signs of hepatitis start to develop including anorexia, nausea, vomiting and hepatic tenderness. These may progress to clinically evident jaundice, hypoglycemia, coagulopathy and hepatic encephalopathy. In some cases, fulminant hepatic failure (Ch. 2.11) follows. If the patient survives, the liver usually recovers completely.

Management

Gut decontamination using activated charcoal is used in patients who present within 4 hours of ingestion and who have taken more than 100 mg/kg.

All patients at risk of hepatotoxicity should have an acetaminophen level measured as well as a baseline full blood count, electrolytes, calcium, urea and creatinine, liver function tests, blood glucose and coagulation studies. These are repeated once or twice daily until stable.

The antidote *N*-acetylcysteine is a glutathione precursor and an antioxidant which can completely prevent toxicity if started within 8 hours of ingestion. Acetylcysteine treatment started after 8 hours reduces mortality but does not prevent hepatotoxicity. When available, the i.v. form is preferable. The dose is:

- 150 mg/kg in 200 ml of 5% dextrose over 15–60 minutes, then
- 10 mg/kg·h for 4 hours, then
- 7 mg/kg·h for 20 hours (if delay <10 hours); 32 hours (if delay 10–16 hours) or 72 hours (if delay >16 hours).

Treatment is continued for longer than 72 hours in the presence of encephalopathy. If the i.v. form of *N*-acetylcysteine is unavailable, the oral 20% solution is used. After an oral loading dose of 140 mg/kg, doses of 70 mg/kg are given 4-hourly for 72 hours. The solution is unpalatable, and one part should be mixed with three parts of fruit juice. Antiemetics may be required.

About 5–10% of patients experience dose-related anaphylactoid reactions due to histamine release by *N*-acetylcysteine.

Supportive treatment of fulminant hepatic failure is given as required (Ch. 2.11).

BETA-BLOCKERS

Stimulation of β_1 receptors causes increased
- heart rate and force of myocardial contraction
- AV node conduction velocity
- renin secretion

Stimulation of β_2-receptors causes:

- relaxation of smooth muscle in bronchi, blood vessels, gastrointestinal and genitourinary tracts
- gluconeogenesis in the liver
- glycolysis in the liver and skeletal muscle

Beta-blockers act by competing with catecholamines at β-receptor sites. The various beta-blockers have different activity according to their:

- β_1 selectivity
- intrinsic sympathomimetic agonist activity
- lipid solubility
- class I and III antiarrhythmic effects

They are generally well absorbed from the small intestine with peak levels being reached within 1–2 hours and a half-life of less than 12 hours.

These drugs tend to have moderate to large volumes of distribution because of their lipid solubility, which also determines the degree of CNS penetration.

In poisoning, the major clinical problems relate to cardiovascular effects. Seizures are common with lipophilic beta-blockers and may precipitate cardiac complications. In toxic doses, β_1 and β_2 selectivity is usually lost and partial β-agonist activity will tend to protect from rather than worsen toxicity.

Hypotension is caused by a combination of bradycardia and myocardial depression. The bradycardia may be due to sinus bradycardia, heart block, or junctional or ventricular bradycardia, and may lead to asystole. Maneuvers such as inducing vomiting or performing gastric lavage, which may cause vagal stimulation, should be avoided. With severe toxicity QRS and QT prolongation may occur, especially with sotalol.

Delirium, coma and seizures may occur with lipid-soluble beta-blocking drugs such as propanolol. Other effects may include bronchospasm in asthmatic patients and hypoglycemia because of inhibition of gluconeogenesis and glycogenolysis.

Management

The prognosis correlates best with the degree of heart block or bradycardia remembering that deterioration can be sudden and rapid. Induced emesis and gastric lavage both may cause sudden deterioration associated with vagal stimulation. Activated charcoal is the decontamination method of choice. Repeated doses of charcoal may be useful, especially with sustained-release drugs.

Intravenous access should be secured so that dextrose and/or volume expanders can be given after electrolytes and blood glucose levels have been measured. The ECG and blood pressure should be continuously monitored. Blood levels of beta-blockers are not helpful in management decisions.

Atropine should be tried in all patients with bradycardia. It should be given prior to intubation or any other procedure that might increase vagal tone.

Glucagon should be used in combination with volume expansion, atropine and catecholamines to treat the cardiovascular effects. Intravenous glucagon increases heart rate, myocardial contractility and atrioventricular conduction. It increases cyclic AMP and activates myosin kinase independently of β-receptors. Doses of 0.05–0.2 mg/kg (maximum 10 mg) i.v. as a bolus given over 1 minute have been suggested. This is followed by an infusion, starting at 5 mg/h, titrated against heart rate and blood pressure. The amount required is variable with no clear upper limit, so that availability of glucagon in the desired quantities may be a problem.

If there is an inadequate response to pharmacologic therapy then more aggressive cardiorespiratory support such as pacemakers and even cardiopulmonary bypass may be indicated as supportive therapy until the beta-blocker has been metabolized.

Seizures generally should be treated with intravenous dextrose even if the blood glucose level is normal. If they do not respond then conventional anticonvulsants such as diazepam, phenobarbital (phenobarbitone) or phenytoin should be used. Bronchoconstriction should be treated with inhaled β$_2$-agonists.

CALCIUM CHANNEL BLOCKERS

All calcium antagonists are rapidly absorbed from the small intestine with peak levels usually achieved within 1–2 hours. They have large volumes of distribution with moderate CNS penetration and are metabolized in the liver. There may be significant enterohepatic circulation. Sustained-release preparations may produce both delayed and prolonged toxicity.

Morbidity and mortality are generally the result of cardiovascular toxicity due to peripheral vasodilatation, myocardial depression and impaired myocardial conduction. Prognosis correlates best with the degree of heart block. Hypotension due to vasodilatation without heart block usually responds to fluid loading.

Other effects include nausea, vomiting, ileus, CNS depression and seizures.

Management

Intravenous access with continuous ECG monitoring should be established. Induced emesis and gas-

tric lavage should be avoided as they may stimulate vagal tone and worsen bradycardia. Atropine should be given prior to any procedure that may increase vagal tone, e.g. intubation. Repeated doses of activated charcoal should be given. Patients who have taken sustained-release preparations may benefit from whole bowel irrigation.

Calcium is probably the most effective agent in the treatment of significant poisoning. Atropine, isoproterenol (isoprenaline) and glucagon are probably useful second-line therapies.

The treatment of hypotension without heart block can usually be managed with volume expansion and vasopressors. Calcium is primarily indicated in patients with heart block. The patient should be given 0.5 ml/kg of 10% calcium gluconate or 0.2 ml/kg of calcium chloride initially and then further increments every few minutes if there is no response in blood pressure or pulse rate. Continuous infusions may be effective. Serum calcium should be measured (recognizing that hypercalcemia may be appropriate).

Glucagon is a well-accepted antidote for beta-blocker poisoning that may also be effective in calcium channel blocker poisoning, as it activates myosin kinase independently of calcium flux.

Isoproterenol (isoprenaline) can be used to increase the heart rate but may be ineffective if there is a high degree of conduction block, as it predominantly acts through increasing the frequency of the sinoatrial node impulses.

Cardiac pacing can also be used to increase heart rate. Ventricular rather than atrial pacing may be necessary if the AV node is blocked. In severe poisoning the heart may fail to capture entirely.

Experimental calcium channel agonists may become available as antidotes but are not yet available.

CARBAMAZEPINE

Carbamazepine is an anticonvulsant that is structurally similar to imipramine. In therapeutic doses carbamazepine is well absorbed, with peak levels occurring 4–8 hours after ingestion. In overdose, absorption can be significantly delayed. It is protein-bound with a small volume of distribution of 1 L/kg. Carbamazepine is metabolized in the liver with about two-thirds excreted renally and one-third in the feces. Erythromycin competes for the same metabolic pathway and elevates carbamazepine levels.

Carbamazepine poisoning has many anticholinergic effects. Clinical features include tachycardia, dysrhythmias, myocardial depression, hypotension, mydriasis, ileus, drowsiness, ataxia, seizures, coma and respiratory depression. Hyponatremia and hypothermia develop, and heart block can occur.

Management

Ensure adequacy of the airway, breathing and circulation. Measure the serum level. Repeated doses of activated charcoal should be given to reduce absorption and enhance clearance. Hypotension should be treated with volume expansion, possibly with the addition of vasoactive drugs such as dopamine or norepinephrine (noradrenaline). If seizures persist they should be treated with diazepam followed by phenobarbital (phenobarbitone) or phenytoin. Heart block responds to isoproterenol (isoprenaline).

DIGOXIN

Only 1% of body digoxin stores are in plasma. The rest is tissue-bound, mostly in the heart, where digoxin concentrations are 30 times the plasma concentration. Most digoxin is excreted by the kidneys. There is some enterohepatic circulation.

Acute poisoning causes nausea, vomiting, hyperkalemia and cardiac dysrhythmias, especially sinus bradycardia, sinus arrest, heart block, ventricular extrasystoles, ventricular tachycardia, ventricular or atrial fibrillation and supraventricular tachycardia.

Management

Digoxin levels may not correlate with tissue levels. They can confirm a poisoning but are a poor guide to the need for treatment.

A significantly poisoned child requires i.v. access and ECG monitoring. Induced vomiting and gastric lavage should be avoided as both can cause vagal stimulation which exacerbates the bradycar-

dia. Activated charcoal is used for gut decontamination, and electrolyte abnormalities (especially hypokalemia, hyperkalemia and hypomagnesemia) should be corrected. If dysrhythmias are potentially life-threatening, digoxin immune Fab fragments should be given in the following dose:

> No. of digoxin Fab vials = serum digoxin (ng/ml) × body wt (kg) ÷ 100
> or
> No. of digoxin Fab vials = no. of tablets (0.25 mg) ingested × 0.34

Measured digoxin levels rise rapidly after administration of digoxin Fab fragments, but free (i.e. active) digoxin levels fall. The inactive Fab–digoxin complex is excreted in the urine.

If digoxin Fab fragments are unavailable, intravenous magnesium sulfate is effective for treating tachyarrhythmias, but may worsen the AV block in bradyarrhythmias. Lidocaine (lignocaine) or phenytoin may be used for tachyarrhythmias (Ch. 3.2), but quinidine and bretylium should be avoided.

IRON

Iron tablets are often available in households with toddlers. Iron is transported in the blood by transferrin: toxicity develops when serum iron levels exceed the iron-binding capacity of transferrin and free iron causes direct cellular damage. There is minimal iron elimination other than by gastrointestinal cell loss and blood loss.

The four phases of severe iron poisoning are:

1. A severe hemorrhagic gastroenteritis occurs within a few hours of ingestion. Vomiting occurs in virtually all severely poisoned children. Massive blood or fluid loss or bowel perforation may cause early death.
2. The survivors of the first phase apparently improve for 4–12 hours.
3. Multiorgan failure then ensues, including circulatory collapse, consumptive coagulopathy, metabolic acidosis, coma and seizures, as well as renal and liver failure.

4. Gastric and pyloric scarring occasionally causes obstruction 1–2 months later.

Iron poisoning can be confused with severe infective gastroenteritis, sepsis or diabetic ketoacidosis. Abdominal X-rays may identify radio-opaque tablets but their absence does not exclude iron overdose. Baseline investigations including a full blood count and coagulation studies, electrolytes, urea, creatinine and blood glucose should be performed at presentation. If the abdominal X-ray is normal and vomiting, leukocytosis and hyperglycemia are absent, serious iron poisoning is unlikely.

The toxicity can be estimated from the dose (Table 4.5.4: beware inaccurate assessment of tablet numbers) or from serum iron levels more than 4 hours after the dose (Table 4.5.5).

Management

After the airway, breathing and circulation are secured and baseline investigations are under way, the next priority is gastrointestinal decontamination. *Iron is not adsorbed by charcoal*, so patients with confirmed exposure to a potentially toxic dose should have whole bowel lavage if they:

- present within 4 hours
- have undissolved tablets on abdominal X-ray
- have taken sustained-release or enteric-coated iron tablets

Deferoxamine (Desferrioxamine) chelates the free iron and the resulting complex is excreted in the urine or by dialysis. If the patient has severe clinical signs, deferoxamine therapy (15 mg/kg·h i.v.) should be commenced without waiting for reports of serum iron levels. If iron-deferoxamine complexes are present in the urine it changes to a *'vin rosé'* color. Treatment should be continued until serum iron levels fall below 60 μmol/L and the urine has returned to its normal color.

TABLE 4.5.4 Estimation of toxicity from the dose of elemental iron ingested

Estimated dose (mg/kg)	Likelihood of toxicity
20–60	Potentially toxic
60–120	Toxic but death unlikely
>120	Can be fatal

TABLE 4.5.5 The use of serum iron levels for prognosis and treatment

Serum iron (μmol/L)	Likely toxicity	Use deferoxamine (desferrioxamine)?
10–30	Normal range	No
30–60	Unlikely	No
60–90	Possible toxicity	Yes if symptomatic
>90	Severe toxicity	Yes: all patients
>180	May be fatal	Yes: all patients

Intensive care treatment involves the supportive management of massive blood and fluid loss (Ch. 2.3) and multiorgan failure (Ch. 2.12).

METHANOL

Methanol is rapidly absorbed from the gastrointestinal tract but may also reach toxic levels though the skin and lungs. Like ethanol, methanol itself produces CNS depression, but it is also oxidized by alcohol dehydrogenase to formaldehyde and then converted by aldehyde dehydrogenase to formic acid which causes most of the toxicity.

Clinical features include visual, CNS and gastrointestinal effects. Victims may complain of blurred vision or seeing spots ('like a snowstorm') that may lead on to blindness. They may complain of nausea, vomiting and abdominal pain. The CNS effects may range from lethargy to seizures, coma and apnea. Hypotension and bradycardia are late findings with a poor prognosis. Laboratory investigations may demonstrate severe metabolic acidosis with a widened anion gap (due to formic acid and possibly lactic acid). A widened osmolal gap may also be found (the measured serum osmolality minus the calculated serum osmolality). The calculated osmolality is equal to 2[Na+] + [glucose] + [urea] (values in mmol/L). An osmolal gap of greater than 10 suggests the presence of low molecular weight solutes such as methanol, ethanol, ethylene glycol or mannitol.

Management

Supportive measures should be instituted. Methanol is rapidly absorbed from the gut but is not well adsorbed by charcoal. Hemodialysis effectively removes both methanol and formate as well as correcting metabolic acidosis. Folic acid has been used to enhance the metabolism of formic acid. Compared with methanol, ethanol has about a hundred times greater affinity for alcohol dehydrogenase. It can be given orally or intravenously to saturate the enzyme system and thus prevent the formation of methanol's toxic metabolites and allow unaltered methanol to be excreted via the lungs and kidneys. A loading dose of 700 mg/kg (600 mg/kg adult) of a 10% ethanol solution i.v. (50% if po) is given. The i.v. loading dose (over 20–40 minutes) is followed by a maintenance dose of 125 mg/kg·h to achieve a serum level of between 100 mg and 150 mg per 100 ml (22–33 mmol/L). (Hemodialysis will also remove ethanol so that an increase in the dose is likely to be required during dialysis) The blood glucose level must be closely monitored as hypoglycemia is a common complication of ethanol administration in children.

ORGANOPHOSPHATES

Organophosphates are an extremely toxic group of compounds which include nerve gases as well as industrial and domestic insecticides. They are rapidly absorbed via the skin, lungs and gastrointestinal tract. Organophosphate compounds bind irreversibly to acetylcholinesterase causing an accumulation of acetylcholine and overstimulation at postganglionic parasympathetic nerve endings (muscarinic receptors), parasympathetic and sympathetic ganglia (nicotinic receptors), neuromuscular junctions (nicotinic receptors) and some sites within the CNS.

The signs and symptoms of organophosphate poisoning are listed in the 'Cholinergic' toxidrome in Table 4.5.3. Inhaled organophosphates may also cause chemical pneumonitis because of hydrocarbon solvents. The severity of the clinical presentation is determined by the degree of anti-cholinesterase inhibition. Death is usually due to cardiorespiratory failure. Hypoventilation from weakness and CNS depression is compounded by increased bronchial secretions, bronchospasm, atelectasis and pulmonary edema. The balance of nicotinic and muscarinic stimulation can produce both tachycardia or bradycardia as well as hypertension or hypotension. More severe toxicity may produce conduction blocks and ventricular dysrhythmias. An intermediate syndrome, developing 1–4 days after the acute cholinergic effects, has

been described in some patients. The features may include proximal muscle weakness, decreased tendon reflexes, cranial nerve lesions and respiratory failure. Long-term neurotoxicity may include peripheral neuropathies due to axonal degeneration, and neuropsychiatric features such as depression, personality changes and memory loss.

Plasma cholinesterase (PChE) is a sensitive indicator of exposure but not of the seriousness of the exposure. Red blood cell cholinesterase is a better indicator of tissue acetylcholinesterase inhibition and correlates well with both severity and prognosis.

Management

Initial management should include removal of the patient's clothes and decontamination of the skin with soap and water. Staff should gown and glove for self-protection. Support of the airway, breathing and circulation should be followed by gut decontamination with repeated doses of activated charcoal.

Specific antidotes are available (see Table 4.5.2). Atropine will block the muscarinic effects but not the neuromuscular junction blockade. Pralidoxime binds to organophosphates and competes with acetylcholinesterase if irreversible binding has not yet occurred. Newly synthesized acetylcholinesterase may be protected in this way. Pralidoxime is most effective if given in the first 48 hours after exposure. The pralidoxime–organophosphate complex is water soluble and renally excreted.

SALICYLATES

Salicylate is well absorbed from the stomach and small intestine. Tablet dissolution may be extremely slow. In overdose, large tablet aggregates may delay absorption. Metabolic pathways in the liver become saturated and the kidneys are the major route of elimination. Clearance is greatly increased in alkaline urine.

Salicylate poisoning causes uncoupling of oxidative phosphorylation and interference with carbohydrate, amino acid and lipid metabolism. This increases the metabolic rate, oxygen consumption, carbon dioxide production, heat production and glucose utilization. Metabolic acidosis is caused in part by the presence of the salicylic acid but more importantly by the increased production of CO_2, lactate, pyruvate and ketone bodies. Salicylates directly stimulate the respiratory center leading to hyperventilation and a respiratory alkalosis. The acid–base disturbance seen may therefore be a mixed picture of respiratory alkalosis, metabolic acidosis or even respiratory acidosis if CNS depression is present.

Poisoning from chronic salicylate ingestion is now more common than acute ingestions. It is usually more severe because of the saturation of hepatic elimination and because the slower onset of symptoms leads to later presentation. Clinical features of poisoning include pyrexia, nausea and vomiting. Epigastric pain and hematemesis are uncommon. Central nervous system disturbances range from confusion and hyperventilation to cerebral edema with seizures and coma.

Vomiting may cause metabolic alkalosis, hyponatremia, hypokalemia and dehydration. The syndrome of innapropriate ADH secretion may develop. Hyperglycemia is often seen early, but life-threatening hypoglycemia may develop in the later stages. Hypokalemia is common because of increased renal excretion and intracellular shift of potassium. Hypocalcemia may be induced by the respiratory alkalosis or by administration of alkali to promote alkaline diuresis. Salicylates competitively inhibit vitamin K-dependent synthesis of factors II, VII, IX and X. Occasionally non-cardiogenic pulmonary edema or an increase in hepatic transaminases occurs in severe poisoning.

Indicators of the likely severity of toxicity include:

- the dose ingested (Table 4.5.6)
- the serum salicylate level
- clinical and laboratory indicators of organ dysfunction

In chronic poisoning the toxicity can vary widely for the same dose. Salicylate absorption can be very variable and levels should be measured to confirm the ingestion and monitor the effectiveness of clearance.

Management

Gastric lavage is often used because of delayed gastric emptying, but activated charcoal is the mainstay of decontamination. Whole bowel lavage is used after ingestion of enteric-coated salicylate.

Supportive therapy includes correction of hypoglycemia and electrolyte disturbances while ensuring adequate renal perfusion (urine output of at least 1.5–2 ml/kg·h) to promote renal excretion. Care must be taken to prevent rapid fluid and electrolyte shifts that might worsen cerebral edema. Bicarbonate (1 mmol/kg·h) is titrated to maintain a urine pH above 7.5. Bicarbonate, which remains extracellular, traps the ionized salicylate outside the cell and enhances elimination.

Hyperthermia should be treated with external cooling, using water spray and fans (Ch. 4.7) and an adequate circulating blood volume maintained. Seizures (Ch. 2.5) are treated with diazepam while specific precipitants such as hypoglycemia or hyponatremia are sought and treated. A prolonged prothrombin time should be treated with vitamin K.

Hemodialysis, hemofiltration and hemoperfusion all enhance salicylate clearance, but hemodialysis or hemofiltration are preferred as they also correct acidosis, as well as fluid and electrolyte disturbances. Indications for hemodialysis or filtration include any clinically serious toxicity, particularly if there is renal failure, severe acidosis and electrolyte disturbances or pulmonary edema. High salicylate levels (> 9.4 mmol/L in acute ingestions or > 4.5 mmol/L in chronic intoxication) also warrant consideration of hemodialysis or hemofiltration.

THEOPHYLLINE

Theophylline is readily available and has a narrow therapeutic index. Its metabolism varies significantly between individuals. Peak concentrations are reached within 2–4 hours of ingestion. With sustained-release preparations, the peak concentration is usually reached between 2–18 hours (occasionally up to 24 hours) after presentation.

TABLE 4.5.6 **Dose and toxicity of salicylates**	
Dose (mg/kg)	**Toxicity**
< 150	Toxicity unlikely
150–300	Some toxicity likely
300–500	Severe toxicity likely
> 500	Potentially fatal

The volume of distribution for theophylline is about 0.5 L/kg. Its clearance increases after the neonatal period, peaks during early childhood and declines to adult levels by adolescence. Absorbed theophylline is metabolized by the liver, then excreted in the urine. Theophylline overdose saturates the hepatic metabolism, prolonging the half-life. Viral illnesses, hepatic and renal disease, congestive cardiac failure and drugs such as erythromycin also prolong theophylline's half-life.

The clinical effects of theophylline poisoning are due to β-adrenergic overactivity:

- smooth muscle relaxation
- peripheral vasodilatation
- cardiac and CNS stimulation
- hyperglycemia, hypokalemia and metabolic acidosis

In poisoning due to chronic ingestion, toxicity occurs at lower theophylline levels than in acute ingestions and signs of minor toxicity may not precede severe toxicity. Nausea and vomiting are usual in both acute and chronic poisoning, while diarrhea and gastrointestinal hemorrhage occur less often. Cardiac dysrhythmias range from sinus tachycardia to ventricular fibrillation. Hypotension due to β_2-receptor mediated vasodilatation is seen in severe acute poisoning and may be compounded by gastrointestinal fluid losses. Signs of CNS toxicity include hyperventilation, agitation, hyperreflexia, seizures and coma.

Theophylline levels are a useful guide to toxicity (Table 4.5.7) and can be used to monitor drug clearance during the acute and recovery phases, but because of wide variations in responses to similar levels they cannot be relied upon to predict toxicity. In children, lower levels than those in Table 4.5.7 have been associated with major toxicity.

Management

Support the airway, breathing and circulation. Gut decontamination should be commenced with repeated doses of activated charcoal. Whole bowel irrigation is especially useful after ingestion of sustained-release theophylline. Vomiting requiring antiemetic treatment with ondansetron may complicate the use of charcoal or bowel irrigation. Extracorporeal removal by hemodialysis, hemofiltration or charcoal hemoperfusion is used for:

- severely symptomatic overdoses
- theophylline levels over 550 μmol/L with moderate toxicity after acute ingestions
- levels over 330 μmol/L and moderate toxicity after chronic poisoning
- deterioration despite repeated doses of charcoal therapy
- markedly impaired liver or hepatic clearance

Seizures are treated with diazepam and phenobarbital (phenobarbitone) but may be difficult to control. Hypotension is treated by volume expansion; beta-blocking agents such as propranolol may correct the vasodilatation but may provoke wheezing in an asthmatic child, so a short-acting β_1-selective agent (e.g. esmolol infused at 50 mg/kg·min) may be more appropriate.

Treat hypoxia, acid-base status and electrolyte abnormalities which may exacerbate dysrhythmias. Control supraventricular dysrhythmias with beta-blockers or verapamil if hypotension is present. Treat ventricular tachyarrhythmias with lidocaine (lignocaine) or beta-blockers; the latter may also help correct the hypokalemia, hyperglycemia and acidosis.

Hyperglycemia and hypokalemia do not usually need treatment.

TABLE 4.5.7 **Serum theophylline level and toxicity in adults**	
Level (μmol/L)	**Toxicity**
> 220	Risk of chronic toxicity
> 550	Risk of seizures and dysrhythmias after acute ingestion
> 825	Severe risk of seizures and dysrhythmias

FURTHER READING

1. Litovitz T, Manoguerra A. Comparison of pediatric poisoning hazards: an analysis of 3.8 million exposure incidents. Paediatrics 1992; 89: 999–1006
   - (*A large series from the American Association of Poison Control Centers that puts the degree of hazard into perspective*)

2. Sibert JR, Routledge PA. Accidental poisoning in children: can we admit fewer children with safety? Arch Dis Child 1991; 66: 263–266
   – *(A British perspective)*

3. Pond SM. Extracorporeal techniques in the treatment of poisoned patients. Med J Aust. 1991; 154: 617–622
   – *(Good summary of extracorporeal techniques)*

4. Banner W Jr, Timmons OD, Vernon DD. Advances in the critical care of poisoned paediatric patients. Drug Safety 1994; 10: 83–92
   – *(A review of management of severe poisoning)*

5. Woolf AD, Berkowitz ID, Liebelt E, Rogers MC. Poisoning and the critically ill child. In: Rogers MC, editor. Textbook of pediatric intensive care, 3rd editor. Baltimore: Williams & Wilkins; 1996: pp. 1315–1391
   – *(Excellent discussion of pediatric poisoning with detailed description of important toxins)*

6. Kulig K. Initial management of ingestions of toxic substances. N Engl J Med 1992; 326(25): 1677–1681

4.6   Hypothermia and cold stress

Andrew J. Macnab

Hypothermia occurs when a child's core temperature falls below 35°C (95°F). Presentation depends on the cause and the core temperature. Four grades of hypothermia are recognized, from mild to profound. Significant effects occur once temperatures fall below the normal homeostatic levels set by the body's control mechanisms. Symptoms that result include shivering, tachycardia, tachypnea, vasoconstriction, and signs of impaired neurological function.

The main cold-related conditions are hypothermia and frostbite. The following children are at particular risk of cold stress:

1. infants (small mass, large surface area, limited energy stores); in particular newborns and babies delivered at home
2. children suffering immersion injury, prolonged exposure to the cold, trauma, shock or burns
3. children with impaired thyroid, adrenal or CNS function
4. patients undergoing prolonged resuscitation or treatment with paralyzing agents
5. children in coma—medically induced or drug-related, e.g. phenobarbital (phenobarbitone), carbamazepine, phenothiazine, narcotics

PHYSIOLOGY

Heat is lost to the environment by radiation, convection, conduction and evaporation. When heat loss exceeds heat production, or there is impairment of temperature control mechanisms, body temperature will fall. Initially, there is stimulation of the sympathetic nervous system with increased catecholamine release and heat generation through shivering. Importantly, the ability to shiver is lost at approximately 30°C.

The systemic effects of hypothermia are summarized in Table 4.6.1.

CARDIOVASCULAR SYSTEM

Initially there is tachycardia, vasoconstriction and cardiac output increases. With continued cooling, cardiac output falls, blood pressure becomes depressed and arrhythmias develop (atrial fibrillation is common from 34°C). The ECG shows prolongation of all phases of the cardiac cycle and J waves (elevation of the ST segment) may be seen between 32°C and 34°C. Severe bradyarrhythmias occur—supraventricular between 30°C and 33°C and ventricular below 30°C. The disorders of rhythm respond primarily to rewarming rather than medication. If ventricular fibrillation is present when core temperature is 32°C or lower consider one DC shock (2 J/kg, nonsynchronized mode).

RESPIRATORY SYSTEM

Tachypnea occurs initially. An associated respiratory alkalosis develops. Depression of respiration occurs as temperature falls. Below 30°C, hypoventilation is present. Infants commonly have apnea with mild degrees of hypothermia. All children become apneic between 26°C and 28°C.

NERVOUS SYSTEM

Initial symptoms are impaired coordination with slurring of speech and confusion. Below 32°C, conscious level falls progressively and the pupils tend to dilate (30–33°C). Rigidity of the muscles also occurs at these temperatures. The child is in coma below 26°C and the pupillary light reflex is lost.

Eventually the EEG becomes isoelectric. Brain death cannot be diagnosed in this situation. Rewarming of core temperature to at least 35°C is essential before the clinical signs of brain death can be relied on.

DIAGNOSIS

Consider the possibility of hypothermia or cold stress in the situations listed above.

TABLE 4.6.1 **Systemic effects of hypothermia**

Hypothermia grade	Core temp. (°C)	Cardiac	Neurological	Respiratory	Other
Mild	35	Increased HR	Confusion	Increased RR	Increased shivering
		Vasoconstriction	Decreased coordination		Increased catecholamines
		Increased cardiac output	Clumsy speech	Increased apnea (infants)	Increased oxygen consumption
		Atrial fibrillation	Muscle stiffness		
		ECG J waves	Pupil dilation		Alkalosis
Moderate	32	Increased arrhrythmias (supraventricular)			
		Decreased HR		Decreased RR	
					Oximeter Sa_{O_2} reliable >31°C
	29	Increased arrhythmias (ventricular)	Coma		Shivering stops
					Increased sensitivity to epinephrine (adrenaline) (>26°C)
					'Cold diuresis'
		Decreased BP			K+ may increase or decrease
				Apnea (all children)	Blood viscosity (Hct) increases
Severe	26	Ventricular fibrillation			
			Muscle relaxation		Neutrophils decrease
			No pupillary light reflex		
					Decreased sensitivity to epinephrine (adrenaline) (<26°C)
	23				Decreased oxygen consumption
Profound		Loss of effective output			
	20	Asystole			

BP, blood pressure; ECG, electrocardiogram; Hct, hematocrit; HR, heart rate; RR, respiratory rate.

Use a low-reading rectal thermometer to determine core temperature accurately. In children, hypothermia is most often a complication that is secondary to another incident or underlying illness. Address the underlying cause as well as the symptoms of cold stress.

The primary differential diagnosis in the hypothermic child is death. In all acute situations or where doubt exists that death preceded the fall in body temperature, resuscitation should continue until the core temperature is at least 33°C and preferably 35°C.

MANAGEMENT

PRE-HOSPITAL CARE

Prevention of further heat loss involves:

- the provision of shelter (insulation and covering—protect from wind and body contact with cold surfaces)
- removal of wet clothing
- drying the skin surface
- insulation with blankets
- transport to a medical facility (raise the temperature inside the vehicle)

Medical intervention consists of attention to airway, breathing and circulation. If equipment is available, provide oxygen and monitor temperature, heart rate, rhythm, blood pressure, and respiratory rate).

HOSPITAL CARE

Core temperature over 32°C:

1. Address airway, breathing and circulation.
2. Administer oxygen by mask, using a cascade humidifier to warm inspired gas where possible (the desired temperature to avoid burning is 42–44°C).
3. Prevent further heat loss by using measures listed under prehospital care.
4. Rewarm the patient:
   - raise ambient room temperature
   - cover with warm blankets
   - consider use of infrared radiant heaters
   - use external heating devices (hot-water bottles and heating pads) with caution (alternatives are preferable as there is a risk of traumatizing poorly perfused skin and extremities and accelerating the return of acidotic and hyperkalemic blood from the periphery)
   - warm intravenous solutions (e.g. with a blood-warming water bath, for exchange transfusion); the desired temperature to avoid hemolysis is 37–41°C
5. Limit exposure during resuscitation and other procedures.
6. Monitor, investigate (Table 4.6.2), triage.

Core temperature less than 32°C

1. Initiate CPR if in arrest (Ch. 2.2). *Note*—the arrhythmias present will be resistant to cardioversion until rewarming occurs. The cardiac effects of epinephrine (adrenaline) are enhanced above 26°C and depressed below this temperature. The myocardium is also more sensitive to potassium and calcium.
2. Assess adequacies of ABC (intubation is likely to be required, but may precipitate ventricular dysrhythmia).

TABLE 4.6.2 Investigation and monitoring

- Monitor core temperature, BP (consider transducing an arterial line), CVP, ECG, urine output, oxygen saturation and the temperature of warmed, inspired gases, i.v. solutions, dialysate
- Laboratory—CBC (platelets), electrolytes, blood gases, glucose, BUN, creatinine, serum osmolarity, urinalysis (consider coagulation screen, drug screen and endocrine function, e.g. thyroid, amylase, AST and ALT
- Other—chest X-ray (consider EEG), NG tube, urinary catheter (consider pulmonary artery catheter if circulation unstable)

---

3. Ventilate with warmed humidified oxygen (avoid hyperventilation) anticipate pulmonary edema.
4. Place a central venous line.
5. Correct hypovolemia.
6. Begin treatment of metabolic acidosis.
7. Rewarm the patient (as for less hypo-thermic group above):
   - consider gastric (or rectal, or bladder) lavage: the temperature of the solution should not exceed 45°C; and sodium chloride is the solution of choice. Large volumes of solution may be absorbed. Follow electrolyte values with care
   - in severe cases, consider peritoneal lavage with dialysate solution warmed to 37–43°C; continuous lavage via dual catheters is desirable (if dwell times are used, 15 minutes is the suggested maximum)
   - if available, rewarming can also be achieved by partial arteriovenous bypass (heart-lung machine) or arteriovenous hemodialysis; in addition to rewarming, the heart-lung machine facilitates correction of acid–base disturbance and is the ultimate means of cardiac support
8. Catheterize the bladder ,and pass a nasogastric tube (defer the latter procedure until the core temperature is above 30°C to lower the risk of arrhythmia).
9. Monitor, investigate (Table 4.6.2), triage.

Risks of rewarming

The major risks encountered are hypovolemia, acidosis, hypokalemia and hypoglycemia. Attention should also be paid to possible skin trauma (burns, pressure sores) if external heating devices are used.

INVESTIGATIONS

Investigations and monitoring that apply in all cases are shown in Table 4.6.2.

CONTROVERSIES IN CARE

Pharmacological management of ventricular arrhythmias may be more effective using bretylium (5–10 mg/kg) rather than lidocaine (lignocaine) (1 mg/kg).

Active rewarming using warming blankets or hot water bottles is of concern because of the risk of burns and acceleration of the return of blood to the central pool that is acid and hyperkalemic.

Oximetric measurement of oxygen saturation is considered unreliable but above 31°C accurate values can be obtained (provided the displayed heart rate on the oximeter tallies with the patient's actual heart rate).

TRIAGE

All patients with a core temperature of 35°C or below require admission. Children who have required resuscitation and those with a core temperature below 32°C should be transported to a facility capable of providing intensive care and the treatment and resuscitation measures listed above.

FROSTBITE

Cold-induced injury to the peripheral tissues can coexist in hypothermia, particularly where there has been prolonged exposure, or local injury may occur separately in extreme climatic conditions. Lesions are usually seen in the extremities, particularly the fingers and toes and on the head, particularly the ears, the tip of the nose, and the lips.

DIAGNOSIS

Frostbite should be suspected where areas of the skin and subcutaneous tissue appear frozen, look white and feel firm. Early signs are pallor or blanching of the skin, mottling and numbness. It is difficult in the early hours of injury to predict the extent of tissue viability.

MANAGEMENT

Initial measures should address restoration of core temperature through prevention of heat loss, drying the skin surface and passive rewarming. When core temperature is in the normal range, the involved extremity should be immersed in warm water (temperature range 37–40°C). Periods of approximately 20 minutes are recommended, followed by gentle drying, reexamination and reassessment. Avoid mechanical trauma to the damaged tissue (do not apply friction or dry heat). The purpose of immersion is to thaw the injured areas. Rewarming is not required if an area is no longer frozen. Thawing is painful and analgesia (i.v. morphine or fentanyl) is justified. As tissues thaw, pallor may resolve and visible flushing may occur. Cover loosely with dry dressings, splint affected extremities and elevate.

TRIAGE

Referral for plastic surgical opinion and debriding of dead tissue is required.

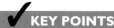 **KEY POINTS**

➤ Prevention of further heat loss is a key element in management
➤ In the hospital setting, the potential for exposure leading to cold stress must be anticipated (e.g. during prolonged resuscitation, paralysis for ventilation, or drug-induced coma)
➤ Hypothermia depresses cardiac function
➤ The rewarming process can be associated with multiple, potentially adverse hypovolemia and metabolic sequelae
➤ Hypothermia mimics death

✗ COMMON ERRORS

➤ Failure to use a low-reading rectal thermometer to measure core temperature

➤ Making a diagnosis of 'brain death' when core temperature is less than 35°C
➤ Attempting to treat cardiac arrhythmias pharmacologically rather than by rewarming
➤ Applying local friction or heat directly to frostbitten tissue

FURTHER READING

1. Macnab AJ, Baker-Brown G, Anderson EE. Oximetry in children recovering from deep hypothermia for cardiac surgery. Crit Care Med 1990; 18: 1006–1069
   – (*A study demonstrating pulse oximeter reliability in children with core temperatures as low as 31°C and toe temperatures as low as 23.5°C*)

2. Curley FJ, Irwin R. Disorders of temperature control: part III. Hyperthermia. Intens Care Med 1986; 1: 270–288
   – (*A good general review of hypothermia*)

4.7 Hyperthermia and heat stress

R. Gregory Delbridge

Heat stress is the sum of environmental and metabolic heat loads and their effects on the body. Heat-related illnesses include:

- heat edema
- heat syncope
- heat cramps
- heat exhaustion
- heatstroke

Many of these conditions are relatively minor, such as heat edema, heat syncope, and heat cramps, but heat exhaustion and heatstroke cause severe metabolic derangement and significant morbidity and mortality.

PHYSIOLOGY

Body temperature is normally maintained within the limits of 36–37.5°C (97–99.5°F) by homeostatic mechanisms controlled by the anterior hypothalamus. During illness, the 'set point' for these mechanisms may be upregulated, causing an actively maintained elevation of body temperature referred to as *fever*. In the absence of fever, body temperature will only rise if the body's ability to dissipate heat is restricted or overwhelmed. When the temperature of blood perfusing the hypothalamus (preoptic nucleus) exceeds the 'set point', an increase in cholinergic sympathetic activity stimulates cutaneous vasodilation, an increase in cutaneous blood flow and sweating. Splanchnic and renal vasoconstriction occur later if the blood pressure cannot be maintained by increasing cardiac output alone. Thus, the capacity to dissipate heat depends on the mechanisms available to manipulate the cardiac output and redistribute the blood volume. In extreme situations, the need to preserve blood pressure by peripheral vasoconstriction may severely limit the body's ability to lose heat. Progressive water and sodium loss in sweat will aggravate these cardiovascular effects and contribute to reduced renal blood flow, poor urine output, electrolyte disturbance and hemoconcentration.

Heat dissipation occurs at body surfaces, especially the skin, with the lungs assuming a lesser role. Under normal circumstances and in order of importance, radiation, convection, evaporation and conduction are the mechanisms by which heat is lost. Active sweating may dramatically increase evaporative heat loss. As the environmental temperature approaches body temperature, the efficiency of radiation, convection and conduction rapidly diminish, leaving evaporation of sweat as the only effective means of heat loss. Ambient humidity above 75% greatly reduces evaporative heat loss and the body's ability to dissipate heat is minimal when the ambient temperature and humidity are both high. The body temperature then rises.

As body temperature approaches 42°C (107.5°F), cellular enzyme dysfunction and failure of oxidative phosphorylation lead to inadequate energy production and inability to maintain membrane integrity. Such effects are catastrophic when metabolic demands are already maximal. All mechanisms to promote heat loss (including sweating) cease functioning. Hyperthermia is now unchecked and tissue necrosis occurs. Most organ and bodily systems are affected, causing acute brain injury, coagulopathy, rhabdomyolysis, renal failure, metabolic acidosis, abnormalities of liver enzymes and of potassium and other electrolytes and acute respiratory distress syndrome (ARDS).

HEAT-RELATED ILLNESSES

HEAT EDEMA

Swelling of the hands, feet and ankles may occur in the early heat acclimatization period and is thought to be due to capillary leak secondary to cutaneous vasodilation. It is not usually seen in children and requires no therapy.

HEAT SYNCOPE

During a period of heat stress the combined effects of venous pooling of blood, mild dehydration and decreased vasomotor tone may sufficiently reduce venous return and cardiac output to stimulate a vasovagal syncopal episode. Consciousness is usually rapidly regained when the child becomes horizontal. Oral rehydration with a salt solution (e.g. commercial oral rehydration fluids containing 50–100 mmol/L of NaCl) may be useful.

HEAT CRAMPS

Most commonly related to exercise in hot conditions, heat cramps are exquisitely painful muscle contractions often involving the most heavily exercised muscles, usually in the calf or hamstring regions. They are probably due to a combination of the partial replacement of sweat losses by fluids with a low salt content, leading to hyponatremia, and the poor perfusion of maximally exercising muscles in a dehydrated person. Treatment consists of rest in the recumbent position, oral rehydration with a salt solution (e.g. commercial oral rehydration fluids as above) and massage of the affected muscles.

HEAT EXHAUSTION

Following heat stress, excessive losses of water and electrolytes may lead to heat exhaustion with symptoms of headache, nausea and vomiting, dizziness, weakness and thirst. Sweating is usually profuse to maximize heat dissipation, hyponatremia or hypernatremia may occur, and the body temperature is less than 40°C (104°F). While the patient may be irritable, anxious or have suffered a syncopal episode, there is no evidence of serious neurological impairment and the patient remains oriented. The presence of disorientation, a rapidly rising temperature, supine hypotension or elevated serum levels of aspartate aminotransferase (AST), alanine aminotransferase (ALT) or lactate dehydrogenase (LDH) suggest heatstroke and the need for immediate appropriate therapy. Treatment of heat exhaustion consists of immediate fluid replacement, by mouth if the child is fully alert, otherwise intravenously with 0.9% sodium chloride (20 ml/kg initially over 2 to 4 hours). Close monitoring is advisable during rapid intravenous rehydration as rapid peripheral cooling may redistribute considerable amounts of blood centrally,

leading to pulmonary edema. Body temperatures approaching 40°C (104°F) should be lowered by moving the patient to a shaded area and fanning exposed areas as they are sprayed with a water mist. Spraying is not needed if the child is still able to sweat.

HEATSTROKE

Heatstroke is a life-threatening emergency characterized by a body temperature (rectal) over 40°C (104°F), seriously altered mental status (delirium, stupor, coma, seizures) and history of exposure to heat stress. Such a presentation demands that immediate cooling maneuvers take precedence over further history-taking and examination. Note that the body temperature may be somewhat lower if effective cooling has commenced before presentation to hospital, and in this setting the mental status may be improving.

The cause may be nonexertional (classical) and is usually due to a combination of a very hot and humid environment and a person who is either unable to escape the conditions (very old or very young) or has a limited ability to dissipate heat (disease or drug-related). The onset is relatively slow and sweating is often absent. On the other hand, exertional heatstroke typically occurs in healthy people who exercise vigorously in a hot and humid environment and persist beyond reasonable limits (adolescent, competitiveness, under orders). The child may deteriorate very rapidly, sweating is often present and the body temperature may be very high—up to 45°C (113°F).

The most common clinical and laboratory features of heatstroke are: tachycardia, hypotension, signs of acute brain injury, coagulopathy, rhabdomyolysis, renal failure, lactic acidosis, increased or decreased serum sodium and potassium levels, hypocalcemia, hypophosphatemia, elevated liver enzymes and ARDS (Table 4.7.1).

DIFFERENTIAL DIAGNOSIS

Since patients with heatstroke have a high body temperature, systemic illness and multiorgan involvement, the possibility of other major illnesses must always be considered, although the start of aggressive cooling must not be delayed.

TABLE 4.7.1 **Complications of heatstroke**

Cardiovascular
- Hypotension
- Lactic acidosis
- Dysrhythmias (electrolyte imbalance)

Hematological
- Coagulopathy
- Hemorrhage
- Thrombocytopenia

Hepatic
- Liver failure (late)

Metabolic
- Hypoglycemia
- Hypokalemia
- Hyperkalemia
- Hypernatremia
- Hypocalcemia
- Hypophosphatemia

Neurological
- Seizures
- Encephalopathy
- Permanent neurological damage (late)

Pulmonary
- Pulmonary edema
- Acute respiratory distress syndrome

Renal failure

Rhabdomyolysis

Altered mental status suggests bacterial meningitis or septic shock and may warrant a septic screen, cerebral CT scan, lumbar puncture (immediate or delayed) and empirical antibiotic therapy. Nonspecific pleocytosis has been reported in the cerebrospinal fluid of heatstroke patients. Unwitnessed prolonged seizures complicating an acute systemic illness may mimic the presentation of heatstroke. In children, drugs such as anticholinergics, salicylates, amphetamines and sympathomimetics may cause elevated body temperature with altered mental status. Occasionally, hyperthyroidism or pheochromocytoma may be responsible for a similar presentation.

Very rarely, idiosyncratic reaction to neuroleptic drugs, especially haloperidol (neuroleptic malignant syndrome) or genetic susceptibility (malignant hyperthermia) to halogenated volatile anesthetic agents and succinylcholine (suxamethonium) cause severe hyperthermia. Both of these conditions should be predictable from the circumstances and both are characterized by severe muscle rigidity. Treatment of these conditions involves removal of the drug, aggressive cooling, and use of intravenous dantrolene sodium.

MANAGEMENT OF HEATSTROKE

PREHOSPITAL CARE

Early treatment consists of removal of all clothing, aggressive cooling by available means (water spray and air flow, ice-packs to groin and axillae, wet sheet) while an adequate airway and breathing are secured. The child should be transferred urgently to hospital; oxygen should be given and assisted ventilation may be required. Ventilation via mask or tracheal tube is effective but may further reduce systemic venous return and worsen hypotension. Vascular access should be gained as soon as possible (the intraosseous route may be needed if aggressive cooling has caused vasoconstriction) and blood glucose estimated. Hypoglycemia is common, check for it and treat immediately.

EMERGENCY ROOM

While cooling continues, other serious acid–base, electrolyte and coagulation abnormalities are sought and treated. Fluid loading is primarily aimed at rapidly restoring adequate circulating blood volume but should be done with care as rapid peripheral cooling may relocate blood to the central compartment and pulmonary edema may result. However, rhabdomyolysis is very common and to minimize the risk of associated renal failure a large urine flow must be maintained. For these reasons, invasive monitoring of blood pressure by arterial catheter and of central venous pressure are needed. A urinary catheter and a nasogastric tube should also be inserted. Standard cerebral resuscitation techniques are indicated for acute brain injury (Ch. 2.6) and should be instituted immediately unless rapid CNS improvement has been already noted with cooling.

Cooling

Many methods of cooling have been recommended (Table 4.7.2). Useful techniques must be capable of lowering body temperature by at least

---

TABLE 4.7.2 Cooling techniques

Efficient

An effective technique should be able to lower elevated body temperature in a heatstroke patient by more than 0.1°C (0.18°F) per minute

- Iced water/iced slush immersion
  - very efficient until vasoconstriction and shivering occur
  - monitoring of critically ill patients is difficult
- Water spray with continuous air flow
  - very efficient (evaporation transfers more heat than ice melting)
  - less vasoconstriction and shivering
  - simpler to set up
- Iced-water peritoneal lavage (10°C or 50°F)
  - extremely efficient in animals; unproven in children
  - invasive
  - unknown risks in inexperienced hands
- Extracorporeal circulation
  - most efficient, especially cardiopulmonary bypass
  - expertise becoming more widely available
  - additional risks of heparinization
  - slow to set up

Inefficient

Use only as an adjunct to one of the more efficient methods

- Ice-packs to axillae and groin
- Iced gastric lavage
- Unwarmed humidified ventilator circuits
- Iced enema

0.1°C per minute, thereby achieving a 'safe' body temperature (less than 39°C or 102°F) in under 1 hour. Several techniques can do this but are not always successful in practice.

Iced water immersion had long been advocated as the preferred technique and is certainly effective (as is the use of iced slush) by the above criterion. However, it is difficult to perform safely, monitoring of critical patients is very difficult, and it is likely to cause peripheral vasoconstriction and shivering which are counterproductive. The use of drugs (diazepam, chlorpromazine) to prevent these latter effects cannot be recommended in patients with acute brain injury. Water spray and air flow techniques which use continuous or intermittent spraying of water over the naked patient while fans maintain high-volume air flow over the patient are currently favored. Vasoconstriction and shivering are less common with this technique, which has been shown to be more efficient than iced-water immersion. The evaporation of 1 g of water transfers seven times as much heat as melting 1 g of ice.

Iced-water peritoneal lavage is very efficient but is invasive and carries the risk of perforation of bowel, liver, kidney and other structures as well as infection and fluid and electrolyte disturbances. The use of extracorporeal circulation (venovenous or venoarterial) as a rapid means of cooling may become more common, as many intensive care units now have this expertise which was previously restricted to large cardiothoracic units. Ice-packs applied to the neck, axillae and groin as well as iced gastric lavage, cold intravenous fluids, unwarmed humidified ventilator circuits and iced enemas are not efficient enough to be used as a primary means of cooling, but are useful adjunctive measures. Antipyretics are not indicated as there is no primary abnormality of the hypothalamic 'set point'.

INTENSIVE CARE

When normothermia has been restored, the child requires supportive treatment of multiple organ failure and its complications—in particular, of encephalopathy (Ch. 2.4), ARDS (Ch. 3.1), electrolyte disturbances, acute renal failure (Ch. 2.10) and coagulopathy (Ch. 2.8).

PROGNOSIS

The outlook in children with heatstroke appears to be better than in the elderly. The presence of complications such as renal failure, ARDS and coagulopathy increase the risk of death or permanent disability. Prognosis is related to peak body temperature. A delay in treatment of over 2 hours, prolonged coma (> 3 hours) and AST levels above 1000 U/L are poor prognostic factors. The likelihood of residual brain and liver damage and of cataract formation is related to the duration of hyperthermia.

EPIDEMIOLOGY

Heat-related illness is much less common in children than in adults and is dependent on both geographical and cultural influences. Parts of the world where periods of high temperature and high humidity occur, either seasonally or as 'heat waves' lasting 4–5 days, have a higher incidence of classic heatstroke. 'Heat waves' do not allow sufficient time (1–2 weeks) for heat acclimatization to occur. This physiological adaptive mechanism produces earlier production of more dilute sweat. Some cultural factors, such as the annual pilgrimage to Mecca or, in some societies, the increasing tendency to leave children unattended in closed motor vehicles, may expose many children to a high risk of heat stress. Participation of children in high-intensity or long-duration athletic events (fun runs, triathlons, etc.) increases the risk.

Children are physiologically disadvantaged compared with adults (Table 4.7.3) by having a higher metabolic rate per unit body surface area, less ability to sweat (delayed onset and reduced rate), slower heat acclimatization and a greater tendency for dehydration to affect thermoregulation. Infants and very young children, in particular, are at risk because of their absolute dependence on caregivers. While lack of supervision (neglect) may occasionally be the cause of heat-related illness in this age group, the presence of a caregiver is probably the major reason that the incidence of heat-related illness is so low in children of all ages.

Other risk factors include diseases that alter the ability to sweat or the constituents of sweat (cystic fibrosis, spinal cord injury, anhidrotic ectodermal

TABLE 4.7.3 Factors affecting the child's tolerance of heat stress

Infants and young children
- Lack of supervision
- Higher metabolic rate
- Delayed onset of sweating
- Less sweat produced
- Greater effect of dehydration on thermoregulation

Older children
- Tend to follow instructions
- Neglect by caregivers

dysplasia). Some drugs decrease the ability to sweat (antihistamines, anticholinergics, phenothiazines), while others increase heat production (thyroxine, amphetamines).

PREVENTION

Education of children, parents, caregivers, coaches and trainers can increase awareness of heat stress and the susceptibility of younger children to its related illnesses. Education about the importance of adequate hydration both before and during prolonged or severe exercise, the use of appropriate clothing that can 'breathe', as well as anticipation of the circumstances where heat stress is greater (middle of the day, hot spells, etc.) reduces the risk to vulnerable children. Acclimatization to hot climates or hot weather will take more than a week, even with daily exercise of increasing duration. Particular attention should also be given to the preventable danger of leaving small children in unattended motor vehicles.

✔ KEY POINTS

➤ Promote public education:
  - lack of awareness of caregivers and children's dependence on them is a major cause of heat stress and related illness in childhood
  - beware of weather that is both hot *and* humid
➤ Suspect the diagnosis:
  - lower body temperatures than expected may result from appropriate first aid and may delay consideration of the correct diagnosis
  - seriously altered mental status as part of a heat-related illness is heatstroke until proved otherwise

➤ Delay in commencing aggressive cooling can worsen the prognosis

➤ Water spray and air flow techniques are relatively simple and very efficient at lowering elevated body temperature due to hyperthermia

➤ In heatstroke, aggressive volume loading may not be required as rapid cooling causes redistribution of blood volume to the central compartment

➤ Use of antipyretic medications is not indicated

✗ COMMON ERRORS

➤ Failure to consider heat stress in the differential diagnosis of elevated body temperature and thereby delaying appropriate treatment

➤ Delay in the identification and treatment of the many potentially organ-threatening and life-threatening complications

➤ In heatstroke, excessive volume loading while rapidly cooling the patient resulting in pulmonary edema

FURTHER READING

1. Shibolet S, Lancaster MC, Danon Y. Heatstroke: a review. Aviat Space Environ Med 1976; 47: 280–301
   – *(Classic comprehensive review of heatstroke)*

2. Robinson MD, Seward PN. Heat injury in children. Ped Emerg Care 1987; 3: 114–117
   – *(Pathophysiology and emergency management in children)*

3. Squire DL. Heat illness. Fluid and electrolyte issues for pediatric and adolescent athletes. Pediatr Clin North Am 1990; 37: 1085–1109
   – *(Pathophysiology, prevention and management of sport-related heatstroke in children)*

4. Delaney KA. Heatstroke. Underlying processes and lifesaving management. Postgrad Med 1992; 91: 379–388
   – *(Pathophysiology, prevention and emergency management)*

5. Simon HB. Current concepts: Hyperthermia. N Engl J Med 1993; 329: 483–487
   – *(Brief review of all causes of hyperthermia and its effects)*

4.8 Anaphylaxis and envenomation

Bruce Lister

ANAPHYLAXIS

Anaphylaxis is the acute clinical syndrome caused by exposure to a foreign substance to which a patient has been previously sensitized. Anaphylaxis can be caused by drugs, blood products, plasma substitutes or contrast media, vaccines, latex, exercise, foods or food additives or insect stings. Drug-induced anaphylaxis is most frequently caused by penicillins, analgesics and nonsteroidal antiinflammatory drugs.

PHYSIOLOGY

Anaphylaxis is a type 1 allergic reaction mediated by IgE or IgG. Exogenous antigen binds to immunoglobulin bound to mast cells and basophils which then degranulate, releasing mediators including histamine, bradykinin, serotonin, and both eosinophil and neutrophil chemotactic factors. Other mediators such as leukotrienes, prostaglandins, nitric oxide, tumor necrosis factor and platelet activating factor are also released. Antigen-antibody (IgG) complexes can also activate the complement cascade directly, forming C3a and C5a which can then trigger the release of the same mediators from mast cells and basophils. Nitric oxide activates guanylate-cyclase in vascular smooth muscle which generates cyclic GMP causing vascular smooth muscle relaxation and vasodilation. Prostacyclin, prostaglandin E_1 and other prostaglandins directly stimulate receptors on vascular smooth muscle to produce vasodilation. Platelet activating factor induces platelet aggregation, bronchoconstriction, hypotension and increased vascular permeability. Histamine acts on H_2-receptors to produce vasodilation and on H1-receptors to produce bronchoconstriction and increased vascular permeability.

Some hypertonic solutions can stimulate the release of mediators directly by unknown mechanisms. The term anaphylactoid is used to describe reactions clinically indistinguishable from anaphylactic reactions but which are not mediated (or not known to be mediated) by IgE. In idiopathic anaphylaxis, immediate life-threatening reactions occur in the absence of an identifiable precipitant. The pathophysiology of idiopathic anaphylaxis is unknown: the clinical manifestations may result from episodic release of histamine or other vasoactive substances from mast cells, basophils, or both.

DIAGNOSIS

The clinical signs usually include flushing, urticaria, itching, bronchospasm, hypotension and angioedema involving the face, eyes, tongue and larynx. Edema and itching are critical early symptoms which warn the patient of an impending attack. Stridor, wheezing and dyspnea are caused by bronchospasm and by edema of the upper airway, usually maximal in the supraglottic and infraglottic areas. Hypotension caused by vasodilation and shift of protein-laden fluid from plasma into the extravascular space is the most common life-threatening feature. Increased capillary permeability can lead to loss of 35% of blood volume within 10 minutes of the first symptoms. Tachycardia is often present and may help distinguish anaphylaxis from vasovagal syncope. Asthmatic patients will almost always develop bronchospasm. Although unpredictable, the onset of anaphylaxis is often rapid, reaching maximum intensity within 5–30 minutes, although slower onset of symptoms can occur.

MANAGEMENT

Prehospital care

Life-threatening inadequacy of the airway (Ch. 6.3), breathing (Ch. 2.1) or circulation (Ch. 2.3) is corrected first. Epinephrine (adrenaline), oxygen and intravenous fluids are the mainstays of treatment. Epinephrine increases intracellular levels of c-AMP in leukocytes and mast cells and inhibits further release of histamine and other mediators. It improves myocardial contractility, restores peripheral vascular tone and relaxes bronchial smooth muscle. Give epinephrine 0.01 mg/kg per dose (SC, IM or IV) at 15–20-minute intervals up to × 3. If used early, or in mild reactions involving urticaria and mild wheezing, epinephrine may be given by nebulizer (0.5 mg/kg to a maximum of 4 mg) and is absorbed more rapidly by this route than by subcutaneous injection. Up to 10% of children may require a repeat dose of epinephrine and occasonally several doses may be needed. When treatment has been delayed, and shock or severe dyspnea is present, epinephrine should be given by slow intravenous injection (0.01 mg/kg) or infusion (0.1–1 µg/kg·min).

> If intravenous access cannot be secured quickly, epinephrine (adrenaline) can be given by injection into the tongue or by the intraosseous route

Epinephrine should be used with caution in the presence of halogenated hydrocarbons such as halothane, in hypoxia or hypercarbia, when it may trigger ventricular fibrillation. Arrhythmias are extremely uncommon in children with anaphylactic shock but heart rate (and rhythm) should be carefully monitored.

Oxygen should be given by face mask. Endotracheal intubation may be required to protect the airway and facilitate artificial ventilation, especially if angioedema of the tongue or larynx is present. External cardiac compression may be required if the patient has no palpable pulses, but will only be successful if combined with epinephrine administration and aggressive fluid resuscitation.

Emergency room

Symptoms should begin to abate within minutes of effective treatment, but ongoing fluid and epinephrine (adrenaline) treatment may be needed for some hours, implying the presence of a persistent capillary leak. Airway edema and wheezing may persist for several hours until edema fluid can be resorbed, but immediate improvement should be seen following administration of epinephrine.

An intravenous fluid bolus (20 ml/kg) of a colloidal solution (e.g. 5% albumin in saline, or polygeline infusion) or 40 ml/kg of a crystalloid solution (0.9% saline or Hartmann's solution) must be given rapidly to restore impaired peripheral perfusion followed by repeated boluses of fluid (up to 200 ml/kg in total) if perfusion remains poor. Right atrial pressure monitoring may be useful to guide fluid resuscitation.

Corticosteroids and antihistamines have no role in the acute resuscitation of the child with anaphylactic shock but may be useful in a child with a mild attack consisting only of urticaria, itchy eyes and sneezing. Corticosteroids may be used before exposure to a potential or known antigen to prevent anaphylaxis, or if bronchospasm persists despite epinephrine.

A child requiring treatment for severe anaphylaxis should be monitored for 24 hours after stabilization because late deterioration can occur.

Follow-up

Subsequent anaphylactic reactions may occur in some patients on repeated exposure to the triggering agent. The drug or substance responsible should be determined by skin testing and by immunoassays for specific IgE. An alert bracelet should be worn and the patient should carry a letter outlining the nature and cause of the reaction. Desensitization should be considered when possible. Pretreatment with antihistamines, sympathomimetics and steroids may be effective in preventing subsequent reactions to essential substances such as intravenous contrast media or horse serum antivenoms.

PREVENTION

Further contact with substances known to cause anaphylaxis should be avoided. Children who are at risk of severe anaphylaxis should carry epinephrine (adrenaline) for self-administration. These children or their relatives should be trained to recognize the symptoms and to administer epinephrine by means of prefilled syringes, autoinjectors or metered aerosols.

ENVENOMATION

A number of animals and insects can injure humans with powerful venoms which have evolved to help the animal immobilize and digest its prey. Envenomation is the symptom complex caused by a bite or sting from a venomous creature and causes as many as 50 000–100 000 deaths per year worldwide. In the USA, poisonous snakes cause approximately 8000 bites and 9–15 fatalities annually. In the western hemisphere, most snakebites are caused by members of the families Crotalidae or Elapidae. Crotalidae or pit vipers include the rattlesnake, copperhead and cotton-mouth of North America, the fer-de-lance and bushmaster of Central and South America and the Asiatic pit vipers. Elapidae include cobras, mambas, coral snakes, kraits and all the venomous snakes of Australia. Bites of the Crotalidae usually cause local necrosis and bleeding whereas the Elapidae commonly cause neurological symptoms, particularly paralysis, and can affect coagulation. Venomous spiders, scorpions, jellyfish, cone shells, fish, blue-ringed octopus and even the Australian platypus are also capable of inflicting painful and potentially dangerous venom-related injuries to humans. Venoms contain a complex mixture of proteins with diverse actions on the animal's prey and its human victims. The signs, symptoms and appropriate treatment of the envenomed patient vary according to the composition and potency of the venom and the amount of venom injected. Children are often more severely affected than adults because of the greater amount of venom injected per unit body mass.

Proteinases and other enzymes in venom from crotalid snakes cause local tissue damage producing severe pain and swelling at the bite site and sometimes progressing to tissue necrosis and abscess formation.

Hyaluronidase in venom allows other components to spread beyond the bite site.

Presynaptic neurotoxins based on a phospholipase enzyme irreversibly inhibit the release of neurotransmitter from the presynaptic nerve endings causing muscle paralysis and are probably the most powerful and lethal component of any venom from elapid snakes. They cause a progressive neuromuscular paralysis which may take several days to reach maximal effect and is not reversed by the administration of antivenom. Venom from other elapid snakes contains only postsynaptic neurotoxins which paralyze voluntary muscle by binding to the acetylcholine receptor on the postsynaptic membrane. This competitive blockade may be reversed by the administration of appropriate antivenom. Some spider venoms from *Latrodectus*, *Loxosceles* and *Atrax* species cause the release of acetylcholine from autonomic nerve endings causing muscle fasciculation, local sweating and systemic hypertension. Phospholipase A_2 from crotalid and elapid snakes hydrolyzes lecithin in cell membranes, causing rhabdomyolysis and progressive muscle weakness and pain on movement, with myoglobinuria, hyperkalemia and secondary renal failure. Increased permeability of erythrocyte membranes causes cell swelling and hemolysis with precipitation of free hemoglobin and erythrocyte casts in renal tubules, contributing to renal impairment. Nephrotoxins in venoms may also cause direct toxic effects on the kidney. Some venom components from Elapidae and Viperidae and other species can act as *fibrinolysins* or thrombin activators, causing rapid complete defibrination (within 30 minutes of the bite) and fatal intracranial hemorrhage. Thrombocytopenia may occur in conjunction with disseminated intravascular coagulation or may be due to a direct effect of the venom.

DIAGNOSIS

Panic is a common reaction to a venomous bite. Fear may cause nausea, vomiting, diarrhea, dizziness, fainting, tachycardia, and cold, clammy skin. These autonomic reactions must not be mistaken for systemic symptoms and signs resulting from the bite, leading to unwarranted administration of antivenom. In small children, no history of a bite may be given. The child may be found crying, collapsed and even fitting. Unless bite marks are obvious or looked for, envenomation may not be suspected and diagnosis and appropriate management may be delayed until more serious effects of envenomation appear. Clinical signs of envenomation depend on the toxins involved. The early signs and symptoms of envenomation include:

- pain, redness and swelling at the bite site
- headache

- disturbance of vision
- abdominal pain and vomiting or nausea

Later clinical features include:

- respiratory failure
- coagulopathy
- rhabdomyolysis
- altered level of consciousness
- renal failure

Bite marks are not a good predictor of toxicity. Adenopathy in nodes draining the bite site is an early sign of absorption of venom but does not necessarily indicate systemic envenomation. Vomiting, abdominal pain and neurological signs such as ptosis, diplopia, convulsions, and respiratory distress mean that systemic envenomation has occurred. *The triad of headache, abdominal pain and vomiting is moderately predictive of significant envenomation.* The presence of a coagulopathy, hemolysis, rhabdomyolysis or renal failure implies serious envenomation.

MANAGEMENT

First aid and prehospital care

Half of all snakebites involve people less than 20 years old and 20% of all deaths occur in children under 5 years of age. Some of these deaths could be prevented by simple first aid measures. Any first aid treatment must be safe and easily applied; it should maximize the chance that the patient will reach definitive care by delaying life-threatening effects of the venom, and should minimize complications (Table 4.8.1); and not delay transfer to hospital inappropriately. Although signs and symptoms of envenomation may first appear several hours after the bite, some toxins (e.g. jellyfish venom) cause rapid deterioration which may necessitate cardiopulmonary resuscitation at the scene. Obsolete first aid measures such as arterial tourniquets, incision and suction, cryotherapy and electric shock should be avoided. Snake venom is not absorbed through the dermis so washing the bite site is unnecessary and should be avoided in countries where venom detection kits are available to enable identification of the snake species. If appropriate, local measures can prevent further injection of venom: following a sting from a jellyfish (e.g. Chironex fleckeri), vinegar applied

TABLE 4.8.1 **Envenomation: first aid**
- Resuscitation: ABC
- Immobilize the child (lying down)
- Immobilize the limb (splint)
- Reassure the child
- Apply a pressure immobilization bandage
- Specific measures if appropriate (e.g. vinegar for jellyfish stings)
- Transport the child to hospital

topically will inactivate nematocysts and prevent further discharge.

Transport

It is important to delay the spread of venom until the patient can reach a hospital where antivenom can be given. Snake venom moves centrally via the lymphatic system so a firm *compression bandage* should be applied at the bite site and extended up the bitten limb. The bandage should be firm (enough to support a sprain) without occluding arterial or venous blood flow. Correctly applied, a pressure immobilization bandage can prevent venom movement into the circulation until removed hours later without any threat to limb perfusion; a serious hazard of arterial tourniquets. Release of the compression bandage to assess signs of envenomation allows venom to reach the circulation and should be delayed until the child reaches hospital and antivenom is available at the bedside. The pressure immobilization method of first aid is used for snakebite by all species (although some authors discourage its use in bites of crotalid snakes in which local tissue necrosis can be severe) as well as for bites of some spiders such as the Australian funnel-web, bites by the blue-ringed octopus, cone shells and severe stings by jellyfish (this must not precede vinegar treatment). It cannot be applied to bites on the head, neck or trunk and is not appropriate for bites of spiders such as the North American black widow, brown recluse or the Australian redback (both *Latrodectus mactans*), scorpions or centipedes or stings from venomous fish because local compression may exacerbate the pain at the bite site. The child should lie down and be reassured, the bitten limb should be splinted, and transport expedited.

In children with signs of significant envenoma-tion, an intravenous cannula should be inserted before long interhospital transfers. Antivenom (at least 2 ampoules, depending on the venomous species) should be transported to the child, rather than delay administration until the child reaches a larger hospital.

Emergency room

A detailed history of the envenomation should include the time of the bite, a description of the animal or insect, the treatment already adminis-tered (e.g. use of a tourniquet or compression bandage), previous snakebites and therapy with (and adverse reactions to) horse serum-derived antivenoms. The bite site is inspected for fang marks and regional lymphadenopathy sought. Vital signs and neurological status are recorded. Plasma electrolytes, urea and creatinine, hemoglo-bin and especially the platelet count and a coagula-tion screen are measured 1–4 hourly until the results stabilize (Table 4.8.2). Skin bleeding time may be measured if laboratory facilities are limited. Recognition and management of envenomation relies on awareness of the types of venomous crea-tures prevalent in the area and the characteristics of their venom. Rapid, accurate diagnosis is impor-tant and requires a high index of suspicion.

When the patient arrives in a hospital where it is possible to administer antivenom, a small part of the pressure immobilization bandage may be cut away from the bite site to allow inspection and swabbing of the site. Snake venom detection kits which identify the presence and type of snake venom are now an accepted part of the management of snakebite in many countries. The best sample for testing is a swab from the bite site: even a bite site that has been washed may yield a positive result. Urine is also useful for venom detection but because of plasma protein binding, blood is less useful. Once intravenous access has been obtained, the bandage may be removed and the child observed for signs of envenomation.

When available, antivenom is the best treatment for envenomation but should only be given if there are signs of significant systemic envenomation. Fewer than 20% of patients bitten or stung by dan-

TABLE 4.8.2 **Envenomation: laboratory screening**
• Snake venom detection
• Coagulation studies: PT, APTT, fibrinogen, fibrin degradation products
• Blood film
• Platelet count
• Plasma electrolytes, urea and creatinine
• Creatine kinase
• Urinary hemoglobin and myoglobin

gerously venomous animals develop signs of sys-temic envenomation. Because the amount of venom may vary markedly between patients, the dosage of antivenom should be guided by the severity and progression of local changes, clinical signs and laboratory findings. If a coagulopathy is present, much larger doses of antivenom may be required to neutralize the procoagulant effect of the venom. Attempts at correcting a coagulopathy with blood products should only follow adminis-tration of sufficient antivenom to produce an improvement in clinical signs and coagulation pro-file. A skin test for hypersensitivity to horse serum is unreliable, wastes time and is unnecessary before the administration of antivenom. If anti-venom is not available for the particular species involved, first aid measures must still be applied and management is supportive. Fluid resuscitation and inotropic drugs may be required in shocked children (Ch. 2.3). Intubation and mechanical ven-tilation may be required for airway protection and respiratory failure. Attempts at weaning from ven-tilation should only follow the administration of adequate antivenom. Routine excision of wounds, even those caused by snakes whose venom causes local tissue destruction, should not be first-line treatment. Antivenom limits the amount of local tissue damage and fasciotomy should not be neces-sary if adequate antivenom has been given. Surgical debridement is only indicated for obvious necrosis. Prophylactic antibiotics are not indicated unless a wound infection or abscess is present. Antitetanus prophylaxis should be given unless the patient is currently immunized against tetanus (see Appendix). If there is any doubt regarding the severity of the envenomation, the patient should be monitored in an intensive care unit for at least 24 hours. Hospital care is summarized in Table 4.8.3.

TABLE 4.8.3 Envenomation: hospital management

- Primary survey (Ch. 2.6)
- Resuscitation: ABC
- Obtain venous access
- Assess for signs of envenomation
- Check coagulation and other laboratory investigations
- Premedicate if antivenom required
- Remove pressure immobilization bandage
- Observe for at least 12 hours: reassess for signs of envenomation
- Antivenom if signs of envenomation
- Repeat antivenom if signs or symptoms or coagulopathy persist
- Treat organ failure or seizures
- Antitetanus prophylaxis

Complications of treatment

In Australia, fewer than 5% of patients given antivenom develop adverse reactions, none of which have been life-threatening, although in other studies up to 40% of patients developed severe acute reactions or delayed serum sickness. Premedication with i.v. antihistamine and epinephrine (adrenaline) 0.005 mg/kg subcutaneously before the administration of antivenom reduces the incidence of adverse reactions. Serum sickness manifested by fever, rash, arthralgias, and lymphadenopathy, and in rare cases peripheral neuritis, pericarditis, or encephalitis, may occur approximately 4–14 days after the administration of antivenom. The risk of serum sickness increases with the amount of antivenom used. Prednisolone (1 mg/kg per day) may be given for 5–7 days after the administration of antivenom to prevent serum sickness. Tourniquets applied too tightly or left in place too long have caused limb necrosis requiring amputation.

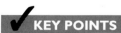

KEY POINTS

ANAPHYLAXIS

➤ Epinephrine (adrenaline) is the treatment of choice for anaphylaxis
➤ Large volumes of plasma expanders are needed in anaphylactic shock

➤ Identification of the allergen, follow-up and education are essential to prevent repeated anaphylactic reactions

ENVENOMATION

➤ Knowledge of local venomous animals and their venoms is vital for management of envenomation
➤ A compression bandage (not tourniquet) prevents venom reaching the circulation by lymphatic (not vascular) compression
➤ Antivenom is the mainstay of treatment but should only be used for significant envenomation

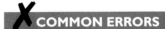

COMMON ERRORS

ANAPHYLAXIS

➤ Insufficient fluid resuscitation
➤ Giving single doses of epinephrine (adrenaline) when multiple doses are required
➤ Use of antihistamines and steroids in severe anaphylaxis

ENVENOMATION

➤ Washing the wound when a snake venom detection kit will be available
➤ Using an arterial tourniquet
➤ Cutting or sucking the wound
➤ Removing the compression bandage to inspect the wound before antivenom and treatment facilities are immediately available

FURTHER READING

1. Fisher M. Treatment of acute anaphylaxis. Br Med J 1995; 311: 731–733
   – (Succinct review of anaphylaxis and its treatment)

2. Meier J, White J, editors. Handbook of clinical toxicology of animal venoms and poisons, Boca Raton: CRC Press; 1995

3. Williamson J, Fenner P, Burnett J, editors. Venomous and poisonous marine animals: a medical and biological handbook. Sydney; University of New South Wales Press; 1996

4.9 Near-drowning

Andrew J. Macnab

Drowning is the second most common cause of death in children aged 1–14 years. 'Drowning' refers to deaths occurring within 24 hours of submersion injury; 'near drowning' means survival, at least temporarily, following asphyxia due to submersion. The lung is the target organ. Aspiration of water depletes surfactant, causing atelectasis and alveolar collapse. Lung compliance is decreased and pulmonary edema develops. Brain injury results from hypoxia, hypercapnia, hypovolemia, acidosis and cardiorespiratory failure. Although many series indicate survival in approximately 50% of cases, the incidence of major neurological sequelae is high (10–24%). Most victims are unattended toddlers. Teenage boys are a second high-risk group; head and neck injury caused by diving is often involved.

PHYSIOLOGY

The clinical severity of drowning relates to the duration of anoxia and hypoperfusion combined with the effects of any underlying cause for the incident (cardiac arrhythmia, convulsion, head and neck injury, drug or alcohol ingestion). The end result of submersion in fresh water or salt water is similar. Most victims (90%) aspirate considerable volumes of fluid. Where no aspiration occurs, laryngospasm or vagally mediated cardiac arrest rapidly follows submersion. The larger the volume of water aspirated, the greater the degree of physiological disturbance: 85% of survivors aspirate 22 ml of water or less per kg of body weight.

Aspirated fresh water depletes surfactant within the alveoli, increasing surface tension. Alveolar collapse and ventilation – perfusion mismatch occur. Water is absorbed rapidly into the circulation with an initial hemodilution and hypervolemia. However, the lung damage rapidly results in pulmonary edema and fluid shifts which effectively result in overall hypovolemia.

Salt water is hypertonic. The effect on surfactant is similar and intrapulmonary shunting occurs followed by edema. There is then migration of water from the intravascular space into the alveoli as a result of hypertonicity which results in hypovolemia.

Hypoxia occurs, from a combination of apnea and respiratory insufficiency, and is aggravated by hypotension, acidosis and hypercarbia. The brain suffers in proportion to the degree and duration of these effects. Children have two protective mechanisms: rapid cooling renders their small body mass hypothermic prior to hypoxic injury, and in infants the primitive diving reflex leads to reflex bradycardia and preferential shunting of blood to the brain and heart from cutaneous and visceral areas.

Abnormal cardiovascular function (bradycardia, reduced myocardial contractility, asystole or ventricular fibrillation) follows changes in arterial oxygen and carbon dioxide tension, pH, blood volume and electrolyte status.

MANAGEMENT

PREHOSPITAL

Cardiopulmonary resuscitation must begin as quickly as possible. Mouth-to-mouth breathing can be initiated in the water (to counteract submersion hypoxemia). If the chest does not move normally when ventilation is attempted, use the standard procedure to position and clear the child's airway. In victims of diving incidents or unwitnessed near-drowning, care must be taken to minimize neck movement at this time, and stabilization of the cervical spine with a semirigid collar or tape and sandbags is important following rescue until X-rays can be performed.

External cardiac compression should begin in the pulseless or bradycardic (rate < 60 beats/min) patient; current recommendations also include those who are hypothermic.

Once equipment becomes available, supplemental oxygen should be administered in all submersion victims; bag-and-mask ventilation initiated where respiratory effort is insufficient and tracheal intubation performed when indicated (Ch. 6.2) to protect/control airway. These procedures should be as rapid as possible to expedite transfer to hospital. A core temperature below 30–32°C increases the risk of ventricular fibrillation. Defibrillation should be attempted, usually only once (2 J/kg nonsynchronized mode). Usually respiratory support, rewarming (> 32°C) and epinephrine (adrenaline) one dose only (Ch. 4.6) are required for this to be effective in hypothermic children. Epinephrine can be given via an endotracheal tube. Access to the circulation may be simplest using the intraosseous route if the patient is cold and peripherally shut down (Ch. 6.1). Shock should be treated with fluid boluses (Ch. 2.3). Rescuers should anticipate regurgitation of stomach contents, as gastric dilatation is common; aspiration is a potent cause of secondary pulmonary insult. Where circumstances allow, nursing the child in a semiprone position is desirable. Once available, suction should be kept close at hand.

Because the devastating effects of hypoxemia continue following rescue, prompt and efficient basic life support at the scene and rapid transport to hospital with advanced life support en route considerably enhance the possibility of recovery.

EMERGENCY ROOM

Many children will arrive pulseless or with symptomatic bradycardia requiring CPR (Ch. 2.2); rewarm hypothermic children (to a core temperature of 32°C and preferably 35°C) before diagnosing brain death and stopping CPR. Most children will have signs of cardiorespiratory and neurological compromise; some will be breathing spontaneously without significant alteration in their conscious level. All require a full history, physical examination, assessment of their level of consciousness using the Glasgow coma scale, exclusion of associated pathology, (particularly injury to the head or cervical spine), appropriate investigation and evaluation of response to emergency treatment (Table 4.9.1). All children should receive additional oxygen until clinical examination, oximetry, blood gas analysis or chest X-ray indicate this is no longer required. Oximetry is reliable in hypothermic patients (core temperature

---

TABLE 4.9.1 Evaluation and diagnosis

History
- Details of submersion
  - type of water (hot, cold, contaminated)
  - duration
  - precipitating circumstances
  - associated injuries
- Status on rescue re:
  - respiratory effort (time to first gasp and to first regular breath)
  - documented asystole (time to detectable heart beat and to effective sinus rhythm)
  - level of consciousness and response
  - past medical history (seizures, drug use)

Physical examination
- Airway
- Respiration (rate and adequacy)
- Pulse, cardiac rhythm, blood pressure (adequacy of circulation)
- Core temperature (use low-reading rectal thermometer)
- Neurological status (Glasgow coma scale score or similar, brain-stem signs)
- Signs of injury

Investigation
- Laboratory
  - blood gas analysis
  - electrolytes, glucose, calcium
  - Hb, blood count
  - urinalysis
  - consider: coagulation screen, liver function, toxic screen
- Radiology
  - CXR (pneumothorax, aspiration/edema/ARDS)
  - consider: cervical spine views, CT scan (possible cerebral injury/edema)
- Other
  - ECG (re arrhythmia)
  - oximetry

> 31°C) and when adequate pulsations occur to generate an accurate pulse rate (maintain SpO_2 > 94%). Vigorously treat hypotension with 20 ml/kg boluses of Ringer-lactate solution. The majority of children should have a nasogastric tube passed to empty their stomach contents, particularly those with any degree of obtundation or diminished ability to protect their airway. Cervical spine X-rays, which include all seven upper vertebrae, are necessary in diving incidents, or where associated head injury is possible (Ch. 2.6).

The major treatment dilemma arises where patients present in a deeply comatose state or with absent vital signs. The controversy regarding resuscitation of these patients is based on reports documenting dismal neurological outcome. Several authors have looked at factors which may predict a hopeless outcome. Unfortunately, no predictor is absolute. Non-reactive pupils in the emergency room and a Glasgow coma scale score of 5 or less on arrival in intensive care are the best independent predictors of poor neurological outcome. However, non-hypothermic patients without vital signs who require CPR can have full neurological recovery. Most authors agree that the change in a patient's neurological examination in the first hours after admission is probably the most valuable predictor of outcome. In this regard, failure to achieve a GCS of 5 or more in the ICU (3.5 ± 1.8 hours after the incident) indicates a poor outcome.

Consequently, whenever a child who suffers submersion requires CPR, this should be instituted on arrival at hospital, while the history is obtained and a physical examination performed. Those children who are in full cardiac arrest or deeply comatose are very likely to die or to have major neurological sequelae; this should be considered where a prompt response to resuscitation does not occur. A similar outcome usually follows if signs of elevated intracranial pressure are evident on admission to intensive care. Survival with good recovery is a strong possibility in those who present awake or with some blunting of conscious level, but are neither comatose nor in full arrest.

Other important aspects of management are:

- always provide support for the family (tremendous guilt and anxiety surround near-drowning incidents)
- triage:
  - admit all children with a history of submersion for observation
  - arrange intensive care for those who required resuscitation, have abnormal blood gases or chest X-ray, or a decreased level of consciousness
- consult with appropriate specialists (share decisions about advisability of continuing resuscitation, optimal supportive care, triage, transfer and ongoing care)
- transfer appropriately

- use an interfacility transport team when available
- communicate early with the receiving hospital about ongoing resuscitation and appropriate preparation for transfer

Interventions that influence outcome are summarized in Table 4.9.2

TRANSPORT CARE

Major secondary problems can compromise the injured brain, particularly during transport by air where ascent to high altitude lowers atmospheric pressure and reduces Pao_2. Call the receiving hospital for advice (Ch. 1.5). Oxygenation and cerebral perfusion must be maintained (have a lower threshold for elective intubation, ensure an adequate oxygen supply to allow for delays). Pneumothorax must be excluded or drained if present (there is an increased risk following submersion). A nasogastric tube and urinary catheter should be placed. Adjust fluid replacement (to maintain normotension but continue overall, postresuscitation fluid restriction). Consider carrying a standby vasopressor infusion, e.g. epinephrine (adrenaline) or dopamine, to maintain adequate cardiac output without giving excessive fluids. Carry medications to continue muscle paralysis, analgesia and sedation. Monitor vital signs (including temperature) and oxygenation (by oximetry). Where possible, allow a parent to accompany the child (to reduce stress for both).

INTENSIVE CARE

Following admission, treatment will depend upon the child's clinical status on reassessment, the extent of the hypoxic ischemic injury on the brain, lung, myocardium, kidney and bowel, and the residual effects of hypothermia. Potential effects of submersion and hypothermia are:

- brain — anoxic neuronal injury
  - decreased cerebral perfusion, increased ICP, cerebral edema
  - impaired autoregulation/metabolism
  - seizures
- lung:

TABLE 4.9.2 **Interventions that influence outcome**

- Full CPR (elevate core temperature > 32°C if arrhythmic)
- Optimal oxygenation (low threshold for intubation)
- Vigorous reversal of hypotension (boluses 20 ml/kg Ringer-lactate solution until normotensive)
- Fluid restriction once normotensive (60% of maintenance)
- Rewarming if < 35°C (avoid rebound above normal body temperature)
- Correction of acidosis (once ventilation established)
- Avoidance of vomiting and aspiration (gastric drainage)
- Avoiding secondary injury to cervical spine
- Promoting venous drainage from head (head elevation 30°)
- Minimizing noxious stimuli (pain, ET suctioning, bladder distention)
- Inserting a Foley catheter
- Monitoring neurological function
- Providing support for the family
- Appropriate triage, arranging intensive care
- Admitting all children with a history of submersion
- Consulting with appropriate specialists
- Transferring appropriately

    – water aspiration, surfactant depletion, hypoventilation, pulmonary edema, ventilation–perfusion mismatch, hypoxia, hypercarbia, apnea
    – aspiration of gastric contents, pneumothorax
    – ARDS
- heart:
    – ischemia, myocardial depression
    – fibrillation, asystole
    – hypotension
- other:
    – vasodilatation on rewarming
    – gastric dilatation, necrosis of bowel mucosa, third spacing of fluid
    – renal tubular necrosis
    – coagulopathy, thrombocytopenia, abnormal platelet function, DIC, hemolysis, electrolyte disturbance, inappropriate ADH secretion, lower resistance to infection (decreased WBC number and activity)

Factors adversely affecting outcome include:

- illness or injury precipitating drowning
- prolonged submersion
- warm water
- no CPR at scene
- delayed hospitalization
- apnea, asystole and/or fixed, dilated pupils on arrival in ER
- inadequate resuscitation in ER

- ongoing hypoxia, hypotension, acidosis, hypercarbia
- elevated intracranial pressure
- low GCS score on admission (< 5)
- deteriorating neurological status

The mainstay of ICU therapy is to support oxygenation and cerebral perfusion via assisted ventilation, muscle paralysis, possibly a slightly lower Pa_{CO_2} (4–4.7 kPa, 30–35 mmHg) on day 1, prompt normalization of blood pressure, inotropic support of myocardial function, mild fluid restriction, control of temperature, sedation or analgesia, and close observation and monitoring to optimize therapy and allow intervention if complications such as cerebral edema, seizures or secondary infection develop. Specific treatment and monitoring measures are listed below.

TREATMENT MEASURES AND MONITORING

General measures

1. Attend to ABCs
2. Give 100% oxygen by non-rebreathing mask (NB evolution of delayed respiratory failure over first 12 hours).

Respiratory status

1. Optimize oxygenation. intubation is required if the Pa_{O_2} is below 13.3 kPA (100 mmHg) or if the Sa_{O_2} is below 90%

when breathing in an FiO_2 of less than 0.6. Also, if CO_2 exceeds 6 kPa (45 mmHg) or when the child is comatose (GCS < 9). For elective intubation, use rapid sequence induction with cerebroprotective medication (Ch. 6.2). Consider mask CPAP (requires correctly fitting mask) for mild respiratory distress in children who are awake, alert, with a $PaCO_2$ of below 45, able to maintain their own airway and not in overt respiratory distress. Initial positive end expiratory pressure for CPAP by mask or in intubated children should be approximately 5 cm water.

2. Sedate and have low threshold for paralysis of the intubated patient.
3. Assisted ventilation with high inspiratory and positive end–expiratory pressures may be required for pulmonary edema, an increased Aa O_2 gradient (normal [35 mmHG] breathing FiO_2 of 1.0) or intrapulmonary shunting – paralysis with pancuronium and sedation is then usual. Anticipate pulmonary edema and pneumothorax, consider mild hyperventilation $PaCO_2$ 4–4.7 kPa (30–35 mmHg) for day 1, $PaCO_2$ 4.7 kPa (35 mmHg) thereafter. Maintain PaO_2 above 13.3 kPa (100 mmHg).
4. Oximetry is required to ensure SaO_2 remains above 90%.
5. Treat acidosis (pH < 7.1), with sodium bicarbonate once effective ventilation is established (slow, half correction).
6. Monitor for and treat bronchospasm.

Circulation

1. Restore spontaneous rhythm.
2. Restore blood pressure by vigorous treatment with fluid boluses (Ringer–lactate, 20 ml/kg) to restore cardiac output and maintain cerebral perfusion. (Hypotension occurs with hypothermia-impaired myocardial function, fluid shifts and vasodilation during rewarming.) Then maintain normotension for age and adequate peripheral perfusion. Use a vasoactive support drug—epinephrine (adrenaline) is the drug of choice, 0.1–1.0 mg/kg·min) (Ch. 7.1).
3. Cardiovascular instability requires assisted ventilation to decrease work of breathing.
4. Maintain normal atrial filling pressures.

Neurological

1. Monitor Glasgow coma scale score (2-hourly); anticipate focal signs of raised intracranial pressure, which should be treated with transient hyperventilation and diuretics (Ch. 2.6).
2. Anticipate seizures; prevent or treat promptly (seizures increase brain oxygen requirement).
3. Protect the cervical spine.
4. Maintain cerebral perfusion pressure. Promote venous drainage (elevate the head of the bed 30°). Minimize noxious stimuli (pain, endotracheal suction, noise, bladder distention): use analgesia, sedation, Foley catheter.

Fluid balance and urine output

1. 40–60 ml/kg are often required for resuscitation; maintenance fluids are then reduced (60%) to lower the risk of cerebral edema.
2. Maintain the urine flow close to 1 ml/kg·h (Foley catheter).

Core temperature

1. Monitor for and treat temperature instability.
2. Maintain the core temperature at 36.5°C to optimize brain oxygen consumption and myocardial function. The diagnosis of brain death is unreliable if the patient is hypothermic. Rewarm or cool, as required (nurse on a cooling or warming blanket). If hypothermic, humidify and warm inspired gases and warm i.v. fluids when required (Ch. 4.6).
3. Treat fever aggressively (elevation increases brain oxygen requirement).

ECG

1. Hypoxia, hypothermia, hypotension and elevated ICP can induce arrhythmias (bradycardia, asystole, fibrillation).
2. Hypercarbia depresses myocardial function.

Laboratory investigations

1. Monitor for and treat rising potassium levels (hyperkalemia => 5.5 mmol/l) (dialysis may be required). (Ch. 2.10).
2. Anticipate hyponatremia (especially in fresh water drowning of children under 1 year old).
3. Follow other electrolyte levels watching for hypokalemia, hyper- or hypoglycaemia, hypocalcemia and hypomagnesemia.
4. Anticipate inappropriate ADH secretion.
5. Monitor for DIC and/or platelet dysfunction and anemia (treatment fresh frozen plasma or packed cells transfusion).

Secondary infection

CXR and sputum

1. A daily examination is needed to check for possible secondary infection. Use broad-spectrum antibacterial agents if therapy is required.

Other

1. A nasogastric tube should be inserted.
2. Control the gastric pH.
3. Support the family.

CONTROVERSIES IN CARE

Brain resuscitation regimens were developed which aggressively intervened in an attempt to reverse the effects of submersion and create the physiological environment most likely to allow recovery. Physicians now question the value of many of these therapies and consider some potentially harmful. This has led to simplified supportive care recognizing that the majority of the primary neuronal injury caused by anoxia is not reversible, and that the objective of postsubmersion therapy must be restitution of optimal oxygen delivery and cerebral perfusion, and measures to reduce the risk of secondary brain insults. Secondary insults are particularly likely where cerebral edema develops, and there is secondary compromise to cerebral blood flow and oxygen delivery.

The treatment measures that are considered controversial are:

- hyperventilation
- hypothermia
- barbiturates
- steroids
- intracranial pressure monitoring
- antibiotics

Routine hyperventilation is no longer practiced. While control of $Paco_2$ is important because of its effect on the caliber of cerebral vessels, excessive hyperventilation can result in vasoconstriction and focal or generalized cerebral oligemia. Hyperventilation ($Pco_2 < 4$ kPA, 30 mmHg) remains an important treatment intervention for proven cerebral edema and raised intracranial pressure, but should not be instituted blindly in all cases of near-drowning.

Hypothermia is only protective prior to the anoxic insult. Rewarming following drowning is important as effective cardiac function will not occur in the hypothermic child. Patients with a core temperature of below 35°C should be rewarmed. It is important, however, to avoid rebound of the core temperature to above 36.5°C, because cerebral oxygen consumption increases significantly where core temperature is above normal. Consequently, stabilization of body temperature and avoidance of fever remain important.

Barbiturate coma to reduce cerebral metabolic activity no longer has a place in therapy. Barbiturates may still be used with phenytoin as part of an anticonvulsant regimen.

Steroids have not been shown to be of any benefit following near-drowning.

Intracranial pressure is rarely elevated, and monitoring ICP does not influence outcome.

Antibiotics are not routinely indicated unless drowning occurs in a heavily contaminated environment; eg. hot tubs, where *Pseudomonas* is prevalent (use ceftazidime 33 mg/kg every 8 hours).

CARE FOLLOWING DISCHARGE

Some temporary developmental regression may occur in the younger child. All victims of catastrophic injury are prone to psychological reactions; children may show transient behavioral problems and their parents may become overprotective. If children have a residual handicap, referral to appropriate agencies for care of their special needs and rehabilitation must be made. The issues of family guilt and grief over the loss of their normal child should also be addressed, perhaps by the family physician. When the incident proves fatal, breaking the bad news should not be delayed; siblings should not be excluded from this process. In incidents when a child dies but others survive, survivor guilt may occur (Ch. 5.8).

EPIDEMIOLOGY

After motor vehicle trauma, drowning is the most common cause of accidental death in children in most countries in the Western world. Part of the difficulty surrounding these deaths is that they tend to be viewed together when treatment and outcome are discussed, rather than examined as individual events. There are unique aspects in the majority of cases. Clearly, the child who develops a fatal arrhythmia when falling into ice-cold water, or the teenager who sustains a massive head injury when diving, will have a different outcome to the small child briefly submerged when swimming while supervised. Similarly, hospital treatment varies, and a major difficulty concerning the prognosis, survival and outcome of these cases has been that important issues such as length of submersion and adequacy of resuscitation at the scene have been virtually impossible to quantify.

Most drownings occur in toddlers, with a peak incidence in the second year of life, and bathtubs, pools and bodies of water close to the home are involved in 85% of cases. Most incidents occur during warm weather and where no gates or fencing are in place. Typically, these infants are found motionless, face down in the water, and mortality is high. Pool covers are implicated in many of these incidents, the children crawling on or under the cover prior to submersion. Incidents at public

swimming pools have a low mortality (6%). The level of supervision is higher and resucitation usually is initiated promptly at the poolside.

Another high-risk group is teenage boys, both swimmers and nonswimmers. Bravado, alcohol and substance abuse are sometimes involved. The association of head and neck injuries is high, secondary to diving. Studies show that although there are some local epidemiological differences, e.g. the incidence of swimming pools in California compared with Sweden, data are generally similar to Kemp's 1-year prospective study in the UK (1988–9). Here, mortality was 48.7%, the male to female ratio was 3:1, 68% of children were under 5 years of age, and 83% were unsupervised by an adult at the time of the injury. Babies and toddlers were most likely to drown in the bath (here the sexes are equally affected), and 4 out of 5 drownings happened when the child was alone or supervised by an older sibling.

In the UK study, 20% of drowning deaths in infants were regarded as unlawful killing by the coroner. Unfortunately, child abuse must now be suspected in drowning incidents, particularly where the history given is contradictory or atypical, or there is a past history of suspicious injury in the family.

Virtually any body of water, no matter how small, is capable of drowning a child. This can include washing machines, pails of water, and roadside ditches. The death rate from drowning varies from 0.7 per 100 000 children under 15 years old in Britain, to 3.1 for Washington State, USA, and 5.2 for Australia. If we consider that incidents resulting in near-drowning are 3–5 times more common than death from drowning, and that many children do not come to hospital as they are saved prior to significant submersion, the full extent of the problem becomes clear.

PREVENTION

All physicians can and should contribute to reducing the incidence and severity of drowning injury in children (Ch. 1.4). They should impress on parents the need for constant supervision of young children around water (particularly during bathtime); draining, covering or fencing garden ponds or pools; teaching children to swim; learning basic life support measures, and employing water safety practices when swimming or boating. Physicians involved with teenagers can promote swimming as a desirable skill, emphasize safe choices when diving, discuss the issue of bravado, drug and alcohol use, and set an example themselves over lifejacket use and equipment safety. Private swimming pools should have fencing and locking gates, and there is a need for improved pool cover design.

✔ KEY POINTS

➤ Prompt, effective cardiopulmonary resuscitation significantly improves prognosis

➤ Near-drowning victims who are pulseless and apneic deserve full resuscitation, including rewarming, on arrival at hospital, while a history is obtained and decisions made

➤ Near-drowning victims with an altered level of consciousness or respiratory compromise should be intubated, ventilated, supported hemodynamically, and transferred promptly to intensive care

➤ Episodes of hypotension, hypoxia or raised intracranial pressure, elevated temperature and seizures will compromise cerebral oxygenation

➤ The possibility of an underlying seizure disorder, cervical spine injury, and nonaccidental injury should be considered

➤ All physicians should promote injury prevention strategies to reduce the incidence of drowning

✗ COMMON ERRORS

➤ Failure to rewarm prior to stopping cardio-pulmonary resuscitation

➤ Failure to protect the cervical spine

➤ Instituting fluid restriction before correction of blood pressure

➤ Excessive hyperventilation

➤ Inadvertent elevation of intracranial pressure through suboptimal intubation, pain, or excessive ET tube suction

➤ Failure to anticipate the adverse effects of rewarming on the circulation and the metabolism

FURTHER READING

1. Levin DL, Morriss FC, Toro LO, Brink LW, Turner GR. Drowning and near drowning. Pediatr Clin North Am 1993; 40(2): 321–336

2. Modell JH. Drowning. N Engl J Med 1993; 328(4): 253–256

– *(Two good general reviews on physiology and management of near-drowning)*

3. Kemp A, Siebert JR. Drowning and near drowning in children in the United Kingdom: lessons for prevention. Br Med J 1992; 304: 1143–1146

– *(A review of epidemiology and potential preventive measures)*

4. Lavelle JM, Shore KN. Near drowning: is emergency department cardiopulmonary resuscitation or intensive care unit cerebral resuscitation indicated? Crit Care Med 1993; 21: 368–373

5. Nichter M, Everett P. Childhood near drownings: is cardiopulmonary resuscitation always indicated? Crit Care Med 1990; 17: 993–995

6. Biggart M, Bohn D. Effect of hypothermia and cardiac arrest on outcome of near drowning accidents in children. J Pediatr 1990; 117: 179–183

– *(Three reports attempting to identify reliable prognostic factors)*

7. Bohn DJ, Biggart WD, Smith CR, Conn AW, Barker GA. Influence of hypothermia, barbiturate therapy, and intracranial pressure monitoring on morbidity and mortality after near drowning. Crit Care Med 1986; 14: 529–534

8. Modell JH. Treatment of near drowning. Is there a role for hypertherapy? Crit Care Med 1986; 14: 593–594

– *(Two papers describing controversial aspects of care)*

Therapeutic principles and practice guidelines for critical care

5

Neil T. Matthews

The use and effects of drugs in critically ill children are modified by the developmental changes in physiology (including liver and kidney function) that occur during childhood, and by the effects of severe illness. These developmental and illness-related changes affect the absorption, distribution, metabolism and excretion of drugs (pharmacokinetics) and the interaction of drugs with their receptors (pharmacodynamics).

Critically ill children usually require the simultaneous use of a large number of potent drugs, which inevitably increases the risk of drug interactions and altered drug effects.

This chapter discusses basic pharmacokinetic principles; developmental pharmacology; effects of critical illness on drug action; therapeutic drug monitoring, and the basis of drug interactions. Indications for and use of individual drugs are mentioned in chapters related to their use (see also Chapters 4.5, 7.1 and 7.2).

Before a drug is given, its benefits should be compared with its risks: the clinical end point to be achieved by its use should be defined and its effectiveness and complications closely monitored.

DEVELOPMENTAL PHARMACOLOGY

The pharmacokinetic and pharmacodynamic data that guide drug therapy in pediatrics are limited, and clinical use is usually based on adult models, clinical experience and therapeutic monitoring.

DRUG ABSORPTION

Gastric acid

In the stomach, the absorption of acidic drugs such as aspirin is favored by low gastric pH, and that of basic drugs by higher pH. Gastric acid is rarely found in the stomachs of neonates of less than 32 weeks' gestation. At birth, gastric pH is between 6 and 8, but falls within a few hours to between 1.5 and 3, and approaches the lower limit of adult values by 3 months of age. The most important factor influencing the secretion of gastric acid in the newborn is initiation of enteral feeding. Penicillins are better absorbed in neonates whose gastric pH is higher than that of older children.

Gastric emptying

Slow gastric emptying reduces or delays the peak concentrations of drugs administered orally. Emptying is slowed by prematurity, gastro-esophageal reflux, respiratory distress syndrome, congenital heart disease, and the presence of long-chain fatty acids, found in many infant feeding formulae. Gastric emptying is accelerated by human milk and by hypoenergetic feeds, but unaffected by posture or the osmolality of feeds. Gastric emptying attains normal adult rates by 6–8 months of age.

Pancreatic function

Exocrine pancreatic function is low at birth and does not achieve adult values until 2 years of age. This may reduce the absorption in infants of oral drugs that require hydrolysis in the bowel lumen.

Drug distribution

The information needed to treat a child with a drug includes:

- the plasma concentration needed to produce the desired effect
- the dose and dose interval needed to achieve that concentration

If a loading dose is not given and the dose interval is less than or equal to the plasma half-life of the drug, it will take five half-lives to reach 96% of the final steady state concentration. A loading dose can be given, which allows the steady state concentration to be reached much more rapidly (e.g. with digoxin or milrinone in a child with heart failure).

Useful calculations:

- loading dose (LD) = $(V \times C_p) \div F$
- loading dose = $(D \times t_{1/2}) \div (I \times 0.693)$
- maintenance dose (D) = $(LD \times I) \div (t_{1/2} \times 1.44)$
- maintenance dose = $(C_{ss} \times V \times I) \div (t_{1/2} \times F \times 1.44)$
- concentration at steady state (C_{ss}) = $(F \times D) \div (Cl \times I)$
- concentration at steady state = $(t_{1/2} \times F \times D) \div (0.693 \times V \times I)$

where:

  LD = loading dose (mg/kg)
  D, maintenance dose (mg/kg)
  I, dose interval (hours)
  V, volume of distribution (L/kg body weight)
  C_p, plasma concentration (mg/L)
  C_{ss}, plasma concentration at steady state (mg/L)
  $t_{1/2}$, plasma half-life (hours)
  F, fraction of dose absorbed (= 1 for i.v. doses)
  Cl, clearance in L/kg·h

Appropriate loading and maintenance doses and dose intervals are given in Chapter 7.1. The volume of distribution, $t_{1/2}$, fractional absorption and clearance are found in standard textbooks (see further reading list), so the other variables can be calculated. When a child's pharmacokinetics are changed (e.g. clearance is reduced by impaired liver or kidney function, or volume of distribution is increased by massive edema), these equations can be used to calculate the appropriate loading and maintenance doses and the dose interval for that child if the change in clearance or volume of distribution can be estimated.

The volume of distribution of a drug determines the loading dose needed to achieve an appropriate plasma concentration (see above). Several important age-dependent variables directly influence volume of distribution. These include the size and composition of body fluid compartments, the extent of protein binding, lipid solubility, membrane permeability and hemodynamic factors such as cardiac output and regional blood flow.

Lipophilic drugs cross cell membranes more readily than hydrophilic drugs and so reach equilibrium concentrations within cells more rapidly. The volume of distribution of highly protein-bound and lipid-bound drugs (especially the latter) can be much greater than the total body water (e.g. 35 L/kg for desipramine). The volume of distribution of lipophilic drugs is lower in neonates because of their lower adipose tissue content.

Body water

The absolute amounts of body water and fat, and the distribution of water between body compartments vary with age (Table 5.1.1).

TABLE 5.1.1 Changes in body water distribution during childhood as a percentage of body weight			
Age	Total body water (%)	Extracellular fluid (%)	Intracellular fluid (%)
3-month fetus	90	65	25
Term neonate	75	35–45	35
4–6 months	60	25	37
12 months	60	25–30	40
Adult	50–60	20	40

Protein binding

Highly protein-bound drugs have a larger volume of distribution and are more slowly filtered at the glomerulus than unbound drugs. Protein binding means less free active drug at any total drug concentration, and longer clearance times. Drug binding to plasma proteins is age-related (Tables 5.1.2, 5.1.3), and depends on:

- plasma protein concentration (varies with illness, e.g. decreased in liver disease)
- the affinity of the drug for the protein
- competition for binding sites, for example with free fatty acids and bilirubin

Differences in protein binding between commonly used drugs are shown in Table 5.1.3.

DRUG METABOLISM

The primary site for drug metabolism is the liver, although the kidney, lung and gut are also involved. Biotransformation of drugs to more water-soluble compounds permits their elimination in urine and bile. The products of liver metabolism are usually inactive or weakly active compounds, but are sometimes active metabolites with pharmacological properties similar to those of the parent compound,

e.g. morphine glucuronide, or with increased toxicity, e.g. normeperidine (norpethidine).

Biotransformation involves oxidation, reduction, hydrolysis and/or conjugation, usually with glucuronic acid (e.g. morphine). Enzymes that catalyze these processes have low activity in the liver in fetal life and in the neonate and infant, although individual enzyme systems mature at different rates. Conjugation is mature at 2–3 months of age. From early infancy until puberty, children metabolize most drugs more rapidly than adults.

DRUG EXCRETION

Most water-soluble drugs and drug metabolites are excreted by the kidney. Smaller amounts are excreted in feces via bile, and in the lungs, sweat and milk. The amount of drug filtered at the glomerulus depends on:

- glomerular filtration rate (GFR), which in turn depends on the renal blood flow (RBF)
- protein binding
- water solubility

At birth, the RBF is 35 ml/m²·min: this doubles by 2 weeks of age and reaches adult values by 2 years. The GFR is 12 ml/m².min at birth, doubles by 2 weeks of age and reaches adult values by 1–2 years. Tubular secretion of drugs attains adult values by 30 weeks of age.

TABLE 5.1.2 Factors that affect protein binding in children, compared with adults			
Variable	Newborn	Infant	Child
Total plasma protein	Lower	Lower	Same
Plasma albumin	Lower	Same	Same
Fetal albumin	Present	Absent	Absent
Plasma globulin	Lower	Lower	Same
Unconjugated bilirubin	Elevated	Same	Same
Free fatty acids	Elevated	Same	Same
Blood pH	Lower	Same	Same

TABLE 5.1.3 Protein binding of common drugs in infancy and adult life (percentage protein-bound)		
Drug	Newborn (%)	Adult (%)
Ampicillin	10	18
Diazepam	84	99
Lidocaine (lignocaine)	20	70
Morphine	46	66
Theophylline	36	56

EFFECT OF CRITICAL ILLNESS

In critically ill children, the function of the liver, kidney and brain and of the cardiovascular and respiratory systems is altered, nutrition is inadequate (Ch. 5.3) and immunity is impaired. Adjustments to drug dosage are often needed to ensure adequate therapy and to avoid toxicity.

DRUG DISTRIBUTION

Hemodynamics

In shock, blood flow redistribution exposes the brain and heart to toxic concentrations of drugs and reduces drug delivery to target organs. The dose and i.v. bolus administration rate of drugs such as thiopental (thiopentone) or phenytoin, which have toxic effects on the brain and heart, should be reduced. Inflammation increases local blood flow and produces high drug concentrations in the inflamed tissue. Changes in pharmacokinetics are difficult to predict in cardiorespiratory illness, and drug concentrations and effects should be monitored carefully. Theophylline clearance increases in asthma, pneumonia and congestive heart failure.

Protein binding

For acidic drugs such as phenytoin and barbiturates, protein binding is significantly reduced in hepatic and renal disease, nephrotic syndrome and protein malnutrition. This increases the volume of distribution and the clearance. The total plasma concentration is reduced but the concentration of free drug remains unchanged and adjustment of dose is usually unnecessary. Basic drugs such as morphine, propranolol and lidocaine (lignocaine) are bound by acute-phase reactants such as α_1-acid glycoprotein which are synthesized in trauma and serious illness: this may decrease the response to the drug dose.

Extravascular fluid collections

Ascitic, pleural and peritoneal fluid may serve as a reservoir of drugs, and reduce the effect of a drug dose or prolong its duration of action.

DRUG ELIMINATION

Renal failure

Renal excretion of drugs is decreased by reduction in vascular volume and renal blood flow. Sepsis and nephrotoxic drugs (Table 5.1.4) also impair drug excretion. In the face of rising serum creatinine levels, the drug dose and dose interval should be adjusted. In a child with significant renal dysfunction (serum creatinine > 0.1 mmol/L), the daily dose of drugs that are excreted by the kidneys must be reduced, either by reducing the dose or by increasing the dose interval. It is possible to calculate a more appropriate dose based on body length and serum creatinine concentration (see below), but the errors in this method are large. Modifications of dose and dose interval of some common drugs in children with renal failure are described in Tables 5.1.5 and 5.1.6. Whenever possible, serum drug levels should be monitored (see below). Renal failure does not affect the loading dose of a drug. Drugs excreted mainly by the kidney include penicillins, cephalosporins, aminoglycosides and vancomycin, digoxin, H_2-antagonists and metoclopramide.

Hepatic failure

Splanchnic vasoconstriction in shock or heart failure reduces drug delivery to the liver, and hypoxemia decreases portal oxygen tension and liver cell metabolism, decreasing the metabolic clearance of drugs. Protein binding and biliary excretion are also reduced. Doses and dose intervals can only be adjusted accurately in liver failure if serum drug levels are monitored. Some drugs should be avoided in children with liver failure: glucocorticoids, tetracyclines and cimetidine can impair liver function. Opiates and sedatives exacerbate hepatic encephalopathy and aspirin analogs such as indomethacin can exacerbate upper gastrointestinal bleeding. Aspirin, acetaminophen (paracetamol), chlorpromazine and erythromycin estolate are themselves hepatotoxic.

PHARMACODYNAMICS

In critically ill children, drug receptor numbers and their affinity for the drug are reduced.

TABLE 5.1.4 **Nephrotoxicity of drugs commonly used in the critically ill child**

Acute renal failure or reduced GFR
Aminoglycosides
Cephalosporins
Tetracyclines
Amphotericin B
Acyclovir
Pentamidine
Aspirin
Indomethacin
Contrast media
Dextran
Cisplatin
Methotrexate
Propranolol
Captopril
Tolazoline
Bismuth compounds
Aminocaproic acid
Phenytoin

Chronic renal failure
Aminoglycosides
Vancomycin
Tetracyclines
Nonsteroidal antiinflammatory drugs
Cyclosporin
Cisplatin
Contrast media

Acute interstitial nephritis
Penicillins and cephalosporins
Aminoglycosides
Antituberculous drugs
Sulfonamides
Trimethoprim and sulfamethoxazole (co-trimoxazole)
Nonsteroidal antiinflammatory drugs
Anticonvulsants
Angiotensin converting enzyme inhibitors
Cimetidine
Propranolol
Azathioprine

Reduced responsiveness of α-adrenergic receptors decreases the efficacy of vasopressors. Insulin resistance follows changes in insulin receptors after burns, sepsis, major surgery and severe trauma. Down-regulation of β-adrenergic receptors in the myocardium in sepsis and heart failure and after 12–24 hours of inotropic drug therapy reduces the efficacy of dopamine and dobutamine, and the infusion rate must often be increased to achieve the same clinical effect.

Drug effects may also be modified by changes in electrolyte concentrations and acid–base status and by endogenous cytokines, catecholamines and adrenal corticosteroids. For example, ventricular arrhythmias caused by digoxin and nephrotoxicity due to aminoglycosides are more common if children are hypokalemic.

Malnutrition

Critically ill patients are usually malnourished. Malnutrition alters drug handling in the body by:

- increasing total body water
- reducing plasma protein concentrations
- decreasing body fat and muscle mass
- decreasing hepatic metabolism and biliary excretion
- reducing cardiac output
- altering renal function

In a malnourished child, the appropriate loading dose of a drug is unchanged; if the liver and kidney function are impaired, the maintenance dose must often be reduced and the dose interval increased. Drug monitoring allows more accurate dosing.

Gastrointestinal function

Serious illness reduces intestinal blood flow, gut motility and drug absorption. Narcotic drugs reduce stomach and bowel motility, and antacids and H_2-receptor antagonists alter the rates of gastric digestion of food. These effects limit the rate of absorption, and delay and reduce peak blood concentrations of orally administered drugs.

THERAPEUTIC DRUG MONITORING

In therapeutic drug monitoring, drug concentrations in plasma or serum are measured, and the dose or dose interval adjusted to achieve the desired concentration. Therapeutic levels and their acceptable limits are set before treatment is started. The two most common approaches to drug therapy in the severely ill are target effect and target concentration.

TARGET EFFECT STRATEGY

The dose is increased until a desired clinical effect is achieved or drug toxicity appears, unless:

- there is no further increase in effect as dose increases
- the desired effect cannot be attained

This approach is most useful for drugs such as catecholamines, H_2-receptor antagonists and neuromuscular blocking agents, oxygen, and vasodilators, whose relationship between blood level and effect—or blood level and toxicity—is very variable from one child to another. For example, the dose of an α-adrenergic agonist is titrated against the desired blood pressure. Signs of toxicity such as skin

---

TABLE 5.1.5 **Drug dosing in renal failure**

- **No change:**
  atracurium
  barbiturates
  benzodiazepines
  calcium channel blockers
  ceftriaxone
  cisatracurium
  fentanyl and its derivatives
  furosemide (frusemide)
  glucocorticoids
  heparin
  phenothiazines
  streptokinase
  warfarin

- **Avoid in severe renal failure:**
  amiloride
  aspirin
  meperidine (pethidine)
  pancuronium
  spironolactone
  succinylcholine (suxamethonium)
  vecuronium

- **Adjust dose and dose interval according to effects:**
  dobutamine
  dopamine
  epinephrine (adrenaline)
  salbutamol (albuterol)
  sodium nitroprusside
  nitroglycerin (glyceryl trinitrate)

- **Adjust dose and dose interval according to levels (see text: target concentration):**
  aminoglycosides
  anticonvulsants
  cyclosporin
  flucytosine
  vancomycin

- **Modify dose or dose interval empirically (see Table 5.1.6)**

TABLE 5.1.6 **Empirical modification of drug dose or dose interval**

Drug	Moderate renal failure (serum creatinine 0.20–1.0 mmol/L)	Severe renal failure (serum creatinine > 1.0 mmol/L)
Aztreonam and imipenem	50% D	50% D, 2 × I
Cefazolin	2 × I	50% D, 8 × I
Cefuroxime	2 × I	70% D, 3 × I
Other cephalosporins	2 × I	4 × I
Ciprofloxacin	75% D	50% D
Acyclovir	2 × I	50% D, 3 × I
Ganciclovir	50% D, 2 × I	50% D, 4 × I
ACE inhibitors (e.g. enalapril)	75% D	50% D
Beta-blockers	Usual dose	75% D
Digoxin	50% D, 2 × I	25% D, 2 × I
Morphine	75% D	50% D
Acetaminophen (paracetamol)	1.5 × I	1.5 × I
H_2-antagonists (e.g. ranitidine)	2 × I	2 × I, 50% D
Metoclopramide	75% D	50% D

D, usual dose; I, usual dose interval.

---

pallor and metabolic acidosis are monitored carefully. In neonates and infants, there may be a 10-fold difference between individuals in the dose of an inotropic drug such as dopamine, dobutamine or epinephrine (adrenaline) needed to produce a given effect. For example, 5 μg/kg of dopamine may be a small dose in one child but a very large dose in another. The appropriate dose is found by titrating the dose against effect and signs of toxicity.

TARGET CONCENTRATION STRATEGY

Plasma or serum levels of the drug are measured and the results compared with an accepted therapeutic range which may be specific to each laboratory. This approach overlooks variations in drug responsiveness between individuals. Identical drug concentrations can produce considerably different responses between patients, or in the same patient when pathophysiology changes during illness. Monitoring drug concentrations in children is useful:

- when the therapeutic index of the drug is small (aminophylline, aminoglycosides or phenytoin)

- when the signs of toxicity are difficult to recognize clinically or to differentiate from those of the underlying disease
- when pharmacokinetics are affected by physiological factors, e.g. if elimination is impaired by liver or renal failure
- if there is therapeutic failure
- in cases of overdose

Monitoring drug concentrations is *not* useful when:

- there is a large therapeutic index (penicillins, cephalosporins)
- the effect is immediate and can be readily measured (diuretic agents, insulin)
- there is no concentration effect (some alkylating agents).

When the toxicity of a drug is related to its *peak* concentration (e.g. theophylline), a blood sample should be taken about 1 hour after the dose (to allow time for redistribution). If the level is high, the appropriate response is usually to reduce the dose. In many cases (e.g. aminoglycosides and flucytosine), toxicity is related to the *mean* concentration. The sample is taken immediately before the dose and if the level is high, the dose interval should be increased. If the level remains high, the dose may have to be reduced.

In most cases, the first sample should be taken after 5 half-lives, to allow time for the plasma concentration to reach a plateau. For very toxic drugs (e.g. aminoglycosides) or when the child's renal and hepatic function are too unstable to predict when a plateau will be reached, the first sample should be taken after one or two doses, and further samples taken regularly, to avoid undetected toxic concentrations of the drug.

When liver or kidney function is impaired, it is possible to calculate the optimal dose interval by measuring plasma drug concentrations 1 hour, 4 hours and 8 hours after a dose and plotting these on a semilog scale (Fig. 5.1.1). The time after which a straight line drawn through these points reaches the desired trough concentration (point 'a') is the appropriate dose interval.

Common errors in applying target concentration strategy include:

- incorrect loading dose

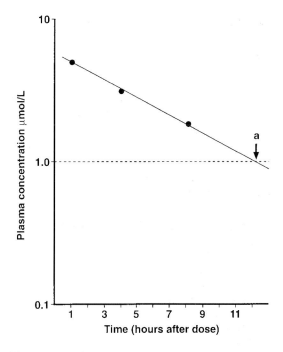

Figure 5.1.1 Semilog plot of plasma concentration of a drug against time after a dose. The appropriate dose interval (12 hours in this case) is the time at which a straight line joining the three points reaches the desired trough level *a* (1 μmol/L in this case): see text

- sampling too early after a dose (before a steady state is reached)
- not considering the half-life when planning the dose interval
- treating the numbers rather than the patient (e.g. maintaining anticonvulsant levels in the 'therapeutic range' at the expense of seizure control)

DRUG INTERACTIONS

It is common for critically ill children to require several drugs simultaneously, often leading to important drug interactions that may affect patient outcome. Such interactions may cause:

- enhancement of the drug effect (e.g. cimetidine increases the effect of theophylline because of inhibition of metabolism)
- inhibition of drug effect (e.g. rifampicin increases the metabolism of phenytoin)

- no change in effect despite alteration in kinetics and metabolism

It is not always possible to predict the effect of a drug given in combination, from its effects given alone. Before starting treatment with a drug, it is important to nominate the acceptable clinical or laboratory limits of toxicity (e.g. tachycardia, serum creatinine level, platelet count), beyond which the drug will be discontinued or the dose reduced.

DIRECT PHYSICAL INTERACTION

Drugs may interact directly, especially in high concentrations. This reduces the effects of each drug, for example heparin and lidocaine (lignocaine) precipitate in solution, reducing the effect of each (although not all physical interactions produce precipitates). Adsorption of drugs, e.g. insulin, fentanyl, sodium nitroprusside and nitroglycerin (glyceryl trinitrate), to glass or plastic reduces the amount of available drug until adsorption sites are saturated. This should be anticipated and the dose or infusion rate adjusted according to effect.

GASTROINTESTINAL ABSORPTION

Interactions may occur in the gut prior to absorption. For example, barbiturates reduce dicumarol (dicoumarol) absorption. Drugs that affect gut motility (e.g. opioids or H_2-antagonists) may inhibit or enhance the absorption of other drugs. Antacids and H_2-antagonists which raise the gastric pH reduce gastric absorption of weak acids such as ketoconazole.

PROTEIN BINDING

Drugs that are highly protein-bound—e.g. phenytoin, valproic acid and furosemide (frusemide)—compete for binding sites, increasing the free drug fraction (and therefore the drug effect) of both drugs, especially of the less tightly bound.

RECEPTOR SITES

Interactions between agonists and antagonists occur at receptor sites, for example opioids and naloxone; benzodiazepines and flumazenil.

INCREASED METABOLISM

Some drugs induce the synthesis of enzyme systems, especially those of the hepatic endoplasmic reticulum, which accelerates their own metabolism and that of other drugs, requiring a compensatory increase in dose. Barbiturates, for example, accelerate the metabolism of phenytoin, carbamazepine induces that of theophylline and phenytoin, and rifampicin that of oral contraceptives, warfarin and theophylline.

REDUCED METABOLISM

Some drugs (e.g. amiodarone, erythromycin, sodium valproate and cimetidine) inhibit the metabolism of other drugs, causing an increased drug concentration and effect. Phenytoin inhibits the metabolism of phenobarbital (phenobarbitone), and H_2-antagonists slow the metabolism of oral anticoagulants, diazepam and carbamazepine.

✓ KEY POINTS

➤ Drug absorption (especially from the gastrointestinal tract), distribution, elimination and drug-receptor interaction are often different in infants compared with older children and adults
➤ Drug absorption (especially from the gastrointestinal tract), distribution, elimination and drug-receptor interaction are often different in severely ill children compared with well children
➤ Drug level monitoring is useful if there is a narrow therapeutic index, liver or kidney failure, or overdose, or if clinical end points are not available
➤ Monitoring of drug concentration is not useful for drugs which have a variable relationship between blood level and effect or toxicity.

FURTHER READING

1. Reed MD, Blumer JL. Therapeutic drug monitoring in the pediatric intensive care unit. Pediatr Clin North Am 1994; 41: 1227–1243
–   *(Review of current pediatric practice)*

2. St Peter WL, Halstenson CE. Pharmacologic approach in patients with renal failure. In: Chernow B, editor. The pharmacologic approach to the critically ill patient, 3rd ed. Baltimore: Williams & Wilkins; 1994
–   *(Detailed summary of available information (mostly adult) on dose modification in renal failure)*

3. Krishnaswarmy K. Drug metabolism and pharmacokinetics in malnutrition. In: Gibaldi M, Prescott L, editors. Handbook of clinical pharmacokinetics. New York: ADIS Health Science Press; 1983
–   *(Review of the effects of malnutrition on drug distribution)*

4. Spector R, Park GD, Johnson GF et al. Therapeutic drug monitoring. Clin Pharmacol Ther 1988; 43: 345
–   *(Overview of drug monitoring in adults and children)*

5. Rudy AC, Brater DC. Drug interactions. In: Chernow B, editor. The pharmacologic approach to the critically ill patient, 3rd ed. Baltimore: Williams & Wilkins; 1994
–   *(Useful reference on interactions between drugs commonly used in the critically ill)*

6. Benet LZ, Kroetz DL, Sheiner LB. Pharmacokinetics. In: Hardman JG, Limbird LE, Molinoff PB, Ruddon RW, editors. Goodman and Gilman's The pharmacological basis of therapeutics, 9th ed. New York: McGraw Hill; 1996
–   *(Succinct summary of the principles of pharmacokinetics)*

5.2 Analgesia and sedation

Ian James and Steven Scuplak

Many critically ill children and nearly all those admitted to a PICU require some form of sedation to alleviate the anxiety and distress that accompany their illness. Anxiety is engendered by fear, parental separation, unfamiliar faces and environment, and ambient noise. Simple matters such as the loss of a normal sleep pattern also make infants irritable and restless, as any parent will affirm. There is also the need for analgesia to relieve the pain associated with trauma or surgery, or the discomfort caused by the illness, the insertion or presence of tubes and drains, and the other invasive procedures involved in treatment. A detailed explanation of the mechanisms of pain production, transmission and blockade is beyond the scope of this chapter. However, patients receiving intensive care are especially susceptible to repeated episodes of high-intensity nociceptive stimulation, which result in prolonged periods of sustained afferent input to the central nervous system. Apart from the immediate issues of discomfort, this can create long-term cellular changes in the dorsal horn, and the development of chronic pain. A cornerstone of the management of sedation and analgesia during critical illness must therefore be the provision of adequate analgesia to all patients, including term and preterm neonates.

PHYSIOLOGY

The physiological response to injury and stress includes a neuroendocrine cascade, many components of which are detrimental to the wellbeing of the critically ill child. Cardiovascular instability, respiratory compromise, increased catabolism and oxygen consumption, sodium retention, splanchnic vasoconstriction and altered immune function are some of these undesirable consequences of stress and are associated with increased morbidity. Obtunding these stress responses with appropriate analgesia and sedation may therefore be important in improving outcome.

It is important to recognize that many of these factors can be alleviated in some measure by non-pharmacological methods. Providing a friendly, child-oriented environment, encouraging normal sleep where possible, paying attention to temperature and clothing, allowing unrestricted parental presence, and where appropriate encouraging parental involvement in procedures, can all be of considerable psychological benefit.

The ideal sedative agent would have the following qualities:

- provides analgesia and sedation
- radid onset and awakening
- multiple delivery options
- wide therapeutic index
- minimal effect on cardiovascular function
- activity unaffected by renal or hepatic disease
- activity unaffected by other drugs
- no active metabolites
- compatible with other infusions
- no tolerance or withdrawal
- safe and inexpensive

No single drug provides optimal sedation and analgesia without significant side-effects, and this is reflected in the wide range of medications currently used (Table 5.2.1). Side-effects can be minimized by the use of combinations of drugs, embodying a balanced approach for the provision of analgesia, sedation and, where necessary, muscle relaxation. *It is essential to ensure that patients given muscle relaxants are fully sedated*, and it is important in all patients not to confuse the need for sedation with the need for analgesia.

AIMS AND ASSESSMENT OF SEDATION

Definitions

- *general anesthesia* refers to a state of unconsciousness plus partial or complete loss of protective reflexes including the inability to independently maintain an airway

TABLE 5.2.1 Suitable medications

Analgesics
- Opioids:
  - morphine
  - fentanyl
  - alfentanil
  - sufentanil
  - remifentanil

Sedatives
- Benzodiazepines:
  - diazepam
  - midazolam
  - lorazepam
- Propofol
- Chloral hydrate
- Barbiturates
- Ketamine
- Phenothiazines:
  - promethazine
  - trimeprazine
- Inhalational agents:
  - nitrous oxide
  - isoflurane

- *neurolepsis* is a state of reduced motor activity, reduced anxiety, and indifference, induced by haloperidol or droperidol; combining opioids with neuroleptics produces neuroleptanalgesia
- *dissociative sedation* is a ketamine-induced state characterized by analgesia, sedation, amnesia, and catalepsy, with preserved ventilatory drive and airway protective reflexes
- *deep sedation* is a state of unconsciousness from which the child is not easily aroused, it may be accompanied by impairment of airway protective reflexes and ventilatory drive
- *light sedation* is a state of lessened awareness and pain perception; the child is able to respond to verbal or physical stimulation, and independently maintain a patent airway and adequate ventilatory drive
- *anxiolysis* is the reduction of apprehension without change in level of awareness

Many children are unable to communicate their pain or anxiety properly because of their young age, their conscious level or the presence of a tracheal tube. This can create problems in establishing the cause of a child's restlessness, and can result in inadequate or inappropriate use of sedation and analgesia in small children. It must be recognized that signs of distress may be due to other readily treated problems such as hunger, colic, a full bladder, headache or pyrexia. More importantly, *restlessness may be a sign of poor cardiac output, hypoxia or inadequate ventilatory support*, and steps must be taken to identify and correct these before starting or increasing sedation.

OBJECTIVES OF SEDATION

What are the objectives of sedation? Clearly, it is important that the individual patient is comfortable, reasonably calm and not so active that tubes and lines are dislodged. Using splints or restraints may at times be necessary, but these should be used as an adjunct to sedation rather than as an alternative. Conversely, apart from a very few specifically indicated situations, it is unnecessary to render a child completely insensitive to the environment and to obtund totally any response to suction. Effectively, the latter is a state of anesthesia and is only indicated when any patient movement may compromise care. Such situations may include difficult airway problems, following complex cardiac or tracheal surgery where it is essential to have optimal physiological stability or avoid accidental dislodgment of the tracheal tube, and where intracranial pressure is acutely elevated and further rises in response to noxious stimuli are to be avoided. However, in these situations it is usually more appropriate to prevent patient movement using neuromuscular blockade as an adjunct to adequate sedation and analgesia.

OPTIMAL SEDATION

Optimal sedation has been described as a state in which the patient is somnolent, responsive to the environment but untroubled by it, and with no excessive motion. In practice, this means a child who is conscious but settled, breathing synchronously with the ventilator, and tolerant of or compliant with other therapeutic procedures. Achieving this state can be difficult, particularly if it is important to be able to reduce the level of sedation readily. Assessment is also a difficult process, often complicated by subjective impression and interobserver variability. While it is generally easy to identify the child who is inadequately sedated or grossly overse-dated, it is notoriously difficult to quantify sensitively and precisely what are essentially descriptive assessments of the gradations between these two extremes. This in turn makes it difficult to prescribe a particular level of sedation and to titrate drugs to achieve this, or to compare the efficacy of different sedative drugs or regimens.

A number of sedation scores have been described, the most commonly used being the Ramsay score (Table 5.2.2) or variants of this. Although the six point Ramsay score is simple, it is essentially a subjective measure of consciousness with three levels when awake and three while asleep. As the asleep levels are assessed by response to a glabellar tap or auditory stimulus, patient stimulation while sedated is required. Furthermore, the levels are neither mutually exclusive nor clearly defined. There is no clear tar-get score for mechanically ventilated patients and with no defined optimum endpoint for sedation, it is unsuitable for comparing different drugs. Many other scores rely on the response to tracheal suc-tion. Such assessments are relatively crude, rely on a potent noxious stimulus, and inaccurately reflect the status of those patients who are otherwise well settled between episodes of suction.

Objective measures of distress or level of seda-tion in paediatric critical care patients have been described and validated. The COMFORT score is a scientifically derived measure of sedative drug efficacy which scores eight empirically derived behavioural and physiological dimensions of patient distress, as assessed by bedside observa-tion. These are somnolence, calmness, respiratory effort, physical movement, blood pressure, heart rate, muscle tone and facial tension. The

Vancouver Sedative Recovery Scale (VSRS) (Table 5.2.3) has a score of 0–22, from unrousable to fully awake, based on conscious responses, eye move-ments and motor coordination. These scores are clearly more complex than the Ramsay scale but should only take approximately 2 minutes to com-plete. It has been shown that the COMFORT score produces a more consistent measure of adequacy of sedation than global assessment by intensive care pediatricians; a score between 17 and 26 is the optimal range. The ability to define a quantifiable target level of sedation using such scales should permit better drug titration in the individual patient, and allow proper studies to assess and compare different sedative agents in children.

PAIN SCORING

Pain scoring is an even more complex issue. Distinguishing pain from agitation is challenging, particularly if the patient is only displaying auto-nomic symptoms of distress. Many pain measure-ment tools are described for infants, though difficulties arise with all of them when they are applied to critically ill children. The psychophysi-ological development of the maturing child is often inadequately taken into account. Many scores assess the cry, which is not applicable to intubated children, and some use oxygenation as a measure which will be unreliable in patients with intracardiac or intrapulmonary shunts and those with advanced pulmonary insufficiency. For neonates on respiratory support, the distress scale for ventilated newborn infants (DSVNI) over-comes some of the problems. Nevertheless, the need to paralyze a critically ill patient renders this tool invalid. Self-report scales (of which there are several) should not be overlooked in children over about 5 years of age who are conscious enough to use them.

AVAILABILITY OF DRUGS FOR CHILDREN

Concern has been raised in recent years about the fact that many drugs lack approval from the licencing authorities for use in children, and are in some cases labeled with disclaimers for such use. This has resulted from the lack of research into use of these drugs in children, and has given rise to

---

TABLE 5.2.2 Sedation scoring: the Ramsay scale

Awake levels
1. Patient anxious and agitated or restless, or both
2. Patient cooperative, oriented and tranquil
3. Patient responds to commands only

Asleep levels—dependent on response to glabellar tap or loud auditory stimulus
4. Brisk response
5. Sluggish response
6. No response

TABLE 5.2.3 **The Vancouver sedative recovery scale. Maximum score is 22 (fully awake); minimum score is 0 (unable to arouse)**

	Score
Response	
A (i) Awake/alert	4
(ii) Awake/drowsy	3
(iii) Asleep/easily aroused	2
(iv) Asleep/difficult to arouse	1
(v) Asleep/unable to arouse	0

Note: if child scores '0' on above, do not proceed

B (i) Responds fully to stimuli in age-appropriate manner	2
(ii) Delayed response to stimuli	1
(iii) Absent response to stimuli	0
C (i) 'Alert' facial expression	1
(ii) 'Flat' facial expression	0
Eyes	
D (i) Bright eyes	1
(ii) Dull eyes; glazed	0
E (i) Looks 'at you'	1
(ii) Looks 'through you'	0
F (i) Accommodates	1
(ii) Does not accommodate	0
G (i) Recognition of stimulus	1
(ii) Limited or no recognition of stimulus	0
H (i) Purposeful and spontaneous eye movement	1
(ii) Little or no spontaneous or purposeful eye movement	0
Movement	
I (i) Spontaneous and varied central activity	4
(ii) Spontaneous and varied peripheral activity	3
(iii) Central activity in response to stimuli	2
(iv) Peripheral activity in response to stimuli	1
(v) No movement	0
J (i) Absence of tremor or ataxia	2
(ii) Minor ataxia or tremor	1
(iii) Major ataxia or tremor	0
K (i) Coordinated spontaneous movement	2
(ii) Weak/coarse spontaneous movement	1
(iii) No purposeful spontaneous movement	0
L (i) Shows age-appropriate manual dexterity	2
(ii) Awkward or clumsy hand movement	1
(iii) No fine hand movement	0

the term 'therapeutic orphans'. This applies to several drugs used for sedation and analgesia, such as midazolam and fentanyl. Lack of approval does not, however, signify disapproval, and use of 'unlicenced' drugs does not constitute improper or illegal use, unless they are specifically contraindicated. However, the lack of comprehensive research studies on these drugs in children does mean that it is difficult to reach proper conclusions about the efficacy, benefits and safety of many agents in children, and to put into proper perspective the inevitable and occasional side-effects that may be encountered.

MANAGEMENT

SPECIFIC PHARMACOLOGICAL AGENTS

The first step in clinical management must be to provide adequate analgesia. The vast majority of children are managed successfully with an opioid, usually morphine, often on its own but more frequently combined with more specific sedating agents, particularly one of the benzodiazepines, or chloral hydrate or propofol (Fig. 5.2.1, Table 5.2.4).

PRE-SEDATION PREPARATION

Emergencies mandate immediate intervention. However, when the clinical situation permits, organized pre-sedation preparation is desirable. Explain the objectives, benefits, risks, and limitations of sedation, the anticipated changes in the child's behavior during and after sedation, and the expected duration of postsedation monitoring.

A relevant history should be taken (medications, allergies, time of last oral intake, history of sedation or anesthesia, and related complications). Consent should be obtained and the degree of physiologic reserve of vital organ functions (cardiovascular, respiratory, and central nervous system) should be assessed.

A physical examination should include vital signs, level of consciousness, weight, and airway evaluation. Note anything that would impede intubation or mask ventilation. Consider the child's physical status according to the American Society of Anesthesiologists (ASA) criteria:

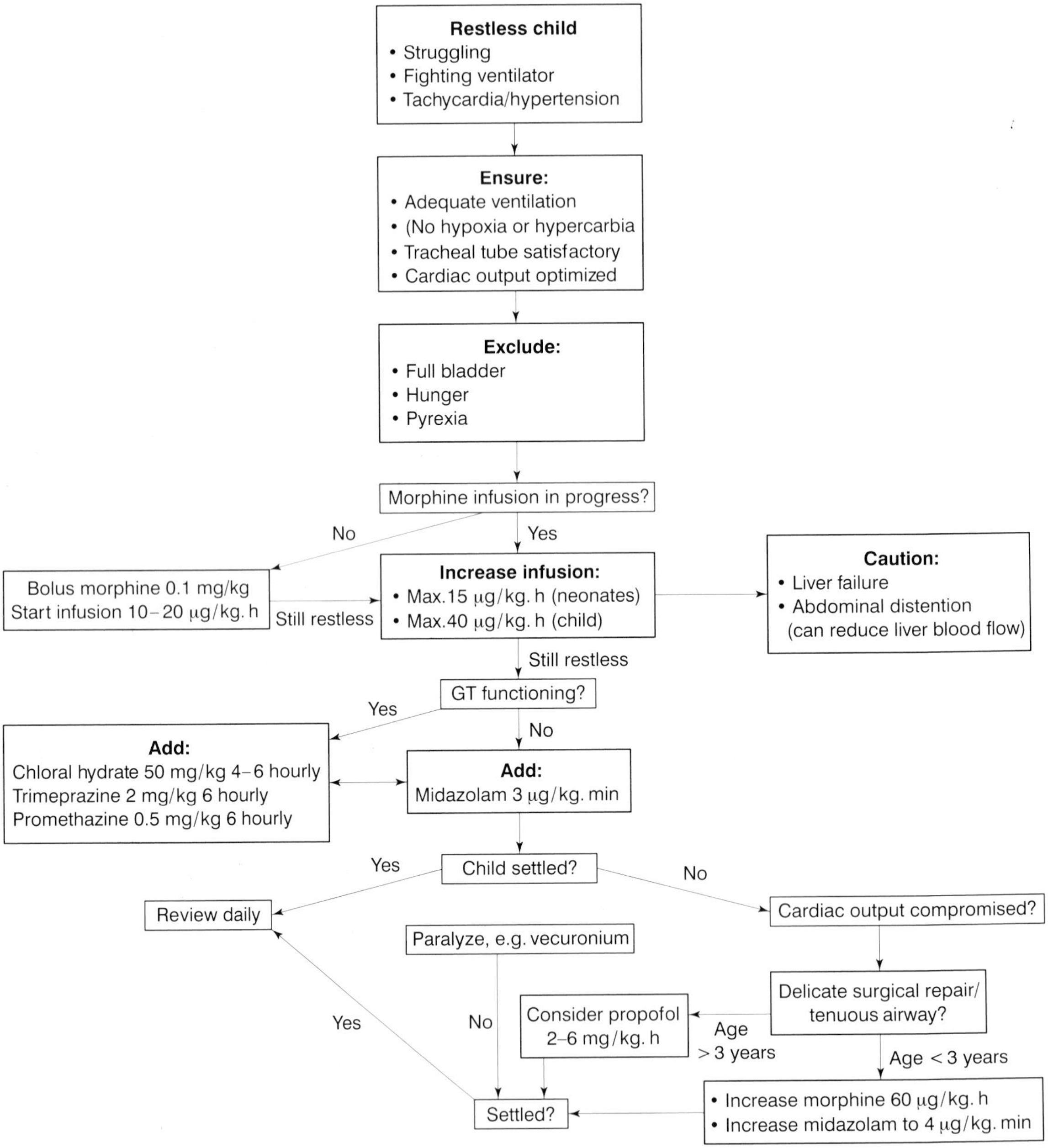

Figure 5.2.1 An algorithm for analgesia or sedation. GIT, gastrointestinal tract

TABLE 5.2.4 **Analgesic and Sedative drug doses**		
Drug	**Route**	**Dose**
Morphine	i.v. bolus (infant)	0.05 mg/kg
	i.v. bolus (child)	0.1–0.2 mg/kg
	i.v. infusion (neonate)	< 15 µg/kg·h
	i.v. infusion (child)	10–40 µg/kg·h
Fentanyl	i.v. bolus	1–2 µg/kg
	i.v. infusion	1–2 µg/kg·h initially (2–4 µg/h may be required)
Chloral hydrate	oral	30–50 mg, 4–6 hourly
Diazepam	i.v. bolus (titrate to effect)	0.1–0.2 mg/kg
	oral	0.5 mg/kg
	rectal	1 mg/kg
Midazolam	i.v. bolus (titrate to effect)	0.04–0.05 mg/kg initially to a maximum of 0.1–0.2 mg/kg
	i.v. infusion	1–3 µg/kg·min
Lorazepam	i.v. bolus	0.05–0.1 mg
Ketamine	i.v. bolus	0.5–2.0 mg/kg

1. Healthy patient
2. Mild systemic disease (no functional limitations)
3. Severe systemic disease (definite functional limitation)
4. Severe systemic disease (a constant threat to life)
5. Moribund patient (not expected to survive without surgery)
6. Brain-dead patient (organs to be removed for donation)

Wherever possible obtain advice and assistance from an anesthesiologist for patients in classes 3–5.

PRE-SEDATION FASTING

Aspiration of gastric contents is a serious potential complication. Fasting before a procedure and the passage of a nasogastric tube decrease aspiration risk. Light sedation with preserved airway reflexes is unlikely to provoke aspiration, but deeper sedation increases the risk.

Physician skills and staffing

Physicians giving sedation and analgesia should understand the pharmacology of the drugs they are administering and be familiar with relevant antagonists. Someone with advanced life support and airway management skills must be present during administration and recovery. An assistant, usually a physician or nurse, has the responsibility to observe airway patency, adequacy of ventilation, vital signs, and any monitoring devices in use.

Equipment and setting

Sedation should be given with the patient monitored. Relevant reversal agents, a pulse oximeter, and a blood pressure cuff or automated blood pressure monitor should be available at the bedside. Suction, oxygen, a nasal cannula, and an age-appropriate oral airway and bag-valve-mask are essential. An intravenous line is always advisable in critical illness, as are a cardiac monitor-defibrillator, a laryngoscope, age-appropriate endotracheal tubes, and a cardiac arrest cart with standard resuscitation drugs.

MONITORING

The degree of monitoring required is proportional to the level of sedation. Patients who remain awake and responsive need no special monitoring. Patients sedated to the extent that their eyes are closed require specific monitoring, which should begin prior to drug administration and continue throughout the recovery phase. Pulse, blood pressure, and respiratory rate should be recorded before and after drug administration, at regular intervals until the patient is awake. During sedation, the physician or support assistant should frequently assess the patient's alertness, response to voice, and if necessary, response to pain, as well as observing the adequacy of ventilation and the color of skin and mucous membranes.

Patients who are sedated to the extent that their eyes are closed should have oxygen saturation monitoring throughout the procedure, preferably using an oximeter that provides a variable pitch beep, reflecting changes in oxygen saturation and pulse rate. Supplemental oxygen is often advisable during sedation.

A sedation record is recommended. Drug administration times and doses should be recorded. Vital signs and oxygen saturation should be charted before drug administration, at least every 5 minutes during the procedure until the patient is fully awake.

DRUG ADMINISTRATION

The specific drug and its dose used will depend on the physician's experience, the clinical situation, and patient factors. If benzodiazepines or opioids are used, the antagonists flumazenil and naloxone should be available at the bedside.

POST-SEDATION CARE

Vital signs and respiratory status should be monitored until the patient is alert. Patients should be observed until airway patency, ventilation, cardiovascular function, and hydration are satisfactory, and the level of consciousness has returned to baseline (for children incapable of the usual responses, the pre-sedation level of responsiveness should be achieved).

ANALGESIC AGENTS

OPIOIDS

Opioids are used not only for their powerful analgesic properties but also because of their sedative effects, and are frequently used as sole agents providing both analgesia and sedation. Morphine and to a lesser extent fentanyl are the agents most commonly used, though alfentanil, sufentanil and the newer remifentanil are also used. Opioids act on specific receptors, of which the mu receptor is the

main site of action for analgesia (both spinal and supraspinal), euphoria, respiratory depression and physical dependence, while the kappa receptor mediates spinal analgesia, sedation and miosis. All clinically useful opioids have significant μ-agonist activity.

Morphine

Morphine, a naturally occurring phenanthrene alkaloid, is the most extensively studied, the most widely used and cheapest opioid available and there is a high level of satisfaction with its efficacy and safety. Its pharmacokinetics and dynamics have been investigated in all age groups, and there is no excuse for denying it to neonates. Plasma half-life and clearance are reduced in neonates but approach adult levels at around the age of 1 month (Table 5.2.5). By 6 months of age both clearance and protein binding are at adult levels. Metabolism is by hepatic glucuronidation, mainly to morphine 3-glucuronide (M3G) and varying amounts of morphine 6-glucuronide (M6G), which is approximately 40 times as active as morphine. Immaturity of the hepatic glucuronidation pathway in neonates may influence the ratio of M6G to M3G and thereby alter the clinical response. Morphine is significantly more hydrophilic than the other fentanyl-based opioids, so the volume of distribution is lower and penetration of the blood-brain barrier is delayed. Morphine produces peripheral venodilation and may predispose to hypotension in hypovolemic patients. This is mediated through histamine release, and caution should also be exercised in patients with severe asthma.

Dosage

Morphine can be given by intermittent intravenous bolus in a dose of 0.1–0.2 mg/kg, but is

TABLE 5.2.5 **Morphine: developmental changes in plasma half-life and clearance**		
	$t_{1/2}$(h)	Clearance (ml/min·kg)
Preterm neonate	9 ± 3.4	2.2 ± 0.7
Term neonate	6.5 ± 2.8	8.1 ± 3.2
Adult	2 ± 1.8	23.6 ± 8.5

most commonly administered by continuous intravenous infusion at 10–40 μg/kg·h. This rate does not usually compromise weaning from mechanical ventilation unless there has been prolonged high-dose administration, when it will often be necessary to reduce the rate. Neonates have a reduced morphine clearance, which may be further reduced if abdominal distention impedes hepatic clearance (convulsions can occur), so it is advisable to maintain the infusion rate in neonates below 15 μg/kg·h. Boluses can easily be given if sedation is inadequate or to cover painful procedures. Intramuscular injections should be avoided wherever possible in critically ill children, as absorption is erratic in the presence of compromised peripheral perfusion. If intravenous access is unavailable, an alternative route is continuous subcutaneous infusion via a small cannula over the abdomen, thorax or deltoid. The site need only be changed at 7-day intervals, unless erythema or leakage occurs.

Intravenous morphine infusions can also be delivered via nurse-controlled or patient-controlled analgesia. Nurse-controlled analgesia (NCA) may be superior to fixed-rate infusions in some circumstances because of safe, readily available bolus dosing for stressful procedures and greater titration of analgesic requirement. It has been used successfully in morphine administration with a maintenance infusion of 10–20 μg/kg·h and bolus doses of 10–20 μg/kg. The use of a long protective lock-out interval is not indicated in the intensive care setting, and 5 minutes seems appropriate, but a 4-hour limit of 400 μg/kg may be required.

Patient-controlled analgesic (PCA) has limited use in the acute management of critically ill children, but may be helpful during the recovery phase in children over the age of about 5 years. A suitable regimen for morphine is 20 μg/kg bolus doses, with a 5-minute lock-out. A combined background infusion of 4 μg/kg·h optimizes pain scores, while minimizing the incidence of side-effects.

Synthetic opioids

Although the first choice of opioid in the majority of cases is usually morphine, because of cost and its proven safety, the synthetic opioids fentanyl, alfentanil and sufentanil have potential benefits in the presence of cardiovascular compromise as they maintain cardiovascular stability over a wide dose range. Fentanyl in particular achieved popularity because of its ability in high dose (20–25 μg/kg) to obtund the stress response and prevent rises in pulmonary artery pressure. This led to its use in some centers as the opioid infusion of choice in patients with (or at risk of) labile pulmonary hypertension, though it is not clear whether the same protection is afforded by the significantly lower doses used in continuous infusion (4–8 μg/kg·min). Nevertheless it remains a useful alternative to morphine.

Fentanyl, alfentanil and sufentanil are synthetic μ-receptor agonists of the anilinopiperidine series. All are lipophilic and readily cross the blood-brain barrier, which explains their significantly greater potency and speedier onset of action compared with morphine. They are metabolized almost entirely by hepatic cytochrome P450 isoenzymes to more hydrophilic compounds with significantly less pharmacological activity, which are renally excreted. Impairment of hepatic function can significantly reduce metabolism and prolong activity. Intravenous fentanyl has a relatively short half-life of less than 1 hour owing to rapid redistribution to peripheral compartments (i.v. bolus dose 1–2 μg/kg). Prolonged infusions saturate the peripheral compartment and the elimination half-life progressively increases up to 16 hours. Most patients will be adequately treated with a fentanyl infusion at a dose of 1–2 μg/kg·h. However, it has been shown that the total body clearance of fentanyl is highly variable and may require a 10-fold variation in infusion rates to achieve similar levels of sedation. It is also clear that there is rapid development of tolerance to fentanyl in neonates, with a high probability of developing dependence and subsequent withdrawal syndrome. It has been shown that a total fentanyl dose of more than 2.5 mg/kg or a duration of infusion exceeding 9 days is 100% predictive of withdrawal problems. It is important therefore to reduce the infusion very slowly after prolonged use.

Alfentanil, which is more commonly used in adults, has a much smaller volume of distribution than fentanyl and the plasma half-life is therefore less dependent on the duration of infusion. The normal infusion rate is 10–20 µg/kg·h. Sufentanil, which is rarely used in children, is some five times more potent than fentanyl (bolus dose 0.1–0.5 µg/kg) with a slightly shorter duration of action. It can produce rapid sedation following intranasal administration.

Remifentanil is a new ultrashort-acting agent with a small volume of distribution and similar analgesic potency to fentanyl. Its elimination half-life is only 8–10 minutes. Metabolism is by plasma and tissue esterases, so accumulation does not occur in hepatic or renal disease, making it a useful agent when these organs are damaged, and its half-life is independent of the rate of infusion. These favorable characteristics allow rapid recovery from the respiratory and sedative effects of the drug, permitting frequent assessment of the patient's underlying level of consciousness. However, accidental interruption of drug delivery may precipitate rapid return of pain, awareness and marked cardiovascular changes. Children with head injury may benefit from its use, as there is no associated increase in intracranial pressure. Remifentanil in bolus doses of 0.5 µg/kg successfully obtunds the effects of respiratory care in children with raised intracranial pressure, although higher doses may precipitate hypotension. Its high cost will probably limit its use at present to patients with renal and hepatic failure, but it may prove in time to offer other benefits to justify its wider use.

Although the intravenous route is the traditional route of administration for opioids in critical illness, other routes such as rectal, nasal and sublingual have been advocated, though these are not routinely employed. Steady state concentrations can be achieved for 72 hours using transdermal fentanyl, though the limitation of choice of drug doses on the patches (25µg, 50µg, 75µg, and 100 µg per hour) means this is only suitable at present for larger children.

Methadone

Where the oral route is the only one available the morphine substitute methadone can be used, oral dose 0.1–0.4 mg/kg to a maximum of 0.7 mg/kg per 24 hours (the plasma half-life is in excess of 24 hours so steady state serum concentrations are maintained). Efficacy has been demonstrated in children older than 3 years. Intravenous methadone has also been used successfully in morphine-tolerant children, restoring adequate analgesia and permitting significant reductions of other sedative agents.

Side-effects

Problems common to all opioids include respiratory depression, dependence, and the enhancement of the gastric retention and ileus associated with critical illness. Chronic opioid administration may also modulate immune function detrimentally, possibly through a novel class of opioid receptor expressed on immune cells, though it is not clear if this a significant clinical problem.

SEDATIVE AGENTS

Although an opioid infusion may provide adequate sedation, there are frequent occasions when this is not enough. The simplest adjunct if the patient's gastrointestinal function permits is *chloral hydrate* orally. There are various formulations, all of which undergo hepatic transformation to the active metabolite trichloroethanol. It is given enterally in a dose of 30–50 mg/kg every 4–6 hours. It has a relatively slow onset of about 30 minutes, but provides gentle, prolonged action (half-life 8–12 hours). Titration of sedation is difficult, but it provides useful background sedation against which shorter-acting agents can operate. Hypotension can occasionally occur in a physiologically unstable child. Alternatives include *trimeprazine* (2 mg/kg 6 hourly), or *promethazine* (0.5–1.0 mg/kg 8–12 hourly), both of which have their advocates. *Barbiturates* are used infrequently on PICUs now, although both thiopental (thiopentone) and pentobarbital (pentobarbitone) infusions may help where fentanyl and midazolam have failed or in the management of otherwise unresponsive status epilepticus. They have beneficial effects on cerebral metabolism and may have a role in the management of raised intracranial pressure, though they can severely compromise cardiac function.

BENZODIAZEPINES

Benzodiazepines are commonly used for sedation, although satisfaction with their efficacy is by no means complete. Benzodiazepines bind to receptors in various regions of the brain and act as CNS depressants by potentiating the inhibitory actions of γ-aminobutyric acid (GABA), thereby reducing cortical activation through the brain-stem reticular formation. Although benzodiazepines have no intrinsic analgesic activity, they may influence nociception and reduce the need for analgesia.

Midazolam is the most widely used benzodiazepine in PICUs in the UK and is also widely used in the USA, although there is also significant usage of diazepam and lorazepam. The mechanism of action is identical for all benzodiazepines, and it is their differing pharmacokinetic profiles that dictate their suitability as titratable sedative agents.

Diazepam

Historically, diazepam has been the favored agent for pediatric sedation. However, its effects are cumulative with prolonged use, owing to the long elimination half-lives of the parent drug and its hypnotically active metabolites desmethyl-diazepam and oxazepam. Administration by continuous intravenous infusion is therefore inappropriate. Intermittent doses of 0.1–0.2 mg/kg intravenously are generally administered, although it can also be given orally (0.5 mg/kg), rectally (1 mg/kg), or nasally (0.2–0.4 mg/kg). The intramuscular route produces unreliable absorption and is painful.

Midazolam

Midazolam is a water-soluble imidazo benzodiazepine derivative. It has an open ring structure that closes at physiological pH, enhancing lipid solubility and ensuring rapid penetration of the blood-brain barrier. The onset of hypnosis is rapid, and this combined with a short elimination half-life of 2–3 hours make it suitable for continuous intravenous infusion for prolonged sedation. The drug is cleared by the P450-dependent mixed function oxidase system of the liver, and the principal metabolite, α-hydroxymidazolam, is also biologically active but with a shorter half-life (less than 1 hour). Tolerance can occur and prolonged sedation can result from the use of midazolam in severely ill patients, as a result of altered pharmacodynamics or kinetics. A reduction in hepatic blood flow will delay metabolism, and prolonged recovery is also seen in renal failure, probably due to the accumulation of active conjugated metabolites. Drugs such as the macrolide antibiotics and anticonvulsants can enhance metabolism by enzyme induction, and erythromycin is reported to inhibit metabolism.

The clearance of midazolam is reduced in children under 2 years old and even more so in neonates. There is considerable interindividual variation in steady state plasma concentrations of midazolam and this probably reflects the varying degree of impairment of the P450 enzyme system by the underlying critical illness. Plasma levels correlate poorly with sedation and tolerance may develop acutely so the application of a uniform dosage regimen is impracticable and *titration to response is essential.* Start with an initial bolus dose of 0.04–0.05 mg/kg. In general, i.v. infusion doses of 1–3 μg/kg·min are used. Midazolam can be absorbed transmucosally, but the oral route limits bioavailability to approximately 50% owing to high liver extraction. The nasal and sublingual routes offer enhanced absorption with a relatively rapid onset of action.

Lorazepam

Lorazepam is a highly potent benzodiazepine with a far greater binding affinity to the receptor site than diazepam or midazolam. Its plasma half-life is 8–25 hours in healthy adults, with elimination principally by hepatic glucuronidation rather than by the P450 enzymes, with renal excretion of a pharmacologically inactive metabolite. This process of elimination is well preserved in the face of severe critical illness and mild liver dysfunction, unlike the elimination of midazolam. The elimination half-life is not prolonged with renal impairment, but may be in the face of severe hepatic dysfunction. The long half-life allows intermittent dosing, either intravenously or orally, although continuous infusions have been successfully employed. Studies on children are limited, but efficacy and hemodynamic stability comparable to midazolam have been demonstrated in adults, and lorazepam is significantly cheaper. The recommended intermittent intravenous administration dose is 0.05–0.1 mg/kg every 4–8 hours, and for continuous infusions a starting rate of 0.025 mg/kg·h (maximum 2 mg/h).

Side-effects

The hemodynamic effects of benzodiazepines are unpredictable. Many studies have revealed no major hemodynamic changes with continuous infusions, but others have noted hypotension in patients after cardiac surgery and falls in cardiac output greater than 20% associated with bolus administration of midazolam. Benzodiazepines have the capacity to reduce sympathetic outflow and thereby reduce systemic vascular resistance and central venous filling pressures. The effect is exaggerated in hypovolemic patients or in the presence of a fixed cardiac output (obstructive cardiac lesions) and may precipitate cardiovascular collapse. Bolus administration of a rapidly acting drug such as midazolam should be used with caution in such critically ill children.

PROPOFOL

Propofol (2,6-disopropylphenol) is a very short-acting intravenous anesthetic agent that has emerged as an alternative to benzodiazepines for sedation in adult patients. It is supplied as an isotonic emulsion containing glycerol, egg phosphatidide, sodium hydroxide, soybean oil and water. Propofol is rapid-acting, producing a dose-related depression of the central nervous system. The mechanism of action is uncertain but probably mediated by inhibiting GABA uptake and potentiating GABA potentials in the central nervous system. There is extensive presystemic metabolism with a hepatic extraction of 82%, so intravenous administration is necessary.

Propofol behaves dissimilarly to benzodiazepines and barbiturates in that clinical recovery from prolonged infusions results primarily from redistribution of the drug rather than metabolism. Its pharmacokinetics are best described by a three-compartment model with central elimination. The central compartment comprises the circulating blood volume and highly perfused tissue with a blood-brain equilibration half-life of 2.9 minutes. The propofol concentration within this compartment corresponds to the clinical sedative response and blood levels above 1 mg/L are required to maintain sleep.

Although recovery results primarily from redistribution, propofol can be eliminated by hepatic conjugation (mainly glucuronidation) and renal excretion of the inactive product. Extrahepatic metabolism has been demonstrated by studies conducted during the anhepatic phase of liver transplantation, the principal alternative site being the gut. A high liver blood flow clearance of propofol ensures rapid elimination by metabolism, with a half-life of 30–60 minutes. On cessation of intravenous infusion, recovery is dependent on the removal of propofol from the central nervous system. Fortunately the rate of ingress of propofol into the peripheral compartments is more rapid than redistribution back into the central compartment, so blood levels fall quickly. Resedation does not occur when propofol slowly leaches out of the large peripheral compartment as subhypnotic concentrations are maintained by the rapid hepatic metabolism.

The efficacy of propofol sedation in mechanically ventilated patients is described in numerous adult studies, pediatric data is limited but short-term use in low dosage can be justified. A relatively simple dosing regimen comprises a 2.5 mg/kg loading dose followed by an infusion of 2.5 mg/kg·h, adjusted incrementally to maintain adequate sedation (it is rarely necessary to exceed 6 mg/kg). Although there is a wide variability in propofol pharmacokinetics, recovery is rapid on termination of infusion, averaging approximately 15 minutes. The consensus is that propofol and midazolam produce adequate and equivalent sedation, but propofol allows easier and more precise titration and time to awakening is significantly shorter for propofol. Although propofol is two to three times more expensive than midazolam, earlier extubation after propofol may redress the balance.

Propofol has other desirable properties, in particular a greater than expected depression in laryngeal sensitivity enabling improved tolerance of a tracheal tube. Rapid alteration of the level of sedation is achievable and intermittent boluses have been shown to reduce significantly the hemodynamic and metabolic stresses caused by physiotherapy. Less desirably, initiation of propofol sedation is frequently associated with hypotension, probably due to inhibition of sympathetic vasoconstriction rather than direct vascular relaxation, particularly if initial bolus doses are employed. It is therefore essential to correct hypovolemia prior to starting propofol.

Unfortunately, unexplained fatal metabolic acidosis has been described in six children with respiratory tract infections who received high-dose propofol infusion, and at present propofol is not recommended for pediatric intensive care sedation in the UK. It continues to be used in the USA in children with good effect. Various neurological complications including fits, abnormal movements and other excitatory manifestations have also been reported, many after discontinuation of propofol, possibly representing a withdrawal phenomenon.

Hypertriacylglycerolemia occurs frequently and may limit the rate of infusion. Total parenteral nutrition requirements should be modified pre-emptively and regular monitoring must be instituted. The availability of a more concentrated formulation (2%) should reduce this problem and reduce excessive volume loads.

CONTRAINDICATIONS

Contraindications for common sedatives and alternative medications are shown in Table 5.2.6.

DISCONTINUATION OF SEDATION

In recent years there has been growing awareness of withdrawal reactions following the use of sedative and analgesic drugs in critically ill children. This is particularly true for both midazolam and fentanyl. The molecular mechanisms underlying tolerance and withdrawal are complex. Opioid tolerance is thought to result from uncoupling of receptor-mediated events, particularly at the level of potassium channel–guanine nucleotide regulatory protein interaction. Actions at nonopioid receptor sites may be contributory, including α_2-adrenergic and N-methyl-D-aspartate (NMDA) receptors, and may influence treatment strategies.

Symptoms of withdrawal include behavioral changes, evidence of neurological excitability, gastrointestinal dysfunction and autonomic hyperactivity which characteristically start within 12 hours of termination of the agent. The probability of withdrawal symptoms approached 100% in infusions lasting more than 9 days. Various strategies have been employed to avoid withdrawal effects but no consensus exists as to the best approach. For patients requiring prolonged sedation, it can be helpful to change the agent every week or so. When this is not possible, it will be necessary to wean the patient very slowly from the drug involved. As noted earlier, methadone may be useful in morphine-tolerant patients, permitting rapid reduction in sedative requirements yet maintaining good analgesia.

Clonidine can be effective in treating and preventing opiate withdrawal symptoms and has been used as a sedative adjunct in intensive care. It is a partial agonist acting centrally on presynaptic α_2-adrenoreceptors, influencing the release of a variety of neurotransmitters and decreasing sympathetic outflow. Its ease of administration make this a logical option, but more research is required.

MISCELLANEOUS AGENTS

Inhalational agents have a limited role owing to problems of drug delivery and environmental pollution. Nitrous oxide has anesthetic and analgesic properties but long-term use leads to inhibition of vitamin B_{12} metabolism and bone marrow suppression. It is poorly effective if given as less than 50–70% of the inhaled gas mixture, so is unsuitable in patients with high oxygen requirements. It can be useful during patient transfer, or for painful procedures such as drain removal.

ISOFLURANE

Isoflurane, a fluorinated inhalational anesthetic agent, provides rapid control of depth of sedation, has been proved to be more effective than midazolam in adults and can be useful in difficult

TABLE 5.2.6 **Contraindications for common sedatives**

Drug	Contraindication	Alternative
Narcotic	Apnea (relative contraindication)	Chloral hydrate
	Hypovolemia	Benzodiazepine, ketamine
	Asthma — avoid morphine and meperidine (pethidine)	Ketamine, fentanyl
	Hemodialysis — avoid morphine	
Ketamine	Increased intracranial pressure	Barbiturate
	Pulmonary artery hypertension	Narcotic, chlorpromazine
	Increased intraocular pressure	Barbiturate
	Seizures (relative contraindication)	Barbiturate, benzodiazepine
	Severe systemic hypertension	Benzodiazepine, morphine
Benzodiazepine	Hepatic failure	Reduce dose, consider narcotic for which the effect can be reversed
Barbiturate	Reduced cardiac reserve	Chloral hydrate
	Porphyria	Benzodiazepine
	Asthma	Ketamine, benzodiazepine, fentanyl
Chloral hydrate	Gastric or rectal irritation	Any

From Levin DL. Essentials of pediatric intensive care (a pocket companion). St Louis: Quality Medical Publishing; 1990.

patients. Prolonged use raises concerns about a rise in plasma inorganic fluoride concentration, though renal toxicity is not a feature. Isoflurane's future in pediatric practice lies particularly in the field of sedation during extracorporeal membrane oxygenation (ECMO), as tolerance can develop rapidly to benzodiazepines and opiates.

KETAMINE

Continuous infusions of ketamine (0.5–1 mg/kg·h) have been successfully given for sedation but are rarely used. Effective analgesia is provided by subanesthetic doses and intermittent i.v. bolus (0.5–2.0 mg/kg) administration is useful to cover painful procedures, particularly in the context of management of victims of disasters in the field, or emergency situations. Burn dressing, bronchoscopy and repetitive radiotherapy are other applications. The advantages of ketamine include cardiovascular stability (by indirect sympathomimetic effects) and bronchodilation, and it has been used successfully in status asthmaticus. Ketamine has the potential to increase intracranial pressure and should be avoided in children at risk of intracranial hypertension. Oral and tracheal secretions may be increased, this effect can be countered by giving atropine. Emergence phenomena, commonly seen in adults, are less frequent in children (1.5%) and can be obtunded with benzodiazepines.

NEUROMUSCULAR BLOCKADE

Although the routine use of muscle relaxation is not advocated here, occasionally specific clinical indications will justify it. It can be provided by intermittent intravenous boluses of any of the nondepolarizing muscle relaxants such as pancuronium (0.1 mg/kg), vecuronium (0.1 mg/kg) or atracurium (0.5 mg/kg). The newer agents rocuronium and particularly cisatracurium may prove to be preferable. It is only necessary to achieve about 50% neuromuscular blockade, but it is essential to ensure complete sedation in paralyzed patients. Higher doses than those quoted can be given but for sustained paralysis it is more convenient to use an infusion, such as vecuronium 2–4 µg/kg·min. Prolonged blockade can occur after long-term use, particularly in the presence of renal failure, probably owing to metabolites. To avoid unnecessary prolonged action a check should be made at least daily of the degree of neuromuscular blockade, using for example a peripheral nerve stimulator. An alternative strategy is to stop the infusion for a short period each day, restarting when there are the first signs of movement. It is important also to be aware that delayed recovery of muscle function may be due to critical illness polyneuropathy (CIP).

REGIONAL ANALGESIA

Various regional anesthetic techniques (e.g. epidural, interpleural and peripheral nerve blockade) can be useful, particularly in patients at risk of multiorgan failure. However, in the critically ill child the possibility of a coagulopathy or bacteremia often limits their use. Equally, the use of NSAIDs is appropriate for the management of pain in many patients, but their adverse effects on platelet function, glomerular function and gastric mucosal integrity may compound critical illness. Topical anesthetic creams can reduce the pain and stress associated with venepuncture and skin perforation. A cream combining lidocaine (lignocaine) and prilocaine (Emla) has been widely used, but the development of tetracaine (amethocaine) gel offers the benefit of a more rapid onset of useful anesthesia (30 minutes compared with more than 60 minutes for Emla).

✔ KEY POINTS

➤ Ensure adequate analgesia for all patients
➤ Morphine is an excellent agent providing good analgesia and sedation
➤ All patients receiving muscle relaxants must be fully sedated
➤ Restlessness may be due to hypoxia, inadequate ventilation or cerebral hypoperfusion; treat the underlying cause before sedating
➤ Never paralyze a restless child without first ensuring the tracheal tube is properly placed, the ventilator is working and the circuit is intact.
➤ Anticipate the possibility of withdrawal following long-term sedation or analgesia, particularly after midazolam and fentanyl
➤ Intravenous titration is the best way to achieve a given end-point
➤ Rapid drug boluses ('i.v. push') are more likely to cause unexpected deterioration than slow administration over 1–2 minutes
➤ Children with cardiorespiratory disease constitute a high-risk group for sedation and analgesia. Any sedative or analgesic can cause cardiorespiratory compromise, and any child can unexpectedly progress to a deeper than desired level of sedation. Hypoventilation, apnea, and hypotension may occur. Do not sedate a patient unless you are confident in your ability to deal with the possible complications

✗ COMMON ERRORS

➤ Using sedatives to provide analgesia
➤ Paralyzing patients without sedation
➤ Oversedating, leading to prolonged recovery
➤ Failure to assess degree of muscle relaxation, particularly in renal failure, leading to prolonged recovery

FURTHER READING

1. Tobias JD, Rasmussen GE. Pain management and sedation in the pediatric intensive care unit. Pediatr Clin North Am 1994; 41(6): 1269–1292
2. Committee on Drugs (American Academy of Pediatrics). Guideline for monitoring and management of pediatric patients during and after sedation for diagnostic and therapeutic procedures. Pediatrics 1992; 89(6): 1110–1115
3. Lloyd-Thomas AR, Howard RF, Llewellyn N. The management of acute and post-operative pain in infancy and childhood. Clin Paediatr 1995; 3(3): 579–600
   – (*Three in-depth reviews*)
4. Morton N. Pain assessment in children. Paed Anaesth 1997; 7: 267–272
   – (*A review of existing methods*)
5. Kuttner L. A child in pain. How to help and what to do. Hartley & Marks, 1996
   – (*A multidimensional text for health care professionals and parents*)
6. Olkkola KT, Hamunen K. Maunuksela EL. Clinical pharmacokinetics and pharmacodynamics of opioid analgesics in infants and children. Clin Pharmacokinet 1995; 28(5): 385–404
   – (*Detailed pharmacological review*)
7. Hansen-Flaschen J, Cowen J, Polomano RC (1994) Beyond the Ramsay scale: need for a validated measure of sedating drug efficacy in the intensive care unit. Crit Care Med 22: 732–733
   – (*Editorial on sedation scoring*)
8. Ambuel B, Hamlett KW, Marx CM et al. Assessing distress in pediatric intensive care environments—the COMFORT scale. J Pediatr Psychol 1992; 17: 95–109
   – (*The development of the COMFORT score for assessing psychological distress*)
9. Marx CM, Smith PG, Lowrie LH et al. Optimal sedation of mechanically ventilated pediatric critical care patients. Crit Care Med 1994; 22: 163–170
   – (*Validating the COMFORT score and deriving a target range for sedation*)

10. Ramsay MAE, Savege TM, Simpson BRJ et al. Controlled sedation with alphaxalone–alphadolone. Br Med J 1974; 2: 656–659
    – (*The Ramsay score*)

11. Macnab AJ, Levine M, Glick N, Phillips N, Susak L, Elliott M. The modified Vancouver Sedative Recovery Scale validation and assessment of reliability of video instruction. Can J Anaesth 1994; 41: 913–918
    – (*Description of Vancouver sedative recovery scale*)

12. Katz R, Kelly WH, Hsi A. Prospective study on the occurrence of withdrawal in critically ill children who receive fentanyl by continuous infusion. Crit Care Med 1994; 22: 763–767
    – (*Describes the high incidence of fentanyl withdrawal symptoms*)

13. Bergman I, Steeves M, Burckart G et al. Reversible neurologic abnormalities associated with prolonged intravenous midazolam and fentanyl administration. J Pediatr 1991; 119: 644–649

14. Macnab AJ, Levine M, Glick N et al. Midazolam following open heart surgery in children: haemodynamic effects of a loading dose. Paed Anaesth 1996; 6: 387–397
    (*Two papers reviewing adverse events following i.v. sedation*)

15. Martin PH, Murthy BVS, Petros AJ. Metabolic, biochemical and haemodynamic effects of infusion of propofol for long-term sedation of children undergoing intensive care. Br J Anaesth 1997; 79: 276–279

16. Parke TJ, Stevens JE, Rice ASC et al. Metabolic acidosis and fatal myocardial failure after propofol infusion in children: five case reports. Br Med J 1992; 305: 613–616
    – (*The report that stopped the use of propofol in young children in the UK*)

17. Reed MD, Yamashita TS, Marx CM et al. A pharmacologically based propofol dosing strategy for sedation of the critically ill, mechanically ventilated pediatric patient. Crit Care Med 1996; 24: 1473–1481
    – (*Large series of children receiving propofol*)

18. Williams PI, Sargunson RE, Ratcliffe JM. Use of methadone in the morphine-tolerant burned paediatric patient. Br J Anaesth 1998; 80: 92–95

19. Bray RJ. Propofol infusion syndrome in children Paed Anaesth 1998; 8: 491–499
    – (*A review of 20 cases with serious unwanted side effects from propofol, showing significant association between long term high dose propofol and myocardial failure*)

5.3 Nutritional management in critical illness

Helen Anthony

Malnutrition appears very early in critical illness and can inhibit recovery. Malnutrition causes:

- an increased risk of infection
- depression of the immune system
- increased surgical mortality
- poor wound healing
- loss of muscle strength, including that of respiratory muscles
- increased length of hospital stay

Nutritional management aims to:

- identify malnourished patients and those at risk of developing acute malnutrition
- provide and monitor appropriate nutritional support designed to maintain nitrogen balance and minimize adverse changes in body composition
- provide micronutrients tailored to meet specific individual requirements

Thirty per cent of patients in a children's hospital display signs of acute or chronic protein-energy malnutrition (PEM) and a quarter of these are in the PICU.

PHYSIOLOGY

THE METABOLIC RESPONSE TO TRAUMA

The stress response (Fig 5.3.1) is the hormonal and metabolic result of the body's attempt to maintain hemodynamic stability after injury, and then to mobilize endogenous substrates as a source of energy for the major organ systems, and maintain immunocompetence. Its effects include glucose intolerance, acid–base disturbance and fluid overload. The stress response is initiated by afferent neural signals and mediated by the hypothalamus.

In the *ebb* or *shock phase*, hypovolemia and low cardiac output reduce the metabolic rate. Resuscitation can reduce the duration and intensity of this phase by maintaining the cardiac output, blood pressure and tissue perfusion and controlling pain. If resuscitation procedures are unsuccessful, the *necrobiosis* phase is entered, oxygen consumption decreases further and death follows.

The duration of the *flow phase* (found to be 3–10 days in adults) depends on the extent of the injury and the success of resuscitation. The flow phase is a period of hypercatabolism with increased oxygen consumption and net protein breakdown as amino acids are mobilized from skeletal muscle for use by visceral tissues. Energy and protein requirements are increased and the provision of exogenous nutrients is essential to minimize catabolism of body tissue. This phase follows a period of relative starvation, and iatrogenic malnutrition rapidly ensues. The final stage is anabolism or recovery, lasting for weeks, especially after major trauma such as extensive burns. Energy, protein and micronutrients must be provided for replenishment of body stores and for catch-up growth.

Infants and children are particularly susceptible to iatrogenic malnutrition because of their relatively high basal metabolic requirements and small endogenous energy reserves. In a starved healthy infant, protein reserves last approximately 6 days; children 8–10 years old have protein reserves for 10–15 days and an average adult for 70 days. Fat stores are also limited by age and body size; children aged 3–10 years deplete their fat reserves most rapidly.

THE METABOLIC RESPONSE TO SEPSIS

Sepsis is a hypermetabolic state triggered by a cascade of reactions involving the release of cytokines, eicosanoids, steroid hormones and other factors. Muscle protein is used as a glucose source and negative nitrogen balance is inevitable. Some of the retained amino acid is used to manufacture acute-phase proteins, rather than for tissue protein synthesis. Poor peripheral glucose utilization usually causes hyperglycemia. Hypoglycemia indicates a failure of gluconeogenesis and is a poor prognostic sign.

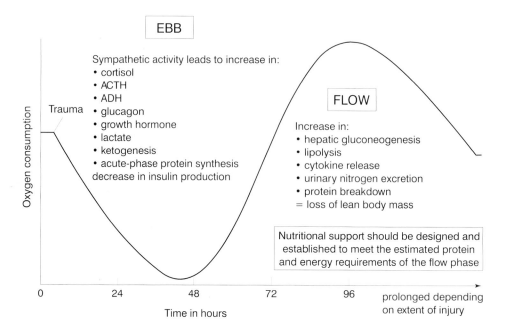

Figure 5.3.1 The metabolic respose to trauma

In adults, supplementation with glutamine, arginine, ω-3 fatty acids and RNA appears to limit post-traumatic depression of immunity. Administration of growth factors enhances protein synthesis and tissue repair. The benefits of dietary supplementation with these substrates have yet to be proved in children.

ASSESSMENT OF NUTRITIONAL STATUS

The nutritional status of children can be rapidly assessed using the measurements listed in Table 5.3.1. Malnutrition in childhood causes growth failure or wasting. Chronic malnutrition is most likely in children under 2 years of age or with a preexisting chronic disease. Children with moderate to severe growth failure are also likely to have micronutrient deficiencies. Risk factors for malnutrition are:

- severe fluid restriction, e.g. after head injury, renal failure and cardiac surgery
- burns
- sepsis syndrome
- multiorgan failure
- long-term ventilator dependency

ASSESSMENT OF NUTRITIONAL REQUIREMENTS

FLUID

See Chapter 2.10.

ENERGY REQUIREMENTS

Recommended energy intakes for healthy children are based on measurements of energy expenditure and allow for optimal growth and normal activity (Table 5.3.2). The provision of energy for growth is not a priority during critical illness. Catch-up growth can be achieved after recovery from critical illness by providing an additional 10–20% of normal energy needs (21 kJ/g of tissue acquired).

Basal energy requirement is the energy expenditure of healthy individuals at rest, in the post-absorptive state in a thermoneutral environment. Basal energy expenditure depends on the body's content of metabolically active tissue. It decreases with age as the body's content of metabolically active tissue per kg body weight decreases (Table 5.3.2).

TABLE 5.3.1 **Rapid assessment of nutritional status**		
	Measurement	**Indication of malnutriton**
Acute malnutrition	Weight for height (%)	< 90% mild, < 70% severe
	Weight for age (%)	< 90% mild, < 60% severe
Chronic malnutrition	Height for age (%)	< 90% mild, < 85% severe
Fat stores	Triceps skinfold thickness	< 5th centile depleted
Protein stores, somatic	Midarm circumference	< 5th centile depleted
Protein stores, visceral	Plasma albumin	< 25 g/L (2.5 g/dl) depleted
	Plasma transferrin	< 1 mg/L (100 µg/dl) depleted
Immune status	Total lymphocyte count	< 1.5 × 10⁹/L (1500/mm³) compromised

Height for age (%) = 100 × child's height/reference height of child of same age.
Weight for height (%) = 100 × child's weight/reference weight for child of same height.
Weight for age (%) = 100 × child's weight/reference weight for child of same age.

TABLE 5.3.2 **Energy requirements per day according to age of the child**					
	Daily energy requirements (kJ/kg)[a]				
	< 1 year	**1–3 years**	**4–6 years**	**7–10 years**	**11–18 years**
Basal[b]	230	238	200	167	125
Maintenance[c]	276	286	241	201	150
Minor stress[d]	322	343	289	241	175
Major stress[e]	413	429	362	301	186
Burns:					
< 20% BSA	345–414	358–429	301–362	251–302	188–225
20–40%	414–510	429–529	362–446	302–372	225–278
> 40%	510–552	529–572	446–482	372–402	278–300
RDI[f]	429	420	376	298	184–210

[a] Recommended daily intakes (RDI) Based on WHO/FAO energy and protein requirements, 1985; 1 kcal = 4.18 kJ.
[b] Deep sedation/muscle relaxants, ebb phase of injury, mechanical ventilation.
[c] Mechanical ventilation, enteral feeding, lying quietly.
[d] Skeletal trauma (long-bone fracture), minor surgery, peritonitis, fever < 39°C.
[e] Multitrauma, large open wound, post head injury, sepsis.
[f] Australian recommended daily intakes.

Activity level and feeding

In critical illness, agitation, seizures, increased work of breathing or increased muscle tone raise the basal energy expenditure by 10–20%. Conversely, a patient who is paralyzed, sedated and ventilated and in the ebb phase of injury may require 10–20% less than estimated basal energy needs. Diet-induced thermogenesis, induced by enteral feeding, increases energy expenditure by 10%. It is the energy cost of digestion, accretion and excretion.

Injury stress factors

The extent and nature of the injury can affect the degree of hypercatabolism (Table 5.3.2).

Drugs

Catecholamines cause a dose-dependent increase in the metabolic rate. Systemic corticosteroids also induce a hypermetabolic response and increase protein catabolism. Opiates, β-blockers, muscle relaxants and barbiturates reduce energy expenditure by 6% to 55%.

Preexisting medical condition

Children with neurological impairment such as cerebral palsy or a chronic disease that affects their nutritional status such as Crohn's disease or AIDS may have different energy needs from those of well-nourished children admitted with critical illness. In obese children, energy requirements are based on ideal weight rather than actual weight. Specialist advice may need to be sought for nutritional management for these patients.

PROTEIN REQUIREMENTS

Protein is used to supply amino acids for growth, for repair of body tissues and for body defenses, including immune function. Protein needs decline with age as growth slows (Table 5.3.3). During critical illness, catabolism induces negative nitrogen balance; the requirement for protein is increased and the need for specific amino acids alters. Glutamine becomes an essential amino acid during critical illness and utilization of the branched-chain amino acids (BCAA) leucine, isoleucine and valine by skeletal muscle increases. This may lead to a reduction in plasma levels of these amino acids, and decrease in protein synthesis. There is some evidence that nutritional status in hepatic failure can be improved using BCAA-enriched feeds.

Oxidation of body protein to supply energy needs after severe injury is inevitable. Exogenous sources of energy and protein must be supplied to minimize this catabolic loss.

Patients with increased losses of protein through large open wounds, burns, protein-losing enteropathies, or severe, protracted diarrhea require extra protein. Nitrogen balance studies can help determine individual requirements. To ensure that protein is used efficiently, sufficient nonprotein energy (NPE) must be supplied in the form of carbohydrate and fat (Table 5.3.3).

Oversupply of protein can cause hyperaminoacidemia and raised serum ammonia levels. Because the ability to excrete protein metabolites via the kidney develops with age, the infant is particularly susceptible. The renal solute load of enteral feeds is important when choosing a feed and is the reason why most adult formulae are not suitable for infants under 2 years of age.

MICRONUTRIENTS

A minimum of the recommended daily allowance should be provided (Table 5.3.4), and additional amounts used when requirements are increased (Table 5.3.5).

MONITORING

BIOCHEMICAL INVESTIGATIONS

On commencement of feeding or parenteral nutrition, and daily until the child is stable, perform urinalysis and measure plasma urea and electrolytes, creatinine, acid–base status, glucose, triacylglycerols, calcium, magnesium and phosphate.

ANTHROPOMETRY

The maintenance of body weight does not necessarily mean adequate nutrition. Fluid retention and edema cause weight gain in critically ill children.

MANAGEMENT

During critical illness, patients may be unwilling or unable to meet their nutritional needs orally. Nutritional support can be provided enterally (by

---

TABLE 5.3.3 Daily protein requirements

Age	Recommended intake (g/kg)	Critical illness (g/kg)	Burns (g/kg)
0–6 months	2.0	2–4.0 max	3
6–12 months	1.6	2–4.0 max	3
1–3 years	1.2	1.5–2.0	3
3–10 years	1.0	1.5–2.0	2.5
10–18 years	1.0	1.5–2.0	2.5
Optimal NPE: N	630–840:1	630:1 (minor stress) 420:1 (major stress)	630:1 (< 10% BSA) 420:1 (> 10% BSA)

NPE: N, ratio of nonprotein energy (kJ) to nitrogen (g). RDI based on WHO/FAO protein and energy requirements, 1985. Initial requirement for burn injury.

TABLE 5.3.4 Recommended daily intakes for micronutrients

Age (years)	Vitamins[a]									Minerals[b]					
	A (mg)	E (mg)	B_1 (mg)	B_2 (mg)	B_6 (mg)	B_{12} (µg)	C (mg)	Niacin (mg)	Folate (µg)	Zinc (mg)	Iron (mg)	Magnesium (mg)	Calcium (mg)	Phosphorus (mg)	Selenium (µg)
0–0.5 (breast fed)	425	2.5	0.15	0.4	0.25	0.3	25	4.0	50	3.0	0.5	40	300	150	10
0–0.5 (formula fed)	425	4.0	0.25	0.4	0.25	0.3	25	4.0	50	3.6	3.0	40	500	150	10
0.6–1	300	4.0	0.35	0.6	0.45	0.7	30	7	75	4.5	9.0	60	550	300	15
1–3	300	5.0	0.5	0.8	0.6–0.9	1.0	30	9–10	100	4.5	6–8	80	700	500	25
4–7	350	6.0	0.7	1.1	0.8–1.3	1.5	30	11–13	100	6.0	6–8	110	800	700	30
boys 8–11	500	8.0	0.9	1.4	1.1–1.6	1.5	30	14–16	150	9.0	6–8	180	800	800	50
girls 8–11	500	8.0	0.9	1.3	1.0–1.5	1.5	30	14–16	150	9.0	6–8	160	900	800	50
boys 12–15	725	10.5	1.2	1.8	1.4–2.1	2.0	30	19–21	200	12	10–13	260	1200	1200	85
girls 12–15	725	9.0	1.0	1.6	1.2–1.8	2.0	30	17–19	200	12	10–13	240	1000	1200	70
boys 16–18	750	11.0	1.2	1.9	1.5–2.2	2.0	40	20–22	200	12	10–13	320	1000	1100	85
girls 16–18	750	8.0	0.9	1.4	1.1–1.6	2.0	30	17–19	200	12	10–13	270	800	1100	70

[a] Vitamin A as retinol equivalents, Vitamin E as α-tocopherol equivalents, niacin as niacin equivalents.

Source: Truswell, AS. (ed) Recommended Nutrient Intakes Australian Papers. Sydney: Australian Professional Publications, 1990.

gastric or jejunal feeding), parenterally or by a combination of both (Fig.5.3.2.)

ENTERAL OR PARENTERAL NUTRITION?

Parenteral nutrition (PN) has been the mainstay of nutritional support in intensive care. It bypasses the gastrointestinal tract and provides macronutrients in the form of dextrose, amino acids and lipid, thus providing energy in a concentrated form which limits the fluid load on the patient. However, the significant metabolic, thrombotic and septic complications associated with PN have increased the popularity of enteral nutrition. Compared with enteral nutrition, parenteral nutrition:

- is more expensive
- may cause cholestasis and hepatocyte dysfunction
- may impair reticuloendothelial function
- may cause gut mucosal atrophy and increase the risk of bacterial translocation across the bowel wall
- increases the risk of systemic sepsis after trauma

ENTERAL NUTRITION

Advantages

An important advantage of enteral nutrition (EN) is the enhancement of gut growth and maturation in neonates, particularly if breast milk is used. Enteral feeding, started early and delivered consistently, helps to maintain gut mucosal structure and function and to reduce the translocation of bacteria and endotoxin from gut lumen to blood in the critically ill.

Delivery

Feed can be directed into the stomach by nasogastric tube or gastrostomy, or into the small bowel by nasojejunal tube or jejunostomy. Nasogastric feeding is preferable. The placement of any feeding tube in a seriously ill child should be checked radiologically before feeding is started.

Large gastric aspirates caused by delayed gastric emptying can retard the progress of the feeding

TABLE 5.3.5 **Disease states that require additional micronutrients**	
Disease	**Increased requirement for**
Burns	Vitamins C, B complex, folate, zinc
HIV/AIDS	Zinc, selenium, iron
Renal failure requiring dialysis procedures	Vitamins C, B complex, folate
Protein–energy malnutrition	Zinc, selenium, iron (assess multivitamin status)
Short bowel syndrome, chronic malabsorption states	Vitamins A, D, E, K, B_{12}, folate, zinc, magnesium, selenium
Liver disease	Vitamins A, D, E, K, B_{12}, zinc, iron
Fistula output, chronic diarrhea	Zinc, magnesium, selenium, folate, vitamin B_{12}, B complex
Pancreatic insufficiency	Vitamins A, D, E, K
Inflamatory bowel disease	Folate, vitamin B_{12}, zinc, iron

plan. This can be treated by reducing the volume of feed, by infusing the feed at low rates continuously, reassessing the concentration of the feed used and assessing gastrointestinal function. A prokinetic agent such as cisapride should be tried but if large gastric aspirates persist, a jejunal tube should be inserted.

Feeding into the small bowel may allow enteral feeding to be started before bowel sounds return. Feeds should be infused continuously, commencing slowly (maximum 10 ml/h) and the rate of delivery increased as tolerated. Failure of jejunal feeding is unusual but if it persists, PN is indicated.

The feeding plan

Standard feeds contain whole proteins and are suitable for up to 80% of patients. *Semi elemental feeds* contain the protein in a hydrolyzed form or as short-chain peptides, and in *elemental feeds* the protein is in the form of amino acids.

Patients with normal gastrointestinal function

Commence EN using an isotonic whole-protein feed in small amounts (1–2 ml/kg) every 2–3 hours. In infants, use expressed breast milk (EBM) or standard-dilution infant formula (2.8 kJ/ml). Ready-to-use pediatric formula (e.g. Pediasure, 4.2 kJ/ml) is suitable for children 1–6 years. If a ready-to-use pediatric formula is not available, infant formula fortified with additional powder and/or a glucose polymer can be used for children 1–2 years of age. An adult formula such as Isocal (4.2 kJ/ml) is suitable for children over 2 years (Table 5.3.6, Fig 5.3.2).

Increase the volume of each feed as feeding is found to be tolerated. Once the maximum volume is reached, if nutritional goals cannot be met, the energy density of the feed may be increased. This can be achieved in infants by adding Human Milk Fortifier to EBM, adding additional powder to infant formula (see Table 5.3.6), or by changing to a 6.3 kJ/ml feed in older children (e.g. Ensure Plus).

Patients with compromised gastrointestinal function

In infants, EBM is still the feed of choice, but if it is not tolerated, change to a semi-elemental formula such as Pregestimil. Neocate is one example of an elemental infant formula and it should only be used in infants who cannot tolerate a semielemental feed. In older children, feeds should be commenced with an isotonic elemental product such as Vivonex Pediatric.

For enteral feeds to be tolerated splanchnic blood flow must be adequate. Intolerance to feeds can be a sensitive marker of sub-optimal gut blood flow (e.g. post cardiac surgery).

Patients with compromised gastrointestinal function often tolerate continuous feeding using a pump. Feeds should commence slowly and run for a maximum of 2–3 hours initially until tolerance to feed is ensured. Rate of delivery can then be increased.

Jejunally fed patients should be initially commenced on a semielemental or elemental formula. The use of whole-protein feeds in these patients remains controversial.

Complications

Diarrhea is often associated with EN but rarely requires cessation of feeds. The cause of the diarrhea should be sought and treated. The most common causes of diarrhea in critically ill children are:

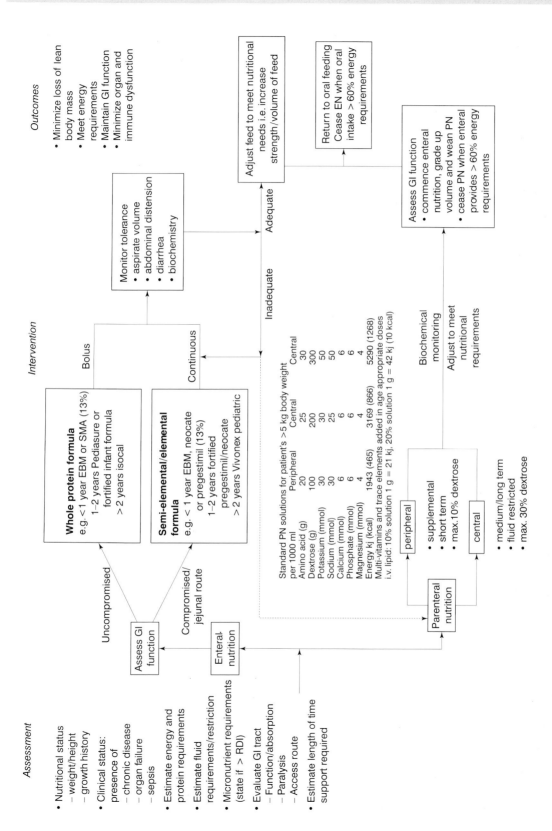

Figure 5.3.2 Planning appropriate nutrition for a critically ill child

TABLE 5.3.6 Examples of enteral feeds

Product name	Manufacturer	Energy (kJ (kcal)/100 ml)	Protein (g/100 ml)	Carbohydrate (g/100 ml)	Fat (g/100 ml)	Osmolality (mosmol/kg)	N: NPE[a]	Protein source	Features
Breast Milk	Wyeth	289 (69)	1.1	7.4[b]	4.2	260	1:1500	Whole protein	The preferred infant feed!
Standard IF:									
SMA (12.8%)	Wyeth	270 (65)	1.5	7.0[b]	3.5	285	1:1027	Demineralized whey	'Standard' IF
Prosobee	MJ	283 (68)	2.0	6.6	3.6	180	1:783	Soy isolate	Non-cow's milk protein IF
O'Lac	MJ	283 (68)	1.5	6.9	3.7	200	1:1098	Milk protein	Lactose-free IF
Pregestimil (13%)	MJ	279 (67)	1.9	6.9	3.8	320	1:827	Hydrolyzed casein	Semielemental IF
Neocate	SHS Inc	292 (70)	1.9	8.1	3.5	353	1:857	Amino acids	Elemental IF
3232A + 6% glucose/fructose	MJ	283 (68)	1.9	9.1	2.9		1:742	Hydrolyzed caesin	Low in phosphate, sodium, potassium
Kindergen PROD	SHS Inc	424 (101)	1.5	12.1	5.2	215	1:1654	Whey	Disaccharide-free IF
Fortified IF:[c]									
Breast milk + FM85 (5%)	Nestlé	365 (87)	2.0	11.0[b]	4.2	452	1:1032	Added whey	Fortified human milk with additional protein, Ca, PO4, energy
breast milk + FM85 + polyjoule (4.2%)	Nestlé Nutricia	432 (103)	2.0	15.4[b]	4.2	499	1:1240	Added whey and maltodextrin	
SMA (16%)[c]	Wyeth	338 (81)	1.9	8.9[b]	4.4	350	1:1009	Demineralized whey	
SMA (16%) + polyjoule (4.2%)	Wyeth Nutricia	405 (97)	1.9	12.9[b]	4.4	397	1:1229	Demineralized whey	
Enteral formula:									
Portagen	MJ	283 (68)	2.4	7.8	3.3	230	1:635	Caseinates	Low LCT, contains 86% fat as MCT
Pediasure	Ross	420 (100)	3.0	11.0	4.9	310	1:766	Whey, casein	Designed for age 1–6 years
Isocal	MJ	440 (100)	3.5	13.5	4.4	300	1:642	Caseinates, soy isolate	'Standard' whole-protein AF
Pulmocare	Ross	630 (150)	6.2	10.6	9.2	475	1:527	Caseinates	Respiratory dysfunction AF
Ensure Plus	Ross	660 (158)	5.6	21.8	5.6	690	1:632	Soy isolate, caseinates	High-energy AF
Twocal HN	Ross	840 (201)	8.4	21.7	9.1	690	1:520	Caseinates	High energy and nitrogen AF
Nepro	Ross	840 (201)	7.0	21.5	9.6	635	1:645	Caseinates	Renal failure AF
Generaid Plus	SHSine	428 (102)	2.4	13.6	4.2	287	1:1005	Amino acids, BCAA	Hepatic failure > 1 year of age
Jevity	Ross	420 (100)	4.4	15.1	3.7	310	1:449	Caseinates	Added fiber AF
Criticare HN	MJ	440 (105)	3.8	22.0	0.53	650	1:617	Amino acids, peptides	High nitrogen, low fat AF
Vital	Ross	420 (100)	4.1	18.5	1.1	500	1:532	Peptides, amino acids	Impaired GI function
Vivonex Pediatric	Novartis	336 (80)	2.4	12.6	2.35	360	1:766	Amino acids	Elemental, impaired GI function AF
Impact	Novartis	420 (100)	5.6	13.2	2.8	375	1:300	Caseinates	Immunonutrition AF

IF, infant formula; AF, Adult formula,

[a] N: NPE, ratio of nitrogen (g) to non-protein energy (kJ)

[b] contains lactose; MJ, Mead Johnson SHS Inc, Scientific Hospital Supplies

[c] nonstandard dilution, extra SMA powder used to increase nutritional value

- antibiotic use
- enteral administration of hypertonic drugs
- hypoalbuminemia
- gastrointestinal tract infection
- rapid infusion of a cold or hypertonic feed

Continuously delivered feeds may be better tolerated than intermittent boluses.

There is a risk of pulmonary aspiration with enteral feeding. This can be minimized by:

- raising the bed head by 45° during and for 1 hour after feeds
- administering feeds as small, frequent boluses or continuous infusion
- using a prokinetic agent such as cisapride (NB. concern re proarrythmic potential)

Jejunal feeding may reduce but does not abolish the risk of regurgitation and aspiration.

PARENTERAL NUTRITION

The conditions for which PN is most often needed in childhood are:

- postoperative care following gastrointestinal surgery
- impaired bowel motility caused by deep sedation, ischemia or sepsis
- aspiration risk associated with enteral feeding
- inability to meet nutritional requirements enterally
- chylothorax
- acute pancreatitis

Delivery

Nutrient solutions are usually infused into a central vein or occasionally a peripheral vein. Peripheral vein administration limits the concentration of dextrose to a 10% solution, and therefore limits energy intake. In the most widely used delivery system, amino acids, dextrose, vitamins and trace elements are mixed in a single bag. The fat emulsion is delivered separately, mixing with the nutrient solution as close as possible to the access point, as some amino acid solutions are incompatible with lipid.

Most hospitals use standard PN solutions (Fig 5.3.2). Specialized solutions are available for patients with unique needs such as hepatic failure. The total

fluid volume per kilogram of body weight per day, the rate of infusion and the number of hours over which the PN will run are ordered for each child.

> PN solutions are incompatible with some drugs —check carefully!

Composition of PN solutions

Protein

Crystalline amino acids are used as the nitrogen source. Estimate protein requirements (see Table 5.3.3); commence at 0.5 g/kg per day, increasing daily in 0.5 g increments until goals are reached. Tolerance to protein can be assessed by measurement of serum ammonia, urea and creatinine.

Nonprotein energy

Aim to provide 30–40% of NPE as lipid emulsion and the rest as dextrose. Lipid solutions containing 10% (300 mosmol/kg) or 20% (350 mosmol/kg) long-chain triacylglycerols (LCTs) are available. These provide 4.2 kJ/ml (1 kcal/ml) and 8.4 kJ/mnl (2 kcal/ml) respectively. A 20% solution such as Intralipid (Kabi Pharmacia) is widely used, as it contains a smaller amount of phospholipid (which inhibits lipoprotein lipase) than a 10% solution.

Tolerance of lipid is measured daily (4 hours after ceasing lipid infusion) by assessing plasma triacylglycerol levels (keep < 2 mmol/L) and turbidity.

Lipid intake can range from 0.5 g/kg to 4 g/kg per day depending on plasma clearance. A minimum of 0.5 g/kg per day of LCTs should prevent deficiency of essential fatty acids. Continuous infusion of a maximum of 0.15 g/kg·min of fat is better tolerated than intermittent boluses.

Dextrose is an important energy source but the amount of glucose that can be directly oxidized is limited. Excess glucose intake causes fat deposition in the liver.

During critical illness, insulin secretion is limited and hyperglycemia can limit the delivery of energy. Infusion rates and dextrose concentration in nutrient solution should be increased slowly to stimulate the production of insulin. This may help prevent glycosuria and osmotic diuresis. Total daily glucose intake should not exceed 18 g/kg. A 10% dextrose solution provides 840 kJ/L (200 kcal/l) and has an osmolality of 277 mosmol/kg.

Glycosuria and serum glucose concentration should be monitored to assess glucose tolerance. Too-rapid infusion rates or high glucose concentrations can lead to excessive carbon dioxide production, which in severe respiratory failure may cause hypercapnia.

When weaning a patient from PN, slowly reduce the rate of infusion to prevent hypoglycemia.

Micronutrients

The micronutrient content (Table 5.3.4) is based on the recommended daily intake of energy and additional amounts are used when requirements are increased (Table 5.3.5).

Complications

Intravenous lipids may impair the function of neutrophils and macrophages and displace conjugated bilirubin from albumin binding sites. Large boluses interfere with pulmonary gas exchange, increase pulmonary vascular resistance and cause thrombocytopenia and coagulopathy. For these reasons the use of lipid should be avoided in acute liver failure and the maximum daily intake limited to 0.5–1 g/kg in children with severe sepsis, respiratory failure, pulmonary hypertension or coagulopathy.

Complications related to PN are severe enough to require its cessation in 5–10% of patients. To minimize the risk of infection, strict aseptic technique should be observed during catheter insertion, bag and line changes.

✓ KEY POINTS

➤ Patients may have a poor nutritional status on admission which limits their fuel reserves and may affect their response to treatment

➤ The metabolic response to trauma leads to a rapid depletion of nutritional reserves which may interfere with recovery

➤ Requirements for nitrogen and energy are increased during sepsis. Catabolic processes may prevent the provision of adequate nutrition. To minimize the nutritional deficit due to sepsis, the most effective measures are
 – surgical drainage of pus
 – appropriate antibiotic therapy

 – vigorous support of the circulation with plasma expanders (Ch. 2.3)

➤ Substrate intolerance, particularly to glucose, combined with fluid overload, acid–base disturbances and the hypermetabolic state impede the provision of adequate nutritional support during critical illness

➤ Use the enteral route whenever possible; access to the small bowel should be planned preoperatively

✗ COMMON ERRORS

➤ Failure to recognize malnourished children and to set goals for energy and protein intake.

➤ Lack of bowel sounds does not preclude enteral feeding. Paralytic ileus does not affect the bowel uniformly and jejunal feeding is often possible despite its presence

FURTHER READING

1. Cuthbertson DP. Observations on the disturbance of metabolism produced by injury to the limbs. Quart J Med 1932; 1: 233–246
 – (*Classic studies describing the stress response*)

2. Mezoff A, Gamm L, Konek S et al. Validation of a nutrition screening tool in children with respiratory syncytial virus admitted to ICU. Pediatrics 1996; 97(4): 543–546
 – (*A rapid method of screening for nutritional risk in ICU*)

3. Greene H, Hambridge K, Schanler R, Tsang R. Guidelines for the use of vitamins, trace elements, calcium, magnesium, phosphorus in infants and children receiving TPN: report to the Subcommittee on Pediatric Parenteral Nutrient Requirements from the Committee on Clinical Practice Issues of the American Society of Clinical Nutrition. Am J Clin Nutr 1988; 48: 1324–1342
 – (*Extensive information on micronutrient requirements in parenteral nutrition*)

4. Wilmore DW, Carpentier YA. (eds) Metabolic support of the critically ill patient. Update in Intensive Care and Emergency Medicine, 17, Berlin: Springer; 1993
 – (*Excellent review of body composition and metabolic changes during critical illness, with chapters on parenteral and enteral nutrition*)

5. Tsang, RC, Lucas A, Uauy R, Zlotzin, S, editors. Nutritional needs of the preterm infant. New York: Caduceus; 1993
 – (*The scientific basis and practical guidelines for feeding preterm infants*)

5.4 Scoring systems and patient audit

Robert I. Ross Russell

SCORING SYSTEMS

THEORY

For many years physicians have recognized the potential value of objectively assessing the severity of illness in their patients. Pediatric intensive care units deal with relatively small numbers of patients with a vast array of different underlying disorders. Individual cases are further complicated by the multisystem involvement of many disease processes. Inevitably the ability to compare groups of patients is severely limited. The diagnosis of asthma, for example, has completely different implications when a child is critically ill from those it might have in a hospital outpatient clinic or in the community. The same disease can vary considerably in severity, and consequently this will affect both the resources needed to treat it and the expected outcome. In theory, effective severity scoring is an immensely powerful tool. It allows groups of patients to be amalgamated in a comparable manner. Protocols for treatment can then be developed and evaluated systematically, comparisons between patient groups or between different institutions can be made, and justification for resources is possible. As these three elements are fundamental to the proper provision of intensive care, it can be seen that the derivation of acceptable and accurate scoring systems is crucial.

Despite this, however, there is little doubt that the tools currently available to effect these comparisons are imperfect. There are two major problems. Firstly, an inaccurate scoring system can give rise to the wrong conclusions. Children who are critically ill frequently pose extremely complex pathological problems, and trying to reflect that complexity in a scoring system will lead to compromise. At one extreme the system might accurately reflect all elements of variability between individual cases. This would require collection of vast numbers of variables, making the process both time-consuming and more open to error. The alternative would be to restrict the variables collected to ensure accuracy and consistency, with a consequent reduction in precision.

The second problem also reflects the difficulties of 'volume'. Because of the relatively small numbers of children requiring intensive care, measuring differences in outcome becomes harder. There is always a substantial variability in the expected outcome for an individual patient, not least because of the limited precision of the tools currently available. To demonstrate 'significant' changes in outcome therefore requires large numbers of patients. In the UK, for example, there is much discussion about the benefits of regionalizing care. Since available measures of long-term morbidity are so limited, the only outcome that can be reliably measured is death. Any discussion on the benefits of one center over another consequently focuses on the mortality rate of children in each unit. Mortality rates in most units lie between 5% and 10%, and so in order to assess whether small units have a different outcome (i.e. mortality) requires participation of many units, and ideally a national study. As the number of units involved in such a study increases, the validity of comparison will decrease owing to the variability between each of those units.

Another important issue is the distinction between population outcomes and individual outcomes. Validation of scoring systems is based on *population* data and as such its predictive value for the individual is limited. In order to extrapolate to individuals there has to be recognition of the variability of the score, and of the individual variation in outcome given a particular score. To date the almost universal consensus is that scoring systems are not precise enough to be used for decisions in individual cases.

Perhaps the most famous scoring system now in use is the APGAR score for newborn babies. This score is now 40 years old and is still widely used to give a moderately objective assessment of an infant's status. In intensive care, most such scoring systems have been designed for an adult population (see below). They use physiological parameters, scored according to their degree of derangement, to give a numerical score that reflects the severity of the illness. This is usually a predictive score for a particular outcome, and the outcome most often predicted is death of the patient.

Most clinicians probably accept the concept of predicting outcome and would subscribe to the collection of such data, but its use must be carefully defined. Severity scoring tools were not developed—and should not be used—for decisions about whether to continue treatment, although they may help in discussing likely outcomes with families.

It is important to explore the definition of 'outcome' a little further. Tools such as the pediatric risk of mortality score (PRISM), any of the many meningococcal predictive scoring systems, or indeed nearly all scoring systems used in intensive care, are designed and weighted to predict death. As such they do not measure severity of illness *except* as it relates to the likelihood of death, which is an extremely crude measure of outcome even in critical illness. In meningococcal disease, for example, survivors are mostly neurologically normal or minimally impaired, compared with survivors of head trauma. However, the physiological derangement seen in meningococcal disease, and consequently the predictive scores seen, are usually far greater than those found following trauma. Scores such as PRISM would be bad predictors of outcome if used to predict long-term outcome rather than survival. The difficulties of developing such predictions can also be seen in the scarcity of models that predict morbidity (short- or long-term), and the assessment of the outcome of intensive care, in its broadest sense requires both premorbid and long-term detailed follow-up data (Ch. 5.11). Of recent reports of morbidity prediction, the most sensitive used a combination of premorbid health status, diagnostic group and severity of illness to crudely predict outcome, which was defined as 'functional', 'compromised' or 'dead'. Neonatal work using the clinical risk index for babies (CRIB) found it to be as good as (but no better than) gestational age and weight in predicting neurological handicap.

So how have the current 'severity of illness' scores been used? Their immediate use (and the

one for which most scores have been designed) is to allow the comparison of patients with (a) varying degrees of the same illness or (b) different illnesses. This can be important in a clinical or organizational setting. The development of 'best practice' in dealing with complex and critical illness requires the ability to compare groups of patients, as described earlier. Severity scoring has therefore been applied to allow the evaluation of treatment regimens in certain conditions. Studies of new antiendotoxin drugs for use in meningococcal disease are using scoring systems to define entry criteria for the study as well as allowing more detailed analysis of results according to different disease severity. At an organizational level, scoring systems are used to justify resource allocation. The famous study by Pollack et al on the improved outcome from pediatric intensive care seen in tertiary compared with nontertiary centers was only possible because of researchers' ability to stratify patients according to mortality risk.

USING SCORING SYSTEMS IN PRACTICE

Severity scoring systems currently available can be divided into four categories: injury scores, severity of illness (case mix adjustment) scores, intervention scores and workload scores.

Injury scores

Injury scores include the Glasgow coma scale, and similar acute scores for specific clinical conditions.

Severity of illness scores

Severity of illness scores are abundant. In pediatric intensive care, PRISM (including PRISM III) is the most relevant and best known. This tool uses 14 physiological variables (17 in PRISM III) measured over the first 24 hours in intensive care. Each variable then receives a weighted score depending on its derangement, and the scores are added together. This total is further adjusted to reflect intrinsic variables, such as patient age and operative status. The PRISM III system is now commercially run, and must therefore be bought, but does offer the potential to compare different units. More recently Shann et al introduced the pediatric index of mortality (PIM) score which appears simpler to apply than PRISM III.

There are a number of problems with existing severity of illness scores. First, each has been developed in a particular population, and so is only directly applicable to that population; to use the score in other circumstances requires further validation. Thus, interpretation of PRISM in the UK is affected by the lack of evaluation in the population. The case mix may be quite different (e.g. in the proportion of trauma that is seen) which may affect the validity of the results. The second problem is that the outcome predicted (death) is limited—even if it is easily defined! Prediction of other outcomes, especially long-term neurological results, may require a completely different approach. Thirdly, the rigors of definition need improving. Variables that are collected need to be exactly defined (e.g. is a reagent strip test equivalent to a blood glucose measurement in the laboratory? Does a calculated bicarbonate value vary from one that is directly measured?). Timing is also relevant (does the period of 'intensive care' start from admission to hospital? ICU? PICU? arrival of a PICU transport team?). The UK Intensive Care National Audit and Research Centre (ICNARC) has begun to define such details and this should greatly enhance the value of these tools.

Intervention scores

Intervention scores are primarily for use in adults. One of the best known of these is the therapeutic intervention scoring system (TISS); this is designed to relate the severity of a patient's illness to the number of medical interventions being conducted. Thus a patient being ventilated will score for that, as well as for other features such as lines, inotropic support, etc. These scores have been used more for financial purposes than for clinical ones. In the UK, many adult intensive care units use a daily TISS score to determine patient charges.

Workload scores

Workload scores differ from intervention scores in that they are designed to look at the amount of personnel support that a patient requires. One

example of this type of tool is Grace Reynolds Adaptation of the System of Peto (GRASP). This method scores each nursing intervention carried out at the bedside, giving a score that reflects the number of nursing hours needed to care for the patient. This may vary from the equivalent intervention score considerably; for example, an intubated patient who is stable may score relatively well on TISS and require little nursing care, whereas the same patient extubated would require far more nursing, but would score less on TISS.

All these methods are becoming more refined with time. Recognition of their development and their intended use is important in defining appropriate groups on which they can be used. In such a context their value is unquestioned.

AUDIT

THEORY

Few clinicians can be unaware by now of the cyclical nature of audit (Fig. 5.4.1). This cycle requires the comparison of current practice against 'standards'. Areas of practice that could be bettered are identified, changed and later audited again to evaluate any improvement. Frequently the most difficult part of the process is the development of standards against which to audit. In

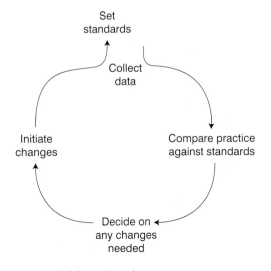

Figure 5.4.1 Audit cycle

intensive care the variability of the workload, the intrinsic differences between different facilities and the sheer complexity of the cases can make productive audit seem almost impossible. There is a vast and generally turgid literature on the subject, but practical guides are rare. Clinicians setting up audit within their departments will often focus a great deal of energy on issues of clinical care: e.g. whether patients with a certain diagnosis received particular forms of care. Classical audit theory, however, looks at the *structure, process* and *outcome* of care. This approach emphasizes the importance of looking at resources (buildings, staff, etc.) and outcomes, as well as the process of care itself.

Audit also needs to be seen on several levels in terms of the areas being reviewed. 'Individual' audit (that is auditing the care of specific patients or diseases) needs to be matched by 'unit' audit, looking at the function of the PICU as a whole, and 'regional' audit, addressing the provision of care for geographic areas. In some circumstances such definitions may require even further expansion. This approach then allows the development of a grid of potential areas for audit (Table 5.4.1).

USING AUDIT IN PRACTICE

If one uses a grid such as that in Table 5.4.1 then the daunting prospect of setting up specific audit projects becomes much easier. Specific topics can be addressed within the grid, such as the examples shown. Once suitable topics have been identified, appropriate standards have to be found or derived. This can be extremely difficult. As a general guide, the more absolute the standard, the easier the audit: for example, if auditing the process of intubation on a unit, it might be reasonable to suggest that 'no elective intubation occurs without formal induction of anesthesia'. While it is possible that there could be situations where such standards were not achieved without there being 'bad practice', the setting of absolute standards will make the identification of cases much easier. Standards that simply recommend a course of action for some circumstances are far more difficult to review. The more exceptions that are allowed for a given standard, the more laborious becomes the task of establishing if each case justified that course of action. A further important aspect of the standard is that the information must be collectable. For example, if auditing communication between doctors and parents on the PICU, it might be reasonable to say that all families present at the bedside should be spoken to by a doctor every day. However, in this situation, information on the residential or visiting status of the parents and on the visit of the doctor would have to be recorded. For most units, such information would be difficult to extract easily from a selection of notes (retrospectively) and so a specific sheet might be needed for the study period.

Standards also require a 'shelf-life', that is a defined date by which the standard should be reviewed. As care strategies evolve, standards will inevitably change too, and so the standards against which we audit need to be reviewed (although not necessarily changed) regularly.

Level of audit	Structure	Process	Outcome
Patient	Bedside equipment	Line sepsis intubations, etc.	Mortality Mortality Social outcome
Unit	Unit design Equipment Staffing levels Training	Efficiency of utilization Readmission rate	Problem-specific outcome (e.g. head injury) Discharge summaries Research
Region	Number of beds Refused admissions Training at local hospitals Communication	Transport service Regional guidelines	Referrals out of region

TABLE 5.4.1 **Breakdown of the categories of audit within an intensive care unit, with examples of audit topics within each category**

TABLE 5.4.2 **Audit timetable**

- Decide audit priorities
  - topic must be relevant and measurable
- Agree standards
  - limit to 3 or 4 only
  - identify 'absolute' standards wherever possible
  - specify 'shelf life'.
- Collect data
  - specify people to collect, method of collection and analysis.
- Compare
  - decide areas of practice that require change
  - all involved staff must agree changes.
- Institute change
  - involve all relevant staff
  - document changes and next review date.
- Review standards and practice
  - revisit the cycle
  - identify the time frames for further review.

A timetable for audit is essential (Table 5.4.2). Each stage of the process must be clearly defined. This stems in great part from the recognition that audit will often entail change. This can seem threatening to many people, and it is therefore important that those involved clearly understand and agree with the process. All those involved (including patients if appropriate) should agree to each stage, so that a democratic consensus can be reached and implemented. Changes are often better 'piloted' for a specific period and then reviewed to ensure acceptability.

SHORTCOMINGS AND CONTROVERSIES

Audit is a powerful and important method of evaluating what we do. It also suffers from a number of weaknesses. The results of audit will only ever be as good as the data on which it is based. When establishing any data collection, it is therefore essential that careful consideration of the process of data collection is given. However good the model or data set, incomplete or inaccurate data will bias the results. This also emphasizes the importance of allowing dedicated time to collect important data. This is essential, and the amount of time required to collect accurate and complete data relating to critically ill children is often underestimated. Finally, results from audit need to be

fed back into the clinical care area. This means that workable changes in practice to address any perceived shortcomings must be *agreed, instituted* and *reviewed over an agreed time frame.*

SUMMARY

Providing more widespread and effective intensive care for critically ill and injured children is a low-volume, high-cost undertaking. Consequently it is essential that we are able to measure our workload accurately, and justify the resources we need. Without the ability to do so, there will be inevitable pressure to limit what is provided, which it will be difficult to resist. The development of severity scoring tools and good audit is not easy, often tedious and a long way from the 'hands on' medicine most of us wish to practice. However, we must all accept the challenge and strive to establish reliable data collection and audit to ensure that we have the means to justify the care our patients need.

 KEY POINTS

- Scoring systems predict outcomes of populations not individual patients
- Performance of intensive care units can only be compared if outcomes are adjusted for disease severity
- Structured audit should be used to evaluate what we do, identify weaknesses and evaluate the changes in practice which result—the *audit cycle*

FURTHER READING

1. Shann F, Pearson G, Slater A, et al. Pediatric index of mortality (PIM): a mortality prediction model for children in intensive care. Intens Care Med 1997; 23: 201–207
2. Pollack MM, Patel KM, Ruttimann UE. PRISM III—an updated pediatric risk of mortality score. Critical Care Med 1996; 24: 743–752
3. Randolph AG. Pediatric index of mortality (PIM): do we need another pediatric mortality prediction score? Intens Care Med 1997; 23: 141–142

5.5 Family support and counseling

Fiona Maxton

It is now recognized that the hospital care of children is greatly enhanced by the presence of their parents. Parents, too, need to be with their ill children, helping them to deal with the change in their lives. This is especially true when the child is critically ill, requiring emergency care and support. Unexpected life-threatening conditions in children are a source of great stress to the parents and to all family members. During the child's illness, parents experience a wide range of emotions, manifested in a variety of ways. It is important that care should focus not only on the critically ill child, but also on the whole family. This notion of family-centered care for children is very different from the philosophy of patient-centered or disease-centered care which underlies the treatment of critically ill adults.

FAMILY-CENTERED CARE

Family-centered care (sometimes known as partnership-in-care or family-oriented care) is the philosophy that should guide the care of sick children worldwide. Its main principle is that the care of children is best carried out by their family members, with varying degrees of assistance from health professionals. In the context of intensive care, most of the technical care is performed by appropriately qualified medical and nursing personnel, but this does not mean that parents should become bystanders in their child's life. The idea of family-centered care is to involve parents and other family members in all steps of care, discussing with them the treatment recommended and their child's prognosis, and taking their wishes into account. It is important to identify who 'the family' consists of. It must be remembered that there are now many variations of the family—for example, one-parent and single-sex families and step-parents. The 'extended' family, which in the past was limited to relatives by blood and by marriage, now includes whomever the patient, or the parent of the ill child says it does.

Parent, sibling, aunt, cousin, grandmother, paid nanny or friend could all be 'family'. In this chapter the use of 'family' embraces all of these groups.

FAMILY STRESS

Parents experience stress of many kinds when their child becomes critically ill.

Change in their role as parents

Parents often have feelings of confusion and inadequacy when their child becomes critically ill. They are unsure of their role, particularly in the technical environment necessary to help their child. Often this confusion is expressed as anger, guilt, aggression and feelings of helplessness or inadequacy as a parent. They also feel a loss of control, particularly in decision-making. It is not possible to relieve their distress completely, but it can be made manageable by listening to them, giving them as much control as possible over decisions about their child's treatment and by establishing roles for them in physical aspects of care such as feeding, bathing and passive limb movements.

Fear that their child may die

This fear is often justified. Honesty at this time is essential. Parents need to be given accurate and truthful information to prepare them for the possibility of their child's death.

Separation from their child

This anxiety is greatest in the first 24 hours after the child becomes critically ill, during which time the child may be transferred to another hospital, to the operating room or to other hospital departments for scans and invasive diagnostic procedures. Parents' separation from their child should be minimized; where possible they should be notified of plans to move their child—this includes relocation of their child within the ward or unit or hospital (not finding their child in the expected bed or space implies an unexpected emergency or even death to the parent).

Altered appearance of their child

Facial swelling, immobility, drains, catheters, infusions and intubation equipment disfigure the child in the eyes of the parent. Even the fact that their child may smell differently from normal can be distressing. Parents are understandably afraid of the alien environment and unfamiliar equipment used to stabilize a critically ill child. Once again, discussion and support from staff is of great importance particularly during the first 24 hours. The role of the equipment in use, particularly those items connected to the child should be explained, and parents should be encouraged to maintain contact by touching their child's hand or foot.

FAMILY NEEDS

To help families cope, recognize their need to be with their child. This includes the stabilization phase before transfer to a specialist unit and may include active resuscitation. Stabilization often requires traumatic procedures, such as insertion of a central line, endotracheal tube or chest drain. Although the presence of parents is encouraged increasingly, particularly in PICUs, some medical staff may perform these procedures less confidently with an audience of anxious parents, seeing their presence as a distraction which interferes with the safe, rapid completion of the procedure. In these circumstances, ask the parents to wait in a room nearby, and designate a staff member to report frequently on the progress of their child.

Parents should not be prevented from being present during resuscitation. If there, they must be accompanied by a member of the staff to interact with them, explain what is happening and why, and to take them elsewhere if necessary. There is understandable concern that parents may become so distraught that their emotions would impede the actions of the staff, resulting in ineffective resuscitation. In practice this rarely occurs, but if it does, the family should be asked to wait in another area. Also, parents may recognize that they need 'time out', but feel that they need permission to leave.

Ideally, the support person should be someone who is not directly involved in the resuscitation procedure. This gives parents an opportunity to talk and ask questions. A senior nurse, chaplain or social worker is usually the ideal person for this role. By being present during resuscitation, the parents can see that everything possible has been done for their child and can say goodbye to the child if death is inevitable.

Information and discussion

Proposed treatment must be discussed with the parents (Ch. 5.7). Health professionals often make the mistake of assuming that all decisions are theirs to make. The short-term (next few hours) and long-term (next few days to weeks) plan of treatment should be discussed regularly. Families need frequent, accurate and truthful information (Table 5.5.1). The faith of parents in hospital staff during the initial phase of their child's illness is maintained by such explanations. The discussions should include the child's condition, prognosis and pros and cons of treatment, and should be couched in everyday language, avoiding medical jargon and unnecessary detail. This is best done in a quiet room, away from the distractions of immediate care. Updates should be offered frequently (at least once a day) or whenever the condition of the child changes. A 'debriefing' visit or phone discussion is much appreciated by many parents following a child's critical illness. This adds an element of closure for families and a learning opportunity for staff.

If the prognosis of a critically ill child is hopeless and the parents wish to withdraw treatment, every effort should be made to accommodate their wishes. In some cases, disagreement will arise between parents and hospital staff about the discontinuation of treatment or more commonly about the timing of such action. Have further regular discussions to allow both parties to reassess the situation. Usually, this ends in agreement on the best course of action, but sometimes, especially when the parents want to cease treatment but the staff feel this to be unethical, other medical opinions may be sought (e.g. from the regional PICU [if the child has not been transferred] or a comparable hospital). Sometimes the support provided by such enquiry is all that is required for agreement, but occasionally care of the child may have to be transferred.

TABLE 5.5.1 Guidelines for optimizing communication with families

- On leaving the treatment area, take a moment to collect yourself and set priorities for what you are going to say to the parents. Also, remove your mask, gloves, and gown (which may be bloodstained), so that you are both physically and mentally prepared
- Take another member of staff with you, preferably one who has met the family. This staff member can introduce you to the family and continue the family support when it is necessary for you to leave to return to the patient
- On entering the room, confirm that you are speaking to the correct family, and identify the appropriate family members (e.g. child's mother and or father) to whom you should be addressing your comments. Check the relevant names in advance so that you are appropriately informed. Ensure that you know what information the family has already been given so you can reemphasize key points, but avoid unnecessary repetition. Also, be sure that you have the correct name and gender of the patient so that you can refer to the child appropriately
- When you enter the room in which the family is waiting, introduce yourself, say who you are and what your role is in the child's care, close the door and sit down near the patient's closest family member (standing holding the door handle gives the impression that you do not have time to listen and that the dialog is not important)
- Look at the person you are talking to, be honest and direct, and keep sentences short and information simple. If there is no sign of understanding on the recipient's face, repeat the information using simpler language. Be prepared to emphasize and repeat the main points, but avoid excessive repetition and technical information. If death is a distinct possibility, say so. Families will forgive you if their child survives, but are always unhappy if a child dies without the possibility having been raised with them
- Pause between delivering items of information, particularly when you are giving bad news or a poor prognosis. A few moments of silence allow the facts to sink in. Invite parents to ask for further information if they are unclear, and give them time to phrase questions that may be difficult for them
- Be prepared for a variety of emotional responses or reactions. Some people may remain on one emotional plane during the interview, whereas others can go through several phases of grieving, demonstrating anger, denial, bargaining and other reactions. Do not be embarrassed by parents' crying; provide tissues and give parents time to make themselves presentable before continuing. Reassure them that tears are not inappropriate. Do not feel badly if your information upsets the family; they appreciate the truth and your honest empathy. Do not say more than is necessary; there is a tendency for those inexperienced in sharing bad news to want to add reassurance. This should only be done if it is appropriate

- Remember that a genuine desire to understand, provide information, support the family and relieve anxiety is communicated nonverbally, and is a great asset
- Touch is natural comfort between human beings. Touching or holding the hand of a relative is not inappropriate, but more demonstrative touch, particularly hugging patients, can be misconstrued. There are a variety of social and cultural factors that influence the appropriateness of touching but generally speaking hand-to-hand contact, if it feels natural, is probably right
- During the dialog, your own feelings need not be completely hidden. Professional composure is necessary to serve the family by presenting an air of competence, experience and skill. However, showing your human side and some signs of emotion are not inappropriate and help relatives to realize that you have genuine concern about their child's situation and will do your best for the child
- Avoid platitudes and false sympathy. In spite of what we think, we do not know what it is like for parents. It is better to reflect back to their emotions and say 'it must be hard for you' or 'this must feel very unreal' rather than saying 'I know what it is like' or 'I understand what you are feeling', or making other inappropriate comments
- Encourage and be prepared for questions. These may indicate the need for more information, or disclose misunderstanding that needs correcting. This presents the chance to reemphasize key points of your message. Reassurance about the skill of the staff, the frequency with which children recover and the expertise of the hospital can be helpful. Never be afraid to tell the parents that you do not know the answer to a particular question
- A visit for the parents to their child should be discussed. Wherever possible, the parents should be given an early opportunity to touch and speak to their child. This often reassures them by providing an opportunity to see the team interacting with and caring for the child. Seeing the monitors and support equipment may help them to realize the reality of their child's condition, and can reassure them that everything possible is being done. If necessary, it also provides an opportunity for the parents to say goodbye to their child, which becomes extremely important should the child not survive. During such a visit parents' priorities are inevitably focused on their child, hence the necessity of exchanging key factual information beforehand
- Indicate when the parents will have further information from you, and how they should obtain other relevant information. Provide any written material that is relevant (phone numbers, orientation maps, accommodation and cafeteria details, parking and waiting rooms)

Modified from Macnab AJ, Richards J, Green G. Family oriented care during pediatric interhospital transport: Patient Education and Counselling, 1999; 36: 3247–3257

Parents often need considerable time with their child before and after death. Family members should not feel rushed into leaving their dead child and should be offered the opportunity to return to the hospital to visit the child again if this is desired. Although this is a highly stressful time for staff, the parents' interests must come first, and staff should then discuss and address their own feelings.

Siblings

Siblings of the critically ill child should be encouraged to visit. Often young children have frightening fantasies about what has happened to their brother or sister. These fears are often far worse than reality and may be alleviated by visiting their sibling. If the child dies, it is important that siblings be given the opportunity to say goodbye, although parents are often reluctant to allow this for fear of upsetting them. During these visits, support and an appropriate explanation should be given by the parents and by a physician, nurse or social worker. While it is important for children to see their sick sister or brother, they also need the security of a normal routine in their lives. While parents are preoccupied at the hospital, there may be no appropriate family members available to care for their other children. The social worker should arrange for other family or friends to perform this role.

Jealousy in siblings over the length of time parents are spending with an ill child can result in anger, regression and other attention-seeking behavior. This may need to be explained, and once the immediate danger is past, parents should be encouraged to allocate 'special' times to be with their other children. Discussion with a social worker may help parents to understand these aspects of their child's illness, and provide an opportunity for them to talk about a variety of their own symptoms, concerns and behaviors in a constructive way. The more parents understand and the better they feel about themselves, the greater the likelihood that they can contribute to the care and wellbeing of their child.

Transport

When a critically ill child is transferred to another hospital, a parent should accompany the child in the transport vehicle whenever possible (Ch. 1.5). The parent should be helped to contact other family members for additional support (e.g. care of other children at home). In many PICUs, 'family packs' are given to parents. Provision of these packs, which include basic items such as maps, local information, a toothbrush, comb, soap and a telephone card, is a practical way in which the PICU can support families during this critical early phase of the child's stay in hospital.

Visiting

In most PICUs, open visiting is the norm. This philosophy should be applied in any area temporarily involved in the care of a critically ill child, such as a referring adult ICU or emergency department. Staff in such areas must recognize the special needs of the child and parents and offer flexible visiting arrangements as much as possible.

Parents should be able to be near their child. If there is no relatives' room available, they should be given the option to stay at their child's bedside. They should also be given 'permission' (tactfully) to spend necessary time away from the bedside. Some parents cannot be present as much as others, because they reside a long distance from the hospital or have commitments to other siblings. These people should not be made to feel guilty that their time with their child is limited. Special efforts should ensure that a doctor or senior nurse contacts them daily to provide an update.

Additional stresses on parents of critically ill children

It is important to recognize that the parents and child do not exist in a vacuum and that external pressures are often acting on families of severely ill children.

Financial

It is easy for health professionals to lose sight of the bigger picture. We should take the time to consider whether the parents are out of work, self-employed or earn wages on a commission basis. Loss of earnings while they are unable to work is a major source of added stress. Parents may not be able to afford even the minimal expenses of living in hospital accommodation. A letter to employers from a senior doctor is usually helpful to explain the details of the child's condition and the reasons why the parent is unable to work. Even this may not be sufficient to provide parents with adequate funding, but the hospital social worker can often assist in submitting claims for assistance with daily living expenses and transport costs.

Relationship issues

Family members react to stress and grief in different ways. Often while one parent is grieving openly, the other is trying to maintain control of his or her feelings, to be strong for the other, or may express grief by exhibiting anger, distrust or disbelief. These differences in the ways individuals react can be a source of conflict in their relationship. Health professionals should recognize this potential conflict, explain its normality, and try to alleviate it through talking with parents. Allow parents time to grieve, help them to understand the feelings of their partner and support them in their own feelings. For parents who are experiencing extreme stress, professional assistance should be offered, for instance from a psychologist or counselor.

Social

Parents of a critically ill or dying child may experience alienation from their regular social network. Friends and family often avoid contact, because they doubt their ability to say the right thing. Once again, it is our responsibility to speak to the 'extended' family (if that is the parents' wish); to explain the parent's need for support from family and friends and offer suggestions of how this might be given. We also need to respect a parent's wish to be alone with their child. Nursing staff can help parents in this regard and restrict visitors at these times to avoid family disagreements. It is important in the context of open visiting that any information regarding a child's condition is given first to the parents, who may then consent for it to be given to others subsequently.

AFTER THE DEATH OF A CHILD

If a child dies, appropriate follow-up should be arranged or suggested to the parents. In most pediatric hospitals, family and friends are given the opportunity to visit the child again the following day. Booklets are often given to the parents which contain a footprint or handprint and a lock of hair from their child. The booklets identify a contact person who was present during the child's death or during the hospital stay. The booklets, which can be obtained from the social work department of most pediatric hospitals, describe some of the emotions commonly experienced by bereaved families and give the contact names and addresses of local bereavement support groups (e.g. Sudden Infant Death Association, Trauma Association or Oncology groups). These support groups are usually formed by parents who have experienced the death of a child and are often very helpful to other bereaved parents. The hospital social worker should also maintain contact with the family until they feel able to break that contact. It is usually through the social worker or contact nurse that funeral details will be given to staff if the parents wish them to be present. If they do not offer these details, no attempt should be made to attend.

STAFF NEEDS

Although it is important to meet the needs of the families, staff have needs too. Staff who care for the critically ill may experience considerable stress, particularly if their hospital or department does not treat critically ill children frequently. Following stabilization, resuscitation (successful or not) or transfer of the child to another hospital, all the staff involved need the chance to express their feelings in their own way. Although this is frequently done in an informal way, it may be helpful in some instances to organize a formal supportive debriefing session in particular cases. Hospital counselors, chaplains or social workers make ideal facilitators.

It is also helpful to receive follow-up information on the child's condition after transfer to another hospital. A staff member should be nominated to provide this and be the regular communication link between the hospitals.

✓ KEY POINTS

➤ Consider the philosophy of family-centered care

➤ The child is an inalienable part of the parents' world and vice versa. Always take the time to let family members know what you are doing

➤ Provide support staff to be with family members if possible

➤ Take time to identify parents' *individual* needs

➤ Involve siblings by helping them see their sick brother or sister

➤ Keep family members informed on the condition and treatment of the child and especially about any changes

➤ Consider other pressures on families (e.g. financial employer related, social or personal relationships) which may contribute to their distress

➤ If the child dies, the social worker should provide support for the family for as long as they require it

➤ After a death, resuscitation or transfer, the staff need the opportunity to debrief and reflect. News about the progress of parents whose child has died is important

➤ After a transfer, a nominated person should regularly contact the receiving hospital for information on the child's progress

✗ COMMON ERRORS

➤ Never give information to other members of the family that you have not already given to the parents

➤ In most circumstances, do not prevent parents from being present during procedures, resuscitation or transport

FURTHER READING

1. Darbyshire P. Living with a sick child in hospital. The experiences of parents and nurses. London: Chapman & Hall; 1994
   – (A profound insight into the experiences of parenting a sick child in hospital: suitable for doctors, nurses and lay people alike)

2. Amico J, Davidhizer R. Supporting families of critically ill children. J Clin Nurs 1994; 3: 213–218

3. Back K. Sudden, unexpected pediatric death: caring for the parents. Pediatr Nurs 1991; 17: 571–574

4. Coulter M. The needs of family members of patients in intensive care units. Intens Care Nurs 1989; 5: 4–10

5. Farrell M. Parents of critically ill children have their needs too! A literature review. Intens Care Nurs 1989; 5: 123–128
   – (Four indepth studies of parental needs and stressors and the available means of assistance from the perspectives of parents and health professionals)

5.6 Staff interactions

Karen Ryall, Aileen Britton and Liz Smith

Pediatric intensive care provides care for critically ill children ranging in age from newborn to adolescence. A unique environment and a variety of health professionals with specialized skills are required to provide optimal care for these children and their families. In hospitals where there is no PICU, care must be provided by those individuals with the best skill level available and coordinated by senior staff who are in contact with a center with PICU expertise. Where there is a PICU, this is usually the most intensive area of the hospital in relation to activity, labor, and resource usage per patient, and one of the few patient care settings where a range of specialties can be called upon to act simultaneously.

THE UNIT

WHO'S IN CHARGE

Hospitals utilize different management models. The organizational structure and level of centralization will influence the roles and relationships among the intensive care staff. In general, however, a PICU requires a medical director who is accountable for the clinical issues and quality of care that is provided. Other responsibilities include quality improvement activities, overseeing physician competence and being a resource throughout the organization in relation to the care of critically ill children, or children at risk of becoming critically ill. There is also a head nurse, nurse manager or program director who works with the medical director to provide administrative leadership. As nurses are the primary caregivers and outnumber other staff, it is beneficial if the program director has a nursing background.

THE STAFF

The physician staff working in the pediatric intensive care unit (PICU) are intensive care physicians who have completed both a residency in pediatrics or other specialty such as surgery or anesthesia, and a critical care fellowship. These physicians provide direct patient care, do research related to critical care, teach and are available for hospital-wide and regional consultation. In addition there are fellows/registrars in training, and in some units, residents from post-graduate programs, e.g. anesthetics, pediatrics or adult intensive care, who are there to gain experience in the management of critically ill children.

Nurses coordinate and provide patient care and liaise with families and other health care professionals. The nursing staff are registered nurses with either in-house, postbasic or postgraduate education or qualifications in pediatric intensive care. The need for tertiary education has led to the development of specialized courses such as a postgraduate diploma in pediatric intensive care, available through universities, colleges and technical institutions.

The relationship between medical and nursing staff is constantly evolving. Nurses have increased their level of education and pursued professional development. In the PICU setting they have developed a broader skill base and moved into areas of practice once seen as medical. An example of this is the advanced nursing practice role, which commenced in North America but is gaining momentum in other countries. 'Advanced nursing practice refers to the role of a nurse working within a specialty area where superior clinical skills and judgment are acquired through a combination of experience and education. Advanced nursing practice integrates research-based theory with expert nursing in a clinical specialty, and combines the role of practitioner, teacher, consultant and researcher' (statement by the Canadian Nurses' Association, 1997).

Other key personnel work in PICUs. Many units in North America employ respiratory therapists who have the role of maintaining endotracheal tubes, assisting with intubations and extubations, and managing ventilatory and oxygen therapy, and aerosol treatments. Other units employ biomedical technologists to provide technical support and training, and to support research and technological development. A large range of therapeutic agents are used in PICUs, so attachment of pharmacy staff who have a comprehensive knowledge of drug doses, actions and interactions is important. These pharmacists often direct the monitoring of drug levels, act as auditors of drug therapy used in the unit, and help minimize therapeutic errors. Most units are served by support staff such as social workers, pastoral care workers and clinical psychologists. In Canada, child life specialists work to minimize psychological trauma in children admitted to PICUs and to promote optimum wellbeing.

STAFF AND NEW TECHNOLOGIES

New technologies should be introduced in a way that ensures that care evolves in a safe and effective manner. Achieving this requires communication and skill development. In the face of poor knowledge and skills, or a lack of communication, staff feel out of their depth and may work against the implementation of new agents, equipment or procedures.

Prior to implementation, there should be review of the topic and discussion among the physicians and managers on the viability of the technology and its optimal implementation. Discussion with staff in other units, who have experience of the technology in question, can help in the planning process. One individual should act as the facilitator for the project. A schedule should be prepared to ensure comprehensive staff orientation. Once the new procedure is implemented, communication should provide continuing information, support and evaluation of the program. Provision for ongoing training of staff should be made. The minimum level of theoretical knowledge and practical skill required must be defined, and assessment made that this level of skill has been achieved before staff use the technology independently. 'Nursing competencies' are being developed in some countries in an attempt to provide a way to assess such skills.

In addition to the theoretical and practical skills required for a new technique, training may need to cover areas such as the ethical and legal requirements of the procedure. Training should be multidisciplinary, and to prevent elitism should be a collaborative initiative.

INTERDEPARTMENTAL RELATIONSHIPS

Each PICU develops an identity and routine of its own, and care must be taken to foster collaboration with other specialists who visit and consult. It is helpful if patient management rounds are conducted collaboratively. The individuals ultimately responsible for care decisions must be clearly identified for each patient. Usually this responsibility falls to the ICU physician or the principal specialist concerned with the patient's management, e.g. the cardiac surgeon. For successful care, it is important that the roles and working relationships of each member of the team are understood by all the staff providing care. For example, the role of a nurse caring for a dying child is likely to overlap with those of the chaplain and the social worker. Each will play a greater or lesser role, depending on the unique set of circumstances that exist. Interdisciplinary relationships should be enriching and cooperative, adding to rather than detracting from care. Staff from different disciplines must be able to communicate openly with each other, within the unit and outside. As staff must make quick decisions in stressful situations, mutual trust is a key attribute. Where conflict or disagreement occurs, this should be addressed in a timely manner. Discussion following disagreement, away from the bedside, will often suffice. When senior staff need to be involved, each person should be listened to and whenever possible a consensus reached. Where agreement is not possible, policies should be set to manage similar situations in the future in the most constructive manner.

POLICIES AND PROCEDURES

Senior medical and nursing staff create the policies, procedures and organizational structure necessary to produce optimal patient outcome. Where possible, these policies should equate with 'best practice' in a national or international context, and provide staff with guidelines that are clear and consistent with those of the overall organization to which they belong.

Because PICU care is often emergent; such policies need to be reviewed as part of continuing education, and should be flexible enough to meet the needs of all the patients, families and staff in the unit. The PICU works at the leading edge of medical practice, and staff should be encouraged to be innovative in their approach to care. All units need regular management and planning meetings and review processes (e.g. 'continuous quality improvement') in addition to local, state or national standards review processes. Through these mechanisms, practices can be reviewed regularly in the context of patient outcomes. Patient databases containing a comprehensive bank of information should be developed (Ch. 5.4). These assist with the evaluation of overall performance and particular forms of treatment. Other important forums for review are morbidity and mortality audits and multidisciplinary case reviews.

STAFF DEVELOPMENT

Support and staff development through comprehensive orientation, the use of preceptorship and research and education programs are extremely important. Having a clinical nurse educator/specialist to support education and research is beneficial; new staff coming to the unit are oriented more effectively, and clinical competence and credibility are maintained by this approach. In many countries national or state staffing criteria exist and should be adopted by all units.

Regular evaluation and review of staff performance are important. This process assists staff to set professional goals and provides them with individual feedback. The evaluation process could include a mechanism for retraining, counseling and support, should the need occur. A stress management program should be in place to deal with adverse effects of critical incidents, and to prevent staff 'burn-out'. Such a program should identify resource personnel and can use formal or informal defusing or debriefing sessions, or peer support.

INTERACTIONS WITH FAMILIES

Children are often admitted to a PICU unexpectedly or with life-threatening conditions. Families find such situations and the environment very stressful. Each family member may react to this stress differently, perhaps displaying anger, shock or stoicism, and staff need to help them experience their emotions as constructively as possible. No child in a PICU should ever be cared for in isolation from the family unit; all elements of care should be family-oriented. For this care to be most effective, parents must be made welcome and encouraged to be part of the care process from the moment the child is admitted. Family-centered care practices are being actively implemented in many units; these practices acknowledge the central role of the family and describe care based on the promotion of policies, programs, and practices that support rather than supplant the family (Ch 5.5).

In the past, visiting hours in PICUs were very restrictive. Open visiting can be beneficial to both the child and the family. Some rationalization may be necessary (such as a limit on the number of people visiting at one time) to ensure the environment is kept comfortable and appropriate for other patients, their families and staff. Families also need to know who the hospital staff members are and that there may be a great many people involved in their child's care. Knowing the main roles of the different individuals is important too if parents are to understand how their child's care is being delivered, and have their questions answered effectively.

Some families retain the view that anything a doctor believes to be necessary is acceptable, but this view is being increasingly questioned. Most parents want to hear about the treatment options available and do not agree to medical action being undertaken without their knowledge except in an absolute emergency.

The question of control is often a big issue for parents in a time of crisis, yet it is at just these times that control effectively sits with the medical team and not with the parents themselves. Although parents can in theory reject any form of treatment, their lack of knowledge and experience usually means that they rely on the judgment of hospital staff. Thus the sharing of information is extremely important; families who have frequent, informative and easily understood updates from medical and nursing staff are more likely to trust the medical team and feel able to share the decision-making process on behalf of their child. The more critical the situation, the more important it is to have one physician who is the principal communicator on all key issues to reduce the chance of misinformation or conflicting information being given, and families need to know how to contact this individual when questions arise.

To provide continuity of care, the same nurse should ideally be assigned to a patient on consecutive days, even though the rostering of 12-hour shifts does limit the number of days each nurse is available. For long-term patients, primary nurses should be identified so that one or two nurses oversee the child's care. For families who have difficulty with the language, using staff who speak the family's native language, asking relatives to visit who can translate and making use of interpreter services should be encouraged. Communication is also important when families cannot stay with their children. Units should have a policy for regular telephone calls to be made to update parents on their child's condition. When families are from out of town it is reassuring to know regular updates will occur and that long-distance charges for the family will be kept to a minimum.

The issue of informed consent is important (Ch. 5.7). Although signing a generic consent form implies that a parent agrees with their child receiving care, when does consent for individual procedures start and end? For example, should an intraarterial monitoring line be inserted with or without additional specific consent? How these issues are addressed will differ depending on the cultural norms and legal practices of the country concerned, but it is an issue of practice increasingly under question. Research consent is another issue. Parents should not feel pressured to enroll their child in research but equally should not fail to realize that the care they are receiving has probably evolved from research. Again, trust based on conscientious communication is a key element in obtaining truly informed consent.

Another challenge to traditional patterns of practice concerns the presence of parents in the unit during major procedures, including resuscitation. Research indicates several potentially positive elements to parents being present during a variety of procedures, and some parents are reluctant to leave during resuscitation of their child. This can present difficulties for staff, many of whom believe they will experience 'performance anxiety' or do not feel comfortable with parents observing difficult procedures or cardiopulmonary resuscitation. There are a number of ways of approaching this. Try to achieve a compromise between the needs of the parents and maintaining an environment where staff feel able to provide effective treatment or resuscitation. One solution is to have parents supported by a nurse, pastoral care worker or social worker, watching from a discreet distance. For resuscitation in the emergency room or during initial care in a smaller hospital the staff must initiate and maintain a dialog with the child's family. Bringing the parents in briefly during resuscitation, and particularly allowing them to be with their child before CPR is terminated if the child is to be declared dead, helps them to comprehend that everything possible has been done (Ch. 5.8).

The diversity of ethnic cultures, complexity of family dynamics and even what constitutes a family today can present difficulties for staff. All the trends and social variations present in modern society will be encountered in the intensive care environment. Parents may have divorced and remarried; guardianship may be shared; there may be extended family or blended family issues; and elements of violence, drug abuse or other social dysfunctions may present themselves. These issues are often long-standing and cannot be changed by the ICU team. The most useful approach is for staff to develop a care plan early in the admission, so that both family and staff know what the care plan involves and what behavior will and will not be acceptable. Some issues should be managed primarily by the social work team or welfare agency; their help should be sought if family discord such as disagreements on treatment options prevent staff from managing the child's illness effectively.

THE PICU AS PART OF THE COMMUNITY SETTING

The PICU is not a unit in isolation but a resource for the hospital as a whole and the community it serves. Inevitably, there is competition for funding in an era of shrinking resources. To maintain an equitable share of the budget, managers must use resources efficiently. There are a number of different tools that can be used to assist with this; such as outcome measures, severity of illness measures, mortality and morbidity measures, comparison between comparable institutions by setting 'benchmarks' and nursing dependency measures.

OUTREACH ACTIVITIES

Tertiary care PICUs provide support to other centers in the community in a number of ways; one way is through telephone advice on management and transport (Ch. 1.5). Another is via outreach education. This will include many topics related to critical care and it is ideal for both physicians and nurses to participate. Particularly important opportunities often follow emergency transfer from one institution to another or situations where the telephone advice process is used.

✔ KEY POINTS

➤ The PICU is a dynamic, ever-changing environment.
➤ Skilled staff from many disciplines must work as a team and should draw on each other's strengths
➤ Trust and flexibility are key elements
➤ Care must be based on sound research and established policies and procedures; strong leadership ensures that this occurs
➤ Care should be family-oriented
➤ Support should be available to alleviate unusual levels of stress
➤ Open communication must be maintained between professionals and with families
➤ Continuing medical education (internal and outreach) is necessary

✘ COMMON ERRORS

➤ Unclear chain of command
➤ Rigidity—failure to recognize evolving therapies and technology
➤ Restrictive practices (e.g. visiting policies, limited roles for parents, narrow or outdated policies)
➤ Suboptimal communication
➤ Greater reliance on technology than on the attributes of personnel

FURTHER READING

1. Fein A. The critical care unit: In search of management. Crit Care Clin 1993; 9(3): 401–413
2. Baggs JG. Intensive care unit use and collaboration between nurses and physicians. Heart Lung 1989;18(4): 332–338
3. Canadian Nurses Association. Canadian clinical nurse specialists standards. Canadian Nurses Association 1997
– (Three papers addressing management and staff interaction strategies and nursing standards)

4. Heuer L. Parental stressors in a pediatric intensive care unit. Pediatr Nurs 1993;19(2): 128–131
5. Letourneau A. Family focus/family support: policy and resource issues. Aims Perspect 1988; 2: 2–3
6. Hanson C, Strawser D. Family presence during cardiopulmonary resuscitation: Foote Hospital emergency department's nine-year perspective. J Emerg Nurs 1992; 18(2): 104–106
7. Adams S, Whitlock M, Baskett P, Bloomfield P, Higgs R. Should relatives be allowed to watch resuscitation? Br Med J 1994; 308(6945): 1687–1689
8. Bauchner H, Vinci R, May A. Teaching parents how to comfort their children during common medical procedures. Arch Dis Child 1994; 70: 548–550
9. Macnab AJ, Emerton-Downey J, Phillips N, Susak L. The purpose of family photographs displayed in the pediatric ICU. Heart Lung 1997; 26: 68–75
– (Six publications on the role of families in critical care, their participation in resuscitation and measures that can be recommended to them to involve them constructively in their child's care and their families' sense of wellbeing)

10. Jefferson R, Northway T. Staff helping staff— establishment of a critical incident stress management team in a tertiary care centre. Offic J CACCN 1996; 7(1): 19–22
– (Support strategy for staff stress management in critical care)

5.7   Ethical, legal and social aspects of care

Adrianus J. van Vught, Reinoud J.B.J. Gemke and Theo van Willigenburg

The purpose of intensive care is to use personnel and equipment to monitor, support and if necessary take over vital functions, with the aim of preventing death and gaining time for further medical or surgical treatment or for spontaneous recovery (Ch. 1.1). Treatment of critically ill children can be started or continued even when failure of respiration or circulation would normally have ended life in situations outside a formal intensive care unit.

Ultimately, however, care in a PICU is usually a prerequisite for a successful outcome unless only short-term care is required. Support of failing vital functions should not merely prevent death but should act as a bridge to recovery. However, in critical illness recovery may not follow, may be incomplete, or the patient may remain dependent on life support. Merely keeping the patient alive may result in an unacceptable level of recovery, with life below the minimum acceptable limits of quality, comfort and happiness. Also, the physical or mental toll of the treatment may come to exceed the gain of health and happiness. These limits, a minimum acceptable quality of life and a maximum acceptable level of physical and mental burden to a patient, are very difficult to assess. Differing medical and ethical views about these limits confront us with the question of patient autonomy.

Intensive care is increasingly expensive. To justify this expense, care must be effective and efficient (Ch. 5.11), with realistic aims achieved within acceptable costs. To do this goals must be clearly defined. The ultimate goal of intensive care is to bridge critical failure of vital functions in a cost-effective way, to allow as many patients as possible to survive to live a life of acceptable quality. What is an acceptable life for each child must be determined within a framework of patient autonomy according to the subjective and possibly diverging views of the hospital staff and the child's family. In children this assessment is complicated by legal issues such as the competence of the child, and the rights and competence of the parents or other caregivers to decide on vital questions, and by the particular emotional relationships that surround the child.

WORKING IN A MULTIDISCIPLINARY TEAM

Successful management of a critically ill child involves the collaboration of many people with different professional backgrounds (Ch. 5.6). Communication within the team is pivotal and lines of communication must be clearly defined (Ch. 1.1). Conflicts must be identified promptly and resolved effectively.

Frustration within the treatment team occurs because of:

- lack of a clear treatment plan
- responsibilities that are not clearly defined or not fully accepted
- unfulfilled expectations of involvement of other team members

INFORMED CONSENT

Quality intensive care involves good communication. At each stage of treatment, all available, relevant information must be provided in terms that can be readily understood to allow the family to comprehend and accept difficult decisions. This is the moral right of the parents and a formal legal obligation of the physician in charge. Complex information is explained and assimilated differently by different people. This can confuse parents and cause distrust, especially if they seek and are given opinions by several staff members. Hence the need for one member of the team to be primarily responsible for keeping parents appropriately informed (Ch. 5.6).

By law in democracies, a patient must be completely informed about the aims and possible consequences of any medical treatment, and must give full and voluntary consent, whether this treatment is routine or experimental. This is indicated by the term 'informed consent'. In an emergency, if no one is available to give consent, the physician may assume consent to treat the patient in the patient's best interests, but actual consent must be obtained at the first opportunity. Informed consent implies a *legally competent* patient: that is, one who is capable of understanding the information, can assess its significance, can base a treatment decision upon it, and can assess the merits of alternative treatments. By law, competence to give consent for medical treatment requires a minimum age, which varies under different judicial systems. If a person is not competent to give informed consent, this must be given by a competent legal surrogate. For children, the usual surrogate is a parent or a legal guardian. Treating physicians are morally obliged to provide full information. Information should be expressed in simple, everyday terms and must not be selective or presented in such a way that there is no real choice. The patient and parents must be free and also *feel* free to decide whether they want the proposed treatment or not (Table 5.7.1).

STARTING, CONTINUING AND FORGOING TREATMENT

The justification for intensive care treatment (supporting life to achieve survival with an acceptable quality of existence) assumes that the results of the treatment (both mortality and long-term morbidity) are known. Predictions of the results of treat-

---

TABLE 5.7.1 **Informed consent**
• Is the patient legally competent?
• If not, who is the legal guardian?
• Is the patient, regardless of legal competence, able to:
– understand the information?
– use the information to make a free decision?
– understand the significance of alternative options?
• Has all relevant information been given in an understandable way?
• Is the decision freely made and do the child and parents feel free to make their own decision?

---

ment must be based on corroborated studies on large numbers of patients; personal experience alone is insufficient. For most diseases where admission to the PICU is considered essential and treatment is straightforward, the complication rate and outcome are good. On the other hand, for some diseases there is a significant risk of a poor or undesired outcome, and for others, likely outcome is not yet known. In some conditions where prognosis has been bad in the past, new treatments may be available, but without sufficient data for the results to be fully evaluated (e.g. the Norwood operation for hypoplastic left heart syndrome). The decision to treat or not to treat such conditions has to be based on the best outcome data available.

The benefits and risks of treatment and whether these are acceptable or unacceptable have to be evaluated for each individual. This introduces additional questions:

- what is acceptable for the child (will treatment and the future be bearable)?
- what is acceptable for the parents (what is their opinion about the best interests of their child?

The answers to these two questions are not necessarily the same. Other considerations are:

- what is acceptable in terms of cost or resource utilization?
- what is acceptable to the treatment team?
- who should take the final decision and on what grounds?

An element of subjectivity in such judgments is inevitable and therefore differences of opinion occur. A process (ideally a protocol) must be available to deal with disagreement within the team or between the team and the patient or parents (Table 5.7.2).

Clearly, decisions concerning starting or forgoing treatment must follow discussion involving the members of the treatment team from inside and outside the PICU, the patient and the parents or guardian. The PICU medical and nursing staff play a central role in this discussion, because of their knowledge of what life-supporting treatments can and cannot achieve, what they involve, and because of their role in delivering the child's care.

TABLE 5.7.2 **Is starting or continuing life support in the best interests of the child?**
<ul><li>What is the probable outcome?</li><li>If complete recovery is not a realistic expectation, what could the anticipated handicaps mean<ul><li>– for the child, in terms of pain and suffering, self-sufficiency, communication</li><li>– for this particular family, in terms of emotional, social and financial burden given the available support</li></ul></li><li>Given the probability of a particular outcome for this child and family, should treatment be started, continued or withdrawn?<ul><li>– is there consensus within the PICU team?</li><li>– are the parents well informed, and do they agree with the arguments and conclusions?</li><li>– what are the relevant legal regulations in this situation?</li></ul></li><li>Would a second opinion be helpful?</li><li>Is transfer to another unit an option?</li><li>Is a child protection order necessary or appropriate?</li><li>Who will take the final decision?</li><li>If treatment will be withdrawn, how will discomfort be prevented?</li><li>Who will care for the child and the family after they leave the PICU?</li></ul>

Frequently, emergency treatment is started assuming a good prognosis, but it becomes evident during subsequent care that the outlook is worse than expected. A full discussion of possible outcomes is often not undertaken, with most physicians tending to give their patients the benefit of the doubt, even when outcomes are uncertain. Ethicists and lawyers now agree that in practical terms there is no difference between not starting a treatment (because it is useless or inappropriate), and withdrawing a treatment that in retrospect should not have been started (because it turned out to be useless or inappropriate). However, many caregivers do tend to regard these two situations as being different. Although they often do so on emotional and nonrational grounds, this should not be allowed to influence decisions regarding whether or not to continue treatment when the prospect of acceptable survival has disappeared.

DNR ORDERS

The first published and openly discussed limitation of treatment in severely ill patients was through the 'do not resuscitate' (DNR) orders in 1979 from Massachusetts General Hospital and Beth Israel Hospital in Boston. It was the first clear recognition that limits can and must be set on the treatment of such patients in a technologically advanced environment. However, DNR orders raise a large number of questions. First, what exactly is meant by resuscitation? Does it mean chest compression or i.v. epinephrine (adrenaline)? What about tracheal suctioning and mask ventilation? To what extent is other supportive treatment indicated? What does resuscitation mean in a patient who is already aggressively supported by ventilation and high doses of inotropes? A DNR order which is not specified further is open to interpretation in a variety of ways, even within the same unit, with the result that appropriate or desired treatments may be waived inappropriately.

Second, is informed consent required for a DNR order, and if consent is not available, should a patient always be resuscitated with all available treatment instituted whatever the expected outcome or cost? Resuscitation is now regarded as a medical treatment for which there must be an indication (considering its aims, benefits, risks and results), rather than a mere terminal formality. Informed consent is not needed to forgo treatments that are not indicated, including resuscitation. For this reason it has been proposed that 'cardiopulmonary resuscitation not indicated' orders should be substituted for DNR orders.

Even 'resuscitation not indicated' orders can be improved upon, and ideally *care plans* should replace them on written orders in which the resuscitation and comfort treatments that are indicated for that patient are clearly set out, as well as those that are not. These care plans should be based on realistic outcome expectations and designed to provide maximum comfort for the patient even when curative treatment is futile. The plan must be fully communicated to the child and/or family, unequivocally set out in the medical orders, and the process documented in the records.

INTRAVENOUS FLUIDS AND TUBE FEEDING

In patients who have no realistic prospect of an acceptable level of intact survival, a decision must be made regarding intravenous fluid administration and tube feeding. Both are medical treatments, for which there must be an indication. The fact that these treatments are simple to institute is irrelevant. The decision to start or continue parenteral fluids or tube feeding must meet the same criteria as any other medical treatment. The following questions need to be addressed:

- what is the aim of treatment?
- will i.v. fluids and tube feeding achieve that aim?
- what are their expected benefits, risks and the expected outcome?
- do the patient, parents or guardian agree to further treatment?

Forgoing i.v. fluids and tube feeding does not imply forgoing the care needed to maintain comfort. If there is concern that hunger may cause discomfort, such discomfort must be prevented by analgesia or sedation or by the provision of feeds. It always remains the responsibility of the physician to relieve discomfort by any available means.

EUTHANASIA

Euthanasia (derived from the Greek word meaning 'a good death') is defined as the purposeful ending of the life of a competent person with insight into his or her own physical and psychological condition, on his or her own voluntary, serious and repeated request. In nearly all countries euthanasia is against the law, but in some countries it may remain unpunished, if a number of strict conditions are met:

- advanced stage and severity of illness
- unacceptable degree of suffering
- lack of effective alternative treatment
- agreement of an independent second opinion
- adequate documentation and legal testability

Because euthanasia involves the purposeful ending of life on the repeated request of the patient, it is seldom appropriate or applicable in children. The deliberate termination of life of severely handicapped, legally incompetent infants goes unpunished in some societies because there is no reasonable alternative to severe suffering and no likelihood of a meaningful life, but this should be distinguished from euthanasia in the defined (legal) sense.

'Passive euthanasia' is an outdated term which refers to withholding, withdrawal or limitation of futile life-lengthening therapy. Throughout the history of medicine this has been regarded as appropriate. Discussions on withholding, withdrawing or limiting life-prolonging therapy, or purposeful termination of life, are situations which are highly emotionally charged and often confused by misunderstanding, unspoken feelings and subjective opinions. Such discussions are also often hampered by ill-defined or inaccurately used terminology, misunderstanding of the law or legal procedures and poorly documented earlier decisions.

ETHICAL DISCUSSION AND DECISION-MAKING

The overriding consideration in decisions about starting, forgoing, continuing or withdrawing treatment (Table 5.7.3) is what is in the best interests of the patient (see Table 5.7.2). The opinion of the well-informed patient and family should carry great weight in the discussion process (see Table 5.7.1). If there is no consensus within the treat-

---

TABLE 5.7.3 Treatment options for the critically ill

- Full unlimited treatment: Admit to or stay in the PICU
- Full treatment until vital functions fail: Stay in the general ward, for i.v. fluids, tube feeding, physiotherapy, oxygen, antibiotics and comfort care
- No additional treatment beyond that now being given: stay either in the ward or in the PICU
- Withdraw life-supporting treatment: if appropriate, transfer to the ward or home for full comfort care

Note—a DNR order is not specified as an option

ment team or between the team and the patient or parents, the next step is to reach agreement by negotiation.

The ethical implications of the different options are the usual source of disagreement. In a society (and PICU) where moral freedom is fundamental and moral pluralism an inevitable fact, a basic ethical discussion is often required. The aim of an ethical discussion is to clarify in moral terms the arguments for and against a given decision and its alternatives, in order to reach agreement by persuasion. In a free ethical discussion, four points are essential:

- discussion is based on generally accepted moral principles about what is good or bad, and acceptable or not acceptable
- the discussion must be nondogmatic, i.e. not based on moral authorities or fixed precepts
- discussion is based on argument and reason
- all views are considered seriously

In most ethical textbooks and discussions four fundamental moral principles are generally accepted:

- principle of nonmaleficence: *do no harm*
- principle of beneficence: *do good*
- principle of self-determination: *respect the autonomy of child and family*
- principle of justice: *distribute scarce good fairly*

These four principles are not always considered to be of equal weight in all circumstances and may sometimes conflict. In any ethical discussion the principles involved must be explicitly stated. In the case of conflict between these principles, priorities must be allocated among them. For example, if acceding to one family's demand for a heart transplant would consume funds needed to save 100 lives by immunization, staff may decide that the principle of justice takes precedence over the principle of autonomy. If after ample discussion there is still no consensus, some solution must be reached. This may be a compromise, a decision by the majority or by the physician with overall responsibility, or a procedure that respects and does justice to the moral feelings of all involved. Whatever the outcome of the discussion, the process must be clear, open and fully documented.

It is remarkable that if the patient or the parents are kept well informed at all stages of the illness and participate in the decision-making process, there is usually no deep conflict between their expectations and opinions and those of the treatment team. Any disagreement is usually emotionally based and caused by nonacceptance of bad news, which requires more time, or occurs because of suboptimal communication which requires further explanation and discussion. It is necessary to recognize the emotional nature of the process and the underlying problems of acceptance. If after full explanation, analysis and discussion, the disagreement remains, a protocol for proper settlement of the conflict must be available. This may involve a second opinion, transfer of the patient to another center or, as a last resort, the legal system may be used to sanction a management plan contrary to one party's wishes. Once again this process must be clear, open and well-documented.

✓ KEY POINTS

- ➤ Establish well-defined lines of communication and decision-making
- ➤ Designate one physician as primarily responsible for communication with the family
- ➤ Futile therapies should be discontinued
- ➤ Dyspnea, pain, anxiety and other discomfort must be relieved, even if this accelerates death
- ➤ There is no ethical or (in most countries) legal difference between withholding and withdrawing treatment
- ➤ Replace DNR orders with a detailed plan for treatment and comfort care, including listing exactly what forms of resuscitation are and are not indicated
- ➤ Tube feeding and i.v. fluids are medical procedures and are only used if justified
- ➤ Discussions regarding withholding, limiting and withdrawing treatment are necessary, need time and good communication, and must be transparent, open and documented
- ➤ A well-defined process is necessary to address any ethical disagreement within the PICU team or with the parents
- ➤ Ethical standards change over time to reflect the technological, social and cultural norms current in society

FURTHER READING

1. Beauchamps TL, Childress JF. Principles of bio-medical ethics. Oxford University Press, 1994
   – *(A standard textbook of ethics, with a thorough discussion of the moral principles and ethical methods as applied to biomedical practice)*

2. Truog R, Burns J, Rogers MC. Ethics. In: Tibboel D, van der Voort E, editors. Intensive care in childhood; a challenge to the future. Update in Intensive Care and Emergency Medicine 25. Berlin: Springer; 1996

3. Carnevale FA. 'Good' medicine: ethics and pediatric critical care. In: Tibboel D, van der Voort E, editors. Intensive care in childhood; a challenge to the future. Update in Intensive Care and Emergency Medicine 25. Berlin: Springer; 1996

   – *(Two reviews of current ethical and legal questions in pediatric intensive care, with extensive lists of references)*

4. Waller DA, Todres ID, Cassem NH, Anderten A. Coping with poor prognosis in the pediatric intensive care unit. Am J Dis Child 1979; 133: 1121–1125
   – *(A discussion of parental denial of their child's bad prognosis)*

5. Luce JM. Physicians do not have a responsibility to provide futile or unreasonable care if a patient or family insists. Crit Care Med 1995; 23: 760–766
   – *(A review of the literature and position papers which concludes that compelling ethical principles exist which support this position)*

5.8   Death, brain death and related decisions

Mary M. Bennett

The death of a patient, particularly a child, is always a distressing event. Physicians in the emergency room or PICU will be more involved with death than most. The majority of the deaths in a pediatric hospital will occur in the PICU; studies have shown that the units usually have a mortality rate of 5–10%, depending on size, patient population and patient numbers.

DEATH

Death may occur in a number of ways:

- it may be expected
- it may occur instantaneously (as in trauma)
- it may occur unexpectedly, with or without preceding illness or injury, and with or without the opportunity to prepare

Mechanisms include:

- failure of cardiopulmonary resuscitation
- declaration of brain death
- active withdrawal of support
- a decision not to resuscitate

No matter what the mode of a child's death, the physician's role must be that of advisor and support to the family. Death may be sudden and unexpected or the result of a long illness, but the finality is common. The duty of the practitioner is not only to provide good medical treatment but also to provide a good death. Often this requires physicians to come to terms with their own feelings of anger, frustration and impotence at their inability to prevent a death. However, once death occurs or is inevitable for whatever reason, the focus of care must change from provision of support to the patient, to provision of support to the family. Some families may prefer their child to die during a prolonged attempt at CPR (and some hospitals encourage parents to witness this), but in most situations the chance to say goodbye (ideally in peaceful surroundings) is very important. The family needs to have information conveyed in as compassionate a manner as possible. Assurances that the child will be or has been kept as comfortable as possible are very important. If possible, one physician should take responsibility for all major communication with the family. The child should be in or be moved to as private a place as possible, at least a curtained corner cubicle, and preferably a private room. Religious or cultural practices should be encouraged so long as they are not harmful to the child.

When death is inevitable it should not be prolonged, particularly if withdrawal of support is planned, but time should be made for visits by relatives (and friends). The parents should be encouraged to hold the child. Mistakenly, this is often discouraged out of concern that it may hasten the death, particularly if the child is cardiovascularly unstable, but such considerations do not make sense. Interventions should be minimized. Unless absolutely necessary, suctioning and other medical handling of the child except for comfort care should be minimized. Monitors should be turned down or monitoring discontinued altogether if this does not distress parents. A single heart-rate monitor can be helpful, but none is preferable.

Parents should be prepared as much as possible for the realities and medical necessities of death. If a child has been declared brain dead, there is often some urgency to go to the operating room. The parents should be made aware of this during discussions of organ donation. If ventilation is being withdrawn the families can be offered the opportunity to remain with the child or return once the child has died. If they wish to stay, they should be told how the child will look, including the possibility of terminal gasping. Assurances that this is a nonpainful reflex are important.

The presence of a nurse, and often a physician, in the room during the dying process is important and can be helpful. Drugs may be used if the patient appears uncomfortable but doses should be consistent with sedative doses and all doses should be documented in the patient's chart. Active euthanasia is not legal in most countries so correct dosage is important. When using sedative doses, it may be that death is hastened but this is acceptable for provision of comfort—the principle of double effect. Morphine in titrated doses of 0.1 mg/kg per dose, or as an infusion is probably the most commonly used sedative and pain reliever. There is no place for paralyzing agents at the time of treatment withdrawal. In children with multi-organ failure and decreased drug metabolism, there is much ethical argument as to whether all muscle relaxant effects from drugs given previously must have worn off prior to withdrawal. This is likely to prolong the dying process by hours or days, and approximately 50% of PICU physicians would not wait. However, a comparable number would feel that the presence of any muscle relaxant contraindicates withdrawal.

Whether or not the parents have been present at the death, they should be encouraged to spend time with the child after death. Depending on the legal circumstances, as many tubes and lines should be removed as possible, particularly from the face. For autopsy purposes, the coroner and pathologist may dictate what can be removed. This should be clarified in each institution. Removal of tape marks, blood, etc., to make the child look more normal is always appreciated. Some religions and cultural traditions are very specific about who should wash and dress the body after death and these customs should always be respected wherever possible.

Postmortem examinations are useful for the physicians and for the family. Many physicians feel uncomfortable asking for an autopsy. If possible, the question of autopsy should be brought up prior to the death of the child. In coroner's cases, an autopsy may be a legal requirement. The parents should have this discussed with them and their agreement obtained if possible. Rules for reporting to the coroner will vary from jurisdiction to jurisdiction but will generally include any sudden, unexpected deaths at home, death within 24 hours of hospitalization or surgery, and any deaths with legal ramifications (child abuse, homicide, suicide).

In cases of death occurring after a long illness, parents are often reluctant to have any more done to the child. If the cause of death is obvious and

nonsuspicious and parents refuse autopsy, the physician can do no more than ask. Often a discussion of what might be learned from an autopsy and an offer of a limited autopsy (e.g. the cardiovascular system in a cardiac patient) will be persuasive. If the physician feels unable to sign the death certificate because of uncertainty about the cause of death, the coroner should be notified. A decision will then be made as to whether an autopsy will be ordered.

There are many cultures that generally do not allow autopsy, but the situation should always be explained and the request made. Studies have shown that the main cause for low autopsy rates is a low request rate. Enlisting another caregiver, for example a family physician who knows the family well, may also help with obtaining parental consent.

Once the child's body has been removed, support should continue from social work, pastoral care, and other services as appropriate. Many units have bereavement plans, including mementos of the child, and follow-up checks at specified intervals in ongoing support of the families. This is important because, while medical staff move onto the next patient, death is only the beginning of a long process for the family.

BRAIN DEATH

The diagnosis of brain death has been a relatively recent advance. The need for a definition of brain death has arisen owing to the rapid expansion of transplant medicine and the increase in medical technology. In the past, death occurred when either the patient stopped breathing or the heart stopped beating. With intensive care, ventilators and inotropes, the body can be supported long after evidence of CNS function has ceased. This is important in the maintenance of organs for transplant, but has given rise to controversy about how to define and diagnose death. Many questions surround brain death criteria, particularly in infants and children. Some important questions include whether or not ancillary tests are necessary (or more valid) to establish brain death (beyond history, physical examination and exclusion of confounding variables), and if certain time intervals must be observed between triggering events, physical examination for signs of brain death and pronouncement.

Brain death criteria are all in agreement that there must be a known diagnosis for the cessation of CNS function (e.g. hypoxic ischemic encephalopathy secondary to cardiac or respiratory arrest, severe head injury), demonstration of irreversibility of state, and a lack of confounding factors such as hypothermia, shock or drug effects. In other respects different brain death criteria do have small variations. (Tables 5.8.1, 5.8.2). You should be aware of those in place in your jurisdiction. Most authors now agree that except in very immature preterm newborns, the same criteria of brain death apply to fullterm newborns, infants more than 7 days old, children and adults.

One of the most controversial areas in brain death testing is the use of corroborative studies to give an objective definition for brain death. Most people now agree that these are useful in the patient with confounding factors such as hypothermia or barbiturates, but in the absence of any such factors, reliance on clinical brain death determination is adequate.

Some of the commonly used corroborative tests include EEG, cerebral angiography and radionuclide flow studies. An EEG was initially required by the Harvard criteria. These can be technically difficult to perform on infants and small children. There may also be EEG activity in patients who fulfill all clinical brain death criteria (all such patients have subsequently died). Conversely, the EEG may be suppressed in many other clinical settings; e.g. shock, hypothermia and drug intoxication. The EEG must be interpreted with caution in premature

---

TABLE 5.8.2 Medical consultants to the President's Commission on Brain Death Criteria (1982)

- Absence of hypothermia, shock, drug intoxication
- Cerebral unresponsiveness
- Apnea with $P_{CO_2} > 8$ kPa (60 mmHg) and O_2 insufflation
- Absent brain-stem reflexes – pupillary, corneal, oculovestibular, oculocephalic, oropharyngeal
- Observation for 6 hours if corroborative testing is used
- Observation for 12 hours if corroborative testing is not used
- Corroborative tests may include EEG, cerebral angiography, radionuclide flow study

These criteria were not recommended for use in children under 5 years old

---

neonates. Therefore, although this test is easily done, the information provided may not be conclusive. Other authors feel that the demonstration of absent intracranial circulation is the best confirmation of brain death; as absent cerebral flow is incompatible with neuronal survival. Radionuclide Tc 99m flow studies and four-vessel angiography have both been used. Both techniques have limitations and are often technically difficult to interpret in infants; they also entail moving patients who are often unstable to areas where these tests can be performed. Evoked potential (EP) studies (brain-stem auditory EP, visual EP, somatosensory EP) have also been used as corroborative tests, but have limitations. None of these corroborative tests has been found to be consistent and foolproof and their use has fallen out of favor for declaration of brain death for this reason.

Most jurisdictions now accept clinical brain death criteria (but this will vary from hospital to hospital). A generally accepted brain death examination includes:

- examination by two separate physicians from the neurology or neurosurgery departments or the PICU
- known cause for brain death
- observation period of at least 12 hours for older children, 24 hours for infants: a single examination is acceptable for older children after 12 hours, two examinations 12 hours apart may be done in children less than 1 year of age

---

TABLE 5.8.1 The Harvard brain death criteria (1968)

- Unresponsiveness, temperature > 32.2°C
- Absence of depressant drugs
- No spontaneous movements
- Apnea off ventilator for 3 minutes at room air
- No reflexes, including: decerebrate or decorticate posturing, pupils fixed and dilated, swallowing, vocalization, corneal and pharyngeal reflexes, stretch and deep tendon reflexes
- Isoelectric EEG

All of the above should be repeated after 24 hours

- normothermia with core temperature above 33°C
- absence of sedative drugs, reversal of all muscle relaxants and confirmation with nerve stimulator if any doubt
- cerebral unresponsiveness
- absence of brain-stem reflexes—doll's eye, gag, cough, cold caloric, corneal and pupillary reflexes
- apnea with a rise in P_{CO_2} to 8 kPa (60 mmHg) (this will generally take at least 5 minutes); the patient must be nonhypoxic which is ensured by insufflation of oxygen down the endotracheal tube
- absence of deep tendon reflexes (some spinal reflexes may be seen)

If there is absence of response to these tests, the diagnosis of brain death is confirmed. Corroborative testing is not used because of the limitations discussed above.

Once brain death is confirmed, if the patient is to be an organ donor, the formal time of death is documented as the time of brain death and the procedures for organ donation can continue. In many places, the coroner must be informed and permission for organ donation obtained.

If the patient is not a donor, the parents are informed. At that point discussion of discontinuation of therapy can occur. It must be remembered that some cultures do not accept the diagnosis of brain death. These can be difficult situations, and occasionally allowing the family to be present at brain death testing will be helpful. A patient who has become brain dead will show increasing cardiac instability usually over the following 12–36 hours, and the need for active withdrawal of support may be obviated. In situations in which the family continues to be unable to accept the diagnosis, ethics committee assistance may be useful. However, once a diagnosis of brain death exists, a physician is not obliged to continue therapy and the goal of an appropriate withdrawal of therapy should be pursued.

THE DECISION TO RESUSCITATE

Cardiopulmonary resuscitation is a relatively recent addition to medicine. With advances in technology, it is now possible to resuscitate most patients with severe illness. The use of such technology should be appropriate (Ch. 5.7). In most hospitals, the policy is that CPR is a standing order and all patients will receive it unless the orders for medical care specifically exclude this measure. Resuscitation should be undertaken with any patient where the diagnosis is unclear. However, there are situations when other orders are appropriate. Ethicists (e.g. the Bioethics Committee of the Canadian Paediatric Society) endorse withholding or withdrawing therapy under the following conditions, and the same principles should guide the writing of orders to clarify whether CPR does or does not constitute part of the child's care plan. The conditions for withholding CPR are:

- there is irreversible progression of a known terminal disease and death is imminent
- treatment will clearly be ineffective or harmful
- life will be severely shortened regardless of treatment, and abandoning treatment will allow a greater degree of caring and comfort
- the patient's life is filled with intolerable or intractable pain and suffering

A clear care plan should be written in the medical orders. Orders excluding resuscitation are appropriate in situations in which the burden of aggressive therapy outweighs the benefit of such therapy to the child, and it is felt that resuscitation is not in the child's best interest. The care plan approach is preferable to the previous practice of writing 'do not resuscitate' orders (Ch. 5.7).

Decisions about resuscitation status are made jointly by the caregivers and the child's surrogate decision-makers, usually the parents. If there is disagreement between the two, the presumption is usually made in favor of resuscitation, but no physician is bound to provide futile care. Ethics committees may be helpful in such situations.

Orders excluding resuscitation are not synonymous with withdrawal of support, and will usually be used to set a limit to aggressive management. The notorious 'slow code' or 'partial code' where the patient may be given bag-mask ventilation and chest compressions but not drugs or intubation or any such variation is totally inappropriate. Timely and clear decision-making about a patient's resuscitation status and the writing of explicit orders are absolutely necessary, and 'slow codes' should be actively discouraged.

Decisions about CPR status should be addressed early in management of children with clearly progressive degenerating illnesses or those in whom life expectancy is likely to be less than normal. Many adults have advance directives but there are generally no such documents for children. However, early and timely discussion with the family about limits of therapy can avoid hurried and inappropriate decision-making. It will also allow a child a more dignified and comfortable death.

 KEY POINTS

BRAIN DEATH

➤ Brain death can only be established after sufficient observation with all criteria fulfilled
➤ Good history-taking is essential, especially as to drugs administered at other hospitals, so appropriate levels can be checked
➤ 'Brain death' is a legal designation and may not be accepted by some cultures
➤ The time of death in the chart should be noted as the time at which brain death was certified in organ donation patients

'DO NOT RESUSCITATE'

➤ Early discussion is essential in patients in whom resuscitation would be inappropriate.
➤ 'Partial' or 'slow' codes are not appropriate
➤ Orders that do not include resuscitation do not mean withdrawal of any therapy or comfort measures, unless these have also been specifically agreed upon by parents and caregivers and included in the ordered care plan

✗ COMMON ERRORS

BRAIN DEATH

➤ Presence of sedative or muscle relaxant: (levels should be therapeutic and 'train of four' muscle stimulation confirmed prior to testing)
➤ Pronouncing brain death in a hypothermic patient: (core temperature should be greater than 33°C)
➤ Mistaking spinal reflex for higher activity: (spinal reflexes can be quite disturbing but are only reflex activity)
➤ Starting an apnea test with P_{CO_2} levels below 4.6–5.3 kPa (35–40 mmHg). A rise in P_{CO_2} of 2 kPa (15 mmHg) to 7.3 kPa (55 mmHg) must be shown
➤ Allowing hypoxia to develop during apnea testing
➤ Failure to observe the eyes for movement for at least 10 seconds during caloric testing; (ice water should be used)
➤ Not observing the patient for a sufficient time

FURTHER READING

1. Farrell MB, Levin DL. Brain death in the pediatric patient: historical, sociological, medical, religious, cultural, legal, and ethical considerations. Crit Care Med 1993; 21 (12): 1951–1965
   – (*Excellent review of brain death controversies and criteria in the pediatric setting*)
2. Vernon DD, Grant MJ, Setzer NA. Brain death, organ donation, and withdrawal of life support. In: Mark C. Rogers, editor. Textbook of paediatric intensive care, 3rd ed, Baltimore: Williams & Wilkins, 1996
   – (*Good reference list for further reading*)
3. Canadian Paediatric Society, Bioethics Committee. Treatment decision for infants and children. Can Med Assoc J 1986; 135: 447–448
4. Multi-Society Task Force on PVS. Medical aspects of the persistent vegetative state. Part I: N Engl J Med 1994; 330(21): 1499–1508; Part II: N Engl Med 1994; 330(22): 1572–1579
   – (*Consensus statement summarizing current knowledge of the persistent vegetative state in adults and children*)

5.9 Organ donation and care of the organ donor

Warwick Butt

Transplantation has become a standard therapeutic option for end-stage organ failure: transplants of heart, lung, kidney, liver and cornea are performed frequently, while those of pancreas and bowel are increasingly common.

Transplantation of solid organs for end-stage organ failure is associated with 1- and 5-year survival rates greater than 70% for most patients. The shortage of organs means that many Australian children (approximately 30%) will die on the waiting list. Increasing public awareness through education is vital, and legislation for 'opt-out' rather than 'opt-in' donation has been effective in some countries.

ETHICS OF TRANSPLANTATION

There are several different types of potential organ donor

BEATING HEART

Brain-dead donors

The concept of brain death must be acceptable to the family and to the society as a whole and the diagnosis of brain death must be clearly defined, with acceptable criteria (Ch. 5.8).

Living donors: related and unrelated

It is essential to obtain formal consent from the donor after ensuring that the donor fully understands the risks of the procedure. These donations are made to specific individuals and immunological compatibility is essential. Payment for organs is unlawful in many countries and is regarded as ethically unacceptable in most Western societies.

Anencephalic donors

Anencephalic infants have no capacity for cognition or sensory experience. Although no cerebrum is present, they have an intact brain stem and are

thus not brain dead by current criteria, so they may not become organ donors.

NONBEATING HEART

In terminally ill patients who are *not* brain dead, organs can be donated after death (e.g. removal of organs 2 minutes after cardiopulmonary arrest). Warm ischemia time may be decreased by rapidly cooling the donor before or after death (with or without cardiopulmonary bypass). After a request has been made for withdrawal of life-sustaining treatment, discussion of this procedure can be undertaken with the family of the donor.

ANIMAL DONORS

Advances in immunosuppression may make xenotransplantation more practicable, although many people regard the breeding of primates for organ donation as unacceptable.

MANAGEMENT OF A POTENTIAL ORGAN DONOR

RECOGNITION OF A POTENTIAL DONOR

Any patient who is likely to become brain dead is a potential organ donor. There are a few absolute contraindications to donation:

- disseminated malignancy
- infections such as HIV infection, hepatitis, tuberculosis, fungemia or disseminated herpes simplex
- certain inherited metabolic diseases including the mucopolysaccharidoses and primary lactic acidosis
- active autoimmune disease such as systemic lupus erythematosus
- dysfunction of the proposed donor organ (Table 5.9.1).

Because there is a shortage of donors, relative contraindications such as septicemia, or head injury

TABLE 5.9.1 **Criteria for the acceptability of individual donor organs**

Heart
- Structurally normal heart on echocardiogram
- Systolic BP > 75% of normal for age
- Cardiac index $\geq$ 2 L/min·m^2
- No metabolic acidosis
- Moderate doses of catecholamines used
  - dopamine $\leq$ 10 μg/kg·min *or*
  - epinephrine (adrenaline) $\leq$ 0.5 μg/kg·min

Lung
- Normal chest radiograph
- Pao_2 > 300 mmHg if Fio_2 = 1.0

Kidney
- Normal plasma creatinine
- Urine output $\geq$ 1 ml/kg·hr

Liver
- Normal liver function tests (other than mild changes due to terminal illness).

Pancreas
- No history of acute or chronic pancreatitis
- No history of diabetes
- No direct pancreatic trauma

Cornea
- No history of eye disease or eye surgery
- No corneal ulceration
- Age > 2 years

and cardiac arrest due to child abuse, need to be considered case by case. In a child with bacterial septicemia, for example, organisms are often cleared from the blood within 12–24 hours of the start of antibiotic treatment and that child's organs can then be transplanted safely.

For renal transplantation, one can be more selective than for heart or lung transplantation, as the child can be supported by dialysis until a suitable organ becomes available.

DIAGNOSIS OF BRAIN DEATH

The diagnosis of brain death is discussed in Chapter 5.8.

DISCUSSION WITH THE FAMILY

The potential organ donor has usually suffered an acute intracranial illness (trauma, hemorrhage or infection). Initial counseling will mention the concern about the long-term outcome and the possibility of major handicap or death. As the child's condition worsens and concerns are raised about brain death (because of fixed dilated pupils, hypothermia or polyuria), this possibility should be mentioned to the parents. The most appropriate person to discuss these issues is the senior doctor who has cared for the child during life (often an intensive care specialist), as organ donation should be seen as the final phase of care of the child and family, rather than as opportunistic 'harvesting' of organs by an uncaring team of transplant surgeons. Contact between transplant teams and the donor family is not encouraged.

An experienced nurse, social worker or chaplain will help the family deal with their child's impending death, and help them begin to understand the concept of brain death. Once the first examination for brain death has been performed, the practical realities of brain death must be discussed in detail with the family. A second and final examination will be made 4–8 hours later (perhaps the next morning): this allows the family time to think, and to accept the child's death and prepare for cessation of treatment. After the second examination confirms brain death, the family should be told of this finding and that treatment should cease. The need for a coroner's inquest (if appropriate) and organ donation may then be discussed.

Some families will have already discussed organ donation, either when death was imminent or before the child became ill. The child's wishes on the subject may even be known. In societies in which brain death and organ donation are accepted, it is the right of every family to be given the opportunity to donate the organs of a brain-dead family member. This right and the chance for some good to emerge from an otherwise unmitigated disaster, can be mentioned briefly and tactfully to the family.

Many families are concerned by the idea of mutilation of the body of a beloved child, and by the further delays in the process of cessation of treatment and burial that are imposed by organ donation. These concerns often deter families from donation. Parents can be reassured that organ removal and wound closure are similar to a normal operation. The process of investigation (see below), stabilization, organ removal and cessation of treatment is discussed step by step. Delays should be minimized and the treating medical, nursing and social work staff should be available to support the family during the waiting period.

Throughout these discussions it is best if the physician is concise and direct: at this time the family needs the truth, not to be spared or protected. In explaining brain death it is useful to show to the family the child's lack of respiratory effort and that the child's head is clearly colder than the chest. It is important to explain the difference between brain death and persistent vegetative state as many families believe the two conditions are identical. Once the child goes to the operating room, many families go home. They should be encouraged to return the next day to view the body in the company of a physician or social worker.

CONSENT FOR ORGAN DONATION

Once the second doctor has certified brain death, the patient is declared dead. If consent for organ donation is denied, treatment is discontinued after discussion with the family (Ch. 5.8).

MEDICAL CARE OF THE ORGAN DONOR

When the parents wish to donate one or more of the child's organs, the regional transplant coordinator is notified. The aim of management now changes to ensuring optimal perfusion of organs other than the brain, establishing the suitability of the patient as a donor and selecting recipients. This requires tests including blood grouping, serology for HIV, hepatitis B and C, cytomegalovirus and any other serology thought to be relevant. Permission of the coroner may be required in cases of death from trauma and when there is doubt about the diagnosis.

PROBLEMS IN MANAGEMENT OF BEATING-HEART, BRAIN-DEAD DONORS

CARDIOVASCULAR

The most common problem is hypotension due to a combination of hypovolemia (caused by fluid restriction and excess water loss due to diuretics or diabetes insipidus), vasodilation (sepsis or loss of sympathetic tone) and myocardial dysfunction.

Initially, boluses of crystalloid or colloid should be given (Ch. 2.3); invasive monitoring of arterial and central venous pressure is essential. A balloon-tipped pulmonary artery catheter can be used to estimate ventricular performance and filling pressure of the left heart, but is rarely used in these circumstances in children. Echocardiography gives a better estimate of cardiac filling and an adequate estimate of cardiac performance, noninvasively. Hypotension with a large pulse pressure means vasodilation is present and vasopressors such as norepinephrine (noradrenaline), at least 0.1 µg/kg·min may be required. If the pulse pressure is narrow (less than a third of systolic pressure), fluid resuscitation (Ch. 2.3) or inotropes such as dopamine (5–15 µg/kg·min) or epinephrine (adrenaline), at least 0.1 µg/kg·min should be used. Occasionally hemodynamic instability persists: in these circumstances, infusion of vasopressin (0.0003 units/kg·min) improves blood pressure control and urine output, and can maintain stability for up to 6 weeks (compared with 2 days with epinephrine alone). Adrenal dysfunction or hemorrhage may also contribute to hemodynamic instability in brain-dead children. Small doses of hydrocortisone 25–50 mg may correct this hypotension.

Severe, paroxysmal, centrally mediated hypertension and tachycardia in critically ill children with raised intracranial pressure can cause myocardial necrosis and damage to other organs and may require antihypertensive treatment. Blockade of adrenergic α- and β-receptors using a single drug such as labetalol, or a combination of a beta-blocker such as esmolol or atenolol and either an alpha-blocker such as phentolamine or a direct vasodilator such as sodium nitroprusside by infusion, stabilizes the blood pressure and prevents organ damage. Arrhythmias are less common in children than in adults but may occur because of electrolyte disturbance, metabolic acidosis and catecholamine use.

RESPIRATORY

Mechanical ventilation is always needed (a child who can breathe is not brain dead). The aim of intermittent positive pressure ventilation is to achieve normal arterial P_{O_2} and P_{CO_2}. Lung injury is often minimal. Carbon dioxide production is reduced because of the decrease in body and cerebral metabolism after brain death, so minimal ventilation is needed. It is important to maintain a normal functional residual capacity by using positive end-expiratory pressure (PEEP, Ch. 6.4) to prevent atelectasis with its risk of secondary bacterial infection. Fluid resuscitation is usually needed to maintain organ perfusion but fluid overload should be avoided by monitoring central venous pressure and the response to 10 ml/kg i.v. boluses of fluid. Inhalation injury due to gastric contents, saliva or smoke may be associated with cerebral injury. Infections secondary to aspiration often involve Gram-positive aerobic or anaerobic bacteria which are sensitive to penicillin G (benzyl penicillin). Corticosteroids, bronchoalveolar lavage and physiotherapy have no role in the management of acute aspiration.

Hypoxemia may occur occasionally because of cardiac or neurogenic pulmonary edema. More commonly, pulmonary edema is part of the acute respiratory distress syndrome due to the shock associated with the original injury. The use of PEEP improves gas exchange in all forms of pulmonary edema.

TEMPERATURE INSTABILITY

Loss of hypothalamic control abolishes the normal neural and endocrine response to heat loss from the child's large body surface area. The child's temperature can rapidly fall towards that of the environment. Heat loss can be minimized by the use of radiant heaters, insulation including a head bonnet, thermal mattresses and warming the inspired gases.

FLUIDS AND ELECTROLYTES

Brain-dead children are often hypovolemic but the usual clinical signs of heart rate, respiratory rate, blood pressure, capillary refill and urine output may be difficult to interpret because of impaired autonomic control. Monitoring accurate fluid balance charts is more useful than repeated weighing. Diabetes insipidus occurs in 40% of brain-dead children. Polyuria (exceeding 3 ml/kg·h (not due to

diuretic therapy) and urine osmolality less than 290 mOsm/kg (specific gravity < 1.010) associated with serum osmolality in excess of 300 mOsm/kg imply the presence of diabetes insipidus. Treatment in organ donors requires rapid replacement of fluid volume deficits, replacement of ongoing losses and administration of antidiuretic hormone. Vasopressin in oil can be given i.m., but replacement of the previous hour's urine output with 0.45% saline (or 4% dextrose and 0.18% saline) containing 2 units of aqueous vasopressin per liter is a self-regulating system which gives much more rapid and accurate control of plasma electrolytes, body water and blood pressure. Hyperglycemia is common after brain death because of glucose administration in intravenous replacement fluids and insulin resistance due to circulating catecholamines. Insulin infusion (0.1 units/kg·hr) may be needed to maintain normoglycemia.

Electrolyte abnormalities including hypernatremia, hyperkalemia and hypocalcemia occur frequently. Hypophosphatemia and hypomagnesemia develop owing to large urinary losses in diabetes insipidus. Citrate in large-volume blood transfusion causes a transient (hours) reduction in ionized calcium concentration. Hyponatremia is uncommon but is sometimes caused by administration of hypotonic fluids and vasopressin or by hypoadrenal or hypothyroid states.

COAGULATION

Coagulopathy, especially disseminated intravascular coagulation, with decreased platelet count, prolonged clotting times (PT, PTT) and increased fibrinolysis (D-dimers) is common in severe brain injury because of associated shock or the exposure of blood to tissue thromboplastins from the injured brain. Platelets and clotting factors are also reduced by dilution during massive transfusion or fluid resuscitation and are consumed by major hemorrhage. Clotting factors should be replaced (Ch. 2.8) and if there is active bleeding the platelet count should be maintained above 50×10^9/L.

ENDOCRINE

Hormone deficiencies are inconsistently found in brain-dead children and adults. Following brain death there is a rapid depletion of ADH, thyroxine, cortisol and insulin, and replacement of these hormones may improve cardiac and renal function.

TRANSPORT OF THE BRAIN-DEAD CHILD

The child's vital signs should be stabilized before transport. Adequate ventilation should be confirmed (preferably with the aid of a chest radiograph and blood gas analysis). The blood pressure and circulation should be secured as described above: if necessary with the aid of fluid resuscitation and infusions of vasopressin and inotropic drugs, and injections of hydrocortisone (1 mg/kg i.v. 8-hourly) and thyroxine.

If possible, plasma electrolytes and glucose should be assessed, and if necessary, corrective measures commenced before departure for any abnormalities found (see above). A urine catheter should be inserted, using a sterile technique and the urine volume monitored. The transport team should be prepared to begin treatment for hypotension or diabetes insipidus which may appear during transfer.

The rectal temperature is monitored and the child carefully insulated during the retrieval. The vehicle cabin temperature may have to be raised to prevent hypothermia. If formal tests have already shown that the child is brain dead and the parents have been informed and have agreed to transfer for the express purpose of organ donation, the transplant coordinator should be informed before departure of the child's condition, age, weight, height and blood group to minimize the waiting time for the family before active treatment is withdrawn.

REMOVAL OF ORGANS

While the condition of the brain-dead patient is stabilized, the transplant coordinator organizes and co-ordinates the removal of organs. Once the blood group and results of viral serology are known, a decision is made on which organs are suitable for transplantation. The various recipients are notified and the order of organ removal decided upon. The timing of surgery is arranged and the patient transferred to the operating room in the normal way. Many anesthesiologists give muscle relaxants to prevent movement due to spinal reflexes during surgery.

✔ **KEY POINTS**

➤ The senior treating doctor discusses donation with the family
➤ Families have the right to be asked if they wish to donate the organs of a brain-dead child
➤ The lungs are usually normal and ventilation requirements minimal
➤ Stabilizing the blood pressure may require fluid resuscitation, inotropes and vasopressin infusion
➤ Consider giving replacement doses of hydrocortisone, thyroxine and vasopressin
➤ Prevent heat loss
➤ Try to minimize delays and other sources of distress to the family

✗ **COMMON ERRORS**

➤ Failing to discuss organ donation with the family of a brain-dead child
➤ Discussion of organ donation before brain death is confirmed
➤ Permitting hypotension, hypothermia and pulmonary atelectasis
➤ Allowing the family to feel abandoned after treatment is withdrawn

FURTHER READING

1. Brink LW, Ballew A. Care of the pediatric organ donor. Am J Dis Child 1992; 146: 1045–1050
   – (Review of medical problems of pediatric organ donors and their management)

2. Klufas CI, Powner DJ, Darby JM, Stein KL, Grenvik A. Organ donor categories and management. In: Ayres SM, Grenvik A, Holbrook PR, Shoemaker WC, editors. Textbook of critical care, 3rd ed. Philadelphia: WB Saunders; 1995
   – (Review of the various types of organ donor, their problems and management: adult and pediatric)

3. Ralston C, Butt W. Continuous vasopressin replacement in diabetes insipidus. Arch Dis Child 1990; 65: 896–897
   – (Description of the technique)

4. Scheinkestel CD, Tuxen DV, Cooper DJ, Butt W. Medical management of the (potential) organ donor. Anaesth Intens Care 1995; 23: 51–59
– (*Review of medical problems and management: adult and pediatric*)

5. Yoshioka T, Sugimoto H, Uenishi M, Sakamoto D, Sakano T, Sugimoto T. Prolonged haemodynamic maintenance by the combined administration of vasopressin and epinephrine in brain death: a clinical study. Neurosurgery 1986; 18: 565–567
– (*Report of prolonged survival after brain death with vasopressin support*)

6. Koogler T, Costarino AT. The potential benefits of the pediatric nonheartbeating organ donor. Pediatr 1998; 101: 1049–1052
– (*Discussion of the ethical issues and potential increase in organ donation relating to use of nonheartbeating organ donors*)

5.10 Special needs (technology-dependent) children

Robert J. Adderley

Life-sustaining therapies involving the use of mechanical or electronic devices are increasingly available to extend intensive care beyond the PICU, even into the home setting. Patients using these therapies are described as 'technology-dependent'. Special units known as 'technology-dependent units' (TDUs) have evolved to care for these patients, and to manage their transition with their technology back into the community.

Those who are technology-dependent use many diverse therapies (Table 5.10.1). Those most relevant to critical care include home oxygen therapy, home tracheostomy care, and home ventilation, as patients needing these therapies are likely to spend time in the PICU setting initially.

HOME OXYGEN THERAPY

Liquid oxygen has revolutionized home oxygen therapy, introducing a degree of patient mobility denied to patients dependent on heavy tanks with compressed gases. Most patients have a stationary 'base' tank of liquid oxygen from which small, lightweight, portable modules (sometimes known as 'strollers') can be filled. Expensive when used as the sole source, liquid oxygen used judiciously in combination with a stationary (bedside) source such as an oxygen concentrator, can be economical.

TABLE 5.10.1 **Technology dependency**

- Home oxygen therapy
- Home tracheostomy care
- Home ventilation
- Home aerosolized medication
- Home intravenous therapy
- Enteral feeding (gastrostomy, jejunostomy)
- Continuous ambulatory peritoneal dialysis
- Home hemodialysis
- Home parenteral nutrition
- Subcutaneous deferoxamine (desferrioxamine) infusion

TRACHEOSTOMY CARE

Provision of a tracheostomy to facilitate long-term ventilation or to relieve upper airway obstruction, either congenital or acquired, is not new; neither is home tracheostomy care. Appreciation of the complications and risk (cumulative mortality rates of 8–27%) has led to increasing sophistication in predischarge planning and caregiver education.

Tracheostomy definitions:

- temporary tracheostomy – any tracheostomy anticipated to eventually be removed
- acute tracheostomy – a tracheostomy in situ for less than 60 days
- chronic tracheostomy – a tracheostomy in situ for more than 60 days
- permanent tracheostomy – implies laryngeal-tracheal discontinuity (either congenital, e.g. laryngeal atresia, or acquired, e.g. surgical)

Note—a child with a true 'permanent' tracheostomy cannot be intubated by the pharyngeal route.

Unlike adult intensive care units where a temporary tracheostomy to facilitate ventilation is often performed within 7–14 days, most PICUs usually defer tracheostomy for longer than 2 months. The rationale for tracheostomy is usually long-term airway maintenance or ventilatory support.

INDICATIONS

Indications for tracheostomy:

- facilitation of long-term ventilation (30%)
- airway obstruction, congenital or acquired (70%)
- decrease dead space (less than 1%)
- access to airway for pulmonary toilet (no longer usually considered an indication for chronic tracheostomy)

PROBLEMS IN TRACHEOSTOMY CARE

Small tracheostomy tubes obstruct easily with inspissated secretions; consequently, optimal humidification and appropriate suctioning are necessary to ensure airway patency. A baby with a tracheostomy may need instillation and suctioning as often as every 2 hours, whereas a teenager may be able to cough and clear secretions and rarely need suctioning.

The tracheostomy by necessity bypasses and therefore nullifies the protective functions of the nasopharynx, i.e. particle filtration, humidification, warming of inspired air, and cell-mediated and humoral immunity provided by the lymphoid tissues of the nasopharynx.

Prior to discharge home, caregivers of a child with a chronic tracheostomy must be educated (in addition to training in skills such as routine hygiene and suctioning) to recognize and deal with both acute (life-threatening) emergencies, and less serious acute and chronic problems associated with the tracheostomy.

Life-threatening emergencies

Life-threatening emergencies include:

- dislodgment
- obstruction
- catastrophic hemorrhage
- overwhelming infection

Dislodgment

Although many children with a tracheostomy (without mechanical ventilation) can breathe at least briefly through their stoma or their native airway, the signs and symptoms of dislodgment are most often those of obstruction, ie. decreased air flow, stridor, increased respiratory effort, and within a variable time frame cyanosis and eventually bradycardia.

A dislodged tracheostomy tube should be replaced as soon as possible. Usually this is easy to achieve, but occasionally, replacement can be difficult, particularly if the tube has been dislodged for some time. In this situation, the stoma should be gently probed with the blunt end of a well-lubricated feeding tube (water-soluble gel), and then dilated successively with larger tubes until a small tracheostomy tube can be inserted 'over the wire' (Seldinger technique) using the feeding tube as the guide. Once an airway has been established, it is most often prudent to let the child rest and return later to dilate the stoma (under anesthesia) to the appropriate size for the regular tracheostomy tube to be replaced. On occasion recannulation may be impossible and it may be necessary to surgically refashion the tracheostomy.

Obstruction

If an obstructed tracheostomy tube cannot be quickly cleared with instillation of saline and passage of a suction catheter, the tube should be removed and replaced.

Catastrophic hemorrhage

Catastrophic hemorrhage, a fortunately rare occurrence, may be caused by erosion of the tracheostomy tube into the innominate artery (tracheal innominate fistula). With the change from rigid stainless steel or silver tracheostomy tubes to plastic tubes (which soften with body heat and conform to tracheal anatomy), and the development of soft Silastic tracheostomy tubes, catastrophic hemorrhage has become less common. Tracheal innominate fistula is usually fatal with only isolated reports of survival. (In the author's institution there has been one case of innominate artery fistula with a successful outcome. The child lived close to the hospital and the diagnosis was made immediately on admission to the emergency department. The tracheostomy tube was removed and an armored endotracheal tube with a large-volume cuff was inserted through the tracheal stoma and positioned with the tip in the right mainstem bronchus. The cuff was then inflated to tamponade the innominate artery, disappearance of the right radial pulse confirmed adequate placement and the patient was taken to the operating room after resuscitation.)

Overwhelming infection

Overwhelming pulmonary infections may be primary, or secondary to aspiration. Fulminating, rapidly fatal pneumonias have occurred with *Legionella pneumoniae* contaminating humidification, suctioning, or ventilatory equipment.

Acute problems

Acute problems in tracheostomy care include:

- infection:
  - purulent bronchitis
  - stomal infections
- skin erosions (tracheostomy ties too tight)
- minor hemorrhage
- partial obstruction

Infection

Purulent bronchitis is the most common acute problem encountered in tracheostomy care. Caregivers are taught to report changes in odor, color, and volume of secretions, and to seek medical care early. With empiric antibiotics (to cover normal respiratory flora), progression to lower respiratory tract infection is relatively uncommon. *Pseudomonas*, although often present in surveillance cultures, rarely needs treatment, and usually only when serious underlying pulmonary disease is present.

Infections of the stoma are not unusual but occur less frequently after hospital discharge. Candidiasis is common and can be treated topically; a spreading cellulitis should be treated systemically.

Skin erosion

Erosion of tracheostomy ties through skin and even through strap muscles may be very difficult to treat. Prevention—i.e. meticulous attention to appropriate looseness of tracheostomy ties—is paramount and the importance of not tying ties too tightly should be frequently re-inforced; it should be possible to insert one adult finger between the tie and the lateral neck.

Minor erosions can be treated with loosening of the ties and placement of a dressing beneath the ties to distribute pressure over a wider area, allowing the skin to heal. Severe erosions may necessitate PICU (or TDU) admission and sometimes temporary suturing of the tracheostomy tube to the skin while the injured area recovers. Surgical intervention is required in serious cases.

Minor hemorrhage

Minor bleeding from the tracheostomy tube is not infrequent and may accompany viral or bacterial infections which may be overt or subtle. Bleeding may indicate the presence of granulation tissue at the stoma, or the presence of traumatic suction granulomas. These episodes are mostly self-limited and if an infection is suspected, may respond to a course of antibiotics.

A search for a bleeding site in the trachea and large airways may be made by passage of a small fiberoptic bronchoscope through the tracheostomy tube.

Partial obstruction

When a tracheostomy patient presents with wheezing in the absence of an obvious viral infection or previous history or family history of reactive airways disease, partial obstruction of the tracheostomy tube with inspissated secretions should always be considered, and the tube removed and replaced as part of the diagnostic investigation.

Chronic problems

Chronic problems in home tracheostomy care include:

- recurrent serous otitis media—hearing impairment
- speech development (delay)
- bronchial or tracheal stenosis

Stenosis of large airways secondary to trauma to the tracheal or bronchial mucosa by suction catheters is an exceedingly difficult problem to treat but should be avoidable. 'Deep' suctioning should be discouraged; the caregiver and patient should be provided with suction catheters with marked gradations and instructed not to suction more than 0.5–1 cm distal to the tip of the tracheostomy tube.

Traumatic suction granulomas, most commonly at the orifice of the right mainstem bronchus, may produce significant bronchial obstruction, secondary infection, and eventually bronchiectasis.

Megatrachea

Megatrachea is an unusual and difficult tracheostomy problem which may occur in the pentaplegic patient or in patients with high ventilatory pressures due to pulmonary disease (pentaplegia is a term applied to traumatic spinal cord injury patients with a very high lesion, usually at the C-1/C-2 level, often involving the medulla as evidenced by dysfunction of cranial nerves X, XI and XII). These patients may be difficult or impossible to ventilate without a cuffed endotracheal or tracheostomy tube. Typically, over time, increasing amounts of air have to be added to the tracheostomy tube cuff to ensure an adequate seal as the trachea dilates.

Foam-cuffed tracheostomy tubes have been used in such cases with some success. The cuff of the foam-cuffed tube inflates passively, providing a low-pressure seal, and is deflated by applying negative pressure to the pilot tubing. In patients who are developing megatrachea or who require high ventilating pressures, the pilot port of the foam-cuffed tracheostomy tube can be connected to a side port connector inserted into the ventilator circuit, such that the envelope of the foam cuff is further inflated to airway pressure during ventilator systole (providing an adequate seal at high pressures), and deflates passively to the residual foam cuff volume (and low pressure) during ventilator diastole.

TRACHEOSTOMY TUBES

Pediatric tracheostomy tubes are available commercially in many configurations (Table 5.10.2); however, in some children, unusual anatomy and growth changes may necessitate customized tracheostomy tubes.

PLANNED DECANNULATION

Patients with a chronic (temporary) tracheostomy may be admitted for a trial of decannulation, or following decannulation under anesthesia.

Decannulation is usually performed after reevaluation of the airway, either with rigid bron-

---

TABLE 5.10.2 Variations in commercially available tracheostomy tubes

- Size: inside and outside diameters
- Length
- Curvature
- With or without inner cannula
- Uncuffed or cuffed (air or foam)
- Flanges: neonatal, pediatric, adult
- Materials: silver, stainless steel, PVC, Silastic

---

choscopy (usually in the operating room) or with fiberoptic laryngobronchoscopy (in the operating room or at the bedside). If findings are favorable, the tracheostomy tube (sometimes after staged downsizing or intermittent occlusion—'corking') is removed. Failure of decannulation may be immediate, with airway obstruction manifest with stridor and increased respiratory effort, and even profound desaturation and bradycardia. Early failure occurs occasionally following an attempt by the patient to clear secretions, or after a feed. Certain children can be successfully decannulated when awake, but obstruct their airway significantly in sleep (late or delayed failure). In most cases, the stoma functionally closes (but can still be gently probed open) over a few hours; occasionally the tracheostoma remains widely patent and eventually needs to be closed surgically.

The author's practice is to observe children after decannulation for a minimum of 5–7 days, or until they demonstrate lack of significant airway obstruction in deep sleep with the stoma functionally closed. On occasion, when the tracheostoma has remained patent, we have resorted to occluding the stoma with a dressing to simulate tracheostomy healing, before discharge home.

LONG-TERM (HOME) MECHANICAL VENTILATION

Long-term mechanical ventilation gained general acceptance following the poliomyelitis epidemics of the 1950s, initially with negative pressure ventilation ('iron lung') and shortly thereafter with the introduction of positive pressure ventilation (Emerson). Most early experience with home mechanical ventilation and portable ventilators, however, was derived from the adult experience with traumatic spinal cord injury, i.e. the ventilator-dependent quadriplegic patient.

Indications for long-term mechanical ventilation have expanded to include congenital as well as acquired conditions, with the countries most experienced in home mechanical ventilation being the USA and France. These indications include:

- Neurological or neuromuscular diseases:
  - traumatic quadriplegia
  - myopathies and muscular dystrophies
  - spinal muscular atrophy
  - central hypoventilation syndromes (Ondine's curse)
  - obstructive sleep apnea
- Pulmonary disease
  - restrictive lung disease, e.g. uncorrected scoliosis
  - chronic lung disease, e.g. bronchopulmonary dysplasia

In addition to classifying mechanical ventilation by method of delivery, i.e. negative or positive pressure, ventilation may be classified by time-on (24 hour, intermittent, night only), as invasive or non-invasive (tracheostomy or not), or by the machine delivering ventilation.

For the younger child, the current standard is positive pressure ventilation delivered by a conventional home ventilator, with a tracheostomy as the interface between machine and patient.

Most home ventilators are simple, electric (powered by mains supply or an internal or external battery) piston-driven volume ventilators with fresh gas intake from the environment; a pressurized gas source is not necessary. Design innovations include more sophisticated alarm systems, and by incorporation of a pressure relief valve, simulation of pressure-limited ventilation (if desired). The ventilators themselves if well maintained are very reliable and problems with the actual equipment (e.g. ventilator failure) are rare. With better alarm systems, machine-patient interaction problems—in particular accidental disconnection or circuit leaks—are recognized earlier. Adequate humidification of ventilator circuits must be provided, particularly with small tracheostomy tubes. Heated humidifiers are usually incorporated into the bedside or stationary ventilatory circuits and paper condenser humidifiers into portable circuits. Circuits and humidification devices need careful care and cleaning to avoid contamination with hydrophilic bacteria, particularly *Legionella* and *Pseudomonas*.

Recurrent pulmonary infection or tracheostomy complications are the problems most often associated with long-term mechanical ventilation.

NONINVASIVE VENTILATION

Because of the more complex care required, and the problems and complications associated with a tracheostomy, noninvasive methods of ventilation (Table 5.10.3) have regained popularity, particularly for patients who require only intermittent or partial (e.g. night-time only) ventilation.

Noninvasive assisted ventilation (NIAV) with face mask or nasal mask as an interface, using either a conventional ventilator, or a ventilation assist device capable of biphasic (continuous positive end-expiratory pressure and inspiratory pressure) assist have enjoyed growing popularity, particularly in those children who need only night-time (sleep) ventilation and have significant daytime mobility. Both NIAV and nasal continuous positive airway pressure by mask have been used successfully with obstructive sleep apnea.

Complications associated with mask ventilation are principally those of mask fit, e.g. pressure sores on the nasal bridge and eye irritation, and have decreased with improved mask technology. As most children are nose breathers, nasal masks (without the need for chin straps) are usually effective. Full face masks are often successful, particularly in children with facial weakness, but carry greater risk, in that these children may be too weak to remove the mask themselves should vomiting occur. A personal alarm system may be provided and gastrostomy feeds should not be continued during full face mask ventilation.

Diaphragmatic pacing, either alone or in combination with intermittent positive pressure ventilation, has been used successfully in many adults and a few children. Advocates point to savings in disposable supplies and improvement in the quality of life. Some patients have even had their tracheostomies closed.

TABLE 5.10.3 **Forms of noninvasive ventilation (without tracheostomy)**	
Positive pressure	**Negative pressure**
Face mask with conventional ventilator	Cuirass
Face mask with ventilation assist device	'Iron lung' (Kevlar lung in the 1990s)
	Pneumobelt
	Phrenic pacemaker (may continue to require tracheostomy)
	Rocking bed

THE VENTILATOR DEPENDENT QUADRIPLEGIC CHILD

Of all the technology-dependent patients, children and young adults with traumatic high spinal cord injury resulting in quadriplegia and ventilator dependency require the most complex care. In addition to the problems of full-time mechanical ventilation and tracheostomy care, loss of motor, sensory and autonomic nervous system functions create unusual and complex problems. These include:

- loss of voluntary motor control
- respiration problems
- spasticity
- cardiovascular instability—orthostatic hypotension
- neurogenic bowel and bladder
- thermoregulation
- autonomic dysreflexia
- decubitus ulcers
- osteoporosis—pathologic fractures

The most apparent manifestation of high spinal cord injury is lack of voluntary motor control. Even when the lesion is sufficiently high to cause loss of diaphragmatic movement, the patient may still have residual voluntary movement in the upper limbs, neck, and face, which allow the use of sophisticated communication devices, and specialized switches (e.g. to operate a self-propelled wheelchair and thus provide a degree of independent mobility). However, such children for the most part remain dependent on trained caregivers for their activities of daily living. Although occasionally the care of a ventilator-dependent quadriplegic child is undertaken solely by the immediate family, most children will have at least a portion of their care provided by specially trained attendants. Both groups of caregivers are usually devoted to the child and in turn are trusted by the child.

Many adult ventilator-dependent quadriplegic patients learn to breathe for variable periods of time with accessory muscles of respiration, i.e. neck muscles ('frog' breathing). Some may even develop this ability to the extent that they can be ventilator-independent during waking hours, and only require assisted ventilation in sleep. Younger children manage this rarely however, and usually not until they are older. Therefore young children with high traumatic spinal cord lesions are most often 'truly' totally ventilator-dependent.

All patients with spinal cord injury undergo a period of flaccid paralysis initially, replaced gradually by hyperreflexia and spasticity, and often have spontaneous episodic muscle spasms. The severity of spasticity increases with the level of the original lesion; all ventilator-dependent quadriplegic patients demonstrate spasticity which sometimes can be sufficiently severe to interfere with seating, and even ventilation. Antispasmodic medications have had only minor success; some patients have been treated successfully with intrathecal continuous baclofen. On occasion rhizotomies may be required. Particular care is necessary to prevent contractures, with therapy programs for range of movement and splinting. During hospital admission, range of movement and splinting previously prescribed should be continued.

Because of poor sympathetic nervous system response, quadriplegic patients may experience significant orthostatic hypotension even with a change in their position from lying to sitting.

Ventilator-dependent quadriplegic patients have been described as poikilothermic, i.e. their body temperature (because of the inability to shiver or sweat, or peripherally vasodilate or vasoconstrict appropriately) is heavily influenced by environment. It is not unusual for these patients to develop either hyper- or hypothermia, particularly in the first few years following injury, and they may even require urgent hospital admission to control their temperature (on average the ventilator-dependent quadriplegic patient's core temperature is 1°C below the norm).

Although any severely ill patient unable to move appropriately may develop pressure sores or decubitus ulcers, the ventilator-dependent quadriplegic patient without sensation and without the ability to spontaneously shift body position, can develop serious pressure sores rapidly unless meticulous care is provided.

Osteoporosis (a consequence of immobility) may result in pathological fractures, and because of lack of sensation, diagnosis may be delayed. Life-threatening fat embolus may occur with what initially appears to be minor trauma.

All patients have abnormal bowel and bladder function, and urinary complications—e.g. recurrent urinary tract infections, pyelonephritis and renal calculi—are frequent. These patients will have a home bowel and bladder routine which should be adhered to. It is important to ensure that these patients do not develop constipation or urinary retention (see below).

Autonomic dysreflexia is a phenomenon thought to be due to an overactive sympathetic response above the level of the spinal lesion with a delayed response of the parasympathetic system. 'Attacks' are manifested by a sudden increase in blood pressure, pounding headaches, flushing, and profuse sweating of the face and neck, and often bradycardia. Autonomic dysreflexia is triggered by a stimulus below the spinal lesion, most often by stool impaction or urinary distention. It can also occur in response to range of motion exercises, cutaneous stretch, spontaneous muscle spasm, or in response to surgical or diagnostic procedures (labor in the pregnant female). The attack may precipitate a life-threatening cerebrovascular accident and must be treated promptly, using the following measures:

- induce postural hypotension
  - if the patient is in a wheelchair, return the patient to bed
  - elevate the head of the bed or hold the patient in a sitting position
- remove causative stimuli if possible, e.g. relieve distended bladder; disimpact rectum; stop procedure, etc.

- systemic hypotensive medications should be given when conservative measures fail

Autonomic dysreflexia occurs generally in patients with a lesion of T-5 (thoracic level V) or higher, with the number of episodes per year increasing, the higher the lesion. A child with a lesion sufficiently high to cause ventilator-dependent quadriplegia will experience autonomic dysreflexia at least once a year and often more frequently.

CARING FOR THE TECHNOLOGY-DEPENDENT CHILD IN THE ICU

Respiratory technology-dependent children may (and often do) require hospitalization either acutely with intercurrent (usually respiratory tract) illness or for planned, elective surgical procedures.

Children with tracheostomies (who require positive pressure ventilation) who develop serious respiratory tract illness, or need surgery may require substitution of a cuffed tracheostomy tube for their regular uncuffed tube. Previously many centers intubated (where possible) these children either orally or nasally, and temporarily discontinued their tracheostomy, or in some cases intubated the stoma with a cuffed endotracheal tube. For safety while undergoing anesthesia, uncuffed tracheostomy tubes would sometimes be sutured to the skin so that they would not be dislodged under the drapes. However, with the advent of small cuffed (both air and foam) tracheostomy tubes (in sizes suitable for neonates to young adults), provision of a temporary cuffed tube is now possible for virtually every patient with a tracheostomy. Usually a tube one size smaller allows the increase in diameter created by the deflated cuff to be accommodated. Insertion and removal of a cuffed tube is uncomfortable and should be performed under anesthesia.

With intercurrent illness or postoperative care, a more sophisticated ventilator than the one used at home may be required (capable of different ventilation modes and variable PEEP). However, because most ventilator-dependent patients are used to their own individual ventilator, unless their condition necessitates sophisticated ventilator support, the patient's own home ventilator should be used. Reinstating the patient's own equipment as soon as possible should always be the goal.

Technology-dependent children often have enteral support devices such as gastrostomy tubes, gastrostomy buttons, or jejunostomy tubes. Many of these appliances have built-in one-way valves to prevent spillage, and even when apparently open may not adequately decompress the stomach. When gastric paresis or ileus is suspected, either a nasogastric tube should be passed or the enteral device should be 'opened' with an appropriate decompression attachment.

Many children, in particular those with ventilator-dependent quadriplegia, have devoted attendant caregivers whom they trust and who know the child intimately. Hospital policies should be such that these attendants can continue to care, at least partially, for their children alongside hospital personnel (particularly after admission to a PICU or TDU).

Many chronically ventilated patients will present with blood gases showing mild to moderate chronic overventilation (P_{CO_2} 4–4.7 kPa, 30–35 mm Hg) and will become air hungry should a well-meaning physician attempt to 'normalize' their blood gases. When prescribing ventilator parameters for a chronically ventilated patient, enquire as to patient comfort. Remember, they know how they feel better than we do!

✓ KEY POINTS

➤ Children with home respiratory technology, tracheostomy or ventilator dependency are few in number but have a significant and specific morbidity

➤ The problems and complications in this group are unusual and often complex

➤ The patient or caregivers are most often more knowledgeable than the physicians they encounter

FURTHER READING

1. Duncan BW, Howell LJ, deLorimier AA et al. Tracheostomy in children with emphasis on home care. J Pediatr Surg 1992; 27(4): 432–435
2. Messines A, Giusti F, Naine S et al. The safety of home tracheostomy care for children. J Pediatr Surg 1995; 30(8): 1246–1248
– (Two references on home tracheostomy care)

3. Zejdlik CP. Management of spinal cord injury, 2nd ed. Boston: Jones & Bartlett, 1992
– (A comprehensive review of traumatic spinal cord injury and rehabilitation)

4. Bach JR. Pulmonary rehabilitation: the obstructive and paralytic conditions. St Louis: Mosby; 1996
5. Fauroux B, Sadet A, Foret D. Home treatment for chronic respiratory failure in children: a prospective study. Eur Respir J 1995; 8(12): 2062–2066
– (Two references on home ventilation)

5.11   Outcome following intensive care

Reinoud J. B. J. Gemke

Intensive care can often increase the likelihood and quality of survival in severely ill children. On the other hand, the nature and severity of disorders causing critical illness mean that the prognosis is often uncertain. Because intensive treatment often requires a large amount of scarce resources, its merits must be assessed. Systematic evaluation of the outcome and quality of intensive care medicine has become essential.

The goal of intensive care medicine is to prevent avoidable death and to restore previous health status. Comparison of outcome in different ICUs is hampered by differences in severity of illness and in case mix patterns. To take account of these differences, clinical scoring systems have been developed, which are used to adjust the mortality rate in a PICU, a city or a country objectively according to severity of illness in order to address questions of effectiveness, efficiency and quality of care. As mortality is not the only criterion by which effectiveness of care is judged, indices of health status or health-related quality of life have been introduced. For survivors it is the final outcome that counts, although it is not always possible to separate the contributions of different aspects of a complex therapy, in which ICU treatment may have only an ancillary role.

MEASURING OUTCOME

The outcome measured and the timing of measurement should be appropriate to the treatment being assessed. Outcome indicators may be clear-cut, short-term indicators, such as mortality rate corrected for severity of illness, or long-term indicators such as residual morbidity and quality of life. Appropriate outcome markers should be measurable and clearly attributable to the care delivered. They should reflect health status and the patient's preferences.

Outcomes of health care are multidimensional. Which dimensions should be evaluated depends on the context and the purpose of the assessment.

Outcomes measured from the patient's perspective are now recognized as the most appropriate means to evaluate effectiveness of health care in terms of length and quality of survival.

EFFECTIVENESS

Effectiveness and efficiency (Table 5.11.1) are the attributes of treatment that outcome and quality measurements aim to assess. The *effectiveness* of a treatment can be defined as its results compared with those of another treatment or a 'gold standard'. One should remember that a treatment that is effective under controlled conditions, e.g. in a clinical trial, may not be effective in daily practice. In the case of potentially life-saving treatments, comparison with alternative options is frequently hampered or precluded on ethical grounds.

There are few large randomized studies comparing intensive care with normal ward care, and the effectiveness of intensive care may be disputed. Some patients may be too ill to benefit from intensive care, while others may not be ill enough to justify ICU admission. The effectiveness of intensive care is frequently expressed as the ratio of observed mortality and expected mortality, adjusted for severity of illness. This is the standardized mortality rate (SMR), which compares the effectiveness of care (or of the whole ICU) with that in a large reference population of similar populations in different ICUs. If the observed mortality is lower than the expected mortality, adjusted for severity of illness (SMR < 1), this suggests a superior performance in the study group compared with the reference PICU population. Most importantly, in several studies substantial higher SMRs were found in non-tertiary PICUs. In these units, the severity of illness adjusted odds ratio for dying was at least two times higher than in tertiary PICUs.

Several factors hamper the assessment of effectiveness of pediatric intensive care:

1. The *diversity* of patient groups—to solve this problem, robust clinical scoring

TABLE 5.11.1 **Attributes of outcome and quality assessment**		
	Definition	**Outcome measure**
Effectiveness	Does the treatment achieve the desired result?	Improved health
Efficiency	The relationship between costs and consequences	Ratio of marginal costs to marginal benefits
Cost-benefit	Comparison of costs with a monetary measure of health outcome	Monetary units
Cost-utility	Comparison of costs with length and quality of survival	Quality-adjusted life years
Cost-effectiveness	Comparison of costs with improved health	Health events

systems for objective and uniform assessment of severity of illness in ICU patients have been developed which enable comparison to be made of patients of different ages, diagnoses and with differing racial and social backgrounds and differing preexisting illnesses.

2. Patients who are admitted to the ICU following an *acute insult* are different from those admitted after major elective surgery. It may be difficult to separate the contribution of pre-ICU treatment from that of ICU treatment.

3. The *heterogeneity* of pediatric ICUs—in specialized tertiary care PICUs, all advanced treatment options are usually available. This is not always the case in nontertiary hospitals where ICUs may also act as postoperative recovery areas, admitting patients mainly for monitoring.

4. In many countries, children are admitted to multidisciplinary 'adult' ICUs, each of which admits few children and is less expert in their care than in that of adults.

EFFICIENCY AND COST EFFECTIVENESS

Because of its high costs, intensive care must be employed efficiently as well as being effective. The efficiency of a health care program is the relationship between its costs and its consequences (benefits or drawbacks). The essential question is: 'Do the marginal (incremental) benefits attributable to the programme outweigh its marginal costs?' A particular PICU can be considered cost-effective if it uses fewer resources, but produces the same results (in terms of mortality rates adjusted for severity of illness) as other units. Similarly, if the same adjusted mortality rate can be achieved by

non-ICU care as by ICU care, the former is usually more cost-effective. To assess the results obtained in an ICU with the resources available (expressed as ICU bed-days), objective criteria are adopted to assess the appropriateness of admission or stay in the ICU.

1. Admission to the ICU can be regarded as efficient if the patient's risk of mortality exceeds an arbitrary value or if the patient undergoes at least one ICU-dependent therapy (Table 5.11.2) on the day of admission. An ICU-dependent therapy is one which generally can only be delivered in the ICU.

2. Stay in the ICU for a day can be regarded as efficient if the patient underwent at least one ICU-dependent therapy on that day. Many children, especially in Western countries, are admitted to ICUs for safety reasons when it appears that they may develop a substantial risk of dying or may require an ICU-dependent therapy. In retrospect, these patients only use monitoring facilities and standard care. Because this uncertainty can never be eliminated completely, unnecessary pediatric ICU admissions occur and may contribute significantly to the cost of health care.

Studies in adult ICU populations have found that most resources are spent on a small subgroup of patients whose outcome is likely to be poor. On the other hand, however, in neonatal intensive care, many infants are admitted with respiratory distress syndrome, a reversible disorder with' a good chance of acceptable functional recovery, and infant nonsurvivors tend to have a shorter hospital course than adult nonsurvivors.

TABLE 5.11.2 Examples of ICU-dependent therapies

- Cardiopulmonary resuscitation or DC countershock
- Mechanical ventilation
- Endotracheal intubation
- Continuous positive airway pressure
- Extracorporeal life support
- Nitric oxide administration
- Continuous infusion of vasoactive drugs
- Cardioversion for arrhythmias
- Intraaortic balloon assist
- Acute (external) pacing
- Acute renal replacement therapy
- Pressurized blood transfusions
- Frequent blood transfusions (> 20 ml/kg per day)
- Active diuresis for cerebral edema or fluid overload
- Induced hypothermia
- Balloon tamponade of varices
- Lavage of acute gastrointestinal tract bleeding
- Emergency thoraco- or pericardiocentesis
- Therapy for convulsions or metabolic encephalopathy

Little information is available about cost-effectiveness and resource utilization in PICUs and the results are divergent. Some authors have suggested that a high proportion of average daily and total ICU resource utilization per admission is determined by characteristics such as severity of illness, surgical status, the presence of substantial chronic illness, emergency admission and transfer from another hospital. High resource utilization may be warranted in high-risk patients if the effectiveness of prolonged intensive therapy can be demonstrated.

TRIAGE

Selection of patients for admission to a pediatric ICU has a major effect on outcome. In a child with failure or potential failure of vital organs, the benefits and drawbacks of intensive care should be considered: admission is justified if it is likely that intensive therapy, including temporary support of vital functions, will contribute to restoration of preexisting health or to meaningful recovery.

When there is serious doubt about the expected effectiveness of therapy, treatment can be started if there is also agreement that it should be stopped when it fails to meet the expected goals.

Sometimes ICU admission is considered in children who develop failure of vital functions while suffering from a preexisting chronic disease known to have a bad prognosis (e.g. respiratory insufficiency in cystic fibrosis). In these cases, the child's poor long-term prognosis should be discussed with the patient, parents and the primary medical specialist involved in the child's care. Consultation with an intensive care pediatrician may be helpful. The discussion should take place when the child is relatively well, but in practice is often postponed until the child is acutely ill and ICU admission is requested, at which time discussion of the pros and cons of treatment may be overtaken by the immediate need to preserve life.

MORTALITY

Crude PICU mortality rates in multicenter studies are mostly about 10%, with large variations between units. On average, these figures are lower than those found in neonatal and adult ICUs, whose mean mortality rates vary around 20%. Late mortality (after hospital discharge) in children is also substantially lower than in adults. Children who die in the ICU are younger on average than survivors. The mean length of ICU stay of both groups is usually comparable, but in nonsurvivors intensity of treatment, as assessed by the therapeutic intervention scoring system (TISS), is usually twice as high as in survivors. A more useful indicator of quality of care is the severity-of-illness-adjusted mortality rate which uses clinical scoring systems such as the pediatric risk of mortality score (PRISM) and the pediatric index of mortality (PIM). The contribution of each clinical variable (e.g. systolic blood pressure or pupil response to light) to the total mortality risk can be objectively weighted by means of logistic regression modeling. The validity of these models has been established in several studies, although it is recommended to check its validity for a particular PICU should be checked before a model is adopted.

Other possible causes of discrepancies between observed and expected mortality rates may include underlying chronic illness, and local differences in practice in withholding and withdrawal of treatment. Circumstances under which children in a PICU die may differ between units and between countries. Some children die despite maximal treatment, because the criteria for brain death are met or because resuscitation is unsuccessful. Other children may die because in consultation between the physicians, nurses and the parents, it is decided to withhold or withdraw certain treatments, or a patient may die after a do not resuscitate (DNR) order has been written. In daily intensive care practice the meaning of a DNR order may not be obvious, and these orders should be replaced by a care plan (Ch. 5.8). What is resuscitation in an unstable, mechanically ventilated patient receiving high doses of inotropic drugs? What are the merits of chest compressions in these cases: when should they be considered potentially effective and when are they merely a ritual before the patient dies? In intensive care patients it seems more appropriate to set well-defined therapeutic goals and the type of care by which these may be achieved. In US, Canadian and Dutch studies assessing the circumstances of dying in pediatric ICUs, it was found that between 25% and 50% of children died after treatment was withdrawn or was withheld because of the virtual certainty of severe disability (due to the acute disease or an underlying chronic disease).

RESIDUAL MORBIDITY

Residual morbidity is persistence of a chronic disorder after discharge from intensive care. Examples of residual morbidity include:

- barotrauma or volutrauma and oxygen toxicity after intermittent positive-pressure ventilation (e.g. bronchopulmonary dysplasia in newborns)
- bronchial hyperreactivity following viral bronchiolitis
- upper airway complications following intubation or tracheostomy (vocal cord granuloma, postintubation laryngeal edema)
- necrosis of digits following septic shock due to *Neisseria meningitides* or other organisms
- functional and cosmetic lesions due to burns
- posthypoxic encephalopathy (e.g. after near-drowning or cardiac arrest)

Organ failure may persist after discharge from the ICU: examples are chronic renal failure requiring dialysis after hemolytic–uremic syndrome; respiratory failure requiring ventilator therapy in cervical spinal cord lesions, and cardiac failure requiring prolonged inotropic support in cardiomyopathy. After an acute hypoxic incident, a patient may survive in a persistent vegetative state. Critical illness polyneuropathy, found in some patients with septic shock and multiorgan system failure, greatly prolongs weaning from mechanical ventilation and leads to months of marked muscle weakness and sensory changes. Abstinence syndromes after prolonged high-dose treatment with opiates or benzodiazepines often complicate recovery after ICU discharge. Substitution of alternative drugs and psychological support may be required.

Residual psychological morbidity

Children who have been admitted to an ICU can develop post-traumatic emotional disturbances, the symptoms of which include:

- recall of the traumatic incident
- anxiety triggered by ICU-like incidents (beeping alarms)
- extreme fear of separation from parents
- persistent night terrors
- persistent state of arousal (extreme irritability and disturbances of sleep, eating and concentration)
- regressive or infantile behavior.

These symptoms should be anticipated and recognized early in children who have been admitted to an ICU. Consultation with a psychologist or psychiatrist may be helpful.

The patient's family is also at risk of developing psychological problems during or after a child's acute ICU admission for a life-threatening event. Parents of survivors and nonsurvivors have indicated that counseling by nursing and medical staff directly involved in the care for their child was very useful in helping them deal with the ICU period and the days or weeks after discharge (Ch. 5.5).

HEALTH-RELATED QUALITY OF LIFE

Although intensive care has probably reduced the acute short-term mortality rate of many illnesses, survival to ICU or hospital discharge is not the only end point of effectiveness of advanced medical care. Decreased mortality may be accompanied by an increasing proportion of patients with chronic residual morbidity, so functional outcome and longitudinal assessment of length and quality of survival have become important supplementary measures of outcome after intensive care. Ultimately children and their families regard survival and health-related quality of life as the measures by which medical care should be judged. There are several domains of health status which should be considered:

- *physical*, including viability, functional limitations and pain
- *cognitive*
- *emotional* and mental health
- *social* integration and relationships
- *roles*, including employment and economic independency in adults and school attendance in children
- *self-perceived* health status

Generic health status (as opposed to disease-specific) measures are appropriate to measure health-related quality of life in such a broad population as ICU patients with a wide range of health problems. Some well-established generic health status classification systems for adults are the Nottingham health profile, the quality of life index, the sickness impact profile, the quality of well-being and the Short Form 36 (SF-36).

Several generic health status measures are available for outcome assessment of heterogeneous groups of children undergoing intensive care (Table 5.11.3) The functional status II and the pediatric performance categories (overall and cerebral) are suitable for all ages, although their coarseness may hamper broader application. More comprehensive health status measures are the health utilities index (mark 3) and the child health questionnaire. A drawback of the latter two measures is that they cannot be used for children under 5 years of age.

Before one of these measures is adopted, its reliability (agreement between observers and between repeated-tests), validity and responsiveness should be established. Validity means applicability, appropriate length, simplicity and lack of potential inherent bias. As there is no 'gold standard' of health status, the validity of the criteria used in each measure cannot be assessed. To assess changes in health status over time or due to specific interventions, the measure should also be sensitive to change.

Table 5.11.4 shows an example of a multi-attribute health status measure. Any combination of domain levels constitutes a health status. This example, the health utility index (HUI), has been used to assess the health status of survivors of neonatal intensive care and childhood cancer and to assess changes in health status in pediatric ICU patients. By weighting and aggregating the scores of all domains a health status score can be produced, and the number of quality-adjusted life years (QALYs) gained by a particular intervention estimated for cost-utility analysis. Despite the attractiveness of a single summary score for health status, compression of the seven domains of the HUI into a single number makes interpretation hazardous, particularly in nonepidemiologic use. In a prospective Dutch study assessing survival and health status 1 year after discharge of 468 children admitted to an ICU, Gemke et al found an ICU mortality rate of 7.5%, a cumulative hospital mortality rate of 8.3% and a 1-year mortality rate of 10.5%. Hospital mortality was mainly found in previously healthy children suffering from an acute, devastating illness. With the HUI, health status before admission and after 1 year was assessed. A high proportion of patients (68%) had experienced some form of health deficit before ICU admission. However, after 1 year, overall health status was better than or equal to their health before admission, cumulative 1-year survival was favorable, and health status was preserved in three-quarters of the children. In a retrospective Australian study assessing long-term outcome of admission to pediatric ICU, Butt et al found a cumulative mortality rate of 14.3% and overall health impairment on follow-up in 58%. Health status remained unchanged in 69%, deteriorated in 8.3% and improved in 8.7% compared with preadmission status.

CONCLUSION

Intensive care has substantially reduced mortality in acutely ill children and is increasingly offered to

TABLE 5.11.3 **Health status measures in children**

Measure	Type	Mode of administration
Functional status II	Descriptive	Parental interview
Pediatric performance scales	Descriptive	Nurse assessment
Health utilities index	Descriptive and valued	Patient and parent questionnaire plus physician classification
Child health questionnaire	Descriptive	Patient and parent questionnaire

TABLE 5.11.4 **Example of a system of health status classification**

Attribute	Level	Description
Sensation	1	Able to see, hear, and speak normally for age
	2	Requires equipment to see or hear or speak
	3	Sees, hears or speaks with limitations, even with equipment
	4	Blind, deaf or mute
Mobility	1	Able to walk, bend, lift, jump, and run normally for age
	2	Walks, bends, lifts, jumps, or runs with some limitations but does not require help
	3	Requires mechanical equipment (such as canes, crutches, braces, or wheelchair) to walk or get around independently
	4	Requires the help of another person to walk or get around and requires mechanical equipment as well
	5	Unable to control or use arms and legs
Emotion	1	Generally happy and free from worry
	2	Occasionally fretful, angry, irritable, anxious, depressed, or suffering night terrors
	3	Often fretful, angry, irritable, anxious, depressed, or suffering night terrors
	4	Almost always fretful, angry, irritable, anxious, depressed
	5	Extremely fretful, angry, irritable, or depressed usually requiring hospitalization or psychiatric institutional care
Cognition	1	Learns and remembers school work normally for age
	2	Learns and remembers school work more slowly than classmates as judged by parents and/or teachers
	3	Learns and remembers very slowly and usually requires special educational assistance
	4	Unable to learn and remember
Self-care	1	Eats, bathes, dresses, and uses the toilet normally for age
	2	Eats, bathes, dresses, or uses the toilet independently (for age) but with difficulty
	3	Requires mechanical equipment to eat, bathe, dress, or use the toilet independently (for age)
	4	Requires (for age more than normal) help of another person to eat, bathe, dress, or use the toilet
Pain	1	Free of pain and discomfort
	2	Occasional pain. Discomfort relieved by nonprescription drugs or self-control activity without disruption of normal activities.
	3	Frequent pain. Discomfort relieved by oral medicines with the occasional disruption of normal activities
	4	Frequent pain; frequent disruption of normal activities. Discomfort requires prescription narcotics for relief
	5	Severe pain. Pain not relieved by drugs and constantly disrupts normal activities

Reprinted with permission from Feeny D, Furlong W, Boyle M, Torrance G. Multi-attribute health status classifications. Pharmacoeconomics 1995; 7: 490–502.

children with complex chronic diseases. In this latter population, the merits of intensive care are far less obvious. Comprehensive studies assessing the merits of advanced medical care should include not only ICU or hospital mortality rates but also late mortality and health-related quality of life measures.

✔ **KEY POINTS**

➤ Outcome is better assessed from the perspective of the patient than from that of the hospital or its staff

➤ The effectiveness of intensive care is the ratio of observed to expected mortality rates, adjusted for severity of illness

➤ Discussions with the family of a child with a severe chronic illness about the advisability of intensive care should take place when the child is well, not when the child becomes critically ill

➤ Assessment of intensive care should include late mortality and health-related quality of life as well as ICU and hospital mortality rates

FURTHER READING

1. Butt W, Shann F, Tibballs J et al. Long-term outcome of children after intensive care. Crit Care Med 1990; 18: 961–965

2. Boyle MH, Torrance GW, Sinclair JC, Horwood SP. Economic evaluation of neonatal intensive care of very-low-birth-weight infants. N Engl J Med 1983; 308: 1330–1338

3. Fiser DH. Assessing the outcome of pediatric intensive care. J Pediatr 1992; 121: 68–72

4. Gemke RJBJ, Bonsel GJ, van Vught AJ. Outcome assessment and quality assurance in pediatric intensive care: In: Tibboel D, van der Voort E, editors. Yearbook on intensive care and emergency medicine. Berlin: Springer; 1996; pp. 284–293

5. Gemke RJBJ. Centralisation of paediatric intensive care to improve outcome. Lancet 1997; 349: 1187–1188

– *(General papers on outcome assessment of pediatric intensive care)*

6. Feeny D, Furlong W, Boyle M, Torrance G. Multi-attribute health status classifications. Pharmacoeconomics 1995; 7: 490–502

7. Fitzpatrick R, Flechter A, Gore S, Jones D, Spiegelhalter D, Cox D. Quality of life measures in health care. Br Med J 1992; 305: 1074–1077, 1145–1148, 1205–1209

8. Froberg DG, Kane RL. Methodology for measuring health state preferences. J Clin Epidem 1989; 142: 345–354, 459–471, 585–592, 675–685

9. Patrick DL, Erickson P. Health status and health policy: quality of life in health care evaluation and resource allocation. Oxford University Press; 1993.

– *(General papers on assessment of health-related quality of life)*

5.12 Medicolegal aspects of care

Andrew J. Macnab and Arthur F. Cogswell

Management of critical illness inevitably brings physicians, other caregivers, families and children into situations in which there are legal consequences. Quite apart from issues discussed elsewhere such as human rights, ethics, consent, the legal definition of death, the role of the coroner, confidentiality, and withdrawing life support, there is the question of the potential for caregivers to have to appear in court. Court proceedings usually involve caregivers in one of two ways:

- they are called to give evidence:
  - as a witness to events that occurred
  - as an expert witness to interpret events in a case they have not managed
- they are the subject of a malpractice claim

Reviews of malpractice claims against physicians indicate that the major reasons for litigation regarding care of critically ill children are:

- a failure to correctly diagnose
- a failure to treat appropriately
- poor communication
  - with parents as to what has occurred
  - through adverse comments from peers or other staff

Suits usually relate to whether care has been negligent. In this regard what has occurred is compared with the accepted 'standard of care' for that condition, at the time in question and at a comparable institution to the one where care was provided.

In any legal proceedings the chart is the key document. From the chart a picture is built up of what history was taken, what examination occurred, what differential diagnosis was arrived at, what tests were ordered, what treatment was given, what interpretation was made of the tests and response to treatment, what consultation, triage and disposition occurred and what was communicated to the patient and family regarding the above.

It is immediately clear that the documentation that exists is deemed to reflect what was done, what was not done, why things were done, and the overall quality of the process. A clear, concise, logical record that describes the actions taken, the reasons behind them, any adverse events that occurred and what was communicated is the best method for a physician to prove that the expected standard of care has been met. Your case records need to indicate that you have provided comprehensive, logical and appropriate care in response to the high-risk elements of the patient's problem. Notes can be brief, but must not have any important omissions. In this regard, the record must contain documentation on:

- the high-risk issues of the child's condition
- pertinent past history
- risk factors relevant to the presenting complaint
- the key positive *and* negative findings in relation to the major risk factors
- vital signs
- child's level of alertness and behavior
- probable and possible differential diagnoses
- investigations
- treatment
- the patient's response to resuscitation and emergency procedures
- clear explanation of deviation from conventional process or practice
- consultation, triage and continuing care arrangements

With regard to subsequent chart entries, major errors include:

- failure to document progress (or lack of progress) and response to treatment
- failure to comment on major changes in vital signs or significant test results
- pursuing a diagnosis, treatment or investigation that is not logical when compared with the documented history, physical signs and test results
- failure to comment on inconsistencies in your record with entries made by others

(e.g. you write, 'patient looks stable', nurse writes, 'patient looks toxic')

- not setting parameters for initiating change in treatment or management interventions
- not recording what has been told to whom in the family
- the time and date of each entry and your signature

The issue is not usually the absolute correctness of the diagnosis but rather the logic of the decisions arrived at; hence the need for documentation of the path between information, physical signs, study results and treatment. The record can omit negatives that add nothing to confirming or eliminating high-risk diagnostic considerations.

In critical situations unusual and sometimes adverse circumstances often occur. These should be recorded in detail. If there is concern that a mistake has been made, collect all the available information, and enter a full and detailed note in the chart, preferably signed by all concerned. If opinions as to what occurred are discrepant, write both down. Report the facts to your senior medical, nursing and management colleagues and discuss what has occurred with the patient and/or the family. Never go back and make changes to a chart but do add a postscript regarding new information, new thoughts or a changed decision.

Dictated records are often more complete but need to be clear regarding the times at which events occurred and when the record was dictated. There is no substitute for a brief note written at the time. However, comprehensive dictation, particularly when errors occur, provides an important record of events which may well be forgotten, or have become vague, by the time legal review ultimately occurs.

APPEARING IN COURT

GIVING EVIDENCE

The basis of a professional presentation in court lies in having made good, detailed notes at the time and reviewing them in detail prior to appearing in court. Remember you are there to help the court interpret the facts. Try to relax, take things slowly, and present the facts in a neutral manner. Do not hesitate to refer back to the chart or ask for time to read through documents produced. This avoids hurried answers or being forced into an ill-advised position by pressure from a lawyer. It is important to distinguish between your role when giving evidence and your role as an expert witness. When giving evidence your testimony is limited to the events that occurred and actions taken, or not taken, at the time. You are neither expected nor wanted to interpret the ramifications of the events or guide the court regarding comparable cases in the literature. Other excellent practical advice which will help diminish courtroom-induced anxiety is contained in the Further Reading section of Chapter 4.3.

ACTING AS AN EXPERT WITNESS

In the role of an expert witness you will be asked to review the medical records and opinions of other experts in order to guide the court. In a medicolegal case, it is necessary for a plaintiff to:

- establish that a duty of care existed for the patient from the physician sued
- show that the appropriate standard of care for the time, level of knowledge and sophistication of the institution was not given, either through commission or omission
- prove that the failure of duty caused the damage in question

Prior to appearing in court as an expert you will be asked to draft a written report stating your opinion and the facts on which this is based. This report should contain:

- a list of the materials that have been examined in preparing the report
- the facts on which the opinion is based (sometimes these are presented by legal counsel as a statement of fact)
- answers to specific questions posed by legal counsel
- an explanation of the appropriate standard of care applying to the situation in question; this should be capable of support by references to other authorities (texts, published papers)

- an opinion of what occurred and on the standard of care received and provided, and whether this was of an acceptable standard

In court your role is to provide information, respond to the questions of the court and interpret the events in relation to the expected standard of care. Once again you will be relying on the written records to provide the building blocks for your opinion. Your clinical experience and expertise will be reviewed by the court in determining whether you are qualified to act as an expert. The court will ask for your curriculum vitae to support your acting as an expert witness. The court wants your opinion as to what occurred, why it occurred, when it occurred, whether the expected standard of care was met and if the child's current problems were caused by the situation in question. An expert witness must be independent in order to be credible, and being a physician and being in court does not necessarily qualify you to give an expert opinion on everything that you are asked. You should make it clear in the court room if a question addressed to you is outside your area of expertise. As an expert you have an obligation to the parents, the child, your colleagues and the court to give an objective opinion based on the facts of the case, your experience and an up-to-date knowledge of the relevant medical literature. Subjective, judgmental, biased opinions or those based on anecdote, inadequate research or a misguided desire to justify what occurred is neither helpful to the court nor honest. Similarly, if you do not feel qualified to give an expert opinion on a case as a whole, then you should defer to an appropriately qualified expert.

INTERHOSPITAL TRANSPORT

The transport of a child from one institution to another is inevitably associated with a transfer of legal responsibilities. Legal cases testing the law in this area apply various 'gold standards' for care and responsibility in different national jurisdictions. In Australia the sending physician is seen as responsible for the transport care plan. This responsibility strengthens the principles of pre-transport stabilization, but means that emergency procedures that fail in transit imply negligence.

In Europe and North America the referring hospital carries full legal responsibility prior to the involvement of the receiving hospital through a transport request. Similarly, once the child has arrived at the receiving hospital, the legal responsibility for ongoing care defaults to that institution. There are, however, many gray areas in relation to patient transfer. Importantly, the teams providing care are often performing 'delegated medical acts' on behalf of the physician directing the transport. This is of particular importance where paramedical personnel make up the team or the physician accompanying the paramedics is still in training. Once the transport coordinator from the receiving hospital is involved in giving advice and sharing decisions about management and transfer, an element of legal responsibility is seen to rest with the receiving institution, even though the majority remains with the treating hospital. With the arrival of the transport team personnel this element of responsibility increases, and that of the referring institution decreases further. Some variation in these divisions occurs where, for instance, the care plan discussed with the transport coordinator is subsequently changed by the caregivers at the referring institution or where actions prior to involvement of the transport team have long-term sequelae with regard to care or outcome.

Although the 'goodwill' generally inherent in the transport process between institutions means that legal arguments rarely arise, the potential is always there, and costly cases have occurred. Once again, the crucial nature of accurate, comprehensive documentation is paramount. This includes telephone dialog and a number of institutions now record telephone conversations in addition to keeping written notes. Transport records should contain the accurate time sequence of the transport, the names of the individuals involved, as well as the information listed in the earlier part of this chapter regarding patient history, signs, care, investigation and diagnosis. Quality assurance review, training, outreach education and research all contribute to the standard of care expected and records must reflect changing trends to ensure that data captured confirm that the current standard of care was delivered.

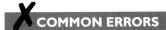

KEY POINTS

➤ Medicolegal problems are most likely to arise because of failure to diagnose, failure to treat, failure to communicate

➤ Your care must meet the expected standard of care

➤ Clear, logical documentation, addressing the high-risk elements of the child's presentation and the 'process' followed by you to enquire, examine, investigate and treat, is the best protection

➤ Physicians have two different roles in court: to provide evidence and to act in the capacity of an expert witness

COMMON ERRORS

➤ Records that are incomplete, particularly with regard to: vital signs, 'high-risk' consequences of the presentation, or significant positive and negative elements of history and physical examination. A differential diagnosis, an explanation if deviation occurred from conventional practice, an absence of progress notes, interpretation of results, and a clear management plan. Consistent documenting of the date and time of actions, and who was involved

FURTHER READING

1. Hull D. A question of negligence. Curr Pediatr 1993; 3(1): 52–55

2. Penick MP. Legal aspects of pediatric intensive care: risk management. In: Levin DL, Morris FC, editors. Essentials of pediatric care, 2nd ed. New York: Churchill Livingstone; 1997; 1069–1070

3. Korgaonkar GJA, Tribe DMR. Acting as a medical expert in medical negligence cases. Br J Hosp Med 1991; 46: 177–178

– *(Three reviews of medicolegal aspects of providing medical care)*

Procedures

6

6.1 Vascular access

Rebecca J. Mawer, Robert Bingham and Andrew J. Macnab

Reliable vascular access is a key component of pediatric critical care and a crucial step in pediatric resuscitation. It is essential for the infusion of fluids in cardiovascular compromise secondary to trauma or sepsis. In many children peripheral venous access either does not provide adequate flow rate, or is difficult to achieve in an emergency owing to poor peripheral circulation because of vessel size, or delay in obtaining access. In these situations insertion of an intraosseous (IO) needle or cannulation of a larger central vein is the procedure of choice. Central venous access must be performed with caution since complications are common in children. The incidence of complications depends on the site of vascular access, the clinical condition of the patient and the experience of the clinician.

The importance of vascular access and the need for physicians to acquire the necessary skills are recognized in current advanced life support training initiatives such as PALS and APLS. The theory taught in these courses is enhanced by practical experience, including use of appropriate 'vascular models'. Figure 6.1.1 is an algorithm for urgent vascular access.

METHODS

Choices for methods of vascular access include:

- percutaneous peripheral venous cannulation
- percutaneous central venous access (femoral, external or internal jugular, or subclavian)
- peripheral venous cut-down
- intraosseous infusion
- arterial line insertion

LOCATION

The location and method of emergency vascular access is determined by the clinical status and the age of the child, plus the skills and experience of the physician. More than one site and/or method are often needed. Regardless of the method and location chosen, the vascular access obtained must be capable of meeting the therapeutic needs of the patient. In some instances, this will be rapid delivery of medications; in other instances, infusion of large volumes of fluid. Frequently both needs exist in the same patient.

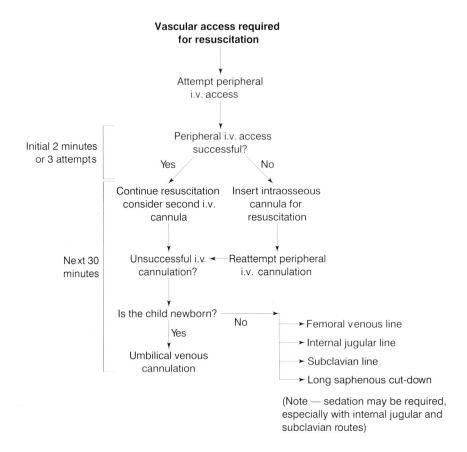

**Vascular access required
for resuscitation**

Attempt peripheral
i.v. access

Peripheral i.v. access
successful?

Initial 2 minutes
or 3 attempts

Yes   No

Continue resuscitation
consider second i.v.
cannula

Insert intraosseous
cannula for
resuscitation

Next 30
minutes

Unsuccessful i.v. ◄— Reattempt peripheral
cannulation?   i.v. cannulation

Is the child newborn? ———————►

No

► Femoral venous line

Yes

► Internal jugular line

Umbilical venous
cannulation

► Subclavian line

► Long saphenous cut-down

(Note — sedation may be required,
especially with internal jugular and
subclavian routes)

Figure 6.1.1 Algorithm for vascular access. Vascular access is crucial in the treatment of critically ill children. The route by which this can be performed is dependent on the age, size and clinical state of the child

PERCUTANEOUS PERIPHERAL VENOUS ACCESS

Percutaneous peripheral venous access has the advantage of being the method that most physicians are familiar with. It is also safe and generally rapid. The options are 'butterfly' needles or over-the-needle cannulas (Table 6.1.1).

In critically ill children, veins are frequently difficult to see. Under these circumstances, choose vessels where the anatomy is relatively constant. Examples are the median cubital vein in the antecubitas fossa, a vessel with the additional advantage of being immobile. It is often easier to palpate than to see. Inflating a blood pressure cuff on the upper arm can make location easier, and gently splinting the elbow across an arm board may also help. In the ankle the long saphenous vein is superficial, anterior to the medial malleolus, and

runs a relatively straight course. An alternative is the dorsal venous arch running across the dorsum of the foot. The saphenous vein tends to be mobile and somewhat more difficult to puncture. These vessels are most readily found after tapping the area gently and with a cuff or loose ligature applied above the knee.

In the hand the 'anesthetist's vein' in the fifth interdigital space on the back of the hand runs parallel to the metacarpals. It is superficial and mobile and easiest to enter if the skin is punctured distal to the vessel and the cannula advanced in a direct line into the vein. Again, tapping the tissues with the fingers, holding the hand in a dependent position and having venous return obstructed with a cuff or ligature on the upper arm can aid access.

Scalp veins are prominent in infants and young children and easy to cannulate with a 25 or 21 gauge butterfly needle. Over-the-needle cannulas are mar-

TABLE 6.1.1 Peripheral venous access		
Commonly used sites	**Age**	**Cannula size (gauge)**
Scalp vein	Up to 12 months	22–24
Ventral wrist vein or foot veins	Preschool	22–24
Hand veins or long saphenous vein	Any age	18–22
Forearm veins	Over 4 years	18–22

ginally more difficult to insert but last longer once in situ. Look first anteriorly over the forehead and then look for vessels behind and above the ear. Shaving small areas of hair improves access. A loose rubber ligature around the head may make vessels more prominent. These vessels are fragile, easy to pass through and rupture with overzealous infusion. Many physicians find access to scalp veins easier when they puncture the skin away from the vessel and hold the needle with the bevel downwards (this makes penetration through the far side of the vein less likely). Entry to scalp veins is easiest to detect using a saline flushed needle without an attached syringe (blood return is immediate on venous entry).

EQUIPMENT

Have available the following equipment:

- appropriately sized cannulas
- skin cleansing agents
- skin lancet
- flush
- connector
- precut tape
- blood test bottles as necessary

PROCEDURE

1. Prepare all the necessary equipment in advance. An experienced assistant is useful.
2. If time allows, anaesthetize the proposed insertion site with topical anesthetic cream.
3. Clean the skin with alcohol and allow to dry.
4. Having assessed the best site, have an assistant immobilize the limb, occlude venous return and, most importantly, keep the skin taut. *Note*—check for distal pulses to ensure only venous occlusion.
5. After cannula placement, flush and attach the connector.
6. Secure the cannula with tape, and if appropriate immobilize the associated joint with a splint.

Technique:

- removal of the hub cap prior to insertion can aid flashback of blood into the cannula hub
- for smaller gauge cannulas, nick the skin with a lancet to avoid damage to the shoulder of the cannula
- if a vessel is transfixed, remove the needle and gently rotate and withdraw the cannula until the tip reenters the vessel, then attempt gentle advancement
- always use Luer connectors
- the long saphenous vein is not always visible but can often be felt just anterior to the medial malleolus; a transfixion technique is the most effective
- consider elbow splints or arm restraints to avoid the child removing the line as conscious level improves

COMPLICATIONS

- Complications include:
  - incorrect placement
  - flush cannula initially with saline to check if placement is correct, and minimize possibility of extravasation injury
  - stop infusion or injections if patient complains of pain or there is evidence of edema or erythema
  - hematoma formation
  - infection (rate approximately 2%)
  - occlusion or kinking of cannula—tape effectively, and provide strain relief to i.v. line
  - intraarterial injection (associated with severe pain, blanching, loss of distal arterial pulses and development of distal ischemia)

ANALGESIA

Vascular access, particularly when technically difficult, is far from pain-free. Consideration should be given to appropriate anesthesia and/or sedation in conscious children. However, the initial vascular access usually has to be obtained urgently. Topical anesthesia using lidocaine (lignocaine) 2.5% and prilocaine 2.5% cream (e.g. Emla) requires up to 1 hour under an occlusive dressing so often cannot be considered prior to a venous puncture. Tetracaine (amethocaine) gel is more rapid (30 minutes). Lidocaine iontophoresis can provide topical anaesthesia of intact skin within 5 to 15 minutes and has been used successfully with peripheral IV line placement in older children. Percutaneous central access, IO access and peripheral cut-down are techniques where local analgesia with lidocaine instilled using a 27 g needle will reduce the discomfort.

IMMOBILIZATION

Immobilization to secure vascular access once obtained has particular relevance when access is difficult. It is also essential prior to transport, either within the hospital or to another institution. In addition to using adhesive tape to directly secure the needle or cannula, ensure that secondary tapes connect the tubing to the limb to act as a strain relief system. Covering the whole site (cannula and distal element of i.v. delivery tubing) with a transparent self-adhesive dressing (e.g. 'Opsite') has great merit. Such dressing provides a secure anchor and allows the site to be inspected for potential infiltration or bleeding.

UMBILICAL VEIN ACCESS

In the newborn the umbilicus can provide emergency access for several days after birth. The umbilical vein can be used as a peripheral drip (hypertonic solutions must not be used), or advanced into the IVC for central venous access. In the latter case, care must be taken to ensure correct positioning by X-ray before administering any medication. Line insertion should be a sterile procedure. A tape or ligature should be applied loosely around the base of the umbilical stump and under aseptic conditions the cord should be shortened to expose the three vessels. With a fresh cord this can

be done by a scalpel cut at right angles across the stump. Where the cord has partially dried, exploration may be necessary at the junction with the skin. Under these circumstances, a ligature (to prevent hemorrhage) cannot be used. Appropriate forceps and dressings to provide occlusion by pressure must be available in case of bleeding. A 3.5 or 5.0 FG catheter with a single end hole and preferably a radio-opaque strip can be inserted into the venous opening (identified as the single, larger, loose-walled of the three vessels). The catheter should be flushed with saline and have a syringe attached prior to insertion. It is advanced gently until a free flow of blood is returned. The optimal catheter position is one where the tip of the catheter has been advanced the shortest distance to obtain easy blood return below the skin. Overzealous insertion can result in disturbance of the hepatic vasculature. The cannula should be anchored securely (with tape to the abdominal wall or a suture through the umbilical stump); inadvertent removal can cause serious hemorrhage. Generally, umbilical venous catheters are used for resuscitative purposes and are replaced with alternative vascular access once the emergency is contained.

EQUIPMENT

Have available the following equipment:

- skin preparation materials, gloves and drapes
- preflushed umbilical venous catheter
- scalpel
- forceps
- syringe and heparinized saline
- umbilical tape, suture

PROCEDURE

1. Prepare and drape the skin and umbilicus.
2. Tie the tape loosely, with one throw, around the base of the umbilicus and cut the umbilicus straight across at 2 cm length with the scalpel.
3. Identify the umbilical vein. If necessary, dilate the vein gently—then pass the flushed catheter into the vein using the forceps and immobilizing the cord by holding it with a sterile swab. If difficulty

is encountered, aiming towards the left shoulder may aid insertion of the catheter.

4. Having checked that it is easy to aspirate and flush, suture the catheter in place by means of a purse-string suture to the base of the umbilical stump, not the adjoining skin.

COMPLICATIONS

Complications include:

- thrombosis
- embolism (air, thrombus)
- local bowel wall necrosis
- infection
- malpositioned catheter—may cause portal vein thrombosis or areas of liver necrosis.
- possible implication in the etiology of necrotizing enterocolitis

CENTRAL VENOUS ACCESS

The femoral vein is the vessel most frequently used during an emergency central venous cannulation in the child because of its consistent anatomy, relative ease of access and low rate of complications (1%). It is particularly useful during resuscitation as cannulation does not interfere with airway, breathing and chest compression procedures. Femoral veins should not be relied on in patients with major pelvic or abdominal trauma owing to the risk of venous trauma or surgical ligation. The second option is the external jugular vein which, although not a true central vein, is large enough to make rapid infusion possible and can allow monitoring of central venous pressure. The Seldinger technique (using a guide wire) can be used to access both vessels. Vascular access through the internal jugular or subclavian vessels in an emergency should be performed ideally by physicians with experience of inserting such lines electively. Central venous cannulation above the diaphragm involves significant complications (pneumothorax, hemothorax, arrhythmia and local hematomas). If the anatomy of a vessel is thought to be unusual or if there have been previous cannulation attempts, an ultrasound examination may help to assess position and patency.

A 'smart' needle prototype exists which incorporates a Doppler sensor into a standard (18 gauge) needle, and there is a practical model for learning Seldinger's technique for femoral access.

SELDINGER TECHNIQUE FOR FEMORAL VEIN ACCESS

The Seldinger technique is optimally employed using a prepackaged kit (e.g. Cook single-lumen, 4 F or 5 F). This should be a sterile technique with the appropriate analgesia.

1. Externally rotate and evert the leg at the hip.
2. Locate the femoral artery one fingerbreadth below the midpoint of the inguinal ligament, which runs between the anterior superior iliac spine and the symphysis pubis.
3. Introduce a thin-walled needle (or over-the-needle cannula) flushed with saline from an attached 3 ml syringe through the skin just medial to the point located for the femoral artery.
4. Advance the needle at an angle of 45° with the tip directed towards the umbilicus. Apply gentle negative pressure via the syringe. A free flow of blood will be obtained as the vessel is entered. If the vessel is transfixed, apply negative pressure again and gently withdraw the needle. Fluid will be obtained as the needle tip reenters the vessel.
5. Remove the syringe from the needle; insert the Seldinger guide wire into the vessel and remove the needle over it. All appropriate techniques to avoid potential air embolism should be followed: apply a thumb over the needle hub on removal of the syringe, and advance the wire during a positive-pressure breath or spontaneous exhalation.
6. If the guide wire does not advance easily, it may have entered a branch of the IVC. Withdraw it a few centimeters and rotate before advancing again. Never advance a guide wire against sustained resistance.
7. Thread the catheter over the wire and advance it into the vessel. If necessary a dilator can be used over the wire prior to inserting the catheter.

8. Remove the wire and secure the catheter in place. Remove any air remaining and connect to infusion. Suture the catheter in place and cover with a transparent dressing.
9. X-ray to confirm correct catheter position.

Complications

Be aware of potential complications:

- vascular tear
- arterial puncture
- air embolism
- infection
- hematoma
- compartment syndrome
- damaged femoral head

INTERNAL JUGULAR VEIN

The internal jugular vein is large and the distance between the skin entry point and the right atrium is small, leading to a high rate of successful placement.

Procedure

1. Position the child 20° head down, with a pad under the shoulders and the head turned away from the side to be cannulated.
2. Prepare the skin and drape. The classical puncture site is at the junction of the sternal and clavicular heads of the sternocleidomastoid muscle. The vessel lies in the carotid sheath, just anterior and lateral to the carotid artery.
3. Inject local anesthetic solution if required and insert the needle or cannula at an angle of 30° to the skin, aiming towards the nipple, advance the needle, aspirating as you go. If the vein has not been reached in 1–2 cm withdraw the needle again, continuing gentle aspiration. It may be necessary to redirect the cannula slightly more laterally or medially to hit the vein.
4. Disconnect the syringe, occluding the needle with a finger to prevent blood loss and air entry, then insert the guide wire. Remove the needle, ensuring that the guide wire stays in the vein, and then advance the central venous catheter over the wire, which is subsequently removed.

5. Secure the catheter in place, once it has been checked that all lumens flush easily and allow blood to be aspirated.
6. Obtain a chest X-ray to confirm position in the superior vena cava or right atrium and exclude a pneumothorax.

Technique

- the internal jugular vein is close to the skin: if it has not been entered in 1–2 cm, redirect the needle or change the puncture site
- it is easy to transfix the vein without realizing it: withdraw the needle slowly, continuing gentle aspiration
- in thin older children, avoid too much head extension, as this tends to flatten the vein
- fixation of catheters should include placement of a suture close to the skin entry point in addition to any 'suture eyes' in the catheter moulding; this ensures that movement of the catheter is minimized, improving catheter life and reducing catheter-associated problems

EXTERNAL JUGULAR VEIN

Procedure

The procedure is the same as for the internal jugular vein, except that an assistant is required to gently compress the visible part of the vein just above the clavicle to distend the vein. The vein is punctured as it is seen crossing the junction of the middle and lower thirds of the sternocleidomastoid muscle.

Problems can be encountered advancing the wire past the valve at the proximal end of the vein, and a 'J' profile wire should be used. In one study only 54% of attempts were successful (more in older children).

SUBCLAVIAN VEIN

The complication rate for the subclavian vein approach is higher than for the internal jugular vein: consider surgical assistance.

Procedure

1. Position the child 20° head down with a pad centrally under the back and the head turned away from the side to be cannulated.

The ipsilateral shoulder should drop posteriorly.

2. Prepare the skin. The puncture point is approximately 1 cm below the midpoint of the clavicle (slightly more in older children).

3. Infiltrate with local anesthetic solution if required and advance the needle between the clavicle and the first rib keeping as superficial as possible and aiming towards the sternal notch. Aspirate continuously with a syringe until the vein is entered.

4. Proceed as for internal jugular cannulation from step 4 onwards.

COMPLICATIONS

Complications of percutaneous central venous cannulation above the diaphragm include:

- pneumothorax
- hematoma (4%), intrathoracic hemorrhage (1%), or vascular damage
- misplacement, arterial puncture up to 10%, or failure of insertion
- infection and sepsis
  - most catheter-related bacteremias occurring shortly after insertion are probably caused by bacteria gaining access to the blood stream by extraluminal migration along the catheter from the skin site
  - infection tracking down the lumen occurs when catheters are in place for long periods
- venous occlusion or thrombosis

INTRAOSSEOUS ACCESS

Intraosseous vascular access is quick and reliable and has important advantages in the critically ill child. The site is readily accessible and even in a state of shock the marrow cavity remains 'uncollapsed'. It is indicated in emergency circumstances when other methods of venous access are unsuccessful or unsuitable, for example in burned patients. The PALS guidelines are that during CPR in children 6 years old and younger, intraosseous access should be obtained if reliable venous access cannot be achieved within three attempts or 90 seconds (whichever comes first). For children over 6 years old intraosseous access has the same advantages as in the younger child or adult, but the anterior tibial marrow is more difficult to access and alternative sites (lower femur, iliac crest or sternum) need to be considered. Devices currently available for adults which accurately determine optimal depth placement in the sternum will probably soon be available for children.

The anterior tibial site is easy to access (even during CPR) and complications are rare (subcutaneous fluid leakage, extravasation from the puncture site, bone damage and infection). The procedure is contraindicated in a fractured extremity. High flow rates can be achieved (particularly when using a syringe to infuse fluid). All resuscitation drugs (except bretylium), crystalloid and blood can be given by this route, as can catecholamines, calcium, antibiotics, digoxin, heparin, lidocaine (lignocaine), phenytoin and neuromuscular blocking agents.

PROCEDURE

Ideally needle insertion is performed as a sterile technique. A variety of custom-designed needles exist and are preferable if available. However, bone marrow aspiration needles are an alternative and in an emergency any 14–20 gauge needle with an internal stylus can be used.

1. Palpate the site of cannulation one or two fingers' breadth (2–3 cm) inferior to the tibial tuberosity on the flat medial surface of the tibia.

2. Prepare the skin and infiltrate with local anesthetic solution (if appropriate)

3. Align the needle at 90° to the tibia and advance it through the bone cortex with firm pressure and a rotary motion (the limb can be supported on a pad and stabilized by holding the lower femur).

4. Entry into the marrow cavity is felt as a 'give' in resistance.

5. Aspiration of bone marrow confirms entry, but may not always be obtained. A secure placement is indicated by an immobile, free-standing needle. Confirm correct placement by flushing with saline (free flow with no evidence of subcutaneous extravasation).

6. Connect to the infusion set. Immobilize with dressing and tension relief using adhesive tape between the infusion set and leg.
7. Obtain venous access once adequate resuscitation is achieved.

Technique:

- use a connector with a short extension and three-way tap to avoid traction on the needle
- blood samples for analysis may be drawn from the interosseous needle prior to infusion but *do not* introduce these samples into a blood gas analyzer as they are too cellular and will obstruct the tubing
- rapid fluid boluses are best given with a syringe as gravity flow may be poor

RELATIVE CONTRAINDICATIONS

The intraosseous route should be avoided if possible in:

- local infection or osteomyelitis
- fractures of the bone to be used
- severe bone disease (particularly osteogenesis imperfecta)

COMPLICATIONS

Complications include:

- infection at the skin site
- osteomyelitis (risk increases with prolonged infusion)
- extravasation of irritant drugs
- fracture

VENOUS CUT-DOWN

Unless the clinician is well practiced in the venous cut-down technique, intraosseous access (which is more rapid) is preferable to gain vascular access in the critically ill child.

PROCEDURE

1. Collect equipment: skin preparation materials, gloves, local anesthetic solution, scalpel, curved hemostats, small, sharp, pointed scissors, cannulas, ties and suture.
2. The assistant immobilizes the limb while the operator identifies the landmarks, prepares the skin and infiltrates local anesthetic solution.
3. Make an incision through the skin alone perpendicular to the vein, and isolate the vein with gentle blunt dissection using the hemostat.
4. Ensure that 1–2 cm of the vein, are exposed and tie one ligature tightly distally and one loosely proximally.
5. Using traction on the distal ligature to stabilize the vessel, make a longitudinal incision in the vein with the pointed scissors and pass the cannula proximally.
6. Flush the cannula and attach a connector to avoid traction on the cannula from the infusion set or syringe. Firmly tie the proximal tie, being careful not to kink the cannula.
7. Suture the wound as necessary and cover with an occlusive dressing.

Landmarks for long saphenous and brachial cut-downs

Long saphenous cut-down

Superior and anterior to medial malleolus by:

- infant: half a finger's breadth
- small child: one finger's breadth
- older child: two fingers' breadth

Brachial cut-down

Lateral to the medial epicondyle of the humerus by:

- infant: one finger's breadth
- small child: two fingers' breadths
- older child: three fingers' breadths

ARTERIAL ACCESS

The priority during resuscitation is to obtain venous access. However, arterial access facilitates resuscitation by:

- allowing serial blood gas analysis, determination of acid-base status, adequacy of respiratory support and completeness of circulatory resuscitation
- providing a means for continuous systemic arterial blood pressure monitoring
- making calculation of cerebral perfusion pressure possible in conjunction with intracranial pressure monitoring

LOCATION

A variety of arterial sites can be used for cannulation. For immediate care of the critically ill child, the radial and femoral vessels are most readily accessed. The radial site can usually be palpated in the wrist as the vessel is an extension of the brachial artery and runs between the tendon of flexor carpi radialis and the distal portion of the radius. Ideally, the adequacy of collateral circulation (via the ulnar artery) should be confirmed by the Allen test, but this is often not possible in an emergency. The femoral artery is readily felt, one finger's breadth below the inguinal ligament at a point halfway between the symphysis pubis and the anterior superior iliac spine. It is relatively superficial at this point and is immediately lateral to the femoral vein and medial to the femoral nerve.

In patients with impalpable pulses location is aided either by the use of a Doppler probe or, in the case of the radial artery, by transillumination from behind the wrist.

PROCEDURE

Two options are available:

- percutaneous cannulation
- cut-down

If unfamiliar with the percutaneous technique, try to obtain assistance, e.g. from an anesthesiologist. The arteries in children are relatively thick-walled, and because of their small diameter a transfixation technique is more often successful in this group than direct cannulation. The cut-down technique allows direct vision for cannulation and is most likely to prove feasible in an emergency (surgical assistance can also be valuable).

Percutaneous cannulation

The site should be immobilized. This is particularly important in the wrist where 25–30° of extension optimizes successful cannulation. The cannula is inserted towards the heart. A sterile procedure should be used and 1% local anesthetic solution without epinephrine (adrenaline) is instilled, sufficient to block pain but not distort the anatomy. A 20–24 G over-the-needle venous catheter should be flushed with heparin. The skin over the point of maximal pulsation should be punctured with a separate needle. The catheter can be inserted by either direct insertion or a transfixion technique. For the direct method, the needle is introduced slowly with the bevel down at a 30° angle to the wrist in the line of the artery, to the point where the catheter hub fills with blood. The catheter is then gently advanced with slight rotation into the vessel. To transfix the artery, the needle is advanced with the bevel up at a steeper angle (45°) and advanced through the artery. The guide needle is then removed and the catheter is gently withdrawn until blood flow is obtained. An alternative is to use a needle catheter and guide wire combination and a modified Seldinger technique. A short, flexible wire is always useful as an adjunct to achieving arterial cannulation. A T connector should be linked to the cannula which is secured with narrow strips of tape to the surrounding skin. A transparent self-adhesive dressing provides additional security.

Cut-down

The landmarks of the chosen vessel are identified and the site is cleaned and draped. Local anesthesia is used as above. Make a transverse incision through the skin at right angles to the artery. Bluntly dissect the subcutaneous tissues and locate the artery. The artery is usually more prominent than the vein even in shock, is not translucent, appears fuller and may pulsate. Elevate the artery with a hemostat and loop stay sutures around the vessel proximally and distally. The vessel should *not* be tied off. Open the forceps below the vessel to stabilize it, and while holding the proximal stay suture, puncture the vessel parallel with its course with a heparinized cannula inserted bevel down. Slow and gentle progress reduces the risk of vessel spasm. Once the cannula is in situ, connect the catheter as for percutaneous insertion. Suture the cannula in place to the surrounding skin after wound closure. Correct placement is confirmed by an arterial pressure wave form via transducer and free aspiration of arterial blood for sampling (inclusion of a three-way stopcock in the line facilitates sampling).

Arterial lines require a pressure infusor to avoid the patient bleeding back, and a slow infusion of heparinized saline to maintain patency. Arterial catheters should not remain in situ longer than required and should be removed immediately if evidence of tissue ischemia develops distally, or if there is extravasation or other major complication (prolonged arterial spasm, thrombosis, infection, bleeding, expanding hematoma, particle emboli). Warming the contralateral extremity can ease vascular spasm (particularly in newborns). *Do not inject or infuse any medications through an arterial line* (except the heparin in the heparinized infusion). Consider anticoagulants or thrombolytic therapy (streptokinase) in the event of thrombosis. Where blood withdrawal becomes difficult, consider irrigation with a dilute solution of lidocaine (lignocaine) in sodium chloride (0.1 ml of 1% lidocaine made up to 1 ml with 0.9% saline).

Technique:

- flushing the cannula prior to insertion with heparinized saline increases the chance of flashback on entering the vessel
- label the line meticulously (to avoid inadvertent arterial injection)
- always use Luer connectors (to avoid hemorrhage from disconnection)

COMPLICATIONS

Complications include:

- incorrect placement (swelling if extraluminal, no spontaneous or nonpulsatile flashback if intravenous)
- hematoma
- infection
- vascular spasm (loss of transduced trace or inability to draw blood)
- thrombosis (risk increases with the number of arterial puncture attempts and with increasing size of cannula)
- embolism (risk increases with vigorous flushing)

- disconnection and associated blood loss
- necrosis of overlying skin

FURTHER READING

1. Textbook of pediatric advanced life support. American Heart Association; Dallas, Texas 1994
2. APLS: The pediatric emergency medicine course, 2nd ed. American Academy of Pediatrics, Elk Grove Village, Illinois; American College of Emergency Physicians, Dallas, Texas, 1993
   – *(Two manuals containing detailed descriptions of the techniques of venous intraosseous and arterial access)*
3. Levin DL, Morriss FC. Essentials of pediatric intensive care, 2nd ed; New York: Churchill Livingstone, 1997
   – *(A comprehensive text containing detailed descriptions of practical procedures and advice for safe procedures and optimal success)*
4. Gauderer MW. Vascular access techniques and devices in the pediatric patient. Surg Clin North Am 1992; 72: 1267–1284
   – *(Comprehensive review article)*
5. Taylor EA, Mowbray MJ, McLellan I. Central venous access in children via the external jugular vein. Anaesthesia 1992; 47: 265–266
6. Hurren JS, Dunn KW. Intraosseous infusion for burns resuscitation. Burns 1995; 21: 285–287
   – *(Two papers on specific techniques)*
7. Stenzel JP, Green TP, Fuhrman BP et al. Percutaneous femoral venous catheterization: a prospective study of complications. J Pediatr 1989; 114: 411–415
8. Shefler A, Gillis J, Lam A et al. Inferior vena cava thrombosis as a complication of femoral vein catheterisation. Arch Dis Child 1995; 72: 343–345
9. Salzman MB, Rubin LG. Intravenous catheter related infections. Adv Ped Infect Dis 1995; 10: 337–368
10. Rosovsky M, Fitzpatrick M, Goldfarb CR et al. Bilateral osteomyelitis due to intraosseous infusion: case report and review of the English language literature. Pediatr Radiol 1994; 24: 72–73
    – *(Four papers reviewing complications of vascular access).*
11. Macnab AJ, Macnab MK. Teaching pediatric procedures: The Vancouver model for instructing Seldinger's technique of central venous access via the femoral vein. Pediatrics 1999; 103(1): electronic pages www.pediatrics.org/cgi/content/full/103/1/e8
    – *(an inexpensive model for practical instruction of central venous access)*
12. Zempsky WT, Anand KJS, Sullivan KM et al. Lidocaine iontophoresis for topical anesthesia before intravenous line placement in children. J Pediatr 1998; 132: 1061–1063
    – *(A double blind, randomized trial of this method of analgesia prior to elective vascular access)*

6.2 Intubation

Frédéric Sage and Robert Bingham

Tracheal intubation of the acutely ill child requires training, experience and preparation. Even experienced operators need to be assisted by a competent, trained assistant. Each case needs careful planning as physiological needs and anatomy of the airway vary with the age of the patient. There is no time to look for missing equipment or an extra pair of hands once the intubation sequence has been initiated.

The numerous indications for tracheal intubation can be broadly separated into:

- protection of the airway
- control of the airway for intermittent positive pressure ventilation (IPPV)
- bypass of upper airway obstruction

ANATOMY

The anatomical differences between the airways of an infant and of a bigger child or near-adult are summarized in Table 6.2.1.

The infant glottis can be difficult to visualize because of the large tongue, high, anterior larynx, narrow and U-shaped epiglottis, small size and soft, mobile structures. Straight laryngoscope blades have been developed to provide a direct view of the patient's glottis by keeping all the intermediate structures aside. The narrowest part of the airway in a young child (less than 8 years old) is at the cricoid ring. This is where the tracheal tube will fit closest to the walls of the airway. In older children, the narrowest part of the airway is at the vocal cords and a cuffed tube may be necessary to form a seal in the trachea and avoid air leak during ventilation.

PHYSIOLOGY

Compared with the adult, the neonate has proportionally a greater oxygen consumption and a small oxygen reserve. Desaturation during apnea occurs rapidly and is shortly followed by bradycardia, unless oxygenation is maintained by artificial means. Bradycardia in children is far more likely to be due to hypoxemia than a primary cardiac cause, and should be managed initially by oxygen administration rather than by atropine or other chronotropic agents.

PREPARATIONS FOR INTUBATION

AIRWAY ASSESSMENT

1. Is supplemental oxygen needed during the preparation for intubation?
2. Evaluate airway patency and the need for airway maneuvers (Ch. 6.3).
3. Identify potential difficulties: anatomical abnormalities, burns, infections, foreign body, obstruction, etc.

EQUIPMENT

The size of the equipment required depends on the age and weight of the child; in unplanned situations, however, the length of the child may be easier to assess than the weight. Suitable measuring tapes are commercially available (e.g. Broselow tape), with drug doses and tube size information given. All areas where emergency care of a child is a possibility should have an allocated trolley, regularly checked, containing the necessary equipment for the range of children's sizes.

TABLE 6.2.1 **Airway anatomy**		
	Infant	**Older child or adult**
Larynx	C3–4 level	C4–5 level
Position	Anterior	Posterior
Shape	Funnel	Parallel
Narrow point	Cricoid cartilage	Vocal cords
Epiglottis	Narrow, U-shaped, projects posteriorly	Wide, flat, horizontal

Intubation equipment includes:

- oxygen supply, working suction
- breathing systems and face masks allowing an F_{IO_2} of 1.0 and positive pressure ventilation
- laryngoscopes and blades (curved or straight)
- bougies—three types are available:
  - soft gum elastic bougies introduced in the trachea to railroad the tracheal tube over it
  - rigid stylet which should not protrude beyond the tip, to shape the tracheal tube
  - flexible light wands which provide enhanced illumination, improving direct vision and providing soft tissue transillumination to assist blind intubation
- Magill forceps to manipulate the tip of the tracheal tube
- tracheal tubes – sizes to suit patient population covered (Table 6.2.2)
- syringes for inflating cuffs of cuffed tubes
- catheter mounts or other suitable connectors for ventilator/breathing circuits
- stethoscope
- monitoring equipment: ECG, pulse oximeter
  - end-tidal CO_2 analyzer to confirm correct position is desirable

Tracheal tubes

Always have a range of tube sizes available at least one size above and one below estimated size. The appropriate tube size for children over 1 year of age can be calculated using the formulae shown below (box).

$$\text{tube internal diameter (mm)} = \frac{\text{age (years)}}{4} + 4$$

$$\text{tube length (cm)} = \text{internal diameter (mm)} \times 3$$
$$\text{(add 3 cm for nasal length)}$$

Oral and nasal tubes can be taped and left uncut for later position adjustment.

TABLE 6.2.2 Tracheal tube sizes

Age range	Tube size: internal diameter (mm)
Premature neonate	2.0–3.0
Term neonate	3.0
Infant (1 year)	4.0
Child (4–8 years)	Uncuffed 5.0–6.5
Child (8 + years)	Cuffed 6.5+
Adult	7.5–10

INTRAVENOUS ACCESS

It is safer and advisable to establish i.v. access before attempting intubation. Awake intubation outside the resuscitation situation (delivery room, cardiac arrest) is no longer standard practice. This technique carries the potential risk of trauma to the airway, laryngospasm, coughing, desaturation, potentially dangerous cardiovascular response and (in prematurity) intraventricular hemorrhage. Sedation or anesthesia with or without neuromuscular blockade is therefore required. It is therefore necessary to be familiar with the cardiovascular effects, pharmacology and side-effects of the anesthetic, analgesic and neuromuscular blocking agents to be used.

DRUGS USED DURING INTUBATION

Atropine

Atropine is used to prevent vagal bradycardic responses to laryngoscopy and reduce secretions. The dose is 20 µg/kg i.m. or i.v.

Sedative, anesthetic and analgesic drugs:

Drugs used and their i.v. pediatric dosages are:

- benzodiazepines: diazepam emulsion or midazolam 100 µg/kg i.v. bolus; repeat as required
- anesthetic agents:
  - thiopental (thiopentone) 3–5 mg/kg *or*
  - propofol (2–4 mg/kg) *or*
  - ketamine 2 mg/kg
- opiates
  - fentanyl 2–10 µg/kg *or*
  - morphine 50–100 µg/kg

Muscle relaxants

Succinylcholine (suxamethonium) is a rapid onset, short-acting depolarizing muscle relaxant providing very good intubating conditions. The dose is 1 mg/kg (2 mg/kg in infants). Give atropine prior to repeat doses as there is a risk of bradycardia and asystole. There are many unwanted side-effects; *do not use in suspected myopathies.*

Nondepolarizing muscle relaxants are listed in Table 6.2.3. Their speed of onset and duration of action may vary and are often inversely related.

TABLE 6.2.3 **Nondepolarizing muscle relaxants**			
	Dose (mg/kg)	**Onset (s)**	**Duration**
Atracurium	0.5	90–120	Intermediate
Pancuronium	0.1	180	Long
Vecuronium	0.08	120	Intermediate
Mivacurium	0.2	90	Short
Rocuronium	0.6	< 60	Intermediate

After intubation

Following intubation sedation and analgesia are essential. Muscle relaxants are not routinely required, except in reduced chest compliance and increased respiratory drive, but may be indicated (Ch. 5.2).

OTHER PREPARATIONS

A trained, competent assistant is essential. The assistant should be able to provide the required equipment to the operator, apply cricoid pressure, assist with the intubation technique and give drugs as requested. Cricoid pressure is applied gently using one fingertip (in infants) or the thumb and index finger (in children). Gentle pressure occludes the esophagus (protects against passive regurgitation) and moves the larynx inferiorly. The cricoid cartilage (the first tracheal ring) is located by feeling for a prominent horizontal band inferior to the thyroid cartilage and cricothyroid membrane.

Except in case of emergency, the patient should be starved, nasogastric feed stopped for 4 hours and the nasogastric tube aspirated.

Monitoring should be started *before* the beginning of the procedure. At the very least pulse oximetry and ECG should be monitored continuously. An end-tidal CO_2 analyzer is desirable and is becoming the standard of care by which successful tracheal tube placement is judged.

THE INTUBATION SEQUENCE

Intubation cannot be learned from a textbook; the best way to learn and maintain skills is in the operating room with an anesthesiologist working on children.

PREPARATION

Prepare the child for the procedure (see above):

- start monitoring
- check equipment, i.v. access, help
- preoxygenation and denitrogenation take a few minutes. In a sick infant, oxygen reserves are low even with preoxygenation
- position the patient

INDUCTION

For intravenous induction give atropine 20 μg/kg i.v. if indicated and induce anesthesia with a combination of benzodiazepine and opiate or an anesthetic induction agent (see above), followed by a muscle relaxant.

Inhalation is safer in cases of airway obstruction or expected difficult laryngoscopy. Consider i.v. or i.m. administration of atropine. Induce with 100% oxygen and an inhalation agent (halothane or sevoflurane). When the patient is asleep, check that the airway is patent and either administer a muscle relaxant or intubate under deep inhalation anesthesia.

As conscious level decreases a child will lose the ability to maintain optimal airway patency and to increase respiratory effort to compensate for hypoxemia, hypercarbia or acidosis (e.g. secondary to shock).

POSITIONING

Neonates and young children have comparatively large heads. When the head is kept in a neutral position with only some extension over the cervical spine, the glottis is already in an adequate position. Placing too large a pillow or wedge under the shoulders to raise the trunk and neck brings the larynx anteriorly and makes laryngoscopy more difficult.

In an older child, the head is smaller compared with the rest of the body. The glottis and trachea are brought into a line of vision by placing a small pillow under the patient's head (neck flexion, head extension) (Fig. 6.2.1)

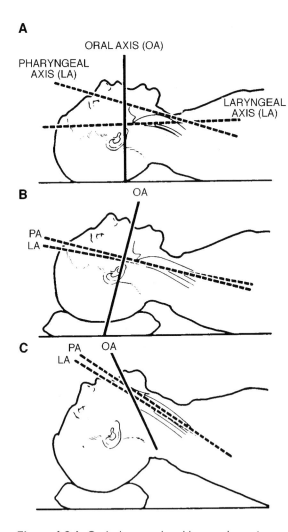

Figure 6.2.1 Oral, pharyngeal, and laryngeal axes in normal supine patient (A), with elevation of the head (B), and with extension at the atlantooccipital joint (C). from Stoelting RK. Endotracheal intubation. In Miller RD, editor. Anesthesia, New York: Churchill Livingstone: 1981. Reproduced with permission

LARYNGOSCOPY

Introduce the laryngoscope blade with care into the right side of the mouth, keeping the tongue to the left. Two types of blade may be used:

- curved (e.g. Mackintosh)
- straight (e.g. Robertshaw)

Intubation technique with curved blade

Slide the laryngoscope blade along the tongue into the vallecula, then an upward movement in the direction of the long axis of the handle lifts the epiglottis from the posterior pharyngeal wall and exposes the larynx. These structures are soft and mobile, and lifting the epiglottis—which often appears narrow, floppy and funneled—may be difficult.

Use gentle posterior pressure at the cricoid level to expose the laryngeal inlet and visualize the cords. Take care not to collapse the airway structures.

Intubation with straight blade

The straight blade laryngoscope is often used in infants. Advance the blade *carefully* in the esophageal inlet, then withdraw slowly. After passing the arytenoid cartilages, the tip of the blade lies against the posterior aspect of the epiglottis, exposing the larynx. Keep a midline position to catch the epiglottis rather than a more lateral structure. In very small patients, the epiglottis may easily slip past the edge of the blade and obstruct the view. The straight blade can also be used as in the same manner as a curved blade, with its tip in the vallecula.

OROTRACHEAL INTUBATION

Use an oral tracheal tube to secure the airway initially, and for short-term intubation or rapid control of the airway. Be sure to see the tip of the tube pass between the cords and advance until the black mark is beyond the larynx.

Fix securely and avoid in and out movements of the tracheal tube, which carry a risk of endobronchial intubation or extubation (see instructions for taping the tube, below).

NASOTRACHEAL INTUBATION

The nasal route is preferred for long-term intubation. It provides a more secure way to fix and maintain the position of the tracheal tube. In a properly positioned patient (neck flexed, head extended), the tracheal tube coming from the nasopharynx will be moving anteriorly whereas the trachea is directed posteriorly. The tip of the tracheal tube can encroach on the anterior aspect of the vocal cords.

Rotate the tube through 360° anticlockwise to swivel the bevel of the tube past the vocal cords, or use the Magill forceps to redirect the tip of the tube. Flexion of the head may also be helpful by placing the tracheal tube in line with the trachea (Table 6.2.4).

AFTER INTUBATION

Attach the patient immediately to a breathing system. Inflate the lungs with oxygen and observe symmetrical chest movements. Check the position of the tracheal tube by listening with a stethoscope over the lung fields and the stomach. Connect an end-tidal CO_2 monitor, if available. Fix the tracheal tube. Pass a nasogastric tube to deflate the stomach if vigorous bag ventilation has been applied.

A leak around the tracheal tube is desirable at a pressure of about 20 cmH_2O to avoid long-term mucosal damage at the subglottic level.

A chest X-ray should be obtained to ensure that the newly placed ET tube is in a satisfactory mid-tracheal position. In neonates, the trachea is short (about 5 cm) and flexion or extension of the head can induce movements of the tube of up to 2 cm.

Position the tracheal tube carefully with the tip in the middle of the trachea so that endobronchial intubation or extubation does not happen during such movements.

A child not responding to intubation should be evaluated as in Table 6.2.5.

ENDOTRACHEAL TUBE TAPING

The purpose of taping the endotracheal tube is to secure it in position to avoid spontaneous extubation or internal migration. You will need the following equipment:

- 15 × 10 mm white adhesive tape
- medicine cup
- compound benzoin tincture (Friars' balsam)
- cotton-wool bud
- two gauze squares (5 cm × 5 cm)
- endotracheal tray set-up
- ruler
- small bottle of sterile water
- scissors
- adhesive (Matisol or similar)

Method for nasotracheal tube

1. With the cotton-wool buds, apply Friars' balsam down the bridge of the nose, on both cheeks and above the upper lip. Allow a few seconds for the balsam to dry and become tacky. Apply adhesive to the same areas.
2. Place the first white tape down the bridge of the nose, around the endotracheal tube

TABLE 6.2.4 **Oral and nasal intubation**		
	ORAL	**NASAL**
Advantages	Easier Less trauma Provides rapid access to the airway	Better fixation More secure Takes less space Easy mouth care Allows reflex sucking Easier suction
Disadvantages	Poor tube fixation Mobile tube Bulky at connector level	Technically more difficult Trauma to nose/adenoids Infection risk Long-term damage to nose

TABLE 6.2.5 **Evaluation of the child not responding following intubation. Most children respond quickly to normal resuscitation techniques, particularly following respiratory arrest. If a child is still cyanosed, pale, obtunded or has an abnormal heart rate after intubation, then a careful examination should be conducted to determine the cause. Check the points listed here**

- Is the endotracheal tube in the trachea?
    - mist should be seen in the tube on expiration
    - chest should expand with positive pressure
    - air entry should be equal and symmetrical over the chest
    - abdomen should not become distended
    - if still in doubt, confirm tube position with laryngoscope and measure end-tidal CO_2
- Are there any mechanical problems with ventilation?
    - check that oxygen source is on
    - check pressure is being delivered; are all circuit connections intact?
    - if using a self-inflating bag, check that reservoir is present and inflated
- Is there right mainstem bronchus intubation?
    - black line on endotracheal tube should be at level of vocal cords
    - air entry should be equal right and left (not decreased on the left side)
- Is there airway obstruction?
    - air entry usually decreased in spite of high pressures (adventitious chest sounds may be present)
    - precordium usually in midline
    - child is more hypercarbic than hypoxic
    - if a blockage is suspected, suction the endotracheal tube; repeat after irrigation with 2 ml 0.9% saline and/or remove tube and reintubate
    - if suspected cause is anatomical or a foreign body, attempt bypassing affected area, advancing tube to near the carina
- Is there acute bleeding or volume depletion?
    - relevant history present?
    - air entry and chest expansion are usually good
    - peripheral perfusion is poor; capillary refill is slow (> 3 s)
    - cold, pale extremities
    - peripheral pulse is difficult to palpate
    - pulse rate relatively rapid
    - heart sounds distant
    - pulse pressure narrow (BP low – late sign)
    - CNS obtunded
    - marked metabolic acidosis is present
- Is infection a possibility?
    - suggestive history?
    - air entry and chest expansion are usually good
    - peripheral perfusion is poor; capillary refill is slow (> 3 s)
    - metabolic acidosis may be present
- Is there a pneumothorax?
    - is precordium in the midline (more likely to be shifted to the left as right-sided pneumothorax is more common during resuscitation)?
    - is air entry asymmetrical (reduced on one side)?
    - does the chest appear hyperinflated?

Modified from Albersheim S, Ling E. In: The Pocket Pediatrician. Seear M. (ed) Cambridge University Press, 1996.

twice, back up on to the tip of the nose and across the cheek

- if the tube is located in the right naris, ensure that the first tape goes down the nose and *around the right side of the tube* first and then on to the right cheek
- if the tube is located in the left naris, ensure that the first tape goes down the nose and around the *left side of the tube first* and then on to the left cheek. This will pull the tube away from the nasal septum and reduce pressure on the septum
- ensure that the tube exits the naris in a downward position, to reduce the chance of iatrogenic nasal notching

3. Place the second white tape down the bridge of the nose, around the endotracheal tube twice (opposite direction to that in step 2), back up onto the tip of the nose and across the untaped cheek.
4. Place a piece of white tape across the bridge of the nose from cheek to cheek to help secure the existing tapes.
5. The fourth tape is placed across the face and around the tube to hold it in a downward position
   - apply this tape from the upper outside corner of the upper lip to the area beneath the naris occupied by the tube
   - twist and wrap the tape around the tube once
   - continue adhering tape onto the upper lip from the midline to the opposite corner of the mouth
6. The fifth tape is used to secure the fourth tape. Measure the length of the endotracheal tube. This measurement *is from the tip of the nose to the end of the tube after the tapes have been applied.*
7. Note the marking on the endotracheal tube at the point where it exits the naris. Place an endotracheal guard around the tube. Secure it in place with two pieces of clear tape. Document in the chart:
   - the mark at which the tube exits the naris
   - the measured length of the tube

8. Restrain the child's arms (e.g. splint arms to prevent elbow flexion but allow movement) and prescribe sedation/analgesia (to avoid self-extubation and distress)

Method for orotracheal tube

1. Apply Friars' balsam and adhesive to the cheek.
2. Apply tapes to the cheek area, wrap twice around the endotracheal tube and secure on adhesive on cheek.
3. Confirm the tube is secure.
4. Note the tube marking at the corner of the mouth.
5. Measure from the point noted in step 4 to the end of the tube.
6. Insert the 'blue' tube connector into the endotracheal tube and attach to humidified gas/ventilator delivery system.
7. Restrain the child's arms (splint elbows) to avoid self-extubation. Sedate.

RAPID SEQUENCE INDUCTION

The rapid sequence induction technique is used when there is a high risk of regurgitation: full stomach, reflux, delayed gastric emptying, and raised intraabdominal pressure. It aims to reduce the length of time between loss of airway reflexes at induction of anesthesia and securing the airway with a tracheal tube. After preoxygenation, induce the patient rapidly with thiopental (thiopentone) 3–5 mg/kg i.v. followed by succinylcholine (suxamethonium) 1 mg/kg i.v. immediately without checking airway patency. Cricoid pressure is applied by an assistant as soon as consciousness is lost. Positive pressure breaths should be avoided between induction and intubation.

> A rapid sequence induction should not be used if the laryngoscopy seems potentially difficult. Positive pressure ventilation may be needed even during a rapid sequence induction if oxygen desaturation occurs. Hypoxia is dangerous.

COMPLICATIONS

IMMEDIATE

Desaturation, hypoxia

Prevent by:

- checking position and equipment before starting
- monitoring oxygen saturation
- confirming hand ventilation is possible before paralyzing

Make oxygenation your priority.

Pneumothorax

Prevent by:

- taking care with bougies and stylets
- checking the position of the tracheal tube
- avoiding high airway pressures

Esophageal intubation

Avoid by:

- intubating trachea under direct vision
- checking position of tracheal tube
- monitoring patient and expired gases

If in doubt, extubate and ventilate with a face mask.

Hemodynamic responses

Neonates can respond to intubation with tachycardia and hypertension. In susceptible patients (premature babies), there may be a risk of intraventricular hemorrhage. Appropriate sedation and anesthesia before intubation will minimize these responses. Avoid vagal stimulation by administration of anticholinergics.

LONG TERM

The following long-term complications may occur:

- vocal cord palsy: direct damage to cricoarytenoid cartilages or joints
- tracheal stenosis, subglottic stenosis—narrowing of the airway after prolonged contact with the tracheal tube

  - the risk is diminished by keeping a leak around the tube and checking it regularly
  - acquired subglottic stenosis in low-birthweight infants may be more common with an oral tracheal tube owing to repeated reintubation and up and down movement of the tube in the trachea
- granuloma formation
- ulceration of nostril
- blocked tube
- infection

✓ KEY POINTS

➤ Oxygenation is the priority

➤ Have everything prepared before starting, including assistance

➤ Use the intubation technique you know best

➤ Do not use specialist equipment (fiberoptic laryngoscope, Bullard laryngoscope, McCoy blade) on difficult patients, unless you are fully familiar with its use

➤ Never lose control of the airway

➤ Intubate orally to secure the airway rapidly and take time to prepare for a nasal intubation

➤ Check you can ventilate the patient manually *before* giving a muscle relaxant and attempting intubation (but see also note on rapid sequence induction)

➤ With proper airway maintenance, low inflation pressures are possible during mask ventilation; high inflation pressures result in gastric distention and increased risk of regurgitation

➤ Beware of cervical spine injury: stabilize the neck if injury is suspected

➤ The main reason for having difficulty in intubating a child is inadequate visibility owing to:
  - overextension of the head and neck
  - overinsertion of the laryngoscope

➤ Leaving the tracheal tube uncut avoids the need for bulky, heavy connectors at the mouth which can kink the tube and cause airway obstruction. As long as the child is ventilated and monitored the effect on airway resistance and rebreathing will be small

FURTHER READING

1. APLS. The pediatric emergency medicine course. Elkgrove: American Academy of Pediatrics, 1993
2. Pediatric advanced life support manual. American Heart Association; Dallas, 1994
3. Geradi MJ, Sacchetti AD, Cantor RM. Rapid sequence intubation of the pediatric patient. Ann Emerg Med 1996; 28(1): 55–74
4. Hung OR Murphy M. Light wands, lighted stylets and blind techniques of intubation. Anesth Clin North Am 1995; 13(2): 477–489
   – *(Four publications providing additional description and illustrations of intubation techniques)*
5. Lubitz DS, Seidel JI, Chameides L et al. A rapid method for estimating weight and resuscitation drug dosages from length in the pediatric age group. Ann Emerg Med 1988; 17: 576
   – *(A description of the Broselow tape)*

6.3 Securing the airway

Frédéric Sage and Robert Bingham

Respiratory problems are a common cause of morbidity in children and many situations can deteriorate rapidly and dramatically. Anticipation of potential problems with airway patency or respiration, early recognition of symptoms and signs, and prompt management of such events are essential.

Many cardiac arrests in children are due to airway obstruction and hypoxia. An asystolic arrest following a period of hypoxia has a very poor prognosis.

THE PEDIATRIC AIRWAY

Neonates have comparatively large tongues and are obligate nose breathers. Obstruction of the nasal passages (e.g. choanal atresia) or exaggeration of the pharyngeal anatomy (e.g. micrognathia) result in airway compromise and respiratory distress.

Infants have airways of small diameter. A minimal reduction in that diameter due to edema for example, produces a large increase in airway resistance. Infants have soft, collapsible airways and compliant chest walls. These anatomical structures collapse with increased respiratory efforts and result in obstruction, stridor and inefficient ventilation.

CAUSES OF AIRWAY PROBLEMS

Many pathological conditions can lead to respiratory compromise or airway obstruction. They may be congenital or acquired, involving the oropharynx, nasopharynx, larynx or tracheobronchial tree. For the purpose of airway management in critical illness and injury, they are discussed here according to their degree of urgency.

AIRWAY EMERGENCIES

Airway assessment and treatment is the first priority in emergency resuscitation of the child or adult. In children, emergency treatment must always include an assessment of the patency of the airway and of the adequacy of oxygen delivery to the lungs. This is particularly important with neonates or premature infants who have a high oxygen consumption and low oxygen reserves (reduced functional residual capacity).

Acute airway emergencies include:

- cardiorespiratory arrest
- depressed conscious level
- infections (epiglottitis, croup, bacterial tracheitis)
- trauma
- edema
- mucus plug
- foreign body aspiration
- pneumothorax
- airway burns

> Beware of epiglottitis: avoid any stimulation and do not leave the child unattended until ready for anesthesia and intubation

NONACUTE AIRWAY MANAGEMENT

Management of the airway can be a chronic problem needing continued treatment.

Upper airway

Continued treatment is needed for infants with anatomical conditions such as Pierre Robin or Treacher Collins syndromes, micrognathia or macroglossia. Patients with cystic hygroma or mucopolysaccharidosis may also be affected.

Lower airway

Patients presenting with laryngomalacia or tracheobronchomalacia, vocal cord palsy, subglottic stenosis, webs, vascular rings or papillomatosis may also require airway support.

Surgical conditions

Gastroesophageal reflux is a cause of airway difficulty and recurrent respiratory problems. Treatment includes nasogastric feeding, prokinetic drugs and surgical correction. Other surgical conditions that may cause airway problems include diaphragmatic hernia and tracheoesophageal fistula. Medical treatment may be needed in some circumstances before the surgical correction can be carried out.

Following extubation

Patients being weaned from ventilation may require some form of airway support such as nasal prongs, continuous positive airway pressure (CPAP) or biphasic positive airway pressure (BIPAP) to assist respiratory efforts and reduce the work of breathing.

AIRWAY MANAGEMENT DURING ANESTHESIA AND SEDATION

> In situations requiring sedation or anesthesia, safe airway management is fundamental

Monitoring of respiration must be started before any drugs are given and should include clinical observation as well as pulse oximetry. Administer supplemental oxygen and provide airway assistance until the patient has fully recovered.

SIGNS OF AIRWAY OBSTRUCTION

As part of the sequential 'ABC' approach of resuscitation, assessment of the patency of the airway only requires a few moments:·

- neurological assessment:
  - is the patient conscious, restless, obtunded or unresponsive?
  - evaluate the ability to talk or feed
- posture:
  - sitting forward gasping for breath (children)
  - mouth open, head extended (infants)

- color:
  - cyanosis, mottling, pallor
- respiratory effort:
  - tachypnea, head bobbing, nasal flaring, tracheal tugging, intercostal, subcostal and suprasternal recession, paradoxical abdominal ventilation
- air entry:
  - look for chest expansion or paradoxical chest movements
  - listen for breath sounds, stridor, grunts, wheezes, gasping
- cardiovascular system:
  - sweating, tachycardia or (in extremis) bradycardia

> In a child who has been fighting to maintain airway and ventilation, the onset of hypotonia and lethargy are ominous signs of fatigue (including failing CNS function) and impending cardiorespiratory arrest

AIRWAY MANAGEMENT MANEUVERS

ACUTE AIRWAY PROBLEMS

Emergency airway maneuvers

These are well described and can be found, for example, in the APLS or PALS manuals. They include:

- airway assessment:
  - look for obstructed respiratory effort
  - listen and feel for air entry
  - look for obvious airway obstruction
- give 100% oxygen throughout
- open the airway:
  - head tilt, chin lift (see Figure 6.3.1) unless suspected cervical spine injury, in which case jaw thrust is used
  - jaw thrust can open the airway without head/neck tilt. Use two or three fingers of each hand at the angle of the jaw to lift it upwards and outwards
  - remove visible foreign body or obstructing debris
  - do *not* do a blind pharyngeal sweep

It is essential to apply pressure only on the mandible and avoid compressing the soft tissues of the submental area, which would make airway obstruction worse

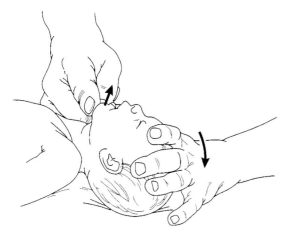

Figure 6.3.1 Opening the airway with head tilt, chin lift

- in suspected foreign body airway obstruction, use techniques to sharply increase intrathoracic pressure:
  - back blows and chest thrusts for infants, with the addition of abdominal thrusts for older children
- if basic maneuvers are successful, give oxygen, maintain airway patency and continue assessment
  - spontaneous ventilation should be easy with unobstructed breaths

Clinical situations evolve: frequently reassess a critically ill child even though the airway was initially patent and respiratory effort adequate

ASSISTED VENTILATION

If no spontaneous breathing is detected, assisted ventilation is provided via a bag-valve and mask system with the highest obtainable inspired oxygen concentration whilst preparations are made to intubate the trachea. The airway is kept clear by placing the fourth and fifth fingers behind the angle of the mandible and thrusting the jaw forward, whilst the first and second fingers apply the

mask firmly to the face and provide an airtight fit. With each slow compression of the bag, the chest should rise equally with minimum inflation pressure. High pressures result in gastric distention.

If the airway remains obstructed, more advanced techniques should be used:

- two operators bag and mask technique: one to hold the airway, the other to compress the bag
- insert an oropharyngeal airway if the patient is unconscious and has lost airway reflexes
- provide respiratory support and CPAP with a bag-and-face mask system
- proceed to endotracheal intubation, which is the definitive airway treatment

PROTECTING THE AIRWAY

Beware of loss of airway protection and risk of vomiting and aspiration. Functioning suction equipment must be available. Cricoid pressure protects against passive regurgitation but not active vomiting. Pressure should be discontinued if vomiting occurs. Esophageal rupture has been reported after cricoid pressure was wrongly applied during vomiting. If active vomiting occurs, place the patient head down on the side and clear the airway with suction.

Equipment

Face masks

Face masks should be preferably clear with soft, deformable rim. Rendell Baker masks have a low dead space but are more difficult to apply properly without a leak (no rim). Some anatomical masks have an inflatable rim which facilitates the seal, but because of their shape, need to be of the correct size to be effective. Circular masks are preferred for neonates as they easily fit their faces.

Airways

Oropharyngeal airways need to be introduced carefully to avoid trauma to the soft tissues. Correctly sized (corner of the mouth to angle of the jaw), the airway keeps the tongue away from the pharyngeal wall and allows an unobstructed path for air entry. A small airway might push the tongue backwards and worsen the obstruction, an oversized airway might stimulate airway reflexes, coughing, laryngospasm or vomiting.

Nasopharyngeal airways are better tolerated in the conscious patient and allow normal feeding and sucking from an infant. They may cause hemorrhage during insertion.

Breathing systems

The bag-valve-mask system (self-inflating bag) is favored for resuscitation as it does not require an oxygen source, does not produce rebreathing (one-way valves) and does not need a perfect seal around the mouth to deliver a breath. Judging the effectiveness of the ventilation, however, is difficult and it is inefficient in the spontaneously breathing patient. A reservoir is required to deliver high oxygen concentrations.

Anesthetic breathing systems (Ayre's T-piece with Jackson-Rees modification, Mapleson C system) require an oxygen source, a gas flow meter and a perfect seal to ensure filling of the reservoir bag. The advantages are that a high concentration of oxygen can be delivered (up to 100%), the absence of valve (T piece) facilitates spontaneous ventilation and the level of airway pressure during insufflation can be adjusted to reinflate collapsed lung, provide CPAP or during physiotherapy. Regular practice is required for safe use.

Other equipment

Oxygen, connectors between face mask and breathing system, suction and full airway resuscitation equipment are also required.

NONACUTE AIRWAY PROBLEMS

Tracheal intubation

Tracheal intubation usually requires nursing, (often respiratory) assistance, sedation and admission to a PICU.

Tracheostomy

A tracheostomy has the advantage of comfort, compliance and ease of care once established. It requires a minimum level of medical supervision, can allow speech and a normal social and psycho-logical development. It can stay in place for many years, until the child grows out of its problem or can undergo a definitive treatment (see Ch. 5.10).

Airway adjuncts

Several techniques are available to help in difficult situations:

- in the short term, an oropharyngeal airway can be taped in place to maintain a clear airway in case of nasal airway obstruction (e.g. choanal atresia)
- a nasopharyngeal airway is indicated if the obstruction is at the level of the oropharynx (e.g. Pierre Robin syndrome)
- CPAP can be applied through nasal prongs or masks and provide a pneumatic splint in laryngo- or tracheomalacia, and to prevent or treat moderate degrees of atelectasis
- The laryngeal mask airway has been successfully used in situations of severe airway compromise where tracheal intubation is impossible. It has been used as the sole means of airway maintenance (complete laryngotracheal cleft) or as an aid to fiberoptic intubation (Pierre Robin, cystic hygroma).

✔ KEY POINTS

- ➤ Always give oxygen
- ➤ Follow 'ABC' procedures; reassess the patient regularly
- ➤ When opening the airway, avoid pressure on the submental area or overextension of the neck as this may worsen obstruction
- ➤ Do not hesitate to ask for assistance (anesthesiologist, intensive care physician, pediatrician, any more experienced individual)
- ➤ Airway support is a practical skill. A theoretical understanding of the principles must be complemented by hands on instruction and skill maintenance. 'Refresher' sessions with an anaesthetist in the OR is the optimal approach

FURTHER READING

See previous chapter

6.4 Assisted ventilation

Robert Henning

In Chapter 2.1, respiratory failure is divided into failure of ventilation (indicated by increased Pa_{CO_2}) and failure of oxygenation (indicated by an increased AaD_{O_2}). That chapter also discusses methods of supporting oxygenation when ventilation is adequate. This chapter discusses the treatment of ventilatory failure with or without impaired oxygenation. Mechanical ventilation and other forms of respiratory support do not cure illness, but merely keep the child alive until the disorder causing respiratory failure is cured by time or some other treatment, so the best form of respiratory support and the best blood gas targets are those that give the greatest chance of survival with the least risk of long-term damage to the lungs or other organs.

If the main cause of hypoventilation is disease of the lower airways or of the lung parenchyma, the static compliance and airways resistance are usually unevenly distributed throughout the lung, so during mechanical ventilation some areas of lung are overinflated while others are underventilated. If high peak inflation pressures (PIP) and large tidal volumes are employed to achieve normal blood gases, this maldistribution of mechanical breaths leads to a greatly increased risk of barotrauma (pneumothorax, pneumomediastinum, pneumoperitoneum and pulmonary interstitial emphysema) and volutrauma (ARDS-like lung injury due to alveolar overdistension in the previously normal, compliant areas of lung).

To minimize this iatrogenic lung damage, a more appropriate strategy is to use only enough ventilation to maintain life: the PIP and tidal volume are restricted to the level needed to maintain the pH above 7.15, and usually the Pa_{CO_2} below 11 kPa (80 mmHg). Peak inflation pressures greater than 35 cmH$_2$O (3.5 kPa) should not be used. Elective, controlled mechanical hypoventilation may require heavy sedation to eliminate distressing dyspnea. Sodium bicarbonate may be infused over 1 hour to maintain the pH above 7.15 in the presence of a metabolic acidosis. Rapid infusion of NaHCO$_3$ may cause an intracellular acidosis, especially when the ability of the lungs to excrete carbon dioxide is limited. The F_{IO_2} is usually kept at 0.5 or below in order to minimize oxygen toxicity to the lung, while the Pa_{O_2} is maintained by positive end-expiratory pressure of 5–15 cmH$_2$O (0.5–1.5 kPa). Pulmonary oxygen toxicity does not occur if the F_{IO_2} is 0.5 or less, but symptoms of chest tightness, followed by reduced vital capacity, tracheitis and all of the pathological changes of ARDS (Ch. 3.1) occur at F_{IO_2} above 0.5, even in previously normal lungs. The higher the F_{IO_2}, the earlier the onset of pathophysiological changes (Fig. 6.4.1).

When alveolar hypoventilation is caused by disease of the central nervous or neuromuscular systems, the lungs are usually compliant, requiring a low PIP for inflation and need little added oxygen to achieve a Pa_{O_2} above 13 kPA (100 mmHg). In this case, it is appropriate to aim for normal blood gases, because significant lung damage due to these low levels of PIP and F_{IO_2} is unlikely.

CONTINUOUS POSITIVE AIRWAYS PRESSURE

Continuous positive airways pressure (CPAP) devices deliver a positive pressure to the child's

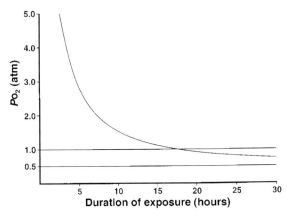

Figure 6.4.1 The time at which signs of significant lung injury appear at different levels of inspired P_{O_2}

airway during inspiration and expiration. The essential features of CPAP delivery are shown in Figure 6.4.2. They are:

- a flow of fresh gas during inspiration and expiration: this flow may be continuous or may be servocontrolled to deliver the desired level of CPAP; fluctuations in airway pressure can be reduced by increasing the fresh gas flow rate
- an expiratory valve which retards gas flow during expiration, creating a positive pressure in the airway
- a pressure measuring device
- a reservoir to prevent pressure fluctuation during inspiration: this may be a pressurized bellows or a large reservoir bag

This type of ventilation may be delivered during spontaneous breathing or may be combined with some form of positive pressure ventilation, when it is known as positive end-expiratory pressure (PEEP). Ventilation using CPAP (or PEEP) can be delivered by an invasive route such as an endotracheal tube or tracheostomy tube, or by a noninvasive route (nasal or nasopharyngeal CPAP) such as a nasal mask, nasal prongs or a nasopharyngeal tube (Ch. 2.1).

BENEFICIAL EFFECTS OF CPAP

1. Continuous positive airway pressure (5–15 cmH$_2$O) splints the upper airway, preventing airway narrowing in conditions such as tracheobronchomalacia and postextubation stridor

2. It splints small airways (e.g. in bronchiolitis, pertussis, and in those cases of asthma in which dynamic expiratory compression of small airways is prominent), preventing their collapse in expiration. This usually requires 5–10 cmH$_2$O (0.5–1 kPa) CPAP. Only a trial of CPAP differentiates responders from nonresponders: success is judged by subjective improvement in dyspnea, by an increase in oxygen saturation, or by a reduction in respiratory rate, $Paco_2$ or the severity of apnea.

3. Collapsed alveoli and small airways are recruited, reducing intrapulmonary shunting and AaDO$_2$, reducing $Paco_2$ and improving oxygen saturation. The use of CPAP is more effective when the intra-pulmonary shunt is due to alveolar edema (e.g. pneumonia or early ARDS) than when it is due to alveolar destruction or fibrosis (e.g. late ARDS or organizing pneumonia).

4. Lung compliance is improved (by increasing the lung volume from section A to section B, Figure 6.4.3), and thereby reducing the work of breathing.

ADVERSE EFFECTS OF CPAP

1. Overdistention of alveoli by CPAP exceeding 5 cmH$_2$O (0.5 kPa) can cause pulmonary barotrauma (pneumothorax, pneumo-mediastinum, pulmonary

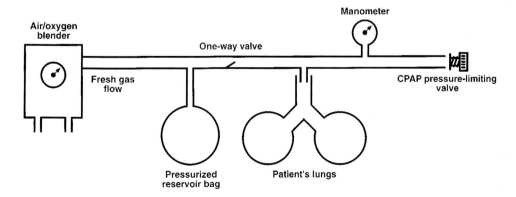

Figure 6.4.2 The essential features of a device for delivering CPAP

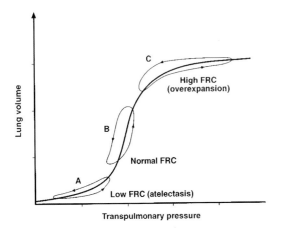

Figure 6.4.3 Lung compliance curve, showing that the change in lung volume per unit change in airway pressure is greatest (B) at the normal functional residual capacity (FRC) and that the lung is much less compliant at low lung volume (A) and when overinflated (C)

interstitial emphysema) it also causes increased ventilation–perfusion mismatch when the raised intraalveolar pressure obstructs the blood flow to some alveoli.

2. Increased work of breathing occurs if CPAP moves the lung onto the flat upper part of the compliance curve (section C in Figure 6.4.3).
3. Pulmonary vascular resistance is increased and pulmonary blood flow reduced when the lungs are very compliant.
4. Exacerbation of gas trapping occurs in some cases of acute asthma (those without dynamic expiratory airways compression), causing increased dyspnea.
5. Intracranial pressure (ICP) is increased in children with intracranial hypertension. In these cases, if PEEP/CPAP is required to maintain adequate oxygenation, the intracranial pressure should be monitored and the level of CPAP titrated against ICP and hemoglobin saturation.
6. Reduced venous return causes reduced cardiac output. The more compliant the lungs, the more the airway pressure is transmitted to the heart, including the right atrium, impairing venous return.
7. Fluid retention results from reduced renal blood flow, reduced production of atrial

natriuretic peptide and increased production of antidiuretic hormone.

POSITIVE PRESSURE VENTILATION

A positive pressure ventilator causes alveolar ventilation by generating a pressure gradient (from a pressurized bellows or reduced from a high-pressure gas cylinder or pipeline) between the ventilator tubing (Fig. 6.4.4) and the alveoli: gas flows into the alveoli down this gradient. The exhalation valve remains closed during inspiration. When it opens, the patient exhales passively via the exhalation valve and a PEEP/CPAP valve.

WHAT INITIATES INSPIRATION?

Inspiration can be initiated by *time* (i.e. breaths are delivered at regular intervals, regardless of the child's breathing) or by *patient effort* (the patient generates a small inspiratory gas flow or a small negative pressure in the ventilator tubing, or abdominal muscle movement is detected by a skin capsule which triggers inspiration). Timed (i.e. nontriggered) onset of inspiration is used for a child who is apneic (e.g. because of muscle relaxant drugs) or who is too small or weak to generate a detectable respiratory effort. Triggered ventilation is more comfortable for the child, and in general requires lower airway pressures and less sedation to achieve the same P_{O_2} and P_{CO_2} as nontriggered ventilation. There is no conclusive evidence that one of the triggered modes (pressure, flow or movement) is better than the others.

WHAT INITIATES EXPIRATION?

This is known as 'cycling':

- *time-cycled*: each breath lasts a fixed time, adjusted by the operator (this is the most common form in modern ventilators)
- *volume-cycled*: inspiration ceases when the set tidal volume has been delivered at the set flow rate or within the set pressure limits
- *pressure-cycled*: the inspiratory phase ceases when the airway pressure reaches a set level

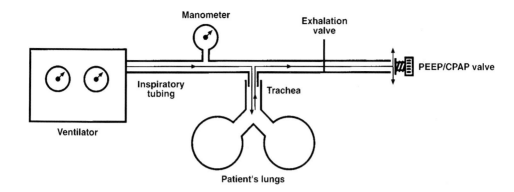

Figure 6.4.4 The essential features of a positive pressure ventilator. During inflation, the exhalation valve closes and gas flows down a pressure gradient into the alveoli. During exhalation, the exhalation valve opens and gas flows passively from the alveoli to atmosphere via the CPAP/PEEP valve

- *flow-cycled*: inspiration ceases when inspiratory gas flow falls to a preset level (e.g. 5% of the initial inspiratory flow)

IS THERE CONTINUOUS FLOW OF GAS THROUGH THE VENTILATOR TUBING DURING EXPIRATION?

Continuous flow is a feature present in most neonatal ventilators and some adult ventilators ('flow by'); it reduces work of breathing by providing gas for spontaneous inspiration between machine breaths without the need to trigger an inspiratory valve. It also permits a much more stable CPAP/PEEP to be maintained. The flow rate used in continuous flow neonatal ventilators is 2–3L/kg·min.

SIZE OF THE VENTILATOR DEAD SPACE

The ventilator dead space is the total gas volume from the tip of the endotracheal tube back to the point in the ventilator circuit where inspired gas is separated from expired gas. Dead space gas is alveolar gas containing CO_2 and is rebreathed. The larger the dead space volume, the higher is the P_{CO_2} for any tidal volume. When setting up a ventilator circuit, one must look very carefully at the way gas flows through the circuit, eliminating any exhalation points (including large leaks) in the *inspiratory* limb of the circuit, as these will lead to rebreathing and CO_2 accumulation.

PRESSURE-LIMITED OR VOLUME-LIMITED VENTILATION

In *volume-limited* ventilation, the operator sets the tidal volume, the PEEP and the inspiratory flow rate (or inspiratory time). The PIP is then dependent on the child's dynamic compliance. The higher the airways resistance or the less compliant the lungs, the higher the PIP that will be reached. In larger patients (> 30 kg), volume-limited ventilation may give more accurate control of gas exchange, provided that there is only a small air leak around the endotracheal tube (Ch. 6.2), as Pa_{CO_2} is inversely related to alveolar ventilation. In smaller patients and especially in those with a large leak of air around the endotracheal tube or into a bronchopleural fistula, the magnitude of the leak often varies markedly with head position, so that the tidal volume delivered to the lungs may vary by 50% or more over a few minutes. The proportion of the set tidal volume that is consumed by stretching of ventilator tubing and compression of gas in the ventilator, humidifier and tubing is quite large in infants, so the adequacy of any set tidal volume must be checked by blood gas analysis (especially Pa_{CO_2}).

In *pressure-limited* ventilation, the PIP is set by the operator. The tidal volume is then dependent on the dynamic compliance of the child's respiratory system—that is, the higher the airways resistance or the lower the static compliance (e.g. in pneumonia or ARDS), the smaller is the tidal volume. The tidal volume for any level of PIP in pressure-limited ventilation can be increased by slowing the inspiratory flow rate.

The pressure delivered to the airway remains constant regardless of leak, and the tidal volume depends only on the lung compliance which is relatively constant (although if the child's respiratory effort is not coordinated with the ventilator, and the child wants to breathe out during machine inspiration, the preset pressure will be reached despite only a small volume of air reaching the lungs.) The best solution to the problem of uncoordinated respiratory effort is triggered, pressure-limited ventilation (i.e. pressure support), although triggered volume-limited ventilation (synchronized intermittent mandatory ventilation, SIMV) or merely increasing the untriggered ventilator rate (entrainment) may be used.

In restrictive lung disease (e.g. pulmonary edema, pneumonia, ARDS or hyaline membrane disease), oxygenation is improved by increasing the *mean* airway pressure (up to the point at which further increases in pressure obstruct blood flow to some alveoli). If all other factors remain constant, increasing the PEEP, increasing the peak inflation pressure or increasing the inspiration:expiration (I:E) ratio increases the mean airway pressure (Fig. 6.4.5).

ADJUSTABLE VARIABLES

The variables that can be adjusted during mechanical ventilation are as follows.

Ventilator rate

Increasing the ventilator rate reduces the arterial P_{CO_2}. For a given total minute ventilation, a high rate and low tidal volume remove less CO_2 than a lower rate and a larger tidal volume (because the dead space is ventilated with each breath), but use a lower peak airway pressure. The ventilator rates used during conventional intermittent positive pressure ventilation (IPPV) are:

- newborn: 30–60 breaths/min
- 6 months old: 25–30 breaths/min
- 1–5 years old: 20–25 breaths/min
- 5–12 years old: 15–20 breaths/min
- >12 years old: 12–15 breaths/min

The ventilator rate determines the cycle time (the time between the start of one inspiration and the start of the next inspiration). At a rate of 30 breaths/min, the cycle time is 2 seconds and at a rate of 20 breaths/min it is 3 seconds.

Tidal volume

Tidal volume (V_T) is adjusted directly in volume-limited mode, but in pressure-limited mode is controlled indirectly by adjusting the inflating pressure (PIP minus PEEP). The arterial P_{CO_2} is inversely proportional to the alveolar ventilation (alveolar ventilation = rate × [tidal volume minus dead space]), so the larger the tidal volume, the lower is the Pa_{CO_2} until alveolar overinflation obstructs pulmonary blood flow. In volume-limited mode, an appropriate tidal volume is 6–10 ml/kg (the PIP should remain below 35 cmH_2O (3.5 kPa), to avoid volutrauma). In pressure-limited mode, PIP and not tidal volume is titrated against the blood gases (especially Pa_{CO_2}).

Inspiratory time or I:E ratio.

The inspiratory time consists of the inflation time (during which gas moves down airways into the lung) and the pause time (during which the lung is held inflated but no gas moves). The remainder of the cycle time consists of the expiratory time. Increasing the I:E ratio increases mean airway pressure (Fig. 6.4.5B) and improves oxygenation in pneumonia, ARDS and other forms of restrictive lung disease. Usually an I:E ratio of 1:1 to 1:3 is appropriate. Too long an inspiratory time causes discomfort in an unsedated child; too short an inspiratory time impairs alveolar recruitment, oxygenation and CO_2 removal, especially in the presence of increased airways resistance (e.g. asthma or bronchiolitis). Too short an expiratory time causes incomplete expiration of each breath, e.g. in asthma or bronchiolitis. Expiratory breath sounds should cease before the next ventilator breath starts.

Peak inflation pressure

The peak inflation pressure is measured in the ventilator tubing, upstream of the patient. If the

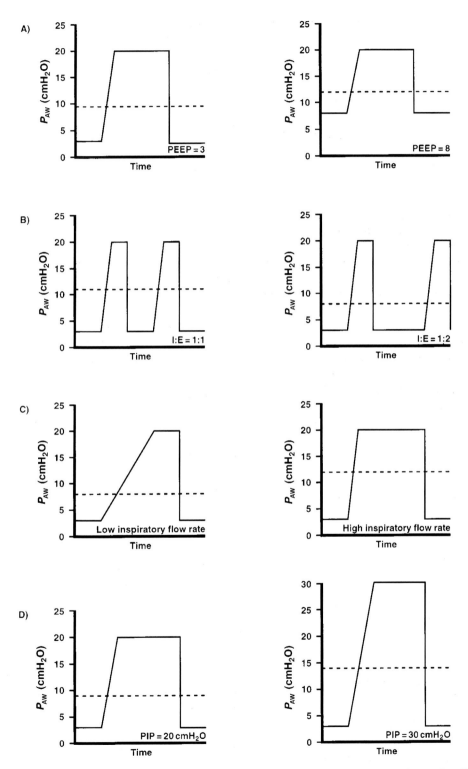

Figure 6.4.5 Changes in airway pressure (P_{AW}, solid line) during positive pressure ventilation showing the effects on mean airway pressure (dotted line) of changes in (A) PEEP; (B) I:E ratio; (C) inspiratory flow rate; and (D) peak inflation pressure

lungs are normal and the inspiratory gas flow rate is low, the child's alveolar pressure will equal the measured PIP at end-inspiration. When a high inspiratory flow rate is used, or when the resistance of the endotracheal tube or of the child's large or small airways is high (e.g. in asthma or tracheal stenosis), the pressure applied to the alveoli will be much lower than that measured. When the airways resistance is unevenly distributed, the alveolar pressure (and hence the ARDS-like lung damage due to alveolar overdistention) will be greater in areas supplied by normal airways than in those supplied by narrowed airways (Fig. 6.4.6). The PIP needed to ventilate normal lungs ranges from 15 cmH$_2$O (1.5 kPa) in an infant to 25 cmH$_2$O (2.5 kPa) in a heavily built teenager. Higher pressures (up to 35 cmH$_2$O or 3.5 kPa) are needed in the presence of lung disease.

PEEP or CPAP

See above.

Inspiratory flow rate or pattern

For any level of PIP, a square pressure wave produced by a rapid initial gas flow rate followed by a pause in inspiration see (Fig. 6.4.5c) gives the highest mean airway pressure (and the best oxygen transfer). This pattern may be uncomfortable, causing an unparalyzed child to cough and struggle.

Trigger sensitivity

A more sensitive setting is appropriate for very small or weak infants, but in larger children, very sensitive settings may cause the ventilator to 'self-trigger', leading to a ventilator rate far higher than the child's spontaneous breathing rate. The movement of pooled water condensing in the expiratory limb of the ventilator has the same effect. Too high a 'flow-by' gas flow rate during expiration may prevent triggering. In practice, if one wants the child to trigger the ventilator, the trigger is made more sensitive until every ventilator breath is triggered (SIMV mode) or until every spontaneous breath triggers a ventilator breath (pressure support mode) without the ventilator autocycling.

A) Normal

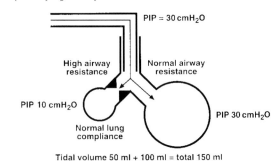

B) Locally high airway resistance

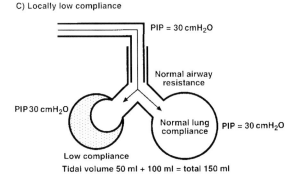

C) Locally low compliance

Figure 6.4.6 The effect of locally increased airway resistance (B) and locally reduced lung compliance (C) on the distribution of tidal volume and alveolar pressure during volume-limited ventilation, compared with normal (A)

MODES OF VENTILATION

CONTROLLED VENTILATION

Controlled ventilation (CV) implies that the child is apneic (often because of muscle relaxant drugs) and that all breaths are ventilator breaths. There is no triggering of breaths, and cycling is usually by time or flow. Breaths may be pressure-limited or volume-limited. This is the most appropriate form of ventilation when the child is making no respiratory effort (e.g. fully paralyzed), when the defect in gas exchange is so severe that other modes of ventilation are unable to achieve adequate blood gas levels, or when other modes (e.g. triggering) are unavailable.

INTERMITTENT MANDATORY VENTILATION

Intermittent mandatory ventilation implies that the patient is taking some spontaneous breaths. In both IMV and SIMV, the ventilator delivers a number (determined by the operator) of breaths per minute, in addition to the patient's spontaneous breaths. In SIMV, these ventilator breaths are triggered by the child's inspiratory effort and are usually volume-limited, although some ventilators can deliver pressure-limited SIMV. The operator must set the size of each breath (PIP or V_t), the inspiratory time, the inspiratory flow pattern, trigger sensitivity and the number of breaths per minute.

Synchronized IMV may be used to ventilate any spontaneously breathing patient. Weaning is by progressive reduction of the SIMV breath rate. This method is preferred to pressure support (or volume support) when the child's respiratory effort is irregular (apnea or bradypnea) or when the triggering is not consistently effective: SIMV ensures that a minimum number of breaths will be delivered each minute even in the absence of patient effort.

PRESSURE SUPPORT

Every spontaneous breath triggers the ventilator to generate a positive pressure in the airway during inspiration. In effect this is triggered, pressure-limited ventilation. Pressure support reduces the work of breathing but allows the patient to exercise the inspiratory muscles. Pressure support is used to wean children from ventilation, especially when the respiratory muscles are weak or the weaning process is likely to take a day or more. The patient is weaned from ventilation by gradual reduction of the PIP: the child can usually be extubated when the PIP is 5 cmH$_2$O (0.5 kPa) above PEEP, but a trial of adequacy of breathing on CPAP

is sometimes used. When the child's respiratory effort is irregular, or if triggering is unreliable (e.g. in a small infant or when the respiratory rate is greater than 100 breaths/min), SIMV may be more appropriate than pressure support.

VOLUME SUPPORT

Every spontaneous breath triggers a volume-limited ventilator breath. This is a weaning mode used when volume-limited ventilation is suitable, with the same reservations mentioned for pressure support.

BIPAP

Available on some ventilators, BiPAP is triggered or timed pressure-limited ventilation, combined with PEEP. Some ventilators permit spontaneous breathing during inspiration and expiration while maintaining constant inspiratory and expiratory pressures. The variables to be set are rate, PIP, PEEP, trigger sensitivity and inspiratory flow/pressure wave shape. BiPAP is appropriate for many forms of lung disease, especially when controlled hypoventilation is used in severe lung disease to minimize the risk of iatrogenic lung injury. Often used for noninvasive ventilation (by nasal or face mask) of patients with chronic lung disease, neuromuscular weakness, *Pneumocystis carinii* pneumonia or recurrent left ventricular failure.

INVERSE RATIO VENTILATION

Inverse ratio ventilation (IRV) is pressure-limited or volume-limited ventilation with an I:E ratio of 1:1 to 4:1 (i.e. prolonged inspiratory hold); it is used to recruit collapsed alveoli and small airways in severe restrictive lung disease such as pneumonia and ARDS. This form of ventilation is extremely uncomfortable: it requires heavy sedation and often muscle relaxation. There is a high incidence of hypotension due to impaired venous return and of pneumothorax.

AIRWAY PRESSURE RELEASE VENTILATION

Airway pressure release ventilation (APRV) is similar to IRV but spontaneous breathing is permitted during ventilator inspiratory and expiratory phases, so APRV is better tolerated than IRV and heavy sedation is not needed. Complications and possible indications are similar to those for IRV. In general, with both IRV and APRV, the PIP is lower and the mean airway pressure higher than would be needed to achieve the same blood gas concentrations with conventional controlled ventilation.

HIGH-FREQUENCY VENTILATION

High-frequency ventilation (HFV) implies the use of ventilator rates greater than 60 breaths/min. The three most common forms of HFV are described below.

High-frequency positive pressure ventilation

High-frequency positive pressure ventilation (HFPPV) uses a conventional neonatal ventilator in pressure-limited mode with rates of 60–120 breaths/min to match the high spontaneous respiratory rate of the neonate with restrictive lung disease and an I:E ratio of 1:3 to 1:4. It needs a fresh gas flow of 5–6 ml/kg·min.

High-frequency oscillation

High-frequency oscillation (HFO) uses a diaphragm, piston or loudspeaker to deliver oscillating pressure to the airway on the background of a mean airway pressure produced by a continuous fresh gas flow past the endotracheal tube, vented via a CPAP-type valve. The tidal volume is 1–3 ml/kg (less than dead space). In infants and children with restrictive lung disease (e.g. severe hyaline membrane disease), oxygenation is directly related to mean airway pressure, while CO_2 removal is directly related to the fresh gas flow and to the magnitude of pressure oscillations and inversely related to frequency. This method can be combined with background IMV, or with nitric oxide or surfactant administration. The most common starting settings are:

- neonates:
  - frequency 10 Hz
  - mean airway pressure 2–5 cm H_2O above that used in CV
  - ΔP 35–40 cmH_2O

- older children: similar to above, but frequency 4–8 Hz

Indications include major air leaks and severe unilateral lung disease. Some children with hyaline membrane disease and some with congenital diaphragmatic hernia or ARDS may benefit from a trial of HFO if gas exchange is inadequate or airway pressures too high with conventional ventilation.

High-frequency jet ventilation

High frequency jet ventilation (HFJV) delivers pulses of pressurized gas into the trachea, entraining extra gas from a bias fresh gas flow. It requires a special triple-lumen endotracheal tube or tube adapter. It is suitable for all sizes of patient from neonate to large adult, for the same indications as for HFO. Although it has not been shown conclusively to be better than CV or HFO, some patients appear to benefit from a trial of HFJV, especially those with major barotrauma (e.g. bronchopleural fistula or severe pulmonary interstitial emphysema).

Frequency range is 3–10 Hz. Peak and mean airway pressures are generally lower than those used with CV or HFO to achieve the same gas exchange. Problems with inadequate humidification, tube blockage and necrotizing laryngotracheitis have been reported.

NEGATIVE PRESSURE VENTILATION

Negative pressure ventilation is a noninvasive method of ventilation by application of intermittent negative pressure to the thorax using a tank or cuirass, which avoids the need for tracheal intubation and its complications. The frequency range is 0–15 Hz. Used for noninvasive long-term ventilation or for weaning from mechanical ventilation of adults and children with chronic lung disease or neuromuscular disorders causing respiratory failure, negative pressure ventilation has also been used for short-term ventilation of patients with severe upper airway obstruction and during laryngeal surgery, and to optimize pulmonary blood flow and cardiac output after the Fontan operation and after correction of tetralogy of

Fallot. Accurate fitting of the cuirass is required to minimize air leaks, with monitoring to change the cuirass size as the child grows. This form of ventilation may be difficult to administer in small infants.

Table 6.4.1 shows appropriate initial ventilator settings during IPPV for children with normal lungs and the common forms of lung disease.

✔ KEY POINTS

➤ When commencing ventilation, choose a tidal volume or PIP that produces visible chest movement, measure blood gases after 15 minutes and adjust the ventilator according to $PaCO_2$ and PaO_2

➤ Pressure-limited ventilation should be used in all children weighing less than 15 kg

➤ Unless the child has normal lungs or a brain injury, use controlled hypoventilation and keep the FIO_2 below 0.5 to avoid iatrogenic lung damage

➤ Triggered ventilation is more comfortable than nontriggered and uses lower airway pressures

➤ Ensure that the apparatus dead space is minimal

➤ Use lightweight tubing in small children to avoid accidental extubation

✗ COMMON ERRORS

➤ Use of excessive tidal volumes, PIP and FIO_2 in an attempt to achieve normal blood gases in children with lung disease

➤ Use of volume-limited ventilation in infants

➤ Use of high-frequency ventilation in children with asthma or bronchiolitis

➤ Use of excessively long inspiratory time in spontaneously breathing children

FURTHER READING

1. Tobin MJ, editor. Principles and practice of mechanical ventilation. New York: McGraw-Hill; 1994
   – (*Comprehensive reference on all aspects of mechanical ventilation*)

2. Kacmarek R, Custer JR, Fugate JH. Mechanical ventilation. In: Todres ID, Fugate JH, editors. Critical care of infants and children. Boston: Little, Brown; 1996
   – (*Practical discussion of the approach to mechanical ventilation in children and its physiological background*)

3. Goldsmith JP, Karotkin EH. Assisted ventilation of the neonate, 3rd ed. Philadelphia: WB Saunders; 1996
   – (*Discussion of issues and approaches relevant to neonates and older infants*)

TABLE 6.4.1 **Suitable initial ventilator settings**

	Normal lungs	Restrictive disease	Obstructive disease
Triggered or timed	Timed if apneic, otherwise triggered	Triggered; timed only as last resort	Triggered; timed only as last resort
Pressure- or volume-limited	< 10 kg: pressure > 10 kg: either	< 10 kg: pressure > 10 kg: either	< 10 kg: pressure > 10 kg: either
Rate	Normal for age (see text)	Normal for age (see text)	Slightly slower than normal for age
PIP	15–25 cmH$_2$O (1.5–2.5 kPa)	≤ 35 cmH$_2$O (3.5 kPa)	≤ 35 cmH$_2$O (3.5 kPa)
PEEP	3–5 cmH$_2$O (0.3–0.5 kPa)	5–15 cmH$_2$O (0.5–1.5 kPa)	3 cmH$_2$O (asthma) 5–15 cmH$_2$O (bronchiolitis)
Tidal volume	6–10 ml/kg	6–10 ml/kg (keep PIP < 35 cmH$_2$O	6–10 ml/kg (keep PIP < 35 cmH$_2$O
Trigger sensitivity	1–2 cmH$_2$O	1–2 cmH$_2$O	1–2 cmH$_2$O
Fresh gas flow	2–3 L/kg·min (neonate) 1–2 L/kg·min (child)	2–3 L/kg·min (neonate) 1–2 L/kg·min (child)	2–3 L/kg·min (neonate) 1–2 L/kg·min (child)
Weaning via:	IMV or pressure support	IMV or pressure support	IMV or pressure support
FIO$_2$	0.21	0.21–0.5	0.21–0.5
Aim for $PaCO_2$	5.3 kPa (40 mmHg)	> 8 kPa (60 mmHg)	> 8 kPa (60 mmHg)
Aim for PaO_2	> 10.5 kPa (80 mmHg)	> 6.5 kPa (50 mmHg)	> 6.5 kPa (50 mmHg)

6.5 Invasive monitoring

Michael D. Seear

Advances in invasive monitoring have paralleled developments in the specialties of anesthesia and subsequently adult and pediatric intensive care. Blood pressure monitoring was introduced at the beginning of the twentieth century as anesthetists began to realize the cardiovascular side-effects of anesthetic drugs. It was not until the early 1950s, however, that intraarterial monitoring became a regular practice. Cannulation of the deep veins was pioneered by Forssman after he catheterized himself in 1929 (for which he was dismissed from his job). Lagerlof's description of the measurement of pulmonary capillary wedge pressure and Fegler's measurement of cardiac output by thermodilution paved the way for the balloon-tipped pulmonary artery catheter described by Swan and Ganz in 1970.

The history of intracranial monitoring follows much the same pattern. The measurement of cerebral blood flow using nitrous oxide as an indicator was introduced by Kety and Schmidt in 1945. The use of jugular venous blood sampling of oxygen content and lactic acid was introduced at the same time because of the need for jugular venous samples in the above technique. Jugular bulb catheters have recently been rediscovered and their use is increasing again. The development of noninvasive techniques for measuring cerebral blood flow such as Doppler, ultrasound and xenon CT scanning have made the Kety–Schmidt technique obsolete. The measurement of intracranial pressure was first described by Lundberg in 1960. The measurement can be made directly via ventriculostomy, from the subdural space or from the brain parenchyma. It has become a routine procedure in most intensive care units.

Although invasive monitoring has been around for several decades, there is still considerable controversy about the need for these procedures. The information gained certainly brightens up a dull ward round, but is this information worth the inevitable expense and side-effects? Enthusiasts will argue that invasive measurements provide early warning of impending trouble and allow subsequent management to be tailored to the primary problem. Opponents argue that the techniques are riddled with errors and there is usually little evidence to suggest that the information gained from hemodynamic monitoring affects outcome in any way. They also mention the practical difficulties in small children and usually finish with some well-chosen comments about side-effects and expense.

In reality, black and white arguments are of little value and each child must be judged individually. The potential value of the invasive technique should be weighed carefully against the known risk of major side-effects. The final decision should also be based on a realistic assessment of measurement and interpretation errors involved in the particular technique. It should be mentioned that errors are usually underestimated, particularly when complex derived variables are calculated based on a single hemodynamic measurement.

PRINCIPLES OF MEASURING PRESSURE

Converting a high-frequency, low-pressure arterial pulse in a neonate to a continuous tracing on a computer screen is such a common procedure in any ICU that the complexity of the task is rarely appreciated. The list of potential problems due to human, electronic and mechanical errors is lengthy and considerable errors in the displayed signal can be introduced quite easily. Since major management decisions are frequently based on pressure displays, it is important that all intensive care clinicians should have a good understanding of the principles involved in pressure transduction. Before embarking on aggressive treatments for high intracranial pressure or low mean arterial pressure, the first question should always be, 'is this number accurate?'

The components required to monitor the pressure signal consist of a catheter, pressure tubing, one or two stopcocks, a transducer, a flushing device, an amplifier and a suitable monitor. Recent advances in transducer and monitor design have made pressure measuring easier, but the characteristics of the system should still be understood.

MECHANICAL SYSTEM

Frequency response

At certain frequencies, any mechanical system will resonate, depending upon its physical properties. Signals at this frequency will tend to be amplified artificially. At other frequencies, the signal may be reduced or attenuated artificially, depending upon the properties of the system. For ideal measurement, the system's amplitude response should be flat over the intended measuring frequency range. Most systems will have a flat response curve to 10 times the measurement frequency. Physiological measurements are often made in the range of 1–2 Hz so band widths of 20 Hz or more are commonly used. The fundamental frequency of a fluid-filled system depends mainly on the tubing length and diameter, the fluid density and its viscosity (Equation 1). The only variable which can be changed easily is tubing length, which should be kept as short as possible.

EQUATION I Fundamental frequency F_n

$F_n = (d/8) \sqrt{(3/\pi L \rho V_d)}$

where d is the tubing diameter, L its length, ρ the fluid viscosity and V_d the transducer fluid volume displacement

---

Damping

The damping of a system refers to the rate at which induced oscillations are damped down. The damping of a system depends on the same physical characteristics as the frequency response, although arranged in a slightly different formula (Equation 2). Excessive distortion in the pressure

---

EQUATION 2 Damping coefficient ζ

$\zeta = (16n/d^3) \sqrt{(3LV_d/\pi \rho)}$

where d is the tubing diameter, L its length, ρ the fluid viscosity, V_d the transducer fluid volume displacement, and n the fluid viscosity

---

signal can be damped by altering the physical characteristics of the tubing. Small air bubbles can be introduced into the line, but they can lead to a loss of detail, underestimation of the pressure and also entail a small risk of embolization. Commercial devices exist which allow finer control of damping if needed.

Fast flush test

The dynamic parameters of transducer plumbing systems can easily be measured at the bedside with a fast flush test. Open the fast flush device and then allow it to snap shut. The subsequent pressure tracing will give an indication of the frequency response of the system and its damping characteristics if a fast strip chart recording is made of the period. Following the flush, the pressure recording should overshoot once and then resume the normal blood pressure tracing. If the system is underdamped or the frequency response is incorrect, there will be excessive oscillation and ringing in the signal.

PRESSURE TRANSDUCERS

The small movement of the fluid column is transmitted to a thin diaphragm within the transducer. Several techniques can be used to convert this movement to a voltage (strain gauge, inductance gauge and capacitance gauge). Older, reusable transducers had to be calibrated prior to each measurement. Modern, disposable transducers are made to tight specifications and have a standard diaphragm displacement for a given pressure. If changing to a new manufacturer, it is a good idea to have the transducers checked by the biomedical engineering department, but this is not necessary in daily clinical practice. However, the transducer does need to have a reference point on the body which is accepted as a zero point. Cardiovascular measurements are usually referenced to the midaxillary line. Errors in zeroing are probably the most common source of pressure transduction problems. When a stopcock is opened at the correct position, it must be remembered that it is the position of the stopcock, not the position of the transducer, that is important. Modern transducers do not drift very much, but should still be zeroed each 12-hour shift.

ELECTRONIC MONITORING

The fluctuating voltage signal requires a good deal of manipulation, including filtering, amplification and display. Errors in this system are the concern of professional biomedical engineers, but the monitor display is under the control of the bedside staff and, once again, is open to human error. Read the instruction manual before pushing buttons at random.

PRINCIPLES OF MEASURING FLOW

The search for a perfect measure of cardiac output has been pursued with vigor. The value certainly provides some insight to the heart's function but gives information only on the supply side of the oxygen consumption–delivery relationship. Measures, that can express the balance between supply and demand of the adequacy of oxygen transport are currently the object of much research. Gastric tonometry and near-infrared spectroscopy are undoubtedly the first steps towards the future direction of intensive care monitoring.

It should be stressed that, even under the best conditions, the errors of the available techniques are considerable, but in the absence of an absolute measure of cardiac output, the true error will remain unknown. Methods are consequently assessed by their reproducibility which, although it may be good, is not the same as accuracy. It has been observed that as long as we all measure the same artifact, true accuracy can be ignored. The following techniques are commonly used:

FICK TECHNIQUE

Fick's method has been used for over a century and is commonly quoted as a 'gold standard' against which other techniques should be measured. Any soluble gas can be used as the indicator but oxygen is the one that is usually used. The cardiac output is calculated from the oxygen consumption, divided by the difference in arterial and mixed venous oxygen content (Equation 3). Depending on the method used to measure oxygen consumption, the technique requires the calculation of up to nine individual variables (inspired and expired oxygen fraction, venous and arterial oxygen saturation, venous and arter-ial partial pressure of oxygen, hemoglobin, barometric pressure and minute ven-

---

EQUATION 3 Fick equation

$$Q = (\dot{V}O_2 / CaO_2 - C\bar{v}O_2)$$

where $\dot{V}O_2$ is the oxygen consumption, CaO_2 is the arterial oxygen content and $C\bar{v}O_2$ is the mixed venous oxygen content

---

EQUATION 4 Oxygen consumption

$$VO_2 = V_{min} (FIO_2 - FEO_2)$$

where V_{min} is the minute ventilation, FIO_2 is the inspired oxygen fraction and FEO_2 is the expired oxygen fraction

---

EQUATION 5 Oxygen content

$$CxO_2 = (1.34 \times Hb \times SxO_2) + (0.003 \times PxO_2)$$

where Hb is the hemoglobin level, SxO_2 is the saturation of arterial or venous blood, and PxO_2 is the partial pressure of oxygen in arterial or venous blood

---

tilation). The cumulative error of the final calculation can be large. While the measurements are being made, time passes and the final value can only be considered as an average cardiac output over a period of about 5 minutes; the technique is therefore only applicable to a stable patient. Attempts have been made to substitute venous samples from the right atrium or vena cava in place of mixed pulmonary artery blood, but the final result is only of value as a trend. Modern bedside metabolic monitors allow a continuous measurement of oxygen consumption to be made. Most will calculate a Fick-derived cardiac output following manual insertion of venous and arterial oxygen content values. Some monitors will also accept continuous input from arterial and mixed venous oxygen saturation devices so that a continuous calculation of cardiac output can be displayed. An adjustment for dissolved oxygen is necessary since this causes considerable error at high levels of arterial partial pressure. Attempts have been made to bypass the need for VO_2 measurements with the use of standardized tables. These are of little value: if you are going to guess the oxygen consumption, you might as well guess the cardiac output. Carbon dioxide production is easier to measure than oxygen consumption. If the CO_2 output is known, it can be converted to VO_2 using an estimated respiratory quotient (Equation 6). This is known as a CO_2 Fick and is occasionally calculated.

> **EQUATION 6 Respiratory quotient (RQ)**
>
> $RQ = (V_{O_2}/V_{CO_2})$
>
> where V_{CO_2} is the carbon dioxide production and V_{O_2} is the oxygen consumption

INDICATOR DILUTION TECHNIQUES

The indicator dilution method consists of injecting a known amount of a marker, then following its concentration change some distance downstream. Cardiac output is derived from a knowledge of the initial concentration and the curve of downstream concentration against time using the Stewart-Hamilton equation (Equation 7). In the past, a

> **EQUATION 7 Stewart–Hamilton equation for dye dilution**
>
> $Q = (I/\int C.dt)$
>
> where I is the initial amount of indicator, and $\int C.dt$ is the integrated concentration over time

venous injection of green dye was sampled downstream by withdrawing an arterial sample through a peripheral artery. The change in concentration was assessed by a spectrophotometer. The equipment was cumbersome and the patient was also exposed to an injection of dye. The subsequent development of saline dilution has made the green dye technique largely obsolete. The development of accurate thermistors has allowed temperature change to be used as a marker. The calculation is otherwise identical (Equation 8). The list of potential errors is extensive and includes mechanical problems due to intracardiac shunts, valvular regurgitation, clots on the thermistor and variations in cardiac output with respiration. Injection errors depend on the speed of injection, temperature and volume of the cold saline. With careful attention, the reproducibility of three consecutive measurements can be brought to about 5%. However, reproducibility should not be confused

> **EQUATION 8 Stewart-Hamilton equation for thermodilution**
>
> $Q = (V (T_B - T_I).k/\int \Delta T.dt$
>
> where V is the volume of injectate, $T_B - T_I$ is the initial temperature difference, k is the content, and $\int \Delta T.dt$ is the integrated temperature change over time

with accuracy. The common practice of averaging three reproducible values from five injections gives some idea of the accuracy that can be expected.

OTHER METHODS

If the ascending aorta is assumed to be a circular cylinder, its cross-sectional area can be calculated by measuring the aortic diameter using two dimensional echocardiography. If it is further assumed that this diameter remains constant, then the cardiac output can be calculated as the product of aortic cross-sectional area and the mean velocity of blood flowing up the ascending aorta. Mean velocity can be calculated by a Doppler probe placed in the xiphisternum (Equation 9). The technique is open to

> **EQUATION 9 Doppler cardiac output**
>
> $Q = (\pi d^2/4) \cdot V$
>
> where d is the aortic root diameter, and V is the mean ascending aortic velocity

a large number of measurement errors and is strongly dependent on operator skill. In addition, it is difficult to obtain accurate readings of the ascending aorta in ventilated patients. Despite initial enthusiasm, this method seems to have fallen into disuse.

Thoracic bioimpedance depends on measuring the variation in impedance caused by changing volumes of blood within the thorax. The technique has had some success in adult patients, but the small cardiac signal is difficult to isolate from the relatively high respiratory frequency found in children. The need for encircling electrodes is another practical problem that has limited its value in children.

TYPES OF INVASIVE MEASUREMENT

There is no body cavity that cannot be reached with a strong right arm and a 16 gauge needle.

(The House of God, Dr Samuel Shem)

With practice, it is usually not difficult to insert catheters into blood vessels. Whether or not these procedures should be performed depends on careful assessment of risk and benefit for each individual patient. The skills are taught in PALS, APLS and similar courses. Outlines for the techniques are given in Chapter 6.1.

INTRAARTERIAL LINES

Arterial access offers continuous reliable measurement of blood pressure, even during shock, and also allows repeated sampling of arterial blood for blood gas estimation. If performed carefully, the risks of vessel thrombosis or infection are small and the threshold for inserting arterial lines is low in most units. The risk of thrombosis is higher with traumatic insertion, large catheters, prolonged cannulation and low blood pressure. The prognosis for arterial recannulation following thrombosis is good. The arteries most commonly used are the radial and femoral arteries although several other sites in the body are accessible. The superficial temporal artery should not be used except in special cases because of the risk of emboli to scalp, face and even the cerebral cortex.

CENTRAL VENOUS PRESSURE

In children the monitoring of central venous pressure is only a minor reason for the placement of central venous lines, which are usually inserted for reliable venous access and to give irritating substances (such as chemotherapy and hyperalimentation) with fewer peripheral side-effects. The child is also spared the pain of repeated reinsertions of peripheral catheters. Several designs of catheter are available, including two- and three-lumen Silastic devices, long, flexible Silastic catheters that can be fed into a central vein from a peripheral access point, and permanent indwelling lines. The principal side-effects include line sepsis and thrombosis. Obtaining exact figures for the incidence of these side-effects is difficult because of wide clinical variations between patients. However, it is fair to say that in very sick children with low venous flows and catheters that have been placed for more than 1 week, the chances of sepsis or thrombosis are significant.

The most common sites of access are the internal jugular and femoral veins. Central venous lines are rarely inserted simply to measure venous pressure—this measurement is usually a bonus of catheter placement. Since low values are involved, it is important to measure them as accurately as possible. Zeroing errors will have a significant effect on the measured pressure. An internal jugular line will give a good approximation to right atrial pressure, but it should be remembered that there are a ventricle and two lungs between the catheter and the left atrium, so very little information is obtained about the left side of the heart. The pressure measured in the femoral vein is less reliable because of the effect of abdominal pressure and constriction at the diaphragm.

JUGULAR VENOUS BULB CATHETERS

This specialized form of central venous line consists of passing a catheter in a retrograde direction up the jugular vein so the tip lies in the jugular bulb. This allows samples of mixed cerebral venous blood to be drawn. The technique was popularized in the 1940s and has recently been reintroduced as a means of assessing the existence of cerebral ischemia during hyperventilation. As the cerebral vessels constrict in response to a falling Pa_{CO_2}, the cerebral oxygen extraction increases (Equation 10). A cut-off of 30% is often used to define the presence of ischemia. Simultaneous studies of cerebral blood flow and cerebral oxygen extraction have shown that the test's reliability is poor. The brain drains through two jugular veins and blood flow is often different in these two vessels, especially when there is a catheter in place. Jugular venous flow and oxygen saturation can differ widely between the two vessels.

PULMONARY ARTERY CATHETERS

The use of pulmonary artery catheters varies widely between different units, making it impossible to give firm recommendations on when they might be useful. Opinions vary from 'never' to 'often'. The smallest thermodilution catheter is 4.5 FG. In small children, the proximal injection port may not even be in the neck with the tip in the pulmonary artery. Single-lumen 2.5 FG. thermistor catheters can be inserted into the pul-

---

EQUATION 10 Cerebral oxygen extraction (CE_{O_2})

$$CE_{O_2} = (Ca_{O_2} - Cj_{O_2})/Ca_{O_2}$$

where Ca_{O_2} is the arterial oxygen content, and Cj_{O_2} is the jugular venous oxygen content monary artery at the time of cardiac surgery. Saline injection needs to be given through a different central line. Once in place, the catheter provides information on pulmonary artery pressure, central venous pressure, mixed venous oxygen saturation, cardiac output and pulmonary artery wedge pressure. Balancing the value of this information against potential problems is difficult. Apart from the inevitable risks of thrombosis and sepsis, pulmonary artery catheters carry risks for arrhythmias (including heart block), catheter knotting, pulmonary infarction and occasionally pulmonary artery rupture. Unfortunately, there is no reported study to suggest that insertion of these catheters improves outcome in unstable children, so arguments for their use depend mainly on anecdote. In view of their potential problems, it seems fair to say that these devices should only be inserted by experienced physicians who fully understand the physiology behind the measurements and the errors involved in their estimation.

INTRACRANIAL PRESSURE MONITORING

Knowledge of the pressure within the skull can be used to guide therapy and also offers some degree of prognostic information. Whether this extra knowledge affects outcome is the subject of much debate, but ICP monitoring has a well-established place in most intensive care units. Some estimate of brain compliance is provided by the brain pressure-volume index (Equation 11), but the main use of the catheter is to monitor the cerebral perfusion pressure which is the difference between mean arterial pressure and the intracranial pressure (Equation 12). It is important that both measurements should be referenced to the same zero position. A safe perfusion pressure in children is usually considered to be above 50 mmHg (6.7 kPa). The pressure in the brain can be monitored using subdural bolts, intracerebral catheters or intraven-

---

EQUATION 12 Cerebral perfusion pressure (CPP)

CPP = MAP − ICP

where MAP is the mean arterial pressure and ICP is the intracranial pressure (both referenced to the same zero point)

---

tricular catheters. Intra-ventricular catheters are the hardest to insert and carry a risk of ventriculitis in addition to the dangers of hematoma, catheter breakage and brain injury, but they offer the most reliable pressure recording and also allow small quantities of CSF to be removed to control intracranial pressure rises.

For additional equations and selected normal values/ranges for monitoring see Chapter 7.3.

✔ KEY POINTS

➤ Before using any invasive measurement technique, a realistic assessment should be made of the potential side-effects and errors associated with its use

➤ No matter how interesting the results, if they do not alter management, then do not accept any side-effects in their measurement

➤ Measurement error is usually greatly under-estimated, particularly by the people selling the machine

➤ Before basing any therapeutic change on a measured variable, always ask the question, 'is this number correct?'

FURTHER READING

1. Huttemann F. Monitoring of O_2 transport and tissue oxygenation in paediatric critical care. Paed Anaesth 1995; 5: 281–286
   – (*The physiology behind the monitoring of tissue oxygenation in critically ill children*)

2. Numa A. Assessment of lung function in the intensive care unit. Ped Pulmonol 1995; 19: 118–178
   – (*This article describes the application of respiratory physiology to the practical monitoring of lung function in intubated children*)

3. Pfenninger J. Neurological intensive care in children. Intens Care Med 1993; 19: 243–250
   – (*The management and monitoring of critically ill children with neurological disease*)

EQUATION 11 Brain pressure-volume index (PVI)

PVI = $V/\log (P_1/P_2)$

where V is the volume withdrawn or injected, and P_1 and P_2 are the pressures before and after injection

6.6   Noninvasive monitoring

John Alexander and Andrew J. Macnab

Physiological variables may be monitored invasively or noninvasively. Invasive monitoring can be difficult to establish and may be associated with complications (Ch. 6.5), but is generally considered to be the 'gold standard'. Advances in sensing devices and computing power, in recent years, have resulted in noninvasive monitoring devices that approximate the 'gold standards' established by invasive monitors and are now often considered as reasonable substitutes for these.

RESPIRATORY SYSTEM

PULSE OXIMETRY

Developed in the 1970s, pulse oximetry has become one of the most valuable monitoring techniques in critical care and in anesthesia. Indications for oximetry are shown in Table 6.6.1. The pulse oximeter consists of a sensor placed on a finger, toe or ear-lobe, or in very small infants on the palm or foot. Where there is extensive injury, the sensor can be placed to transilluminate the cheek or tongue. The sensor contains two light-emitting diodes (LED) which sequentially emit light at around 660 nm (red light) and 940 nm (infrared light). A photodiode senses the intensity

---

TABLE 6.6.1 **Indications for oximetry**

- Resuscitation/management of any critical illness or injury
- Interhospital transport
- Intrahospital transport (to operating room, ICU, radiology)
- Prehospital ambulance transport
- CPR
- Patients with potential to desaturate (e.g. asthma, trauma, seizures)
- During procedures capable of producing hypoxemia (e.g. intubation, ET tube suctioning, bronchoscopy)
- Patients receiving oxygen or assisted ventilation where FIO_2 and/or ventilation settings are changed
- Minor procedures done under conscious sedation
- Intra- and postoperative monitoring

---

of the light after it has passed through the tissues. Oxygenated hemoglobin absorbs more red light than does reduced hemoglobin, while the latter absorbs more infrared light. Additionally, there is a pulsatile variation in the overall absorption of light by the tissues which corresponds to the pulse wave. By detecting the pulsatile wave and then measuring the difference in absorption of red and infrared light, the pulse oximeter calculates the oxygen saturation of the blood. This provides a beat-to-beat measure of oxygenation that is reliable between 80% and 100% saturation. It provides a continuous measure of the oxygenation saturation of the blood and reliably detects sudden changes in saturation. Recent improvements in software attempt to provide a measure of peripheral perfusion, but this has not been validated as yet.

Problems with this device (Table 6.6.2) include unreliable values caused by poor peripheral perfusion, vasoconstriction and motion artifact (which disturbs the unit's ability to establish a baseline during diastole). Most monitors have an analog display of the pulse signal, and it is important to confirm a good signal (the value of which correlates with measured heart rate) before accepting the saturation reading. Carboxyhemoglobin and methemoglobin do not absorb red or infrared light and the presence of large amounts of either of these types of hemoglobin will result in an overestimation of the true oxygen saturation. The device detects hypoxia but cannot reliably detect hyperoxia. Its use in neonatal practice should therefore be monitored with arterial or arterialized capillary gas analysis to avoid the complications of hyperoxia, and SpO_2 values in this population are usually maintained at 92–94%.

CAPNOGRAPHY

Capnography is the measurement of carbon dioxide in a gas mixture which in clinical practice consists of expired gases. The technique has had limited value in pediatric practice because of tech-

TABLE 6.6.2 **Situations limiting pulse oximetry measurement or accuracy**

- Motion—unreliable or impossible measurement due to inability to track diastolic reference point
- Light interference
  - high ambient light
  - sunlight (particularly if 'strobed' through rotating helicopter blades)
  - phototherapy, procedure or operating room lights
  - infrared heaters
  - Use light-occluding wrap over sensor
- Abnormal hemoglobin
  - carboxyhemoglobin and methemoglobin lead to significant overestimation
  - major potential for error in burns — use arterial samples and cooximetry
- Pigments—dark skin, black or purple nail polish
- Intravenously administered dyes—methylene blue, indocyanin green, indigo carmine, fluorescein
- Limited perfusion—hypovolemia, extreme vasoconstriction, sphygmomanometer cuff inflation on limb used for Sro_2, extreme hypothermia (core < 31°C). *Note*—if oximeter pulse readout is accurate (as compared with auscultation), oximeter Sro_2 is generally reliable.
- Incorrect probe size, poor attachment—light can be transmitted from diode directly to photosensor (can artificially elevate values in desaturation)
- Low saturation states—measurement becomes less accurate when Spo_2 is < 85%, and at 50% and below measurement is invalid

nical difficulties, but its use is increasing. Carbon dioxide can be measured by mass spectrometry or by an infrared monitor. Mass spectrometry is expensive and not portable, so the infrared capnometer is used more commonly. Inspired and expired CO_2 is measured continuously either by a sensor placed in line between the ventilator circuit and the endotracheal tube or by sampling gas from the endotracheal tube. The sensor is an infrared device that measures the absorption of infrared radiation in the sample gas. This is calibrated against the absorption of the same light by a reference calibration gas containing CO_2. An analog output displays a capnogram which is a continuous display of the CO_2 concentration while a numerical display shows the end-tidal CO_2.

The principle of capnography is based on the assumption that end-tidal CO_2 equals alveolar CO_2 which in turn equals arterial CO_2: this assumes no ventilation–perfusion mismatching. In a healthy adult breathing spontaneously, end-tidal and arterial CO_2 values differ by less than 0.13 kPa (1 mmHg). However, in a ventilated, critically ill patient with significant degrees of dead space ventilation and physiologic shunt in the lung, there is a large discrepancy between the two values. Given these limitations, the instrument has some role in the intensive care unit. It can be used at its most basic level as an extubation or ventilator disconnect alarm.

Carbon dioxide is found in large quantities only in expired gases. Normal air or gas from the stomach contains negligible amounts. Detecting CO_2 in the expired gas confirms that alveolar ventilation has occurred and helps to distinguish tracheal from esophageal intubation. It does not distinguish tracheal from pharyngeal intubation, however, as CO_2 will be detected if alveolar ventilation occurs with pharyngeal intubation.

Although capnography cannot reliably predict arterial CO_2 levels, it is possible to use this technique for monitoring trends in arterial CO_2. This helps avoid progressive hyper- or hypoventilation, and is of particular value with head-injured children, or during interhospital transport. A change in end-tidal CO_2 usually reflects a change in arterial CO_2, but it must be remembered that the reverse is not always true.

The use of CO_2 monitoring has been advocated during cardiopulmonary resuscitation as an indicator of pulmonary perfusion and therefore a measure of the success of the CPR maneuvers in increasing cardiac output. In cardiac arrest, there is no perfusion of the lungs and therefore no excretion of CO_2 from the lungs. With successful CPR, the presence of pulmonary perfusion will be suggested by the presence of CO_2 in the expired gases. Increasing concentration of CO_2 will therefore be an indicator of improving pulmonary perfusion and therefore systemic perfusion.

TRANSCUTANEOUS O_2 AND CO_2 MONITORS

Arterial blood gases can be estimated by electrodes that measure the concentration of gas diffusing out through an area of heated skin. This is only of value in the management of premature infants or newborn babies who have a skin thickness that allows relatively unimpeded diffusion of gases. Even in these patients, transcutaneous monitors only provide trend information and measurement that approximates blood gas values.

RESPIRATORY MECHANICS

Continuous measurement of airway pressure and flow with a pressure transducer and an in-line pneumotachometer allows ventilator function and changes in lung compliance and resistance to be monitored. Using appropriate computer software, it is relatively simple to obtain values for tidal volume and minute ventilation and calculate dynamic compliance and airway resistance. Display of flow volume loops and pressure volume loops allows the continuous monitoring of respiratory mechanics and is of some value in patients with pulmonary conditions that change with time. Interpretation of respiratory function data must be made with care, because significant errors can be introduced by leakage around the endotracheal tube, secretions and collection of fluid in the ventilator circuit.

CARDIOVASCULAR SYSTEM

HEART RATE

Heart rate is monitored continuously with two ECG electrodes placed on the chest wall and one on the abdomen. The rate is determined by detecting QRS complexes and averaging the time taken for three or more beats. Visual display of the waveform allows detection of arrhythmias which should then be confirmed with a formal study. Electrocardiographic monitoring systems often include inductance respiratory plethysmography to detect chest wall movement and determine respiratory rate. Different software exists for pediatric and neonatal monitors, which means that these units can only be used reliably in the population that the software is written for.

BLOOD PRESSURE

Most noninvasive blood pressure measurements rely on the occlusion of an artery with a Riva–Rocci cuff and detection of changes in sound, vessel wall movement or pulsation when the occlusion is gradually eased off. Detection of changes in sound are made by auscultation of the Korotkoff sounds, by amplification of the sounds using a microphone, or by using a Doppler probe. Vessel wall movement can be detected by a Doppler ultrasound probe, while arterial pulsation distal to the cuff can be detected using a piezoelectric crystal or by the oscillometric method. The latter technique is utilized in the widely used Dinamap blood pressure monitor. This has a pressure transducer that detects pressure oscillations within the sphygmomanometer cuff. As the cuff is deflated, pressure oscillations increase suddenly at systolic pressure and continue increasing in amplitude to a maximum which corresponds to the mean arterial pressure. The point at which the oscillations decrease in amplitude is the diastolic pressure. By automating the process, it is possible to obtain measurements at regular intervals that are closely correlated to invasive pressure measurements.

Blood pressure percentiles for age and sex are in Chapter 7.3.

CARDIAC OUTPUT

Echocardiography and Doppler ultrasound measurement of flow velocity in the aorta correlates with invasive measurement of cardiac output, but this technique is not easily applicable at the bedside and requires specialized training. Therefore, estimation of changes in cardiac output remains in the domain of invasive assessment. One or more of a combination of core–toe temperature difference, capillary refill time, urine output and arterial blood gas measurement can be used to estimate peripheral perfusion and hence infer cardiac output, but this approach has frequently been shown not to be consistently reliable.

CENTRAL NERVOUS SYSTEM

The EEG, which is a summation of postsynaptic action potentials can be recorded by electrodes placed on the scalp. This bears a general relationship to cerebral blood flow and oxygen consumption and is important in monitoring seizure activity in patients in status epilepticus. However, this is a cumbersome procedure and not practical for routine monitoring. Derivatives of the EEG which include the cerebral function monitor, the cerebral function activity monitor and the activity of brain monitor have been developed, but have only found application during general anesthesia.

NEAR-INFRARED SPECTROSCOPY

The principles of near-infrared spectroscopy rely on two properties of biological tissues. First, chromophore molecules such as hemoglobin absorb infrared radiation in direct proportion to their concentration. Secondly, infrared radiation penetrates tissues to a depth of 6–8 cm. The brain has only three mobile chromophores (oxyhemoglobin, deoxyhemoglobin and cytochrome oxidase). By measuring the absorption of infrared radiation in the brain, it is possible to estimate the change in concentration of oxyhemoglobin and deoxyhemoglobin and from this calculate cerebral blood flow. Changes in oxyhemoglobin concentrations can also be monitored in the brain during cardiopulmonary bypass, over the stomach and splanchnic bed during resuscitation, and in the spinal cord as a measure of the adequacy of delivery of oxygenated blood. This technique has potential applications in patients with head injury and other conditions where cerebral oxygenation is compromised but is as yet in the stage of research and development.

✓ KEY POINTS

➤ Oximetry is essentially the 'fifth vital sign' in critical care
➤ Oximeter readings of SpO_2 where displayed heart rate is significantly different to actual heart rate are likely to be inaccurate

✗ COMMON ERRORS

➤ Using oximetry in burned patients whose carboxyhemoglobin level artificially elevates SpO_2
➤ Accepting a reassuring SpO_2 value in the face of an abnormal physical examination

FURTHER READING

1. Poets CF, Southall DP. Non-invasive monitoring of oxygenation in infants and children: practical considerations and areas of concern. Pediatrics 1994; 93: 737–746
2. Manab AJ, Baker-Brown G, Anderson EE. Oximetry in children recovering from deep hypothermia for cardiac surgery. Crit Care Med 1990; 18: 1066–1069
3. Hess D. Capnography: technical aspects and clinical applications. In: Kacmarek RM, Hess D, Stoller JK (editors). Monitoring in respiratory care. St Louis: Mosby; 1993; pp. 375–403
4. Chance B, Cooper CE, Delpy DT, Reynolds EOR. Near infra-red spectroscopy and imaging of living systems. Phils Trans Roy Soc Lond B Biol Sci 1997; 352(1354): 643–761
– (*Four reviews of practical clinical issues relating to noninvasive monitoring*)

5. Macnab AJ, Gagnon RE, Gagnon FA. Unresolved instrumentation problems following clinical trials using near infrared spectroscopy. J Biomed Optics 1998; 3(4): 386–390
– (*This paper reviews problems encountered by clinicians with current near infrared spectroscopy equipment in the clinical area*)

6.7 Extracorporeal life support

Allan P. Goldman

Extracorporeal life support (ECLS), also known as extracorporeal membrane oxygenation (ECMO), is a complex life-support technique. Using a modified heart-lung bypass machine, temporary respiratory and if necessary circulatory support is provided to patients with life-threatening but potentially reversible cardiorespiratory failure. It aims to take over the function of the lung and/or heart, allowing time and the milieu for damaged organs to recover while minimizing iatrogenic injury.

Extracorporeal life support requires cannulation of major blood vessels, usually the internal jugular vein and sometimes the carotid artery. Venous blood is drained from the right atrium and pumped through an extracorporeal circuit consisting of an artificial membrane lung, a heat exchanger and the pump itself. Blood is returned either to the arterial circulation, via a cannula placed in the right common carotid artery or femoral artery (venoarterial ECLS), or to the venous circulation, usually via the right internal jugular or femoral veins (venovenous ECLS) (Fig. 6.7.1).

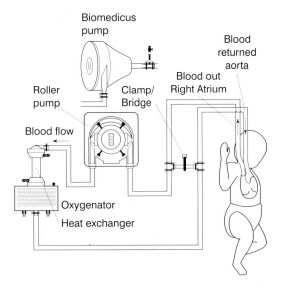

Figure 6.7.1 Typical ECMO circuit with roller pump and centrifugal pump inserted

WHO IS ELIGIBLE FOR ECLS?

Extracorporeal life support is appropriate for patients with high predicted mortality who have potentially reversible disease, in whom:

- conventional non-ECLS treatment is ineffective
- anticoagulation is not contraindicated
- neurological and other organ function is demonstrably intact or recoverable

CLINICAL APPLICATIONS

NEONATAL ECLS

Over 11 000 neonates with severe respiratory failure have been supported on ECLS with an overall survival of 80%, as recorded by the Extracorporeal Life Support Organization (ELSO) registry. The most conclusive evidence for the use of ECLS in severe neonatal respiratory failure over conventional treatment comes from the recent UK collaborative randomized ECLS trial, in which 54 of 92 (59%) neonates allocated conventional treatment died, compared with 30 of 93 (32%) allocated to ECLS.

The most common diagnoses leading to ECLS support in neonates are primary persistent pulmonary hypertension of the newborn (PPHN) and PPHN secondary to meconium aspiration, sepsis, respiratory distress syndrome and congenital diaphragmatic hernia (CDH). Although babies with CDH have a worse survival rate (58%) than other neonates receiving ECMO, the application of ECLS even in these patients appears to be associated with reduced mortality.

The oxygenation index (OI) is a widely used and easily calculated selection criterion for neonatal ECLS eligibility (see box). It reflects the degree of ventilation and inspired oxygen being delivered and the level of patient oxygenation being achieved.

$$\text{Oxygenation index} = \frac{\text{mean airway pressure (cmH}_2\text{O}) \times \text{inspired oxygen (\%)}}{\text{postductal arterial } P\text{O}_2 \text{ (mmHg)}}$$

Most centers use an OI of more than 40 for ECLS consideration, since this has been associated with a mortality in excess of 60% in conventionally treated babies. Premature babies are unsuitable for ECLS both because they are at increased risk of intraventricular hemorrhage and because of technical difficulties cannulating their very small neck vessels.

Consider ECLS referral for severe neonatal respiratory failure if:

- OI more than 40, *or*
- significant barotrauma or air leak syndrome, despite an OI below 40, *or*
- acute deterioration—$Pa\text{O}_2$ less than 4 kPa (30 mmHg) or $Pa\text{CO}_2$ over 12 kPa (90 mmHg)

Provided birthweight was more than 2 kg and gestational age exceeded 35 weeks.

PEDIATRIC ECLS

The technical success of neonatal ECLS has led to an increased interest in the use of ECLS in older patients with severe refractory respiratory failure, with recent improvements in reported survival rates (53% up to 88%). However, there have been no randomized clinical trials of ECLS in this group of patients. The most common critical illnesses for which ECLS has been used in this age group are bacterial, viral and aspiration pneumonias and acute respiratory distress syndrome (ARDS). Some groups report successful management of shock states, such as in meningococcal sepsis, with ECLS. Failure of maximal conventional therapy, severe barotrauma and acute deterioration form the basis of ECLS selection in this group.

Indications

Consider referral for pediatric ECLS if:

- inadequate oxygenation, as evidenced by OI > 35 or $Aa\text{D}\text{O}_2$ > 500 mmHg *or* $Pa\text{O}_2$(mmHg)/$F\text{IO}_2$ < 100 or $Sa\text{O}_2$ < 85%, $Pa\text{O}_2$ < 8 Kpa (60 mmHg), despite appropriate ventilation, and need for:

- $F\text{IO}_2$ > 0.9 for 4 hours
- PEEP > 10 cmH$_2$O for 4 hours
- PIP > 40 cmH$_2$O or MAP > 30 cmH$_2$O high frequency oscillation ventilation (HFOV)
- respiratory acidosis (pH < 7.2) despite appropriate rate, inspiratory time and need for PIP > 40 cmH$_2$O or HFOV
- air leak syndrome or severe barotrauma
- acute deterioration: $Pa\text{O}_2$ < 5.3 kPa (40 mmHg) or $Pa\text{CO}_2$ > 13.3 kPa (100 mmHg)
- large airway disease/disruption making ventilation impossible
- refractory septic shock

CARDIAC ECLS

Prolonged mechanical circulatory support outside the operating room has been widely used in over 1700 congenital heart patients (ELSO registry, 1998) with a reported survival rate of approximately 41%, and in an unknown number of children in pediatric cardiac centers not reporting to this or similar registries. The principal difference in managing the cardiac patient is that in order to achieve the goal of 'heart rest' to maximize myocardial recovery, the left heart must be adequately decompressed and positive inotropic drugs discontinued. This can be achieved by placement of an additional left heart decompression cannula in the left atrium via a median sternotomy, or percutaneously by blade septostomy.

When to consider cardiac ECLS in children

Extracorporeal circulatory support should be considered in the following situations:

- failure to wean from cardiopulmonary bypass after cardiac surgery despite maximal pharmacological support
- progressive and unremitting low cardiac output state following cardiac surgery due to reversible causes including pulmonary hypertension, arrhythmia and/or severely impaired contractility
- progressive or unremitting low cardiac output or shock state due to myocarditis, cardiomyopathy or septic shock

Provided that:

- surgery is complete, appropriate and judged technically successful
- cardiorespiratory recovery is expected
- there is no intractable system or organ dysfunction

In addition, children may benefit from support for severe grades of ARDS complicating cardiac surgery. Some centers undertake ECLS as a bridge to transplantation.

COMPLICATIONS

The most common patient complications of ECLS are bleeding, sepsis and need for hemofiltration, the latter usually for volume overload rather than frank renal failure. Common mechanical complications include cannula problems, including poor drainage, malposition and migration, clots in the circuit, oxygenator failures and leakage or rupture of parts of the extracorporeal circuit (Table 6.7.1). Patients should be urgently removed from ECLS if any of the following events occur:

- air or major clots, especially postmembrane
- cracks, leakage, disconnection or rupture of circuit
- accidental decannulation

LONG-TERM OUTCOME

Instrumentation of major neck vessels and anticoagulation are obviously of concern. In the UK ECLS trial there was an excess of respiratory morbidity in the conventionally treated patients at 1 year of age. One patient in each group had severe impairment, while 71% of survivors in each group showed no sign of impairment or disability, suggesting that neurological morbidity relates more to severity of the underlying illness than to ECLS itself.

There are little data available on the long-term follow-up of pediatric and cardiac survivors; however, current evidence suggests most survivors have a favorable outcome.

TECHNICAL ASPECTS OF ECLS

CANNULATION

The advantages and disadvantages of venovenous (V-V) ECLS and venoarterial (V-A) ECLS are shown in Table 6.7.2. In general, V-V ECLS is regarded as the mode of choice for isolated respiratory failure, while V-A ECLS is chosen for children with significant hemodynamic compromise.

DETERMINING MEMBRANE F_{IO_2}, PUMP AND SWEEP FLOW

The oxygen delivery of the ECLS circuit is the product of the O_2 content in the blood and the pump flow (see box). In addition, the patient's heart will contribute unless pump flows are very high. The oxygen content is optimized by maintaining the hematocrit above 0.4 (40%) and adjusting the F_{IO_2} on the membrane blender to ensure that blood leaving the membrane is fully saturated (usually requires $F_{IO_2} < 0.6$). Once this is achieved, O_2 delivery can only be improved by increasing pump flow. Adequacy of O_2 delivery is assessed by $S\bar{v}_{O_2}$, lactate and absence of metabolic acidosis. During V-A ECLS, aim to keep the mixed venous oxygen saturation ($S\bar{v}_{O_2}$) above 70%; $S\bar{v}_{O_2}$ is not useful in V-V ECLS because of recirculation of oxygenated blood in the right atrium.

> O_2 delivery = O_2 content × cardiac output

The fresh gas flow across the membrane, 'sweep flow', is adjusted to achieve desired CO_2 clearance, a similar function to adjusting mechanical minute ventilation volumes in conventional mechanical ventilation. Never exceed the maximum prescribed for the membrane as there is a risk of membrane rupture with catastrophic air embolus.

Typical 'rest mechanical ventilator settings' used during ECLS to minimize barotrauma, volutrauma and oxygen toxicity while encouraging alveolar recruitment are:

- PIP 20 cmH_2O, PEEP 10 cmH_2O
- F_{IO_2} 0.21
- ventilator rate 10/min
- inspiratory time 1 second

TABLE 6.7.1 **Emergencies and troubleshooting**

EMERGENCY ACTION
- If child needs to come off ECLS urgently (see text for reasons):
    1. Call for assistance, emergency drugs, colloid and blood
    2. Increase emergency ventilator settings/hand ventilate
    3. 'Come off ECLS'—on **roller pump**, remember 'Very Bad Accident':
        V—clamp Venous line above bridge
        B—unclamp Bridge
        A—clamp Arterial line above bridge (circuit will explode if arterial line is clamped first on roller pump)
        On **centrifugal pump**, come off ECLS in opposite order: AB V
    4. Once the patient is off ECLS, turn pump and sweep gas off, transfer infusions to the patient and maintain patient and circuit anticoagulation
    5. Identify and correct problem and recommence ECLS (AB V on roller pump, VBA on centrifugal pump).
- In **accidental decannulation**, apply pressure to cannulation site
- In **power failure**, use the hand crank, adjusting speed to maintain vital signs and perfusion, and if on roller pump, watch and prevent bladder from collapsing

TROUBLESHOOTING
Failing membrane oxygenator
- Signs:
    - falling PO_2 and rising PCO_2 in patient and postmembrane gas
    - rising premembrane pressure and transmembrane pressure gradient
    - increased platelet consumption and labile ACTs (see below) are often the most sensitive signs.
    - reduced CO_2 clearance in the face of normal oxygenation usually indicates a wet rather than a failing membrane
- Action to be taken:
    - increase FiO_2 to 1.0 and sweep flow to maximum for that membrane
    - increase mechanical ventilation as required
    - change membrane
    - in the case of a 'wet membrane', increasing the sweep flow usually corrects the problem

Inadequate systemic oxygenation, despite high ECLS flow (> 150%)
- Is bridge clamp fully occlusive (not overshunting)?
- Are sweep flow and FiO_2 settings on blender correct and is gas tubing connected to membrane gas ports?
- Is membrane failing (see above)?
- If postmembrane gas adequate, is pump delivering desired set flow? Check pump flow matches predicted flow for rev/min and raceway size, and that rollers are adequately occlusive against raceway. If using centrifugal pump, recalibrate flow sensor
- If cannulation is venovenous, check for excessive recirculation of oxygenated blood (blood leaving from and returning to the patient looks a similar color).
- Look for right-to-left shunting at atrial or ductal level (echocardiogram)
- If problem persists despite above, consider patient to have high metabolic rate. Ensure adequate sedation, normothermia, treat sepsis if suspected, and increase pump flow to meet metabolic demands

High postmembrane pressure
- Causes:
    - kinked, clotted, malpositioned or restricted (suture) infusion cannula
    - flow too high for cannula size (check 'M' number of cannula)
    - aortic arch dissection
- CXR and/or echocardiogram may help identify cause

Bladder box alarm sounds, excessive negative prepump pressure on centrifugal pump (below minus 30 mmHg)
- Bladder box sounds an alarm and 'cuts out' power to pump if bladder collapses (below minus 20 mmHg)
    1. First administer fluid challenge, as hypovolemia is most common cause (can temporarily reduce pump flow)
    2. If alarm persists, meticulously examine prepump venous limb for kinks, clots or even misplaced clamp
    3. If the above fails, obtain urgent CXR and echocardiogram to exclude tension pneumothorax, pericardial tamponade or malpositioned/restrictive venous cannula
    4. At this point venous drainage should be optimized by increasing the height of patient above the bladder.
- If all above fails to identify and correct problem, it is likely that the venous cannula is too small, and an additional cannula or replacement for a larger one should be considered

Abnormal activated clotting times
- Sudden change in ACT—repeat test, exclude heparin infusion error
- High ACT—exclude thrombocytopenia, oliguria/renal impairment or heparin infusion error
- Low ACT
    - associated with diuresis and platelet infusion
    - exclude heparin infusion error
- Unstable ACT—exclude membrane/circuit thrombosis, sepsis and faulty syringe drive

TABLE 6.7.2 **Comparison of venovenous and venoarterial ECLS**	
V-V ECLS	**V-A ECLS**
Advantages	
Spares carotid artery	Provides cardiac and respiratory support
Oxygenated blood to lungs	More rapid stabilization
Retains pulsatile flow	Technically easier
Reduced risk of thromboemboli to brain	
Disadvantages	
No direct cardiac support	Necessitates instrumentation of major neck vessels

ANTICOAGULATION AND BLOOD PRODUCTS

A heparin infusion is used for anticoagulation (Table 6.7.3). Also aim to achieve:

- hemoglobin 120 g/L (12g/dl)
- hematocrit > 0.4 (40%)
- plasma Hb < 0.3 g/L (0.03 g/dl)
- fibrinogen > 1.5 g/L (150 mg/dl)

It is usually necessary to increase heparin administration during diuresis and platelet transfusions and reduce it during renal failure and thrombocytopenia. Heparin bonded systems may permit lower levels of anticoagulation to be used.

SEDATION

Sedation is essential during ECLS, as during other forms of intensive care. Rapid lightening of sedation is, however, desirable to facilitate regular neurological assessments. Isoflurane (0.25–1.0%) a volatile anesthetic agent, in addition to routine sedation (opiates or benzodiazepines) is particularly useful in achieving a good but partially reversible level of sedation.

WEANING FROM ECLS

Lung recovery is indicated by improvement in chest compliance, improved aeration seen on chest X-ray and decreased dependence on the membrane oxygenator. In cardiac ECLS, myocardial recovery is indicated by the return of a pulse wave on the arterial trace, improvement of ventricular function on echocardiography, and maintenance of adequate blood pressure, systemic perfusion and normal atrial filling pressures on low ECLS flow.

✔ KEY POINTS

➤ ECLS can successfully support infants and children with intractable but recoverable cardiorespiratory failure

➤ The complexity of ECLS delivery and the limited number of patients needing ECLS require that it should only be practiced in centers with specially trained ECLS teams and pediatric multidisciplinary back-up

➤ Advances in ECLS technology will make the procedure simpler and safer in the future, particularly heparin-bonded ECLS circuitry

FURTHER READING

1. UK collaborative randomised trial of neonatal extracorporeal membrane oxygenation. UK Collaborative ECLS Trial Group. Lancet 1996; 348: 75–82
2. Anderson HL, Snedecor SM, Otsu T, Bartlett RH. Multicenter comparison of conventional venoarterial access versus venovenous double-lumen catheter access in newborn infants undergoing extracorporeal membrane oxygenation. J Pediatr Surg 1993; 28: 530

TABLE 6.7.3 **Guidelines for anticoagulation**		
ECLS	**Activated clotting time (s)**	**Platelets (10^9/L)**
Normal	180–220	> 100
Postoperative thoracotomy or laparotomy	160–180	> 150

3. The Pediatric ECLS Registry of the Extracorporeal Life Support Organization. Ann Arbor: ELSO; 1995

4. Moler RW, Custer JR, Bartlett RH et al. Extracorporeal life support for severe pediatric respiratory failure: an updated experience 1991–1993. J Pediatr 1994; 124: 875–880

5. Farjado E, Dalton H, Palermo NL et al. Outcome and follow up of pediatric ECMO survivors. Tenth National Childrens Medical Centre ECMO Symposium, Keystone, Colorado, Sponsored by The George Washington University Medical Center, 1994

6. Ruzevich SA, Kantor KR, Pennington DG, Swartz MT, McBride LR, Termuhlen DF. Long term follow up of survivors of postcardiotomy circulatory support. Trans Ann Soc Artif Organs 1988; 34: 116–124

Appendices

7.1 Drug dosage and principles of drug administration

John Macready, Claire Aston and Robert Adderley

The information contained in the following table has been obtained from among primary and tertiary reference sources for pediatric intensive care and from the experience obtained at British Columbia's Children's Hospital Pediatric Intensive Care Unit in Vancouver, Canada. We have attempted to provide the most up-to-date information available at the time of publication. It should be recognized that these doses represent guidelines for use in an intensive care area where suitable expertise and technology exist to support vital functions in case of various systems failure. It is incumbent upon the practitioner to modify drug therapy to suit each individual patient. Similarly, it is the ultimate responsibility of the physician in charge to ensure that these recommendations are suitable for use in the particular locality and patient population.

Some information has been included on antidotes for pediatric poisoning. It is recommended that the clinician seek the guidance from a local or regional poison control center.

USING THE TABLE

The information is presented in a three-column format designed to facilitate easy location and interpretation of the data.

DRUG NAME

The drugs are listed by nonproprietary (generic) name. Where applicable we have included a common representative trademark available in Canada. All trademarks are not included and may be different in different areas of the world. A number of standard dose forms and strengths are included to give the reader some sense of the availability of the various pharmaceutical forms of the medications.

INDICATION, DOSAGE AND ROUTE

Indications

Where possible, drug therapy indications are included.

Routes of administration

The abbreviations used are listed in the key.

Intravenous infusion: Where drugs are commonly administered by intravenous infusion, refer to Chapter 7.2.

Drug doses

Doses are mostly indicated in mg/kg per day in divided doses or mg/kg per dose repeated as indicated. Some infusions are indicated in terms of μg/kg or mg/kg per minute or hour. Use care and common sense to determine the correct dose and interval. When the dose calculated on a weight basis exceeds that of a maximum adult dose, the maximum adult dose is used.

Neonates

Some neonatal doses are included but more specific references should be consulted to obtain specialized information to apply to this age group.

REMARKS

Some additional information is given in column 3 about the practical aspects of using and monitoring these drugs, such as minimum dilutions, rates of administration and the more common adverse effects pertinent to critically ill children.

KEY TO ABBREVIATIONS	
AED	antiepileptic drugs
amp	ampoule
bid	twice a day (*bis in die*)
cap	capsule
CHD	congenital heart disease
chewtab	chewable tablets
CR	controlled release
ETT	endotracheal tube
D5W	5% glucose/water solution
D10W	10% glucose/water solution
div	divided
IM	intramuscular
inj	injection
IO	intraosseous
IV	intravenous
IVI	intravenous infusion
liq	liquid
mo	month
NG	nasogastric
NS	normal saline (0.9%)
od	once daily (*omes dies*)
PFS	prefilled syringe
PO	by mouth (*per os*)
PR	rectally (*per rectum*)
prn	when required (*pro re nata*)
qid	four times a day (*quater in die*)
qxh	every *x* hours (*quaque x hora*)
SC	subcutaneous
SL	sublingual
supp	suppository
susp	suspension
SWI	sterile water for injection
tab	tablet
tid	three times a day (*ter in die*)
t½	half life
U	units
yr	year

Drug name	Indication, dose, route	Remarks

Acetaminophen (paracetamol) [Tylenol, Tempra]
 	
tab: 325 mg
chewtab: 80 mg
liq: 32, 80 mg/ml
supp: 120, 325, 650 mg
	Analgesia, antipyresis:
	  10–15 mg/kg per dose PO q4–6 h prn
	  20–25 mg/kg per dose PR q4–6 h prn
	Postsurgical analgesia:
	  20 mg/kg per dose PO or 35 mg/kg per
	    dose PR q6h × 48 h, then reassess
	Max. dose: 90 mg/kg per day, up to 4 g
	  daily PO
		Regular dosing in the postoperative period
		  provides more effective pain relief
		Rectal administration produces inconsistent
		  blood levels and unpredictable dose-
		  response effect.
		Hepatotoxic in acute and chronic overdose
		  —see acetylcysteine for treatment of
		  toxic ingestion, 1 μg/ml = 0.15 mmol/L

Acetazolamide [Diamox] tab: 250 mg liq: compounded individually inj: 500 mg	Metabolic alkalosis: 3–5 mg/kg per dose 2–3 times daily	Carbonic anhydrase inhibitor May cause hypokalemia, metabolic acidosis Avoid in renal insufficiency

Acetylcysteine (N-acetylcysteine) [Mucomyst]
 	
inj: 20% solution (2 g/10 ml)
	Antidote for acetaminophen (paracetamol)
	  toxicity:
	Early presentation (< 16 h after ingestion)
	  with toxic levels or exhibiting signs or
	  symptoms of toxicity:
	  150 mg/kg in 200 ml D5W IV over 1 h
	  then 50 mg/kg in 500 ml D5W IV over 4 h
	  then 100 mg/kg in 1 L D5W IV over 16 h
	Late presentation (> 16 h after ingestion) or
	  prolonged therapy:
	  6.25 mg/kg·h until acetaminophen is
	    undetectable and hepatic recovery is apparent
		Consult poison control center

Acetylsalicylic acid (ASA, aspirin) [many brands]
 	
tab: 325 mg
chewtab: 80 mg
supp: 150, 325, 650 mg
	Platelet inhibition:
	  Surgical shunts/endovascular stents: 2–5 mg/kg
	    per day
	  mechanical heart valves: 5–10 mg/kg
	    per day
	Analgesia:
	  10–15 mg/kg per dose PO/PR q4–6h prn
	Kawasaki's disease:
	  100 mg/kg per day PO div q6h until fever
	    resolves, then 3–5 mg/kg per day PO od
	Antiinflammatory:
	  60–100 mg/kg per day PO div q6–8h
		Therapeutic blood level for Kawasaki's
		  disease 1.5–2 mmol/L
		ASA is associated with Reye's syndrome
		  when used following a febrile illness

Acid citrate dextrose (ACD) solution: see chapter 3.5		

Acyclovir [Zovirax]
 	
tab: 200 mg
liq: 40 ml/ml
inj: 500 mg/vial
	Mucocutaneous HSV:
	  15 mg/kg per day IV div q8h
	  immunocompromised hosts: 30 mg/kg
	    per day IV div q8h
	Varicella-zoster:
	  30 mg/kg per day IV div q8h
	  immunocompromised hosts: 45 mg/kg
	    per day IV div q8h
	HSV encephalitis:
	  < 1 yr: 1500 mg/m^2 per day IV div q8h ×
	    10–21 days
	  > 1 yr: 30 mg/kg per day IV div q8h ×
	    10–21 days
	Doses must be adjusted for renal impairment
	CMV prophylaxis in immunocompromised hosts:
	  50–80 mg/kg per day PO div qid
		Doses must be adjusted for renal failure
		Supplemental doses of 60–100% are
		  necessary after hemodialysis
		Patients must be well hydrated; failure to do
		  so may cause crystallization in renal
		  tubules (seen as fine needle-like crystals in
		  the urine)

Drug name	Indication, dose, route	Remarks
Adenosine [Adenocard] inj: 6 mg/2ml	Supraventricular tachycardia: Neonates: 0.05 mg/kg IV push; may repeat q2min up to 5 total doses Infants/children: 0.05 mg/kg rapid IV push; increase by 0.05 mg/kg every 2 min to max. 0.3 mg/kg Max. 12 mg in a single dose Pulmonary hypertension: 50 μg/kg·min initially and titrate by 50 μg/kg·min q2h to a max of 350 μg/kg·min	Must be given over 10 s, followed by a rapid saline push Contraindicated in heart transplant patients Use with caution in patients with bronchospastic disease A defibrillator must be immediately available
Adrenaline—see epinephrine		
Adrenaline, racemic— see epinephrine, racemic		
Albuterol—see salbutamol		
Alcohol, ethyl—see ethanol		
Allopurinol [Zyloprim] tab: 100, 200, 300 mg susp (compounded): 5 mg/ml	Hyperuricemic states: 10 mg/kg per day PO/IV in 2–3 div doses Max. dose 600 mg per day	Inhibits xanthine oxidase Decrease dose in renal failure Alkaline urine enhances uric acid clearance Injection for investigational use (200 mg vials) requires health protection branch approval in Canada
Alprostadil—see Prostaglandin E₁		
Ateplase—see Tissue Plasminogen Activator		
Aminocaproic acid (EACA) [Amicar] tab: 500 mg liq: 250 mg/ml inj: 250 mg/ml	Antifibrinolytic Acute bleeding: 100 mg/kg IV over 1 h as a single dose, followed by a 33 mg/kg·h infusion or 100 mg/kg per dose PO/IV q4–6h	Tranexamic acid is as effective and one-tenth the cost of aminocaproic acid Contraindicated in DIC, hematuria
Aminophylline (theophylline) [many brands] inj: 500 mg/10 ml amp	Bronchodilator: loading dose 6mg/kg IV over 30 min, followed by an infusion (see age groups), titrated to therapeutic effect and blood levels 1–12 mo: 0.2–0.9 mg/kg·h 1–9 y: 1 mg/kg·h 9–16 y: 0.8 mg/kg·h > 16 y: 0.5 mg/kg·h Apnea of prematurity: 5 mg/kg PO/IV loading dose followed by 2.5–3.75 mg/kg per dose IV/PO q12h	Therapeutic range for bronchospasm: 55–110 mmol/L (Theophylline) Therapeutic range for apnea: 60–80 mmol/L Aminophylline = 80% theophylline Multiple drug interactions
Amiodarone [Cordarone] tab: 200 mg inj: 150 mg/3ml amp	Antiarrhythmic: IV loading dose 5 mg/kg IV over 20–60 min (may be repeated × 2 doses) up to total of 15 mg/kg; then continuous IV solution of 5–15 μg/kg·min PO loading dose 4 mg/kg per dose every 8 h for 1 week, then every 12–24 h	Central line preferable To convert from IV to oral, start tabs, then taper infusion over 5 days IV solution must be diluted to a final concentration between 0.6 mg/ml and 4.8 mg/ml For infusion see Ch. 7.2 Multiple drug interactions It is recommended that pacing wires be in place for loading doses > 5 mg/kg

Drug name	Indication, dose, route	Remarks

Amoxicillin
[Amoxil, Novamoxin]
 	
cap: 250, 500 mg
liq: 50 mg/ml
	Infection due to susceptible organisms:
	   20–60 mg/kg per day PO div q8h
	Prophylaxis in asplenic patients:
	   2–5 y: 20 mg/kg per day PO div q12h
	   > 5 y: 250 mg PO q12h
		Achieves serum levels twice that of oral
		   ampicillin
		Absorption not affected by food

Amphotericin B
[Fungizone]
 	
inj: 50 mg vial
	Antifungal:
	initial dose 0.25–0.5 mg/kg per day IV,
	   increase to 1 mg/kg per day IV on day 2
	   or 3; infused over 4–6 h
	Max. dose 1.5 mg/kg per day IV
	Bladder instillations:
	   15–50 mg per day; diluted to 0.05 mg/ml
	      in SWI as a continuous irrigation over
	      24 h
		Drug is inactivated in lipid; do not add to
		   lipid emulsion
		Test doses of 1 mg are not required. In life-
		   threatening infection, start with 1 mg/kg
		   per day on day 1
		Premedicate with acetaminophen
		   (paracetamol) and add hydrocortisone
		   1 mg/ml of amphotericin B, up to a max.
		   dose of 25 mg hydrocortisone, to prevent
		   immediate reactions in patients who are
		   susceptible

Ampicillin
[many brands]
 	
cap: 250, 500 mg
liq: 50 mg/ml
inj: 125, 250, 500 mg, 1 g and 2 g vials
	Neonates:
	   < 7 days: 50–100 mg/kg per day div q12h
	   > 7 days: 100 mg/kg per day div q8h
	Meningitis:
	   200–400 mg/kg per day IV div q6h
	Other infections:
	   100–200 mg/kg per day IV div q6h *or*
	   50 mg/kg per day PO div q6h
	Usual adult dose 1–2 g IV q6H
		Amoxicillin is the preferred oral drug except
		   if treating *Salmonella* or *Shigella,* where
		   ampicillin is the drug of choice

Amrinone
[Inocor]
 	
inj: 100 mg/20 ml amps
	Acute heart failure:
	   loading dose 0.75–3 mg/kg per dose IV
	      over 5 min, followed by 5–20 µg/kg·min
	      infusion
	Neonates: 3–5 µg/kg·min
		For infusion see Ch. 7.2
		Causes dose/time related reduction in
		   platelets; avoid if platelets < 50 × 10^9/L

Amyl nitrite—see Cyanide antidote kit		

Antithymocyte (equine) globulin
[ALG, lymphocyte immune globulin]
 	
inj: 250 mg/5 ml
	Test dose: 5 µg intradermally
	Renal allograft recipients:
	acute rejection: 10–15 mg/kg per day × 14
	   days (may continue for 21 days if necessary)
	delaying onset of allograph rejection:
	   15 mg/kg per day for 14 days, then every
	      other day for 14 days, starting within
	      24 h of transplant (total of 21 doses)
	Aplastic anemia:
	   10–20 mg/kg per day for 8–21 doses
	Bone marrow transplantation:
	   20 mg/kg per day for 3–11 doses (some
	      protocols use up to 40 mg/kg per day)
		Patients may require pretreatment with
		   acetaminophen, antihistamine, and/or
		   corticosteroid
		Intradermal testing is recommended prior
		   to the administration of the initial dose of
		   ALG with 5 µg/0.1 ml
		Incompatible with dextrose solutions; use
		   0.9% or 0.45% saline
		Infuse via central line

Aspirin—see Acetylsalicylic acid		

Atracurium
[Tracrium]
	Neuromuscular blocker:
	   intubation 0.6 mg/kg per dose
	   neuromuscular blockade 0.3–0.6 mg/kg
	      per dose
		Metabolized by plasma esterases
		Hypotension is secondary to histamine
		   release
		Largely replaced by cisatracurium

Atropine
[many brands]
 	
inj: 0.4, 0.6 mg/ml
	Preoperative:
	   children: 0.01–0.02 mg/kg per dose IV
	   max. single dose 0.4 mg
	   adult: 0.6 mg per dose IV
	CPR (bradycardia):
	   0.02 mg/kg per dose IV q2–5 minutes
	      × 2–3 doses
	   min. single dose 0.1 mg
	   max. single dose pediatric 1 mg
	   max. single dose adolescent 2 mg
	   max. single dose adult 3 mg
	Organophosphate/carbamate poisoning/
	   cholinergic crisis:
	   0.01–0.05 mg/kg IV; repeat q5–10 min
	      until symptoms are reversed. Large
	      doses may be required
		In carbamate poisoning must be used in
		   conjunction with pralidoxime. Atropine
		   alone will not reverse nicotinic
		   manifestations

Drug name	Indication, dose, route	Remarks
Azathioprine [Imuran] tab: 50 mg liq: 10 mg/ml compounded inj: 100 mg/vial	Immunosuppression: initial 3–5 mg/kg per day IV/PO maintenance 1–3 mg/kg per day IV/PO	Reduce dose in renal impairment or concomitant allopurinol administration
Benztropine [Cogentin] tab: 1, 2 mg inj: 2 mg/2ml amp	Drug-induced extrapyramidal disorders: 0.02–0.05 mg/kg per dose PO/IM/IV div od or bid max. dose 0.1 mg/kg per dose or up to 6 mg per day	Anticholinergic side-effects
Bretylium [Bretylol] inj: 500 mg/10 ml vial	CPR (acute ventricular fibrillation): 5–10 mg/kg per dose IV q5min, up to 35 mg/kg	Caution: will cause profound hypotension
Calcium chloride 10% [many brands] inj: 0.68 mmol/ml = 27 mg $elemCa^{2+}$/ml (supplied as 10 ml amp or prefilled syringe)	Hypocalcemia, hyperkalemia, or calcium channel blocker toxicity: 10–20 mg/kg per dose IV or IO (0.1–0.2 ml/kg per dose)	Via central line only: extravasation causes severe tissue damage requiring plastic surgery in some cases
Calcium gluconate 10% [many brands] inj: 0.23 mmol/ml Ca_{2+} = 9 mg $elemCa_{2+}$/ml (supplied as 10 ml vial or prefilled syringe) tab: 650 mg (1.5 mmol Ca_{2+})	Hypocalcemia, hyperkalemia, calcium channel blocker toxicity: 60 mg/kg per dose (0.6 ml/kg per dose) IV	Calcium gluconate is as effective as calcium chloride in acute situations but the dose of gluconate is 3 times the dose of chloride
Calcium disodium EDTA [calcium disodium versenate] inj: 1000 mg/5 ml amp	Chelating agent acute lead intoxication: 1–1.5 g/m^2 per day IV or 50–75 mg/kg per day; administered over 12–24 h × 5 days	Consult poison control center Doses must be adjusted in renal failure. Monitor renal function closely in all patients. A dose of dimercaprol must precede the first dose of calcium disodium EDTA
Calcium polystyrene sulfonate [Resonium Calcium] liq: 0.25 mg/ml in 25% sorbitol powder: suspensions for rectal use can be made with tap water, dextrose solutions, or equal parts water and 2% methylcellulose	Acute hyperkalemia: 1 g/kg per day PO/PR div tid/qid Maintenance: 0.5 g/kg per day PO/PR div tid/qid Max. dose 20 g per dose PO/PR	Exchanges about 1.6 mmol potassium per gram of resin Do not mix with fruit juices containing potassium Rectal route is less effective than oral route due to variable absorption; however, the onset of action is faster. The oral route may have a delayed onset of action of 1–2 days until resin reaches the colon. Exchange will continue until all the resin is voided. Sorbitol-containing suspensions are used for oral administration, but are not recommended for rectal use as they may cause necrosis of bowel wall
Captopril [Capoten] tab: 6.25, 12.5, 25, 50, 100 mg liq: 1 mg/ml (compounded)	Afterload reduction: test dose 0.1 mg/kg per dose; titrate by 0.15 mg/kg increments until effective dose reached (1 mg/kg per dose) max. dose 6 mg/kg per day Adolescents 6.25–12.5 mg per dose q8–12h max. dose 50–75 mg per dose	Reduce dose in renal failure Hypovolemia increases risk of postdose hypotension Can cause hyperkalemia when added to potassium-sparing diuretics or potassium supplements Effective dose should show a transient decrease in systolic blood pressure of 10% (at peak)

Drug name	Indication, dose, route	Remarks

Carbamazepine
[Tegretol, many generic brands]
 	
tab: 200 mg
chewtab: 100, 200 mg
CR tab: 200, 400 mg
liq: 20 mg/ml
	Anticonvulsant:
	  < 20 kg: 50 mg per day; increase by 50 mg
	    per day every 5–7 days up to a
	    maintenance dose of 20 mg/kg or
	    600 mg per day, whichever is less
	Higher doses may be required in some patients
	Divide dose tid for regular tab/chewtab/liq
	  and bid for CR tabs
		Do not crush CR tabs
		Therapeutic range 25–50 μmol/L
		Adjust according to response
		Carbamazepine has many important drug
		  interactions due to induction of
		  cytochrome P450 enzymes, including
		  induction of its own metabolism
		Erythromycin will inhibit the metabolism of
		  carbamazepine

Carnitine (L-carnitine)
[Carnitor]
 	
liq: 100 mg/ml
inj: 1000 mg/5 ml
	Therapeutic nutrient
	Primary carnitine deficiency; secondary carnitine
	  deficiency; associated with valproic acid therapy:
	    50–500 mg/kg per day div 2 or 3 doses
	    higher doses may be required in patients
	    with inborn errors of metabolism,
	    e.g. up to 700 mg/kg per day	

Cefaclor
[Ceclor]
 	
cap: 250 mg
liq: 50 mg/ml
	Oral treatment of infections due to
	  susceptible organisms (not a drug of
	  first choice):
	  40 mg/kg per day PO div q6–12h
	  Adult max. 1.5 g per day
		May cause serum sickness, erythema
		  multiforme, and Stevens–Johnson syndrome

Cefazolin (cephazolin)
[Kefzol, Ancef]
 	
inj: 500 mg, 1 g vials
	Prophylaxis and treatment of infection due
	  to susceptible organisms:
	  50–100 mg/kg per day IM/IV div q8h
	  usual adult dose 1g IV q8h
	  max. dose 2 g IV q8h
	Prophylaxis after cardiopulmonary bypass:
	  120 mg/kg per day IV div q8h
		First-generation cephalosporin

Cefotaxime
[Claforan]
 	
inj: 500 mg, 1 g and 2 g vials
	Neonates > 2000 g:
	  0–7 days: 50 mg/kg per dose IV q12h
	  > 7 days: 50 mg/kg per dose IV q8h
	Infants/children:
	  100–150 mg/kg per day IM/IV div q8h
	Meningitis dose:
	  200 mg/kg per day div q6h
	  usual adult dose 1–2 g IV q8–12h
		Third-generation cephalosporin
		Good CSF penetration
		Doses of 300 mg/kg are recommended in
		  areas with intermediate pneumococcal
		  resistance

Cefoxitin
[Mefoxin]
 	
inj: 1 and 2 g
	Surgical (abdominal/genitourinary)
	  prophylaxis:
	Neonate > 2000 g:
	  < 7 days: 20 mg/kg per dose IV q12h
	  > 7 days: 20 mg/kg per dose IV q8h
	Pediatric:
	  80–160 mg/kg per day IM/IV div q4–6h
	Adult:
	  1–2 g IM/IV div q6h
	  max. adult dose 12 g per day
		Second-generation cephalosporin
		Does not cross blood-brain barrier
		Has aerobic and anaerobic coverage; good
		  for mixed infections

Ceftazidine
[Tazidime, Fortaz]
	Empiric coverage for *Pseudomonas aeruginosa*;
	  infection due to susceptible Gram-negative
	  organisms. Not a drug of first choice
	Neonates > 2000 g:
	  < 7 days: 50 mg/kg per dose IV q12h
	  > 7 days: 50 mg/kg per dose IV q8h
	Pediatric:
	  100–150 mg/kg per day IM/IV q8h
	Cystic fibrosis:
	  200–300 mg/kg per day IV div q8h
	Adult max. dose 6 g per day
		Third-generation cephalosporin with good
		  coverage for *Pseudomonas aeruginosa*
		Reserve for empiric treatment in select
		  populations (e.g. febrile neutropenic
		  patients) or when culture and sensitivity
		  results indicate

Drug name	Indication, dose, route	Remarks
Ceftriaxone [Rocephin] inj: 250 mg, 1 and 2 g vials	Infants/children: 50–100 mg/kg per day IM/IV div od or q12h (higher dose for meningitis – give q12h) Max. dose 4 g per day	Use cefotaxime as drug of first choice (identical spectrum to ceftriaxone) Only advantage is once-daily dosing, making ceftriaxone suitable for IM use and for outpatient IV programs Not used in neonates
Cefuroxime [Zinacef] inj: 750 mg, 1.5 g vials	Pediatric: 100–150 mg/kg per day IM/IV div q8h Adult: 750–1500 mg IM/IV q8h	Second-generation cephalosporin Penetration through blood-brain barrier occurs more slowly than with third-generation cephalosporins; therefore do not use for meningitis
Cephalexin [Keflex, Novalexin] cap: 250 and 500 mg liq: 50 mg/ml	Oral treatment of susceptible infections: Pediatric: mild to moderate infections 25–50 mg/kg per day PO div q6h severe infections 100–150 mg/kg per day PO div q6h Adult dose 1–4 g per day PO div q6h	First-generation cephalosporin Oral equivalent to cefazolin A palatable oral liquid for step-down therapy from IV cloxacillin (instead of oral cloxacillin)
Cephazolin—see cefazolin		
Charcoal (activated charcoal) bottle: 50 g/250 ml aqueous solution	Poison antidote: Pediatric 1–2 g/kg PO/NG initially, then 0.5–1 g/kg PO/NG q4–6h prn Adolescent/adult 30–100 g PO/NG initially, then 25–50 g/kg PO/NG q4–6h prn	Consult poison control center Check for bowel sounds before using Sorbitol-containing preparations are no longer recommended
Chloral hydrate [many brands] liq: 100 mg/ml	Sedation: 25 mg/kg per dose PO/PR prn Hypnotic: 50–75 mg/kg per dose PO/PR; max. dose 1 g per dose or 2 g per day Preprocedural: 50–75 mg/kg per dose PO/PR 60 min prior to procedure Max. dose 100 mg/kg per day or 2 g per day	Oral liquid may be used rectally Generally considered safe Oral liquid should be diluted prior to administration, especially in neonates, due to local irritation (osmolality 3285 mOsm/kg H_2O) Can cause paradoxical excitement
Chloramphenicol [Chloromycetin] inj: 1 g vials eye drops: 0.5% eye ointment: 1%	Neonates > 2000 g: < 7 days: 25 mg/kg IV q24h > 7 days: 25 mg/kg IV q12h Meningitis: 75–100 mg/kg per day IV div q6h Max. dose 4 g per day	Not a drug of first choice in children owing to toxic and idiosyncratic reactions In neonates, close clinical monitoring is required for dose-related and idiosyncratic toxicity Avoid in liver impairment Check with clinical microbiologist if therapeutic monitoring is required: therapeutic level is 15–25 mg/L post dose, 2–10 mg/L predose
Clormethiazole edisylate (emergency release drug in Canada) [Heminevrin] inj: premixed in 500 ml bottles of 0.8% in D4W	Refractory status epilepticus: Dose is highly variable and must be titrated on an individual basis Pediatric: 0.01 ml/kg·min, may be increased every 2–4 h until seizures are abolished Once control has been achieved for 2 days, gradually wean rate every 4–6 h Adult: 5–15 ml/min up to a total dose of 40–100 ml, then 0.5–1 ml/min In countries where clormethiazole is on the market, it can be used for sedation and alcohol withdrawal	Extensively metabolized by the liver Causes respiratory and cardiovascular depression at higher doses Clormethiazole adsorbs to Silastic and PVC tubing; glass, Teflon or polyethylene tubing should be used

Drug name	Indication, dose, route	Remarks
Chlorpromazine [Largactil] tab: 10, 25, 100 mg liq: 5 mg/ml, 20 mg/ml supp: 100 mg inj: 25 mg/ml	Behavioral problems, psychosis, nausea and vomiting: > 6 months: 2.5–6 mg/kg per day IM/IV div q6–8h or 2.5–6 mg/kg per day PO div q4–6h or 1 mg/kg per dose PR q6–8h Max. IM/IV dose: < 5 y: 40 mg per day > 5 y: 75 mg per day	IV route can cause hypotension Can cause drowsiness, arrhythmias, extrapyramidal symptoms
Cimetidine [Tagamet, many brands] tab: 200, 300 mg liq: 60 mg/ml inj: 300 mg/2 ml vial	Neonate > 2000 g: < 7 days: 2–4 mg/kg per dose IV q8h 8–30 days: 2–4 mg/kg per dose IV q6h Pediatric: 20–40 mg/kg per day PO/IV div q6h	Cimetidine is an cytochrome P450 system inhibitor, therefore has many drug interactions, e.g.with phenytoin, warfarin, theophylline
Ciprofloxacin [Cipro] tab: 250, 500 mg inj: 400 mg/40 ml amp	Antibiotic Pediatric: 5–10 mg/kg per day IV div q12h, max. dose 800 mg/24 h or 15–30 mg/kg per day PO div q8–12h, max. dose 1500 mg/24 h	Not recommended for children under 18 years old owing to transient arthropathy (and cartilage damage in immature laboratory animals) May cause seizures—use with caution in patients with underlying neurologic disorders Has multiple drug interactions including warfarin, cyclosporin, theophylline, cimetidine and sucralfate Doses must be adjusted in renal failure
Cisapride [Prepulsid] tab: 10 mg liq: 1 mg/ml	Gastrointestinal prokinetic agent Gastroparesis, GE reflux: neonate: 0.15–0.3 mg/kg per dose PO tid or qid, 15–30 min prior to feeding pediatric: 0.3–0.5 mg/kg per dose PO tid or qid, 15–30 min prior to meals and at bedtime Max. dose 60 mg per day	Similar to metoclopramide or domperidone, but without dopamine antagonist effects or extrapyramidal effects Cases of QT interval prolongation and ventricular arrhythmias (including torsade des pointes), have occurred in susceptible patients. Contraindicated in combination with azole antifungals, the erythromycins, protease inhibitors and nefazodone. Risk of arrythmia increased with concommitant use of certain anti arrythmic agents
Cisatracurium [Nimbex] inj: 20 mg/10 ml vial	Neuromuscular blockade: Intubation: 0.15–0.2 mg/kg IV maintenance of neuromuscular blockade: 0.1 mg/kg per dose IV	Metabolized by plasma esterases Preferable to atracurium because of lower incidence of histamine release
Clarithromycin [Biaxin] tab: 250, 500 mg liq: 125 mg/5 ml	Infection due to susceptible organisms: 15 mg/kg/day div BID Max adult dose: 1000 mg/day	Has less GI side effects than erythromycin Is a C-P450 IIIA4 enzyme inhibitor and use should be avoided with cisapride, astemizole and terfenadine. May increase the sedative effects of benzodiazepines.
Clindamycin [Dalacin] cap: 150, 300 mg liq: 15 mg/ml inj: 300 mg/2 ml vials	Infection due to susceptible organisms: Neonates > 2000 g: < 7 days: 5 mg/kg per dose IV q8h > 7 days: 5 mg/kg per dose IV q6h Infant/pediatric: 20–40 mg/kg per day IV div q6–8h 20–30 mg/kg per day PO div q6h Max. dose 900 mg IV q8h; 450 mg PO q6h	Associated with pseudomembranous colitis Avoid using with erythromycin (antagonistic effect) Can prolong neuromuscular blockade Do not give IV bolus; give over at least 10 min Well absorbed orally (serum levels PO = serum levels IV) Poor CSF penetration

Drug name	Indication, dose, route	Remarks

Clobazam
[Frisium]
 	
tab: 10 mg
liq: 1 mg/ml compounded
	Adjunctive anticonvulsant in refractory
	  epilepsy:
	    < 20 kg: 5 mg per day PO initially,
	      increase by 5 mg per dose at 5 day
	      intervals
	  Usual maintenance dose 0.5–1 mg/kg per
	    day
	    > 20 kg: 10 mg per day PO initially, increase
	      by 5 mg per dose at 5 day intervals
	  Maintenance dose 1 mg/kg per day up to
	    a max. of 50 mg per day
		Sudden withdrawal may exacerbate seizures;
		  do not discontinue therapy abruptly

Clonazepam
[Rivotril]
 	
tab: 0.5, 2 mg
liq: compounded on request
	Anticonvulsant:
	  < 30 kg or < 10 y:
	    initial: 0.01–0.05 mg/kg/day div tid,
	      increase by 0.25 mg every 3–5 days
	  Maintenance dose 0.1–0.2 mg/kg per day
	    PO div tid
	  > 30 kg or > 10 years
	    initial: 0.5 mg per day PO div tid, increase by
	      0.5 mg per day PO every 5 days
	  Max. dose 20 mg per day
		Sudden withdrawal may exacerbate seizures;
		  do not discontinue therapy abruptly

Clonidine
[Dixarit, Catapres]
 	
tab: 0.025, 0.1 and 0.2 mg
	Preoperative:
	  2–3 µg/kg per dose PO to potentiate
	    narcotic analgesia
	Hypertension:
	  5–25 µg/kg per day PO div q6h
		May cause hypotension
		Has multiple indications for use
		  (hypertension, migraine, narcotic
		  withdrawal, Gilles de la Tourette syndrome,
		  ADHD, and growth hormone testing)

Cloxacillin
[Orbenin, Tegopen, Novocloxin]
 	
cap: 250, 500 mg
liq: 25 mg/ml
inj: 250 mg, 500 mg, 2 g vials
	Penicillinase-resistant penicillin
	Neonate:
	  < 7 days: 25 mg/kg per dose IV q12h
	  > 7 days: 25 mg/kg per dose IV q8h
	Infant/child < 20 kg:
	  mild to moderate infections: 50–100
	    mg/kg per day PO/IM/IV div q6h
	  severe infections (meningitis, osteomyelitis,
	    cystic fibrosis, febrile neutropenia):
	    150–200 mg/kg per day IM/IV div q6h
	    up to 6 g per day
		For PO stepdown use oral cephalexin
		Causes thrombophlebitis: give via central
		  line where possible
		Duration of therapy is 4–6 weeks for acute
		  osteomyelitis or endocarditis

Codeine
[many brands]
 	
tab: 15, 30 mg
liq: 15 mg/ml
inj: 30 mg/ml amp
	Analgesic:
	0.5–1 mg/kg per dose PO/IM q4–6h prn
		Do not give IV; has potent antihistamine-
		  releasing action (hypotension, urticaria,
		  bronchoconstriction)

Co-trimoxazole
[Bactrim, Septra, Novotrimel]
 	
tab: combination of 400 mg
  sulfamethoxazole (SMX) and
  80 mg trimethoprim (TMP)
 	
liq: combination of 40 mg SMX and
  8 mg TMP
inj: combination of 800 mg SMX
  and 160 mg TMP per 10 ml vial
	Infants > 1 mo and children:
	  Prophylaxis UTI: 2 mg/kg per day TMP
	  Minor infections: 8 mg//kg per day TMP
	    div q12h
	  Prophylaxis in immunocompromised hosts:
	    4 mg/kg per day TMP div q12h on
	    3 days/week
	  Pneumocystis carinii pneumonia:
	    20 mg/kg per day TMP div q6h
		Intravenous form must be diluted in sufficient
		  volume to prevent microprecipitation of
		  drug and failure of therapy. Ideal volume is
		  at least 1 ml solution in 25 ml total fluid.
		  Fluid-restricted patients can be given 1 ml
		  solution in 15 ml total fluid, but this must
		  be given within 1 h to prevent inactivation
		  of drug
		Dose must be adjusted for renal failure
		  (creatinine clearance < 30 ml/min)
		Do not use in infants < 1 month of age

Drug name	Indication, dose, route	Remarks

Cyanide antidote kit
 	
Contains:
  (1) Amyl nitrite
  (2) Sodium nitrite
  (3) Sodium thiosulfate
	Acute cyanide poisoning:
	1. Crush amyl nitrite capsules and allow patient to inhale contents for 30s out of 60 s while sodium nitrite is being prepared
	2. Stop amyl nitrite and give 10 mg/kg sodium nitrite (0.3 ml/kg of a 3% solution) IV over 2–4 min. Further administration should be based on Hb levels
	3. Through same IV line give 1.65 ml/kg of a 25% sodium thiosulfate solution over 10 min. Further administration is based on Hb levels
		Consult poison control center
		Exceeding recommended dose of sodium nitrite may result in fatal methemoglobinuria (total methemoglobin should not exceed 25%)
		If symptoms persist, half the initial doses of sodium nitrite and sodium thiosulfate may be administered 30 min later
		Cyanide is released in fires in which polyurethanes or plastics have been burned
		All patients should receive 100% oxygen and supportive care

Cyclosporin
[Neoral, Sandimmune]
 	
cap: 25, 50, 100 mg
liq: 100 mg/ml (100 ml bottle)
inj: 50 mg/ml amp
 	
(All newly manufactured oral forms are now Neoral. Presently both forms are available. Conversion is 1:1; however, Neoral doses necessary may be 15% lower than plain cyclosporin)
	Immunosuppressant:
	BMT:
	  3–6 mg/kg per day IV div q8–12h *or*
	  10–15 mg/kg per day PO div q8–12h
	Renal transplant:
	  5–15 mg/kg per day PO div q8–12h
	For some indications continuous infusions may be used
	Also used in liver/heart transplants
		Doses are guidelines only and pharmacokinetic variability is great
		Clearance rates are higher in young children and infants
		Serum levels should be regularly monitored and vary between indications. 'Pre' levels should be taken 0–60 min before a dose renal graft rejection: 25–100 μg/L
		GVHD in BMT, for first 30 days: 150 μg/L
		GVHD in BMT, after 30 days: $\geqslant$ 150 μg/L
		Excessively high levels can cause nephrotoxicity; low levels can cause failure of graft
		Do not draw levels through same lumen that drug was administered through
		Cyclosporin has multiple drug interactions. Check other references for a complete list
		'Rule of thumb': PO doses are 3 times IV doses

Dantrolene
[Dantrium]
 	
cap: 25, 100 mg
liq: compounded
inj: 20 mg vial
	Acute malignant hyperthermia:
	  1 mg/kg IV, may repeat prn up to a maximum cumulative dose of 10 mg/kg, then continue with 4–8 mg/kg per day PO div q6h × 3 days
	Preoperative prophylaxis of malignant hyperthermia:
	  25 mg/kg IV over 1 h (one dose)
		Reconstitute with 60 ml SWI (without bacteriostat) and use within 6 h
		Avoid extravasation; solution has a high pH
		Do not use calcium channel blockers in combination with dantrolene (has caused hyperkalemia and subsequent ventricular fibrillation and cardiovascular collapse)

Deferoxamine (desferrioxamine)
[Desferal]
 	
inj: 500 mg, 2 g vial
	Iron chelating agent
	Acute overdose:
	  15 mg/kg·h until symptoms have resolved *and* radio-opacities are no longer present *and* serum iron is < 63 μmol/L *and* vin rosé urine color has cleared, if present initially
	Chronic iron overload:
	  20–80 mg/kg per day IM/IV/SC titrated based on iron stores/excretion
		1 μmol/L = 27 μg/L
		SC is the preferred route for most chronic overload patients
		IV administration may be preferred in patients with massive iron stores and significant organ damage or for patients who do not comply with SC infusion

Desferrioxamine—see deferoxamine		

Desmopressin (arginine vasopressin)
[DDAVP, Octostim]
 	
intranasal solution: 0.1 mg/ml
intranasal spray: 10 μg/spray
  inj: 4 μg/amp, 15 μg/amp
	Hemostasis:
	  0.3 μg/kg per dose IV/SC
	ADH replacement in central diabetes insipidus:
	  5–20 μg intranasal once daily or divided bid
		Parenteral dose is one-tenth of intranasal dose
		Duration of action 8–12 h
		High concentration nasal spray available on investigational basis (Canada) for Von Willebrand Disease patients
		Beware of hyponatremia

Drug name	Indication, dose, route	Remarks

Dexamethasone [many brands]
 	
 tab: 0.5, 0.75, 4 mg
 liq: 0.5 mg/ml compounded
 inj: 4 mg/ml – 5 ml vial
 eyedrops: 0.1%
 eye ointment: 0.1%
	Steroid
	 Cerebral edema:
	   1–2 mg/kg IM/IV loading dose, then 0.25
	     mg/kg per dose q6h × 5 days, then taper
	 Airway edema:
	   0.3–0.6 mg/kg per dose IM/IV given q6h
	     × 4, starting 12–24 h prior to extubation
	 Acute antiinflammatory:
	   0.03–0.15 mg/kg per day PO/IM/IV div q6–12h
	 Croup:
	   0.3–0.6 mg/kg IV/IM/PO single dose
		25 times more potent than hydrocortisone
		 Taper if treatment period is more than
		   one week

Dextrose 50% [many brands]
 	
 inj: 500 mg/ml—50 ml syringe
	Documented hypoglycemia:
	   0.5–1 g/kg loading dose followed by
	     a continuous infusion not
	     exceeding 0.5 g/kg·h
		Use central line if concentration exceeds
		   12.5%
		 Rapid administration may cause osmotic
		   fluid shifts
		 pH of solution 4.2; osmolality 2.53 mOsm/ml

Diazepam [Valium, Diazemuls]
 	
 tab: 2, 5, 10 mg
 liq: 1 mg/ml
 inj: 5 mg/ml—2 ml
	Status epilepticus:
	   0.3 mg/kg/dose IV over 3 min; may
	     repeat 3 times at 10 min intervals
	 Max. dose:
	   < 5 y: = 5 mg
	   > 5 y. = 10 mg
		May cause hypotension/apnea, especially with
		   rapid IV administration. Respiratory
		   support must be immediately available
		 Administer into a large vein, preferably with
		   a running IV. Diazemuls is formulated in
		   lipid to decrease problem of phlebitis
		 Lorazepam is drug of choice for status
		   epilepticus because of its longer duration
		   of action

Digoxin [Lanoxin]
 	
 tab: 0.0625, 0.125, 0.25 mg
 liq: 0.05 mg/ml
 inj: 0.05, 0.25 mg/ml
	Heart failure:
	 Digitalizing dose given as ½ dose initially,
	   followed by ¼ dose q8h × 2 doses:
	 term infant < 2 mo:
	   20–25 μg/kg over 24 h divided as indicated
	 infant < 2y:
	   30–40 μg/kg over 24 h
	     divided as indicated
	 > 2 y:
	   25–30 μg/kg over 24 h divided as indicated
	 > 12 years:
	   0.5–1 mg over 24 h divided as indicated
	 Maintenance dose:
	 < 2 mo:
	   6–8 μg/kg per day
	 < 2 y:
	   7–9 μg/kg per day
	 2–12 y:
	   6–8 μg/kg per day
	 > 12 y:
	   0.1–0.4 mg/day
		Reduce dose in patients with renal failure
		 Toxicity markedly enhanced by hypokalemia
		   and any drug that disturbs potassium
		   equilibrium
		 Therapeutic levels 1–2.5 nmol/l
		 Has multiple drug interactions
		 Oral doses = IV dose × 1.4

Digoxin Fab [Digibind]
 	
 inj: 40 mg/vial
	Antidote for digoxin toxicity
	 Acute ingestion of unknown quantity of
	   digoxin:
	   dose of Digibind in mg = [serum digoxin
	     in ng/mL] × 5.6 × body weight in kg × 0.0667
	 Acute ingestion of known quantity of digoxin:
	   dose of Digibind in mg = digoxin
	     ingested in mg × 0.8 × 0.0667
	   infuse over 30 min through a 0.22 micron
	     filter, or in an emergency may give over
	     5 min
		40 mg Digibind will bind 0.6 mg digoxin
		 Monitor serum potassium for hypokalemia
		 Except in emergencies the patient should
		   receive a test dose of 1 mg IV or 0.01 mg
		   intradermally
		 Digibind will significantly increase laboratory
		   serum digoxin levels making subsequent
		   levels *uninterpretable*

Drug name	Indication, dose, route	Remarks

Dimenhydrinate
[Gravol, many brands]
 	
tab: 50 mg
liq: 3 mg/ml
supp: 50 mg, 100 mg
inj: IM 50 mg/ml
    IV 10 mg/ml
	Antiemetic:
	1 mg/kg per dose PO/PR/IM/IV q4–6h prn
	Max. dose PO:
	  2–6 y: 75 mg/day
	  6–12 y: 150 mg/day
	  Adults: 400 mg/day
	Max. dose IM/IV: 300 mg/day
		Anticholinergic side-effects
		Paradoxical excitement may occur

Dimercaprol (British antilewisite in oil)
 	
inj: 300 mg/3 ml amp
	Antidote for heavy metal poisoning
	Arsenic, gold, mercury:
	  3–4 mg/kg IM q4–6h for 2 days,
	    then 2.5–3 mg/kg IM q6–12h for 1 day,
	    then 2.5–3 mg/kg IM q12–24h for 10
	    days or until recovery is complete
	Lead:
	  3–4 mg/kg IM q4h (with calcium disodium
	    EDTA), duration dictated by lead levels
		Consult poison control center
		Alkaline urine enhances urinary excretion of
		  chelated metal
		Contraindicated in organic mercury
		  poisoning, G6PD and preexisting hepatic
		  insufficiency
		Symptoms of tachycardia, headache, fever,
		  hypertension, GI upset may be treated
		  with antihistamines
		Must be given by deep IM injection

Diphenhydramine
[Benadryl, many brands]
 	
caps: 25, 50 mg
liq: 2.5 mg/ml
inj: 50 mg/ml
	Antihistamine:
	5 mg/kg per day PO/IM/IV q6–8h
	  Treatment of hypersensitivity reactions,
	    dyskinesias/dystonic reactions and
	    drug-induced extrapyramidal reactions:
	    1-2 mg/kg IV slowly
	Max. dose 300 mg/day
		May cause paradoxical CNS excitation
		Anticholinergic side-effects

Dobutamine
[Dobutrex]
 	
inj: 12.5 mg/ml—20 ml vial
	Sympathomimetic:
	  2–20 µg/kg·min IV infusion; titrate to
	    effect
	Max. dose 40 µg/kg·min
		Give via central line wherever possible
		Extravasation may cause dermal necrosis
		  (see phentolamine)

Dopamine
[Inotropin]
 	
inj: 40 mg/ml—5 ml PFS
    800 µg/ml in D5W-250 and
    500 ml bag
	Sympathomimetic:
	  2–20 µg/kg·min IV infusion; titrate to
	    effect
	Max. dose 50 µg/kg·min
		Low doses used to enhance renal blood flow
		Central line required; extravasation may
		  cause dermal necrosis requiring plastic
		  surgery (see phentolamine)

Droperidol
[Inapsine]
 	
inj: 2.5 mg/ml—2 ml amp
	Antiemetic, sedative, anxiolytic
	Premedication:
	  0.1–0.15 mg/kg IM 30–60 min prior to
	    procedure
	Nausea, vomiting:
	  0.05 mg/kg per dose q4–6h prn
	Adjunct to general anesthesia 0.09–0.17 mg/kg
		May produce extrapyramidal reactions and
		  orthostatic hypotension
		Used alone may produce intense dysphoria

Edrophonium
[Tensilon]
 	
inj: 10 mg/ml
	Diagnosis of myasthenia gravis 0.04 mg/kg
	  over 1 min, followed by 0.16 mg/kg if no
	  response to a total of 5 mg for children
	  < 34 kg and 10 mg for children > 34 kg
		Atropine should be available for treatment
		  of cholinergic reaction

Enalapril
[Vasotec]
 	
tab: 2.5, 5, 10, 20
	Afterload reduction:
	  0.1 mg/kg per day, titrate to effect
	Usual maintenance dose:
	  0.1–0.4 mg/kg per day in 1 or 2 divided
	    doses
		Initiate therapy with lower doses and titrate
		  to effect
		Patient must be adequately hydrated
		May cause hyperkalemia
		A prodrug that undergoes transformation in
		  the liver to the active drug enalaprilat

Enoxaparin
  (low molecular weight heparin)
[Lovenox]
 	
inj: 30 mg/0.3 ml PFS
	Anticoagulation:
	Infants < 1 year:
	  treatment dose 3 mg/kg per day SC
	    div q12h
	  prophylaxis 1.5 mg/kg per day SC div q12h
	> 1 year:
	  treatment dose 2 mg/kg per day SC
	    div q12h
	  prophylaxis 1 mg/kg per day SC div q12h
		Monitor anti-Xa activity; monitoring of
		  PT/PTT not useful
		Therapeutic Xa levels (treatment): 0.5–1 u/mL
		Therapeutic Xa levels (prophylaxis):
		  0.2–0.4 u/ml
		Hematology consult suggested

Drug name	Indication, dose, route	Remarks

Epinephrine (adrenaline) [many brands]
 	
inj: 1:1000 amp (1 mg/ml)
1:1000 30 ml vial for infusion
inj: 1:10 000 syringe with intracardiac needle
	CPR/bradycardia:
	    IV/IO 0.1 ml/kg of 1:10 000
	    ETT: 0.1 ml/kg of 1:1000
	Cardiac arrest:
	    first dose:
	        0.1 ml/kg of 1:10 000 IV/IO
	        q3–5 min
	OR 0.1 ml/kg of 1:1000 via ETT
	    subsequent doses:
	        IV/IO/ET: 0.1 ml/kg 1:1000 q3–5 min
	    Doses as high as 0.2 ml/kg of 1:1000
	        may be effective
	Anaphylaxis:
	    0.01 ml/kg of a 1:1000 or 0.1 ml/kg of a
	    1:10 000 SC q20min up to 3 doses
	CV support:
	    0.1 μg/kg·min and titrate (infusion range
	    0.1–3 μg/kg·min)
	Nebulization for Croup/post extubation stridor:
	    0–6 mon: 2 ml of 1:1000 solution plus 2 ml NS
	    over 6 mon: 4 ml of 1:1000 solution
		For infusion see Ch. 7.2
		Do not use discolored solutions
		Extravasation causes tissue necrosis (see phentolamine)
		Incompatible with sodium bicarbonate solution
		Give IV infusions through a central line only
		Epinephrine 1:1000 solution may be used by nebulizer instead of Racemic Epinephrine as the latter product has not been available from the manufacturer recently

Epinephrine, racemic (adrenaline, racemic)
[Vaponephrine]
solution for inhalation: 2.25%
see epinephrine 1:1000 solutions
	Nebulized for croup/post-extubation stridor:
	    0–20 kg: 0.25 ml/dose in 2 ml NS via nebulizer
	    > 20 kg: 0.5 ml/dose in 2 ml NS via nebulizer
		Sputum may be pink-tinged following inhalation
		(May also substitute undiluted 4 ml 1:1000 epinephrine)
		This product has not been available from the manufacturers recently. Use epinephrine 1:1000 instead

Epoprostenol—see prostacyclin		

Erythromycin [many brands]
 	
tab: 250 mg
sprinkle cap: 250 mg (Eryc)
liq (estolate): 50 mg/ml
inj: 500 mg, 1 g vial
	Neonate:
	    0–7 days: 10 mg/kg q12h
	    > 7 days: 10 mg/kg q8h
	Infants/children:
	    30–50 mg/kg per day PO div q6h
	    or 20–40 mg/kg per day IV div q6h
	    Max. IV dose 4 g/day
	Pertussis:
	    50 mg/kg per day PO/IV div q6h
	Endocarditis prophylaxis in penicillin-allergic patients:
	    20 mg/kg PO 2 h prior to procedure and 6 h later
		Erythromycin is a C-P450IIIA (an isozyme of cytochrome P450 in the liver) enzyme inhibitor, and decreases the clearance of many drugs including cyclosporin, carbamazepine and theophylline
		A GI prokinetic agent, it has been used to treat gastroparesis
		Lactobionate IV salt contains benzyl alcohol which is contraindicated in neonates
		Do not exceed 2 g/day PO
		Reduce dose in renal failure

Erythromycin with sulfisoxazole suspension:
[Pediazole]
erythromycin 200 mg and sulfisoxazole 600 mg/5 ml suspension
	PO (based on the erythromycin component):
	    40 mg/kg per day div q6–8h
	    also 1 ml/kg per day in 4 div doses
		Should not be used in children < 2 months of age because of sulfonamide component
		Consider erythromycin component interactions with astemizole, carbamazepine, cisapride, terfenadine, theophylline and cyclosporin

Erythropoietin (EPO) [Eprex]
 	
inj: 4000 unit vial
	Hematopoietic agent
	Renal failure:
	    initial doses 50–100 U/kg IV/SC
	    3 times weekly, then titrate down by 25 U/kg per dose according to hematocrit
	Refusal of blood products prior to surgery:
	    150 U/kg per dose SC 3 times weekly to
	
	    start, with adjustments made according to hematocrit
	Facilitation of autologous blood collection:
	    600 U/kg IV twice weekly for 3 weeks prior to surgery
		Iron must be coadministered with EPO (3 mg/kg per day elemental iron); consult hematology or pharmacy for complete protocol
		Intraperitoneal administration (with dialysis) are less well absorbed than recommended routes, and may require larger doses
		Also indicated in HIV-related anemia, anemia of malignancy, perisurgically to reduce allogeneic blood exposure and hasten erythroid recovery
		High-cost item

Drug name	Indication, dose, route	Remarks
Esmolol [Brevibloc] inj: 100 mg/10 ml vial	Perioperative hypertension: loading dose 500 mcg/kg over 1 min, then 50–200 µg/kg·min IV infusion	Very short-acting beta-blocker (t½ 9 min) Onset 2–10 min; effects dissipate in 20–30 min Adjust dose for renal dysfunction Central line administration recommended
Ethanol (ethyl alcohol)	Ethylene glycol and methyl alcohol poisoning: dose adjusted to maintain ethyl alcohol levels	For infusion, see chart Blood ethanol in mg/dL = 4.6 × [blood alcohol ethanol in mmol/L]
Ethacrynic acid [Edecrin] tab: 50 mg inj: 50 mg/vial	Initial: 1 mg/kg per day PO once daily, to a max. of 3 mg/kg per day 1 mg/kg per dose IV to a max. of 25 mg per dose; may repeat in 8–12 h Routine dosing not recommended	Use only for patients refractory to other diuretics High ceiling loop diuretic Do not exceed max. rate of 10 mg over 1 min; preferably give over 20–30 min. Rapid IV administration has caused permanent deafness
Fentanyl [Sublimaze] inj: 50 µg/ml—2 and 5 ml amp	Narcotic analgesic: 1–5 µg/kg per dose IV prn IV infusion: 1–6 µg/kg·h (titrate to effect)	May cause chest wall rigidity, especially in larger doses if given too rapidly. Give over 3–5 min. Treatment of overdose: naloxone 0.01 mg/kg IV
Fluconazole [Diflucan] tab: 100 mg inj: 2 mg/mL—50 mL vial	Antifungal Neonate 0–7 days: 6 mg/kg per dose PO/IV q48h Neonate > 7 days: 6 mg/kg per dose PO/IV q24h Pediatric: 3–6 mg/kg per day PO/IV once daily Max. dose 200 mg/day	Fluconazole is a cytochrome P450 enzyme inhibitor and has multiple drug interactions Dose must be adjusted in renal failure Infuse IV over 1–2 h
Flumazenil [Anexate] inj: 0.1 mg/ml, 5 and 10 ml amp	Benzodiazepine antagonist: 10–25 µg/kg per dose IV; may repeat × 2 prn, up to an adult max. of 1 mg Maintenance infusion dose (for long-acting benzodiazepine overdose): 10–50 µg/kg·h	Consult poison control center Indicated for overdose; not to be used for reversal of sedation. Short duration of action, repeat doses may be necessary Can precipitate seizures in susceptible patients or in mixed overdoses involving tricyclic antidepressants, or precipitate withdrawal in dependent patients Has limited usefulness, since most efficacious in reversing sedation, not respiratory depression
Frusemide—see furosemide		
Furosemide (frusemide) [Lasix, many brands] tab: 20, 40 mg liq: 1 mg/ml inj: 10 mg/ml, 2 and 25 ml amp; 4 ml PFS	Diuretic: 0.5–1 mg/kg per dose IV prn IV infusion 0.1–1 mg/kg·h 1–2 mg/kg per dose PO prn (up to q6h)	Give IV doses over 3 min, not to exceed a rate of 0.5 mg/kg·min Rapid IV administration is ototoxic, especially in combination with other ototoxic agents Difficult infusion drug because of long t½
Gabapentin [Neurontin] tab: 100, 300, 400 mg	Oral anticonvulsant: initial dose 300–400 mg/day up to 900–1800 mg/day div tid	Taper dose to prevent withdrawal seizures Dose must be adjusted in renal failure
Ganciclovir [Cytovene] inj: 500 mg/vial	CMV retinitis, CMV pneumonia, prevention of CMV transmission in transplant patients (bone marrow, renal, solid organ): 5 mg/kg per dose IV q12h × 14–21 days, then 5 mg/kg per day IV daily	Causes bone marrow suppression; contraindicated if ANC < 500/mm³ and/or platelet count < 25 × 10⁹/L Use/dispose of as potential mutagen Dose must be adjusted in renal failure

Drug name	Indication, dose, route	Remarks

Gentamicin
[Garamycin]
 	
inj: 10 mg/ml, 40 mg/ml—2 ml vials
	Neonate < 7 days:
	  2.5 mg/kg per dose IV q12h (preterm
	   infants require further increase in
	   interval between doses)
	Infant/pediatric:
	  7.5 mg/kg per day once daily or divided q8h
		Dose must be adjusted in renal failure,
		  according to individual serum levels

Glucagon
 	
inj: 1 mg/vial
	Persistent hypoglycemia (despite glucose
	  infusion):
	neonates:
	  0.5–2 mg/day as a continuous IV
	   infusion or 0.3 mg/kg per dose q4h prn
	pediatric:
	  0.03–0.1 mg/kg per dose IM/SC/IV q5–20
	   min up to a max. dose of 1 mg
	Adult:
	  0.5–1 mg per dose q5–10 min
	Severe beta-blocker overdose (adult data):
	  0.05–0.15 mg/kg IV over 1 min, then
	   0.01–0.05 mg/kg·h titrated to response
		Can cause hypokalemia, nausea, vomiting
		Do not delay glucose administration; works
		  in 5–20 min
		1 IU = 1 mg

Glucose—see dextrose		
Glyceryl trinitrate—see nitroglycerin		

Glycopyrrollate
 	
inj: 0.2 mg/ml amp
	Control upper airway secretions/inhibit
	  salivation:
	  4–10 µg/kg per dose q3–4h prn; up to a
	   max. of 0.2 mg per dose or 0.8 mg/24 h
	Intraoperative: 4 µg/kg IV up to a max. of
	  0.1 mg q2–3 min prn
	Preoperative:
	  < 2 y:
	   4.4–8.8 µg/kg per dose IM 30–60 mg preop
	  > 2 y:
	   4.4 µg/kg per dose IM 30–60 min preop
		Contraindications: paralytic ileus/GI
		  obstruction, tachycardia, acute hemorrhage
		Use with caution in patients with spastic
		  paralysis or brain damage, Down syndrome
		Antidote (for anticholinergic reaction);
		  physostigmine 0.02 mg/kg SC/IV

Haloperidol
[Haldol]
 	
tab: 0.5, 1, 2, 5 mg
liq: 2 mg/ml
inj: 5 mg/ml—1 ml
	Agitation:
	  0.1 mg/kg IM/IV q1h prn; up to a max.
	   single dose of 5 mg
		IM/IV routes have increased incidence of
		  hypotension. IM preferred parenteral
		  route.
		Not recommended in children < 3 years
		Pronounced sedative/anticholinergic effects
		Decreases seizure threshold
		May produce extrapyramidal effects

Halothane
1% solution for inhalation—
  250 ml bottle
	Status asthmaticus refractory to standard
	  treatment:
	  0.5–1% solution continuously via
	   anesthetic machine
		Isoflurane may have fewer complications;
		  adverse reactions include myocardial
		  depression and arrhythmias, can worsen
		  ventilation–perfusion mismatch, sensitizes
		  myocardium to catecholamines, can
		  increase ICP, decrease renal blood flow,
		  and cause hepatotoxicity

Heparin
[many brands]

inj: 1000 units/ml—1 ml amps;
  10 ml vials
  10 000 units/ml—1 ml amps;
   5 ml vials

Anticoagulant:
75 units kg IV bolus; then 20–25 units/
kg·h IV infusion, titrated according to
PTT 1.5–2.5 normal

Adjustment recommendations:

APTT	Bolus (units)	Hold (min)	Rate change	Repeat APTT (h)
< 40	50	0	+ 20%	4
40–49	0	0	+ 10%	4
50–75	0	0	0	4
76–85	0	0	– 10%	4
86–95	0	30	– 10%	4
> 95	0	60	– 15%	4

Antidote: protamine sulfate 1 mg per 100
units heparin received within last 4 h

Drug name	Indication, dose, route	Remarks
Hydralazine [Apresoline] tab: 10, 25, 50 mg inj: 20 mg/ml—1 ml amp	Hypertensive crisis: Pediatric: 0.1–0.5 mg/kg per dose IM/IV q6–8h Adult: 10–50 mg per dose IM/IV q3–6h prn	Give IV hydralazine slowly over 3–5 min
Hydrocortisone [Cortef, Solu-cortef] tab: 10, 20 mg inj: (as sodium succinate) 100, 250, 500 mg vial	Antiinflammatory: 0.8–4 mg/kg per day PO/IV div q6h Status asthmaticus: loading dose 4–8 mg/kg per dose IV maintenance dose 2–4 mg/kg per dose IV q6h Acute adrenal insufficiency: loading dose 70 mg/m^2 per dose IV, followed by 70 mg/m^2 per day IV div q4–6h, then wean to maintenance Physiologic replacement: 14–20 mg/m^2 per day div q8h *or* 0.2 mg/kg per dose IV q8h	4 mg hydrocortisone = 1 mg prednisone
Hydroxyzine [Atarax] cap: 10, 25 mg liq: 2 mg/ml inj: 50 mg/ml amp	Antihistamine/anxiolytic: Pediatric: 0.5–1 mg/kg per dose IM q4–6h prn 2 mg/kg per day PO div q6h Adults: 25–100 mg per dose tid/qid	Used alternating q4h with trimeprazine for itching/sedation in burn patients Not recommended for IV/SC use
Imipenem with cilastatin [Primaxin] inj: 500 mg imipenem, 500 mg cilastatin per vial	Antibiotic: < 3 y: 100 mg/kg per day IV div q6h > 3 y: 40–60 mg/kg per day IV div q6h Cystic fibrosis: 100 mg/kg per day IV div q6h Usual max. dose 2g/day; may go up to 4g/day in special cases	Causes nausea, vomiting, seizures in high doses Broad spectrum of gram-positive, gram-negative and anaerobic coverage High incidence of cross-sensitivity with penicillin Dose must be adjusted in renal failure Meropenem preferred
Insulin, human regular [Humulin-R] 100 u/ml	Diabetic ketoacidosis: IV infusion 0.1 U/kg.h When the patient's blood glucose begins to fall add glucose to the IV fluid in a concentration sufficient to keep the blood glucose at 10–15 mmol/L without altering the insulin infusion rate Hyperkalemia: 0.1 U/kg IV with 0.4 g/kg glucose	No insulin IV bolus is necessary for ketoacidosis For continuous infusion, dilute regular insulin in 0.9% NaCl Monitor blood glucose every 30–60 min Monitor electrolytes and acid/base q2–4h for 24 h Prime IV delivery tubing with *insulin* solution before use
Isoflurane [Forane] bottle: 100 ml	Inhalation anesthesia Status asthmaticus: maintenance 1–2.5% by inhalation	Malignant hyperthermia, hypotension, respiratory depression, arrhythmias, shivering, nausea and vomiting, elevation of WBC and liver function tests
Ipratropium [Atrovent] solution for inhalation: 0.25 mg/ml	Inhalation via nebulizer: 0.5–1 ml q4–6h prn	May be added to salbutamol (albuterol) in nebulizer cup Dilute dose up to 4 ml in nebulizer cup with 0.9% NaCl
Isoprenaline—see isoproterenol		
Isoproterenol (isoprenaline) [Isuprel] inj: 1:5000, 0.2 mg/ml	Bradycardia, heart block, CHF: IV infusion 0.025–2 μg/kg·min	Tachyarrhythmias, hypertension/ hypotension, myocardial ischemia May be infused via a central or peripheral line For infusion see Ch. 7.2

Drug name	Indication, dose, route	Remarks

Ketamine
[Ketalar]
 	
inj: 10, 50 mg/ml
	Dissociative anaesthesia:
	  induction 0.5–2 mg/kg per dose IV over > 1 min
	  infusion 5–20 μg/kg·min
	Bronchodilator in mechanically ventilated
	  patients:
	  infusion 20–40 μg/kg·min
	Oral dose for *conscious* sedation
	  10 mg/kg
		Observe airway during administration as
		  laryngospasm or obstructive apnea may
		  occur
		Duration of effect is about 10 min
		Coadministration of a benzodiazepine will
		  minimize emergence reactions
		Atropine will counteract increased salivation
		For infusion see Ch. 7.2
		IV preparation may be used *orally*

Ketorolac
[Toradol]
 	
inj: 10, 15, 30 mg/ml
	Pain management:
	  loading dose: 1 mg/kg per dose IM/IV
	  maintenance: 0.5 mg/kg per dose IM/IV q6h
	Max. dose:
	  < 50 kg 60 mg/day
	  > 50 kg 120 mg/day
		Nonsteroidal antiinflammatory agent; should
		  be used with caution in patients with
		  renal or hepatic disease
		IM/IV routes are considered comparable in
		  bioavailability

Labetalol
[Trandate]
 	
inj: 5 mg/ml
	Hypertension:
	  IV infusion:
	  1 mg/kg·h
	  increase by 0.5 mg/kg·h every 30
	    min until the desired effect on
	    blood pressure occurs
	  Max. infusion rate 3 mg/kg·h
	  PO 1–2 mg/kg per dose bid and
	    titrate to a desired response
		Use beta-blockers with extreme caution in
		  asthma, cardiogenic shock, heart block
		  and bradycardia
		Caution in patients with hepatic dysfunction
		Monitor heart rate, BP, ECG
		Incompatible with sodium bicarbonate
		For infusion see Ch. 7.2
		Pediatric information is limited for oral
		  labetalol

Lactulose
[Cephulac]
 	
syrup: 667 mg/ml
	Hepatic encephalopathy:
	  Infants:
	    2.5–10 ml/day div 3–4 doses
	  Children:
	    40–90 ml/day in 3–4 divided doses
		Titrate dose to produce 2–3 soft stools per
		  day
		Contraindicated in patients with galactosemia
		Caution in patients with diabetes mellitus
		May cause nausea, vomiting, diarrhea,
		  flatulence, abdominal distention

Lamotrigine
[Lamactil]
 	
tab: 25, 50 mg
	Children 2–12 y:
	PO with valproate:
	  first 2 weeks: 0.2 mg/kg per day
	    once daily
	  weeks 3 and 4: 0.5 mg/kg per day
	    once daily
	  maintenance: 1–5 mg/kg per day div bid
	Without valproate:
	  first 2 weeks: 2 mg/kg per 24 h div bid
	  weeks 3 and 4: 5 mg/kg per day div bid
	  maintenance: 5–15 mg/kg per 24 h PO
	    div bid
		Not approved for use in children
		Half-life decreased with enzyme-inducing
		  agents (carbamazepine) and increased with
		  enzyme inhibitors (valproic acid)
		Other side-effects include diplopia, dizziness,
		  drowsiness, headache, and rash

Lidocaine (lignocaine)
[Xylocaine]
 	
inj: 2%, 20 mg/ml
prefilled syringes, 100 mg/5 ml
  (bolus)
 	
premixed bag for infusion 0.4%
  (1 g/250 ml D5W)
	Ventricular arrhythmias:
	IV loading dose:
	  1 mg/kg per dose q5–10 min until a
	    max. total dose of 3 mg/kg is given
	ETT:
	  1 mg/kg per dose followed with a 5 ml
	    saline flush
	IV Infusion:
	  20–50 μg/kg·min
		Serum concentration monitoring highly
		  recommended
		Therapeutic range 7–29 mmol/L (1.5–6 mg/L)
		Excessive serum concentrations may
		  produce myocardial and CNS depression
		  > 29 mmol/L (7 mg/L)
		Reduce dose in patients with CHF, shock,
		  liver dysfunction
		Contraindicated in complete heart block
		  and wide complex tachycardia
		For infusion see Ch. 7.2

Lignocaine—see lidocaine

Drug name	Indication, dose, route	Remarks
Lorazepam [Ativan] inj: 4 mg/ml tab: SL and PO: 0.5, 1, 2 mg	Status epilepticus: IV: 0.05–0.1 mg/kg per dose q10min for clinical effect Anxiety and sedation: IV, IM, PO, SL: 0.05 mg/kg per dose every 4–8 h when necessary	Lorazepam may produce apnea when combined with other CNS depressants. Be prepared to support ventilation, monitor SaO_2 Give 0.05 mg/kg by IV injection slowly over 2–5 min or at a rate not to exceed 2 mg/min Dilute the dose in an equal volume of IV diluent prior to administration Injection contains benzyl alcohol, propylene glycol and polyethylene glycol which may be toxic to the newborn Longer duration of action than diazepam
Magnesium sulfate inj: 50%, 500 mg/ml, 2 mmol Mg (4 mEq)/ml 50 mg/ml elemental Mg	Hypomagnesemia: IV 0.1–0.2 mmol/kg per dose (25–50 mg/kg per dose) every 4–6 h for 3–4 doses Max. rate 150 mg/min Max. concentration 200 mg/ml	Use with caution in patients with heart block, renal impairment and those on digoxin Rapid administration may cause hypotension, arrhythmias, CNS depression and respiratory depression
Mannitol inj: 25% vials, premixed infusion bag 20% (20 g/100 ml)	Acutely increased intracranial pressure: 0.25 g/kg per dose IV over 3–5 min may repeat at 5 min intervals as needed may increase to 1 g/kg per dose Usually 0.25–0.5 g/kg per dose q4h is sufficient for control of intracranial pressure	Rapid infusions of mannitol may cause hypotension, hyperosmolarity and elevated intracranial pressure For mannitol concentrations > 20%, an in-line 5 μm filter should be used Store solutions in warmer to prevent crystalization
Meperidine (pethidine) [Demerol] inj: 50 mg/ml	Analgesia: IM, IV, SC: 1–2 mg/kg per dose every 3–4 h as needed Continuous infusion: 0.1–0.3 mg/kg.h Fentanyl or morphine is preferred for continuous infusion of narcotics	Give by slow infusion over 5 min at a concentration less than 10 mg/ml Metabolite normeperidine (norpethidine) accumulates in renal impairment and may cause seizures Use cautiously in patients with CNS, renal, cardiac, biliary colic or increased ICP
Meropenem [Merrem] inj: 500 mg, 1 g	Infants and children: over 3 mo: IV: 30–60 mg/kg per day div q8h Febrile neutropenia: IV: 60 mg/kg per day div q8h Meningitis: IV: 120 mg/kg per day div q8h Cystic fibrosis: 75–100 mg/kg per day div q8h Max. dose 2 g IV q8h	Indicated for severe infection with multiple resistant organisms Good penetration into CNS makes drug effective for treatment of meningitis Lower incidence of CNS effects (e.g. seizures, nausea and vomiting) than with imipenem Seizures may occur if dose is not adjusted in renal impairment May give at 50 mg/ml over 10 min in critical care areas
Methylene blue inj: 10 mg/ml	Methemoglobinemia: 1–2 mg/kg IV over several min may repeat in 1 h if necessary	Use cautiously in patients with G6PD as hemolysis may occur Do not inject SC or intrathecally
Methylprednisolone [Solu-Medrol] inj: 40, 125, 500, 1000 mg as sodium succinate	Antiinflammatory/immunosuppressive 'pulse therapy': IV: 15–30 mg/kg per dose or 600 mg/m^2 per day for 3 days Max. single dose 3g Status asthmaticus: IV: 1–2 mg/kg once followed by 2–4 mg/kg per day div q6h Spinal cord injury (< 12 h since injury): 30 mg/kg load followed by 5.4 mg/kg·h for 23 h	Anaphylaxis, sudden death, seizures, atrial fibrillation, transient blindness and fatal varicella have been reported to occur after methylprednisolone administration Ideally given within 12 hrs of spinal cord injury; may have benefits within 48 hrs of injury Maximum concentration and rate for IV push is 125 mg/ml over 1–3 min; for IV infusion 2.5 mg/ml Injection contains benzyl alcohol 9 mg/ml as preservative 4 mg methylprednisolone = 5 mg prednisone

Drug name	Indication, dose, route	Remarks

Metoclopramide [Maxeran]
 	
inj: 5 mg/ml
	Prokinetic agent:
	  IV: 0.1 mg/kg per dose q4–6h prn up
	    to 0.5 mg/kg per day
	Emetogenic chemotherapy:
	  IV: 1–3 mg/kg per dose initially repeat
	    q2–3h for 8–12 h post chemotherapy
	Postsurgical nausea and vomiting:
	  IV: 0.15–0.5 mg/kg per dose q6h prn
		Administer by slow IV push at a max.
		  concentration of 5 mg/ml over 1–2 min.
		  Otherwise infuse at a diluted concentration
		  of 0.2 mg/ml over > 15 min
		Large doses (0.5 mg/kg) may cause acute
		  dystonic reactions especially in children.
		  These can be treated with
		  diphenhydramine 0.5–1 mg/kg per dose
		Methemoglobinemia has occurred in
		  neonates given 1–4 mg/kg per day for
		  more than 1 day

Metolazone [Zaroxolyn]
 	
tab: 2.5, 5 mg
	Diuretic:
	  0.1–0.4 mg/kg per day PO in one daily
	    dose or div bid
		Occasionally combined with furosemide
		  (frusemide) for diuretic-resistant edema
		Metabolic side-effects are similar to
		  thiazide diuretics

Metronidazole [Flagyl]
 	
inj: 500 mg/100 ml premixed bags
 	
tab: 250 mg
 	
Susp: (extemporaneous)
  10–50 mg/ml in chocolate
  cherry syrup
	Anaerobic infections:
	IV Neonates:
	  < 7 days:
	    15 mg/kg IV loading dose then 7.5
	      mg/kg per dose q12h
	  > 7 days:
	    15 mg/kg per dose q12h
	IV Children:
	  7.5 mg/kg per dose IV q6h
	  PO: 30 mg/kg per day PO div q6h
	Antibiotic-associated colitis:
	  20 mg/kg per day PO/IV div q6h
		IV and PO doses are equivalent so use the
		  oral route whenever possible
		Drug of choice for antibiotic-associated
		  colitis
		IV form is prediluted. Avoid further dilution
		  with other IV solutions
		IV solution contains Na 28 mEq/g

Midazolam [Versed]
 	
inj: 5 mg/ml
	Conscious sedation during mechanical
	  ventilation:
	  IV loading dose 0.1–0.2 mg/kg then
	    0.5–6 μg/kg·min or titrate to
	    desired effect
	Preprocedural sedation:
	  oral:
	    0.5–0.75 mg/kg per dose
	    10–15 min prior to procedure
	  Max. dose 20 mg
	  IV:
	    0.05–0.1 mg/kg per dose by slow
	      IV injection over 1–3 min
	    may repeat 0.05 mg/kg boluses
	      × 3 at 2 min intervals to max. 8 mg
		Midazolam is a respiratory and cardiac
		  depressant and may cause respiratory
		  or cardiac arrest especially after rapid
		  administration of large IV doses or use
		  with narcotics
		Benzodiazepines may cause paradoxical
		  excitement in children
		Maximum concentration for IV push is
		  5 mg/ml. May also be diluted to 1–5 mg/ml
		  to control the rate of administration or
		  when drug is given by infusion
		For oral doses use injectable formulation
		  and mix in flavored drink
		For infusion see ch. 7.2

Milrinone [Primacor]
 	
inj: 1 mg (milrinone) ml
	Inotrope/vasodilator for low cardiac output
	  states
	IV loading dose: 50 mcg/kg over 10–15
	  minutes and repeat 25 mcg/kg IV twice
	  if necessary
	IV infusion: 0.25–0.75 mcg/kg/minute
		Arrhythmias (JET), tachycardia after loading
		  dose, thrombocytopenia (less than
		  amrinone), hypotension
		Be prepared to adjust dose in patients with
		  renal impairment
		Contraindicated in patients with outflow
		  tract obstruction

Mivacurium [Mivacron]
 	
inj: 2 mg/ml
(multiple dose vials contain
  benzyl alcohol 9 mg/ml)
	Neuromuscular blockade:
	Children (2–12 y):
	  initial 0.2 mg/kg by rapid IV injection
	    (over 5–15 s)
	maintenance dose 0.1 mg/kg q10 min
	  following initial dose
	continuous infusion 5–10 μg/kg·min
		Rapid onset 1.5–2 min. Short duration:
		  $t^{1/2}$ 1.5–2.5 min, 25% recovery 16–23 min
		Mivacurium administration may result in
		  histamine release with complications such
		  as bronchospasm and anaphylaxis
		To calculate initial dose, use ideal body weight
		Caution in patients with CVS disease, asthma,
		  anaphylactoid reactions or myasthenia
		  gravis
		Give injection undiluted or dilute to 0.5
		  mg/ml for infusions

Drug name	Indication, dose, route	Remarks

Morphine
 	
inj: 10 mg/ml and other concentrations
epidural, no preservative: 5 mg/5ml
oral solution: 1, 5 mg/ml
	Infants 1–12 mo:
	  IV intermittent:
	    0.04–0.1 mg/kg per dose q4h
	  IV continuous infusion:
	    0.01–0.05 mg/kg.h
	Children > 1 yr:
	  IV intermittent:
	    0.05–0.1 mg/kg per dose q3–4h
	  IV continuous infusion:
	    0.02–0.06 mg/kg·h
	Higher doses may be necessary for certain conditions
		IV to PO: oral dose is 3 × IV dose
		Respiratory depression is major concern in nonventilated patients
		Antidote for opiate-induced respiratory depression is naloxone 0.01–0.1 mg/kg per dose IV prn
		Dose adjustment may be required for renal and hepatic impairment
		For IV push, administer at a concentration of 0.05–5 mg/ml over 5 min
		For infusion see Ch. 7.2

Muromonab-cd3
[Orthoclone, OKT3]
 	
inj: 5 mg/5 ml
	Immunosuppressant acute rejection:
	  < 30 kg:
	    0.1 mg/kg per dose IV up to 2.5 mg daily for 10–14 days
	  > 30 kg:
	    5 mg per dose IV once daily for 10–14 days
	Premedicate with methylprednisolone 1 mg/kg before first dose
		Premedication with corticosteroids, diphenhydramine and acetaminophen (paracetamol) will minimize reactions
		Monitor chest X-ray to avoid pulmonary edema
		Monitor vital signs until stable
		Contents of ampoule must be filtered through a 0.2–0.22 μm low protein-binding filter
		Give IV dose undiluted (1 mg/ml) over less than 1 min

Mycophenolate mofetil [CellCept] cap: 250 mg susp: 200 mg/ml	Immunosuppressant Children: renal transplant: 600 mg/m^2 per dose PO bid Adults: PO 1 g bid start within 72 h following transplant	Leukopenia occurs commonly in renal transplant patients and can be severe. Complete blood counts are recommended weekly during the first month of therapy Other side-effects include nausea, vomiting, diarrhea, increased incidence of infections. These respond to dose reduction or extension of dose interval

Nalbuphine
[Nubain]
 	
inj: 10, 20 mg/ml
	Premedication, IV, IM, SC:
	Children:
	  0.2 mg/kg per *dose*
	Adults:
	  10–20 mg to a maximum of 20 mg per dose and 160 mg/day
		Narcotic agonist with partial antagonist activity
		Equivalent mg/mg narcotic agonist potency with morphine

Naloxone
[Narcan]
 	
inj: 0.4, 1 mg/ml and others
	Reversal of narcotic-induced respiratory depression:
	Children < 20 kg:
	  0.01–0.1 mg/kg per dose q3–5 min prn
	Children > 20 kg:
	  2 mg per dose IV q3–5 min prn
	  Give by rapid IV push over < 30 s at a concentration of 0.4–1 mg/ml
	Severe opiate poisoning of infancy:
	  0.04–0.16 mg/kg·h by IV infusion
		Giving 0.1 mg/kg per dose will achieve total reversal of narcotic effects. If only partial reversal is needed, smaller doses (0.01 mg/kg) may be used
		Monitor respiratory rate
		Since the duration of effect of some narcotics may outlast naloxone, repeat doses of naloxone should be given as necessary to maintain reversal of narcotic effect

Naproxen
[Naprosyn]
 	
tab: 125, 250 mg
susp: 25 mg/ml
supp: 500 mg
	Analgesic:
	Children > 2 yr:
	  10 mg/kg per day PO/PR div bid
	  max. 15 mg/kg per day
	Adults:
	  250–500 mg per dose up to q8h
	  max. 1500 mg/day
		Give with food or milk to avoid GI side-effects
		Contraindicated in patients with hypersensitivity to ASA (asthma)
		Use cautiously in patients with GI, renal, cardiac disease or those on anticoagulant therapy

Drug name	Indication, dose, route	Remarks

Neostigmine
[Prostigmin]
 	
inj: 0.5 mg/ml
	Reversal of nondepolarizing neuromuscular blockade:
	    0.025–0.1 mg/kg per dose IV with
	    atropine or glycopyrollate
		Give by slow undiluted IV injection over several minutes
		Onset of action: 1–20 min; duration: 1–2 h
		Atropine (0.01 mg/kg) is an antidote for the cholinergic effects of neostigmine

Nifedipine
[Adalat]
 	
cap: 5, 10 mg
tab: prolonged acting 10, 20 mg
extended release
tab: 30, 60 mg
	Hypertensive emergencies:
	    0.25–0.5 mg/kg per dose PO/SL to
	    q1–3h prn
		For administration of oral doses withdraw contents from capsule with a TB syringe and 27 gauge needle. Measure dose accordingly
		A 5 mg capsule contains 0.1 ml of liquid 50 mg/ml

Nimodipine
[Nimotop]
 	
inj: 0.2 mg/ml, 250 ml bottles
cap: 30 mg
	Neurological deficits post subarachnoid hemorrhage:
	Commence nimodipine within 4 days of diagnosis:
	Coinfusion strategy:
	    nimodipine injection 5 ml/h (1 mg/h)
	      for 2 h with 20 ml/h coinfusion solution.
	      Then 10 ml/h (2 mg/h) with 40 ml/h of
	      coinfusion solution for 7–10 days
	      post diagnosis, then
	orally:
	    60 mg (2 capsules) PO q4h for 21 days
	    doses up to 90 mg PO q4h have been
	    used
	The safety and efficacy of larger doses is not well established
		May improve outcome after recovery from subarachnoid hemorrhage
		Use cautiously in patients with increased ICP
		Hypotension, edema, intestinal pseudoobstruction and heart failure (when combined with beta-blockers) may occur
		Nimodipine injection contains propylene glycol and ethanol
		This drug should be coninfused with D5W, Ringer's, dextran or 0.9% saline in a 1:4 ratio by volume
		Nimodipine is light-sensitive and the capsules should be stored in the original package
		The injection does not need to be protected from light while being infused

Nitrazepam
[Mogadon]
 	
tab: 5 mg
susp (extemporaneous): 1 mg/ml
	Anticonvulsant
	Infantile spasms and myoclonic seizures
	    children up to 30 kg:
	    0.3–3 mg/kg per 24 h PO div tid
		Begin therapy at a low dose and titrate to effect
		May cause drowsiness at higher doses, drooling and aspiration pneumonia

Nitroglycerin (glyceryl trinitrate)
[Nitrostat]
 	
inj: 5 mg/ml
ointment: 2%
	IV infusion:
	    0.5–10 μg/kg·min
	Topical:
	    Not well established in children
	    add up total daily dose on infusion and
	      estimate amount of ointment necessary
	      divide dose in 2–4 daily applications
		Use of non-PVC tubing for IV infusion will minimize loss from adsorption
		For topical administration, 1 cm of 2% ointment contains approximately 7.5 mg of nitroglycerin
		For infusion see Ch. 7.2

Nitroprusside
[Nipride]
 	
inj: 50 mg/vial
	IV infusion:
	    start at the lowest dose and
	      titrate up for clinical effect
	    0.5–8 μg/kg·min
	    if used for more than 24 h max.
	      infusion rate should not exceed
	      4 μg/kg·min
		Nitroprusside administration may result in profound hypotension. Blood pressure should be monitored continuously with a indwelling arterial catheter
		Check thiocyanate levels (< 0.8 mmol/L) with high dose (> 3 μg/kg·min), prolonged infusions (> 48 h) and in renal failure
		Protect infusion bottle and buretrol from light
		Watch for metabolic acidosis due to cyanide toxicity
		For infusion see Ch. 7.2

Drug name	Indication, dose, route	Remarks
Norepinephrine (noradrenaline) [Levophed] inj: 1 mg (base)/ml	IV infusion: 0.01–0.1 μg/kg·min and titrate to blood pressure Max. dose: variable; titrate dose to desired increase in peripheral vascular resistance	Administer by central venous plastic indwelling catheter Dilute in D5W and avoid mixing in 0.9% saline as drug will oxidize Incompatible with alkali Do not use if brown or solution contains a precipitate Extravasation will cause tissue necrosis and skin sloughing. In this case phentolamine infiltration is the antidote For infusion see Ch. 7.2
Octreotide [Sandostatin] inj: 50, 100, 500 μg/ml	IV/SC: 1–10 μg/kg per day div bid or tid Oral: 2 mg orally is approximately equivalent to 50 μg by the subcutaneous route	The subcutaneous route is the preferred route of administration although both intermittent bolus and continuous IV infusions are used Monitor serum glucose levels frequently before and during administration Abdominal distention, anorexia, nausea, vomiting, abdominal pain, bloating and steatorrhea may occur Local reactions such as burning at the site of injection may be minimized by warming solution
Omeprazole [Losec] tab:10, 20 mg cap: 20 mg with enteric-coated granules, some countries susp: in sodium bicarbonate (extemporaneous)	Refractory gastroesophageal reflux disease: 0.7–3.3 mg/kg per day once daily *or:* children < 3 yr: 10 mg/day in the morning children > 3 yr: 20 mg/day in the morning *or:* 40 mg per 1.73 m^2 per day Esophagitis: 0.5 mg/kg per day div bid	Omeprazole has not been approved for use in children and therefore published guidelines are scarce Tablets may be crushed and dissolved in water for administration down feeding tubes A suspension can be made with sodium bicarbonate
Ondansetron [Zofran] inj: 2 mg/ml tab: 4, 8 mg Oral solution: 4 mg/5 ml	Treatment and prevention of chemotherapy-induced nausea and vomiting: IV 0.15 mg/kg per dose PO 0.2 mg/kg per dose First IV dose 30 min (PO dose 60 min) before chemotherapy and then q8h afterwards until 24 h after chemotherapy stops Usual maximum dose 4 mg	For highly emetogenic chemotherapy dexamethasone may be added to enhance antiemetic effect Undiluted injection may be given over 30s to 2 min, or dilute to 0.04 mg/ml in 0.9% saline or D5W and infuse over 15 min
Pancuronium [Pavulon] inj: 2 mg/ml	Neuromuscular blockade: IV 0.05–0.1 mg/kg per dose q30–60 min prn	Long-acting neuromuscular blocker with a 2–3 min onset of action Facilities for age-appropriate intubation and ventilation must be immediately available Tachycardia, hypotension, salivation, rash may occur
Paracetamol—see acetaminophen		
Paraldehyde inj: 1 g/ml	Anticonvulsant: PR: 0.3 ml/kg per dose q2–4h prn up to 5 ml/dose Status epilepticus: IV loading dose: 0.15 ml/kg per dose (0.15 g/kg per dose of paraldehyde) diluted to a 5% solution IV infusion: 0.4 ml/kg·h as a 5% solution in NS or D5W is equivalent to 20 mg/kg·h	For PR use dilute 1:1 in mineral or olive oil Will dissolve plastic and rubber in disposable syringes and IV bags and tubing Administer immediately after preparation PR form causes proctitis IV administration can cause pulmonary hemorrhage and pulmonary edema. Overdose causes metabolic acidosis For infusion see Ch. 7.2. Do not exceed 5% concentration To administer IV as a 5% solution add 2.5 ml paraldehyde to 47.5 ml NS or D5W Change IV solutions every 8 h

Drug name	Indication, dose, route	Remarks

Penicillin G (benzyl penicillin) (sodium and potassium salts)
 	
inj: 1, 5, 10 million units/vial
	Neonates:
	  25 000–50 000 U/kg per dose IV q6h
	Infants and children:
	  100 000–250 000 U/kg per day IV
	    div q4–6h
	Serious infections/meningitis: up to 400 000
	  U/kg per day div q 4–6h
	  or a maximum 24 millions U/day
		Sodium salt provides 1.68 mmol Na per 1 000 000 units
		Adjust dose interval in patients with renal impairment
		Hypersensitivity reactions, interstitial nephritis, electrolyte disorders, seizures, thrombophlebitis, hemolytic anemia may occur

Pentamidine [Pentacarinat]
 	
inj: 200 mg, 300 mg/vial
	Prophylaxis of PCP:
	  Inhalation:
	    > 5 yrs: 60 mg by Respirgard nebulizer
	    q2week or 300 mg q4week
	  IV: 4 mg/kg q2–4 week
	Treatment of PCP:
	  4 mg/kg per day IV for 14–21 days
	Leishmaniasis (visceral):
	  4 mg/kg IV/IM 3 times a week for
	  5–25 weeks (WHO)
	Leishmaniasis (cutaneous):
	  2–4 mg/kg per dose IV/IM once or
	  twice a week until lesions are healed
	Administer IV dose over 60 minutes at a
	  concentration of 1–6 mg/ml
		Prior to initiating prophylaxis, attempts must be made to exclude the presence of active PCP as the prophylactic dose is not sufficient to treat active disease
		Cough and bronchospasm occur with inhalation therapy
		Fatalities due to hypotension, hypoglycemia, acute pancreatitis, and cardiac arrhythmias have been reported with IV administration
		Profound, severe hypotension may occur after one dose
		Other side-effects: abnormal liver function tests, leukopenia, neutropenia, thrombocytopenia
		For inhalation place 300 mg of drug plus 6 ml of sterile water for injection into nebulizer. Nebulize solution until the cup is empty

Phenobarbital (phenobarbitone) [Luminal]
 	
inj: 30, 120 mg/ml
elixir: 5 mg/ml
	Status epilepticus:
	IV loading dose:
	  15–20 mg/kg per dose at max. rate of
	  1 mg/kg·min or 30 mg/min
	  May repeat 5 mg/kg portions to a total
	  loading dose of 30 mg/kg (infants and
	  children) and 40 mg/kg (neonates)
	Maintenance dose:
	  IV/IM/PO: 5 mg/kg once daily or div bid
		Use caution in nonventilated patients as phenobarbital infusions may cause respiratory depression and/or hypotension
		Phenobarbital may increase the clearance of other drugs and reduce their serum concentrations
		Phenytoin and valproate will increase phenobarbital levels
		Long half-life (40–200+ h) in neonates, and will accumulate
		Therapeutic range is 65–170 μmol/L

Phenoxybenzamine [Dibenzyline]
 	
inj: 100 mg/2 ml
	Afterload reduction/alpha-blocker:
	  Loading dose: 1–2 mg/kg IV
	  Maintenance dose: 1–2 mg/kg per day
	    div q6h
		Cardiopulmonary bypass provides a good opportunity for loading doses
		Irreversible inhibitor of α-receptors
		Onset of action 1 h, half-life 24 h, duration 3–4 days
		Have colloid or crystalloid available to counteract hypotension
		Irritating; dilute and infuse slowly (> 1 h) via central line

Phentolamine [Rogitine]
 	
inj: 5 mg/vial
	Phentolamine infiltration protocol
	Dermal necrosis after extravasation of
	  α-adrenergic drugs:
	  Infiltrate area with small amount of
	    solution of phentolamine or give
	    0.1–0.2 mg/kg SC up to 5 mg total
	    into area of extravasation within
	    12 h of exposure
	After load reduction/alpha blocker:
	  loading dose 0.1 mg/kg IV
	Maintenance IV infusion 5–50 μg/kg·min
		Competitive inhibition of α-receptors, brief effect
		Direct IV use of this drug may cause severe hypotension
		Use norepinephrine (noradrenaline) to reverse hypotension
		Reconstitute powder with 5 ml 0.9% saline for injection

Drug name	Indication, dose, route	Remarks
Phenylephrine [Neo-Synephrine] inj: 10 mg/ml	Tetralogy (hypercyanotic spells) IV: 5–20 µg/kg per dose q10–15 min as needed max. 0.5 mg IV infusion: 0.1–0.5 µg/kg·min and titrate as needed max. 4 µg/kg·min Adults: 0.1–0.5 mg/dose q10–15 min infusion: 1–4 mg/kg·min and titrate as needed	Immediate onset, 20–30 min duration For direct injection, dilute to final concentration of 1 mg/ml and give over 30 s Extravasation will cause tissue necrosis—see phentolamine infiltration protocol Tremors, hypertension, angina, arrhythmias, bradycardia may occur Injection contains sulfites which may cause allergic reactions; do not use if solution contains a precipitate or turns brown
Phenytoin [Dilantin] inj: 100 mg/2 ml chew tab: 50 mg cap: 30, 100 mg susp: 125 mg/5 ml	Status epilepticus: IV loading dose: neonates: 20 mg/kg at 0.5 mg/kg.min infants and children: 18 mg/kg infused at 1 mg/kg·min IV/PO maintenance dose: neonates: 2–3 mg/kg per dose q12h infants and children: < 9 yr: 8–15 mg/kg per day div q8h > 9 yr: 4–8 mg/kg per day div q8–12h	Rapid administration causes hypotension, cardiovascular collapse and CNS depression Dilute initial dose to 5 mg/ml in 0.9% saline (phenytoin will precipitate in glucose infusions) and infuse no faster than 1 mg/kg·min or 50 mg/min, or give by direct injection at 50 mg/ml followed by saline flush to avoid vein irritation Dose adjustment may be required for renal or hepatic dysfunction—levels 40–80 µmol/L (10–20 mg/L)
Phytonadione (phytomenadione) [vitamin K] inj: 1 mg/0.5 ml, 10 mg/ml	Hemorrhagic disease of the newborn: Prophylaxis Neonates < 1500 g: 0.5 mg IM/SC Neonates > 1500 g: 1 mg IM/SC within 1 h of birth Treatment: IM, SC 1–2 mg daily Anticoagulant overdose: 0.5–5 mg IV, SC depending upon the need for further anticoagulation and the presence of bleeding Vitamin K deficiency: Infants/children 2–5 mg per 24h PO: 1–2 mg per dose IV, IM, SC	IV administration may cause anaphylactoid-like reactions and therefore the use of this route should be limited to acute care conditions IM or SC routes are preferable for routine use For IV administration, rate should not exceed 1 mg/min For intermittent infusion, dilute to 0.2 mg/ml and infuse over a period of 15–30 min For reversal of bleeding consider the use of FFP (20 ml/kg IV) if significant bleeding is present; 1–2 h may be needed to see improvement in hemostasis The daily requirement for vitamin K deficiency is not well established
Piperacillin [Pipracil] inj: 2, 3, 4 g	Severe infection: 300 mg/kg per day IV div q4–6h Cystic fibrosis: 600 mg/kg per day IV div q4–6h Adult dose: 3–4 g IV q4–6h	Caution in patients with history of sensitivity to penicillin Can cause thrombophlebitis Maximum concentration for IV push 200 mg/ml; infuse over 3–5 min IV infusion: 10–20 mg/ml over 30–60 min Contains 1.85 mmol Na per g
Potassium chloride inj: 2 mmol/ml	Hypokalemia (arteriolar K⁺ mmol/L) < 2.8: 0.5 mmol/kg IV over 1 h Infuse centrally via a syringe pump at a max. concentration of 50 mmol/100 ml (0.5 mmol/ml) **Infusions of high-dose potassium chloride may cause fatal arrhythmias; ECG monitoring is required.**	Maximum rate of delivery is 0.5 mmol/kg·h Maximum concentration via central line is 50 mmol/100 ml Maximum concentration via peripheral line is 6 mmol/100 ml—concentrations > 6 mmol/100 ml will cause phlebitis and must be infused via a central line ECG signs of hyperkalemia include peaked T waves and widening of QRS complex

Drug name	Indication, dose, route	Remarks

Potassium phosphate
 	
inj: 3 mmol P and 4.4 mmol K per ml
Also available as sodium phosphate
	Hypophosphatemia:
	  0.15–0.33 mmol/kg per dose IV
	    infused over 6 h
	Repeat as required to keep P levels over
	  1.3 mmol/L
	Maintenance:
	  0.5–1.5 mmol/kg per day IV by slow
	    continuous infusion
	    dilute in maintenance fluids
		Intravenous infusions should be reserved for
		  severe phosphate depletion syndromes
		Phosphate will precipitate in the presence of
		  calcium. Check with a pharmacist to avoid
		Max. concentration PO_4 is 0.04 mmol/ml
		  peripherally and 0.06 mmol/ml centrally
		Max. infusion rate is 0.05 mmol/kg·h
		Hyperphosphatemia, hyperkalemia,
		  hypocalcemia hypotension, renal failure
		  may occur

Prednisone
[Deltasone]
 	
tab: 5 mg, 50 mg
Extemporaneously compounded
  susp: 5 mg/ml
	Acute asthma:
	  1–2 mg/kg PO once daily or div bid
	    for 3–5 days
	Antiinflammatory, immunosuppressant:
	  0.1–2 mg/kg once daily or div bid–qid
	  Adults: 5–60 mg once daily or in divided doses
	Children/adult replacement:
	  4–5 mg/m² per day
		Prednisone is converted to prednisolone
		  (active drug) in the liver
		Prednisolone is preferred in patients with
		  liver disease
		20 mg hydrocortisone = 5 mg prednisone
		For severe refractory asthma, alternate-day
		  morning therapy is preferred
		Give after meals with food or milk

Prednisolone
[Pediapred]
 	
sol: 5 mg/5 ml prednisolone equivalent
  (as acetate)
	Acute asthma:
	  1–2 mg/kg PO per day in 1–2
	    divided doses for 3–5 days
	Antiinflammatory:
	  0.1–2 mg/kg per day PO in 1–4 divided doses
		Prednisolone is supplied as a solution of
		  prednisolone acetate equivalent to 1 mg/ml
		  prednisolone
		20 mg hydrocortisone = 4 mg prednisolone

Procainamide
[Pronestyl]
 	
inj: 100 mg/ml
cap: 250, 375 mg
	Class Ia antiarrhythmic agent indicated
	  for supraventricular and ventricular
	  arrhythmias:
	Infants:
	  IV loading dose 1 mg/kg q5min up to
	    15 mg/kg or 100 mg in 30 min
	  IV maintenance infusion 20–80 μg/kg·min
	Children:
	  IV loading dose 3–6 mg/kg (max. 100 mg)
	    over 5 min.
	  may repeat q5min up to a total of 15 mg/kg
	  IV maintenance infusion 20–80 μg/kg·min
	Oral: 15–50 mg/kg per 24 h div q3–6h
		IV administration can cause hypotension,
		  AV block, arrhythmias and cardiac arrest
		Monitor ECG, procainamide levels, and for
		  long-term therapy, CBC, differential and
		  platelets
		Monitor serum concentrations to determine
		  a 'target' effective concentration,
		  procainamide 17–43 μmol/L
		Metabolized (acetylated) to
		  N-acetylprocainamide (NAPA)
		$t\frac{1}{2}$ (PCA) 1.7 h (children), 2.5–7 h (adults)
		Some products contain benzyl alcohol which
		  has been associated with the 'fatal
		  gasping syndrome in neonates'
		Adjust dose in renal impairment

Prochlorperazine
[Stemetil]
 	
tab: 5, 10 mg
liq: 1 mg/ml
inj: 5 mg/ml
supp: 10 mg
	Children over 10 kg or > 2 y:
	PO/PR:
	  0.4 mg/kg per 24 h div tid–qid
	  or 2.5 mg per dose q12h (9–14 kg),
	    q8–12h (14–18 kg), q8h (18–39 kg)
	IM:
	  0.1–0.15 mg/kg per dose
	    to a max. of 10 mg per dose
	Adults:
	  PO/IM: 5–10 mg per dose
	IV:
	  2.5–10 mg per dose
	  max: 40 mg per day all routes
	PR: 25 mg per dose bid
		Safety and efficacy have not been established
		  in children < 2 y or < 9 kg
		A high incidence of extrapyramidal side-
		  effects can occur in children
		Sedation, EPE, constipation, hypotension,
		  tachycardia, arrhythmias may occur
		Not recommended by IV route in children;
		  switch to oral as soon as possible
		Not recommended by SC route due to local
		  irritation

Drug name	Indication, dose, route	Remarks
Propafenone [Rythmol] inj: 70 mg/20 ml tab: 150, 300 mg	Class Ic antiarrhythmic agent with sodium, weak beta and calcium channel blocking activity Paroxysmal SVT (60–100% effective), junctional ectopic tachycardia, atrial ectopic tachycardia and chaotic atrial rhythm: PO: oral dose 200 mg/m^2 per day increasing in increments of 100 mg/m^2 per day to 600 mg/m^2 per day or 8–15 mg/kg·day div tid	Well tolerated in young children Proarrhythmic events (2%) may be less common than with other class Ic agents Drug reactions include AV block, bradycardia, CHF Caution: MI, CHF, hepatic/renal dysfunction, asthma may occur
Propofol [Diprivan] inj: 10 mg/ml in soybean oil emulsion	Induction of anesthesia: Children > 1 y: 2–3.5 mg/kg IV over 20–30 s followed by 100–200 µg/kg·min up to 500 µg/kg·min by IV infusion Maintenance of anesthesia: 200–300 µg/kg·min for first 15 min following induction thereafter reduce the dose to 50–100 µg/kg·min Conscious sedation in a ventilated patient: loading dose 1–2 mg/kg IV or 100–150 µg/kg.min for 3–5 min and titrate to the desired level of sedation, then adjust the rate to the desired response (75–100 µg/kg·min)	Safety and efficacy have not been established in pediatric patients less than 3 y old Dosing recommendations only apply to healthy children over 3 yr Max. dose not established but six cases of fatal metabolic acidosis have been reported after prolonged use Dilution of propofol in D5W (to not less than 2 mg/ml) was reported to decrease the incidence of injection site pain in adults Cardiorespiratory depression may occur with bolus doses or rapid increases in the infusion rate: wait 3–5 min between dose adjustments Pain at injection site may be minimized by using a large vein, injecting lidocaine (lignocaine) prior to propofol, or mixing propofol with lidocaine (1 mg lidocaine/ 1 ml propofol emulsion) or storing refrigerated
Propranolol [Inderal] inj: 1 mg/ml tab: 10, 20, 40, 80 mg long-acting 60, 80, 120, 160 mg and others	Arrhythmias: IV: 0.01–0.25 mg/kg per dose q2 min up to 1 mg for infants and 2–3 mg for children; thereafter q4h PO: 2–6 mg/kg per day div q6–8h Hypertension: IV: 0.01–0.15 mg/kg per dose q6h up to 2 mg/kg per day PO: 0.5–1 mg/kg per day div q6–8h; usual dose is 5 mg/kg per day div q6–12h Tetralogy (hyper cyanotic spells) IV: 0.15–0.25 mg/kg per dose by slow IV push; repeat in 15 min Max. dose 1 mg PO: 1–2 mg/kg per dose q6h prn	Intravenous propranolol is used for life-threatening arrhythmias ECG and hemodynamic monitoring are required The rate of administration should not exceed 1 mg/min Propranol is contraindicated in asthma, sinus bradycardia, second-degree heart block, cardiogenic shock and right ventricular failure secondary to pulmonary hypertension Use with caution in patients with Wolff–Parkinson–White syndrome
Prostacyclin (Prostaglandin I$_2$, epoprostenol) [Flolan]	Persistent pulmonary hypertension: IV infusion: 1–5 ng/kg·min	Hypotension Central venous line only Infuse in special diluent only Keep infusion solution at 2–8°C See Ch. 7.2
Prostaglandin E$_1$ (alprostadil) [Prostin VR] inj: 0.5 mg/ml (requires refrigeration)	Maintenance of patent ductus arteriosus: 0.01–0.1 µg/kg·min Pulmonary vasodilation 0.1 µg/kg·min and titrate	Usual starting dose 0.05 µg/kg·min Lower infusion rates (0.025–0.05 µg/kg·min) are often adequate to maintain ductal patency With left-sided obstructive lesions doses up to 0.2 µg/kg·min may be required Reactions include apnea (be prepared to support ventilation), also fever, flushing, hypotension and rarely myoclonic jerks Facilities should be available to support ventilation in the event that apnea occurs For infusion see Ch. 7.2

Drug name	Indication, dose, route	Remarks

Protamine
 	
inj: 50 mg/5 ml
  (requires refrigeration)
	Base dose on amount of heparin used, route of administration and time since last dose or end of infusion
	1 mg protamine per 100 units of heparin over previous 3–4h
	Subsequent doses 1mg/kg per dose up to 25–50 mg protamine
	To neutralize enoxaparin:
	  1 mg protamine per 1 mg enoxaparin
	Max. dose 50 mg/10 min
		Avoid rapid IV administration of protamine because it can cause severe hypotension, bradycardia, flushing and anaphylactic reactions
		May be given by slow direct injection over 1–3 min at a rate no faster than 5 mg/min or dilute in D5W or 0.9% saline
		Doses in excess of 100 mg (adults) may cause paradoxical anticoagulation
		Protamine does not completely reverse the anti-Xa activity of low molecular weight heparin

Pyridoxine
 	
inj: 100 mg/ml
	Deficiency: therapy
	  PO: 5–10 mg per 24 h for 3 weeks
	Seizures in pyridoxine-dependent infants:
	  IM/IV: 100–200 mg (not/kg) IV/IM daily
	Once a clinical response has been established oral therapy should be started:
	  PO 2–100 mg per day
		Can be given IV, IM or SC if oral route is not possible
		Occasionally convulsions have occurred after very large IV doses
		Burning or stinging of the injection site occurs with SC doses
		Respiratory distress has followed administration in neonates

Ranitidine
[Zantac]
 	
inj: 25 mg/ml
tab: 150 mg
liq: 15 mg/ml
	Prophylaxis of stress ulcers:
	intermittent IV injection:
	  3–6 mg/kg per day div q6–8h
	or
	continuous IV infusion:
	  0.03–0.25 mg/kg·h or added to TPN solution
	Max. dose 400 mg per day (adult)
		Rapid infusions (50 mg < 5 min) have caused transient hypotension in adults
		Bradycardia occurred in a neonate 2 h after an infusion of ranitidine
		Dilute to 2.5 mg/ml and give dose over a period of 5 min or a max. rate of 10 mg/min
		Adjust dose in patients with severe renal dysfunction
		Titrate dose to keep intragastric pH > 4

Rifampicin
[Rifadin]
 	
inj: 600 mg powder for reconstitution
cap: 300 mg
susp (extemporaneous): 10 mg/ml
	Hib meningitis prophylaxis:
	  20 mg/kg per day PO daily for 4 days
	Meningococcal meningitis prophylaxis:
	  10 mg per dose PO bid for 4 doses
	IV: 10–20 mg/kg per day
	  divided 8–12 h
		For intravenous infusion, dilute calculated dose in 100–500 mg of D5W or 0.9% saline and infuse over 4 h
		Extravasation can cause local tissue irritation
		Rifampicin will discolor body secretions (sweat, tears and urine)

Rocuronium
[Zemuron]
 	
inj: 10 mg/ml
  refrigerate at 2–8°C until ready to use
	Neuromuscular blockade for intubation:
	  IV: 0.6 mg/kg per dose initially
	For rapid sequence induction:
	  1–2 mg/kg IV
	Maintenance of neuromuscular blockade:
	  0.3 mg/kg·h intermittently
	  0.6 mg/kg·h continuous IVI
		An alternative to succinylcholine (suxamethonium) for rapid sequence intubation
		Rapid onset is 40–60 s and duration of block is 30–45 min
		Age-appropriate facilities to support ventilation must be available

Salbutamol (albuterol)
[Ventolin]
 	
Nebulizer sol: 5 mg/ml and 1.25, 2.5, 5 mg nebules
inj: 0.5 mg/ml
oral sol: 0.4 mg/ml
Metered dose inhaler 100 μg/puff metered doses
	Inhalation for acute asthma:
	> 6 mo:
	  dilute 5 mg (1 ml) in 3 ml 0.9% saline and nebulize over 20 min
	< 6 mo:
	  2.5 mg (0.5 ml) in 3.5 ml 0.9% saline dose is repeated until desired clinical effect is attained or intolerable tachycardia results
	IV infusion: 1–10 μg/kg·min
	MDI: 1–2 puffs qid
	oral: 0.3–0.6 mg/kg per day div tid-qid
		For status asthmaticus continuous nebulization may be required salbutamol may be required
		High-dose salbutamol infusions or inhalations can cause tachycardia, tremor, nervousness, GI symptoms, headaches and hypokalemia
		The use of a spacer device is an alternative to nebulizer in some patients
		For infusion see Ch. 7.2

Drug name	Indication, dose, route	Remarks

Sodium bicarbonate
 	
inj: 8.4%, 1 mmol/ml
50 ml prefilled syringe
 	
inj: 4.2%, 0.5 mmol/ml
10 ml prefilled syringes
	Cardiopulmonary resuscitation:
	    IV, IO: 1–2 mmol/kg per dose
	    repeat q10–15 min according to arterial
	      blood gas analysis
		Routine use in cardiac arrest is not
		   recommended
		NaHCO3 can cause fluid and sodium overload
		   and metabolic alkalosis
		Use 8.4% (1 mmol/ml) concentration for
		   children and 4.2% (0.5 mmol/ml) for
		   neonates and infants and infuse slowly

Sodium nitrite
(also cyanide antidote kit)
 	
inj: 3%, 300 mg/10 ml
Check with poison control center
   for availability and guidance
	Cyanide and nitroprusside poisoning:
	Children < 25 kg:
	    4 mg/kg IV over 5–20 min followed by
	      sodium thiosulfate (below)
	All cyanide-poisoned patients must receive
	    100% oxygen in addition to antidotes
		May repeat half dose after first dose if
		   necessary for severe poisoning
		To minimize hypotensive effect dilute dose
		   in 50–100 ml 0.9% saline and/or reduce
		   the rate of infusion
		Titrate to clinical response but do not
		   exceed 25% methemoglobin concentration

Sodium polystyrene sulfonate
[Kayexalate]
 	
susp: 0.25 g/ml with 25% sorbitol
Suspensions for rectal use can be
   made using water, D10W, or
   equal parts of water and 2%
   methylcellulose
	Children:
	    PO 1 g/kg per dose q6h
	    PR: 1 g/kg per dose q2–6h prn
	Adolescents:
	    PO: 15g 1–4 times a day
	    PR: 30–50 g q6h
		Rectal route has a faster onset but oral
		   route results in a greater reduction in
		   serum potassium
		1 g resin binds 1 mmol potassium
		Sorbitol suspensions may be used for oral
		   but are not recommended for rectal use
		   as they may cause necrosis of bowel wall

Sodium thiosulfate
 	
inj: 10% (100 mg/ml),
   25% (250 mg/ml)
	Cyanide and nitroprusside
	   poisoning:
	Children < 25 kg:
	    410 mg/kg (1.65 ml/kg of a 25%
	      solution) following sodium nitrate—
	      do not exceed 12.5 g (50 ml)
	Children > 25 kg and adults:
	    12.5 g IV (50 ml) after sodium nitrate
	All cyanide-poisoned patients must receive
	    100% oxygen in addition to antidotes
		May repeat half dose if necessary for severe
		   poisonings
		Give by slow IV injection over not less than
		   10 min as may cause hypotension if given
		   rapidly
		Other reactions include hypotension, nausea
		   and vomiting, hyponatremia and osmotic
		   diuresis with large doses
		Consult poison center for guidance

Sotalol
[Sotacor]
 	
tab: 160 mg
susp: (extemporaneous):
   1–5 mg/ml
	Arrhythmias:
	    2–8 mg/kg per day PO (average
	      4 mg/kg per day)
	    or 135 mg/m² per day PO div q12h
	    Treatment should be initiated in the
	      hospital under continuous ECG
	      monitoring
		A beta-blocker with class IV (prolongs the
		   refractory period) antiarrhythmic activity
		Contraindicated in patients with asthma,
		   sinus node dysfunction, sinus bradycardia,
		   second- and third-degree heart block,
		   long QT syndrome, CHF, cardiogenic
		   shock and hypokalemia
		Caution when combined with other drugs
		   which affect cardiac conduction

Spironolactone
[Aldactone]
 	
tab: 25, 100 mg
susp (extemporaneous): 1, 2 mg/ml
	Potassium-sparing diuretic:
	    0.5–3 mg/kg PO once daily or
	      div bid
		Caution: concomitant use of spironolactone
		   with potassium supplements and ACE
		   inhibitors will cause hyperkalemia
		Gastrointestinal irritation, rash, gynecomastia,
		   hyperchloremic metabolic acidosis may
		   occur

Streptokinase
[Streptase]
 	
inj: 250 000, 750 000,
   1 500 000 unit vials
	Systemic thrombolysis:
	Loading dose:
	    4000 units/kg IV over 30 min to max
	      250 000 units
	Maintenance dose:
	    2000 units/kg·h IV
	Max. duration is 24 h
		Bleeding, hypotension, arrhythmias, flushing,
		   fever, urticaria, bronchospasm may occur
		Do not use if recent streptococcal infection
		   or previous use of streptokinase
		Contraindicated in active bleeding disorder,
		   previous major surgery (10 days),
		   neurosurgery within 3 weeks

Drug name	Indication, dose, route	Remarks
Succinylcholine (suxamethonium) [Quelicin] inj: 20 mg/ml (requires refrigeration)	Depolarizing neuromuscular blocker Neuromuscular blockade for emergency intubation: 1–2 mg/kg per dose IV follow IV bolus with a flush of 0.9% saline or D5W Conditions for intubation occur 30–60 s and last 4–6 min after IV administration Maintenance: 0.3–0.6 mg/kg per dose q5–10 min as needed Nondepolarizing agents are preferred for continuous neuromuscular blockade	Facilities for age-appropriate intubation and ventilation must be immediately available Atropine 0.02 mg/kg should be combined with succinylcholine to prevent bradycardia or asystole especially with repeated doses Contraindicated in history of malignant hyperthermia, severe burns, spinal cord injury, neuromuscular disease, crush injury or myopathy
Sucralfate (aluminum sucrose sulfate) [Sucrate] tab: 1000 mg susp: 200 mg/ml	Stress ulcer prophylaxis or peptic ulcer disease: Children < 6 y: 0.5 g PO qid Children > 6 y: 1 g PO qid or 40–80 mg/kg per 24 h div qid Adults: 1 g PO qid	Sucralfate contains aluminum ion which can accumulate in patients with renal impairment Give 1 h before, or 2 hours after meals and at bedtime Constipation, gastric bezoars have been reported in the young
Sufentanil [Sufenta] inj: 50 µg/ml (store at room temperature)	Synthetic narcotic anesthetic agent Intubation/ventilation (combined with NO_2/O_2): 1–2 µg/kg per dose Surgical procedures (combined with NO_2/O_2): 2–8 µg/kg per dose General anesthesia: 8–30 µg/kg per dose	More potent (5–10 times), more rapid onset (1–3 min) and shorter duration (36 min) than fentanyl with minimal cardiovascular effects Will produce sleep and general anesthesia at doses above 8 µg/kg
Tacrolimus (FK506) [Prograf] inj: 5 mg/ml cap: 1 mg	Immuno suppressant Initial dose: IV: 0.03–0.05 mg/kg per day up to 0.15 mg/kg per day as a slow continuous infusion diluted in D5W or 0.9% saline to a concentration of 0.004–0.02 mg/ml PO: 0.15 mg/kg PO q12h on an empty stomach	Pediatric patients without preexisting renal or hepatic dysfunction have required higher doses than adults Substitute oral therapy as soon as possible after IV therapy Oral dose is 3–4 times IV dose Start oral 8–12 h after discontinuing IV Discontinue cyclosporin before starting tacrolimus
Thiopental (thiopentone) [Pentothal] inj: 2.5%, 25 mg/ml	Barbiturate anesthesia: Neonates: 3–4 mg/kg per dose Infants and children: 4–5 mg/kg per dose by steady IV push Intracranial hypertension: variable: 1.5–5 mg/kg, repeat as necessary or 1–5 mg/kg·h by IV infusion	Administer infusion by central line only to avoid extravasation Solution pH is 10–11 Causes hypotension, particularly with hypovolemia and myocardial depression For infusion see Ch. 7.2
Ticarcillin [Ticar] inj: 1, 3, 6 g vials	Extended-spectrum penicillin 200–300 mg/kg per day div q4–6h Cystic fibrosis: 600 mg/kg per day div q6h to max. 24 g per day	Minimum dilution is 100 mg/ml Inject slowly over 5–10 min (thrombophlebitis) Contains 5.2 mmol Na per g
Tissue plasminogen activator (alteplase) [Activase] inj: 50 mg, 100 mg lyophilized powder (reconstitute vial with sterile water for injection, roll to dissolve—do not shake)	Systemic thrombolysis: IV infusion: 0.1–0.6 mg/kg·h for 6 h Low-dose infusion for local venous or catheter-related thrombosis: 0.01–0.05 mg/kg·h For blocked central lines: instill a sufficient volume of alteplase 1 mg/ml to fill lumen of catheter and leave in place for 2 h, aspirate	Before starting therapy measure the major baseline indices for hemostasis: CBC, Hct, Hb, PLT, APTT and INR During therapy monitor for bleeding, fibrinogen, INR, and APTT, and D-Dimer For major bleeds, stop the infusion and give cryoprecipitate (1 bag/5 kg) and other blood products. If the bleeding is life-threatening use tranexamic acid For information on infusion, see Ch. 7.2

Drug name	Indication, dose, route	Remarks
Tobramycin [Nebicin] inj: 40 mg/ml	IV: 7.5 mg/kg per day once daily or div q8h	Once-daily therapy may not be suitable for some patients, e.g. with burns, renal failure or endocarditis
Tranexamic acid [Cyklokapron] inj: 500 mg/ml tab: 500 mg	IV: Antifibrinolytic agent: 10–20 mg/kg per dose bid or tid infused over 15 min PO: 25 mg/kg per dose tid-qid	Reduce dose in patients with renal dysfunction
Urokinase [Abbokinase] inj: 5000 units, 250 000 units/vial	Systemic thrombolytic therapy: IV loading dose: 4000 units/kg IV over 10 min Infusion: 4000 units/kg·h Low-dose local infusion: 200 units/kg·h To clear blocked central lines: 1–1.5 ml of 5000 units/ml solution injected into the line, left for 1–4 h and then aspirated; do not flush See also Alteplase (TPA) to clear central lines	Urokinase is preferred to streptokinase for patients less than 3 mo and those previously given streptokinase Obtain baseline indices of hemostasis before use During therapy monitor bleeding, TCT, fibrinogen, INR, PTT and d-Dimer For major bleeds, stop the infusion and give cryoprecipitate (1 bag/5 kg) and other blood products. If the bleeding is life-threatening use tranexamic acid For infusion, see Ch. 7.2
Valproic acid [Depakene] cap: 250, 500 mg syrup: 50 mg/ml **Divalproex** [Epival] enteric coated tab: 125, 250, 500 mg	Initial: 10 mg/kg per day div tid Increase by 5–10 mg/kg per day to a maintenance 20 mg/kg per day div tid Higher doses may be required for patients on polytherapy	Monitor levels of other anticonvulsants to avoid effects of enzyme inhibition Therapeutic range is 350–750 micro mol/L Avoid children < 2 years and on multiple antiepileptic drugs
Vancomycin [Vancocin] inj: 500 mg/vial	IV: 45–60 mg/kg per day div q8h PO: antibiotic associated colitis 50mg/kg per day div q6h	Monitor serum levels to maintain peak 25–40 mg/L and trough 5–10 mg/L Reduce dose in patients with renal failure Infuse slowly over 1 h to avoid 'red man' syndrome
Vasopressin [Pitressin] inj: 20 units/ml inj: aqueous: 20 units/ml, 5 ml	Diabetes insipidus: Aqueous: 2.5–10 units SC bid to qid IV infusion: 0.00003–0.0003 units/kg·min begin at 0.0003 units/kg·min and titrate *downwards* as control of urine output is achieved GI hemorrhage: 0.002–0.01 units/kg·min and titrate dose as needed	Water intoxication, electrolyte disturbances, cardiac arrhythmias hypertension, chest pain, angina, fever, wheezing may occur For infusion see Ch. 7.2 Side-effects occur more commonly with doses over 0.01 units/kg·min
Vecuronium [Norcuron] inj: 10 mg/vial (requires reconstitution with 10 ml SWI, 0.9% saline, or D5W to make 1 mg/ml	Neuromuscular blockade: 0.1 mg/kg per dose Additional maintenance doses of 0.05–0.1 mg/kg per dose may be given at 25–40 min intervals Continuous infusion: 1 μg/kg·min For infusion see Ch. 7.2	Facilities for age-appropriate intubation and ventilation must be immediately available Conditions for endotracheal intubation generally occur within 1–2 min after administration Less cardiostimulatory effect than pancuronium Give undiluted solution (1 mg/ml) by direct rapid injection
Verapamil [Isoptin IV] inj: 2.5 mg/ml tabs: 50 mg susp: extemporaneous	Children < 1 yr: 0.1–0.2 mg/kg per dose IV q30min prn Children > 1 yr: 0.1–0.3 mg/kg per dose IV to max. 5 mg q30 min prn if stable tid, bid PO: 1.5–3.5 mg/kg per dose tid	Verapamil is a negative inotrope and can cause hypotension, apnea, bradycardia Extreme caution to be taken in infants and those patients with Wolff–Parkinson–White syndrome Antidote is calcium chloride injection, isoprenaline (isoprenaline) and volume Reduce digoxin dose by one third to a half

Drug name	Indication, dose, route	Remarks

Vigabatrin
[Sabril]
 	
tabs: 500 mg
	Initial dose is 40 mg/kg per day
	Increase by 250 mg every 7 days to a
	    maximum of 100 mg/kg per day
	Maintenance: 35–45 mg/kg per day
		Infantile spasms may require doses of up to
		    150 mg/kg per day
		Useful for adjunctive therapy of refractory
		    partial epilepsy
		Drowsiness, insomnia, ataxia, dizziness,
		    headache, hyperactivity may occur

Vitamin K—see Phytonadione		

Warfarin
[Coumadin]
 	
tab: 1, 2, 2.5, 4, 5, 10 mg
	Antithrombotic effect:
	PO: initial dose 0.2 mg/kg, max 10 mg
	Maintenance dose 0.1 mg/kg per day adjusted
	    to keep INR in desired range
	Administer once daily in evening
		Onset of anticoagulant activity, 36–72 h
		INR should be measured every 1–2 days
		    during the first week of therapy
		Fever, skin lesions with necrosis, anorexia,
		    hemorrhage, hemoptysis may occur
		Effect increases with ethacrynic acid,
		    indomethacin, ASA
		Avoid loading does in patients with liver
		    disease or liver congestion secondary to
		    CHD

FURTHER READING

See chapter section following Chapter 7.2

7.2   Continuous infusion drug guidelines

John Macready, Claire Aston and Robert Adderley

The following table has been developed for use in a pediatric intensive care area. It is intended to be used only as a guideline to provide the minimum amount of information necessary to start the most common intravenous infusions. Ultimately, the requirements of the dose and administration of these medications are dictated by each individual clinical situation. For more detailed information on these drugs, the user should consult other comprehensive reference sources. The information is presented in a six-column format, which relates the dilution of the drug given by continuous infusion to the dose delivered.

DEFINITIONS

PATIENT GROUP

These guidelines normally apply to infants and children. Where information is available for neonates, it has been included.

DILUTION

The second column of the table gives the number of milligrams or milliliters of each drug to be added to the diluent up to a total volume of 50 ml. The dilutions represented here are applicable for use in children weighing 5–20 kg. Younger children, i.e. those weighing less than 5 kg, or those who are fluid restricted, may require more concentrated solutions (double to quadruple strength), especially for drugs marked with two asterisks. Older children may tolerate more dilute solutions of these drugs.

Note—For children weighing more than 20 kg, calcium chloride, dopamine, and norepinephrine (noradrenaline) are to be diluted to half strength.

> The dilution and dose recommendations in this table do not apply to neonates for drugs marked with one asterisk. Please consult special neonatal references and use extra care when treating this age group

It should be noted that:

1. The dilution may be indicated as either mg/kg of drug product per 50 ml (e.g. dopamine) or mg or ml of drug product per 50 ml (e.g. aminophylline, alcohol). It is the responsibility of the prescriber and the nurse to verify that the dilution used will deliver the correct dose.
2. Some drugs (e.g. alcohol, diazepam, paraldehyde) are recommended to be given at the fixed concentrations indicated in the dilution column.
3. The maximum recommended infusion concentration of each drug is stated in the comments section. In most cases there is little evidence to substantiate the concentrations recommended for use in this table. Where available a recommendation for central or peripheral line is included.

INFUSION RATE

The rate given in the third column of the table is the standard initial infusion rate.

DOSE DELIVERED

The fourth column lists the dose delivered at the standard infusion rate.

DOSE RANGE

The infusion dose range recommended is given in column 5.

COMMENTS

Other pertinent information pertaining to the infusion of each drug is presented in the 'Comments' column, including:

- loading dose, where applicable
- central or peripheral line recommendations

- protect from light (where noted only)
- maximum recommended concentration for infusion
- solution expiry noted, change tubing at specified time

KEY TO ABBREVIATIONS	
D5W	5% dextrose in water
IV	intravenous
IVI	intravenous infusion
NS	normal saline (0.9%)
prn	when required (*pro re nata*)
qid	four times a day (*quater in die*)
qxh	every *x* hours (*quaque x hora*)
qxmin	every *x* min
SWI	sterile water for injection
s.g.	specific gravity

Drug	Dilution (mg or ml to total of 50 ml IV fluid) or special instructions	Infusion rate	Dose delivered	Dose range	Comments
Adrenaline—see epinephrine					
* **Alcohol, ethyl 99%**	5 ml (to make 10% dilution) NS or SWI	No dialysis: 1.4 ml/kg·h Dialysis: 3.0 ml/kg·h	109 mg/kg·h (s.g. 0.79) 237 mg/kg·h	Titrate IV rate to keep blood ethanol level in range that will block alcohol dehydrogenase (> 22 mmol/L)	− Loading dose is 7.6 ml/kg IV (of 10% solution) over 30 min − To make 10% dilution mix 5 ml ethanol 99% with 45 ml IV fluid − Peripheral or central line − Max. concentration is 10% solution − Consider early hemodialysis, if methanol levels are > 15 mmol/L if acidosis is refractory to $NaHCO_3$ − 24 h
Alprostadil—see prostaglandin E_1					
* **Aminophylline** 25 mg/ml pH 8.6–9.0	50 mg D5W, NS (use as a 1 mg/ml dilution)	1 ml/kg·h	1 mg/kg·h	Reduce dose for children < 1 y, or > 9 y. Titrate to keep theophylline blood level in therapeutic range (55–110 μmol/L)	− Loading dose is 6 mg/kg IV over 20 min − Peripheral or central line − Max. concentration 10 mg/ml − 72 h − 55–110 μmol/L = 10–20 mg/L
Amiodarone 150 mg/3 ml	15 mg/kg D5W only infuse at concentrations 0.6–4.8 mg/ml	1 ml/h	5 μg/kg·min	5–15 μg/kg·min	− Loading dose: 5 mg/kg slow IV over 20–60 min − The duration of injection should *never* be < 3 min N.B. for loading doses > 5 mg/kg pacing wires are recommended − Avoid the use of direct undiluted injections − Central line preferred − Adsorbs to PVC bags and tubing − Change buretrol and tubing at 24 h − Ref. [2, 3, 4]
Amrinone 5 mg/ml pH 3–4	15 mg/kg 0.45%, 0.9% saline only	1 ml/h	5 μg/kg·min	5–10 μg/kg·min Neonates: 3–5 μg/kg·min	− Infuse at a concentration of approx. 1–5 mg/ml − Incompatible with dextrose; however, may be run through a Y-site connector into a line containing dextrose − Peripheral or central lines − 72 h − Ref. [5]

*The dilution and dosage recommendations for these drugs do not apply to neonates.

Drug	Dilution (mg or ml to total of 50 ml IV fluid) or special instructions	Infusion rate	Dose delivered	Dose range	Comments
Calcium chloride 10% 100 mg/ml pH 5.5–7.5 **	150 mg/kg (1.5 ml/kg) CACl$_2$ D5W, NS For children > 20 kg, dilute to half strength	1 ml/h	0.5 mmol/kg per day *or* 1 mEq/kg per day (Ca^{2+})	0.5–1.5 mmol/kg per day *or* 1–3 mEq/kg per day (Ca^{2+})	– Central venous (RA) line only – Avoid extravasation – Max. concentration 10%, 100 mg/ml – 1 mEq = 20 mg Ca^{2+} – 27 mg Ca^{2+} = 1.36 mEq = 0.68 mmol/ml
Calcium gluconate 10% 100 mg/ml pH 6–8.2	Dilute to 20 mg/ml or less and mix in maintenance fluids			Neonates: 200–400 mg/kg (2–4 ml/kg of 10% sol'n) per day Infants, children: 200–1000 mg/kg (2–10 ml/kg of 10% sol'n) per day	– Central line where Ca > 400 mg/100, or peripheral line – Do not give by scalp vein – Max. concentration 20 mg/ml peripherally – 9 mg Ca^{2+} = 0.47 mEq = 0.24 mmol/ml – Ref. [6, 7]
Clormethiazole 8 mg/ml in D4W premixed in 500 ml glass containers Store at 5–8°C	Does not require dilution	0.01 ml/kg·min	0.08 mg/kg·min	0.01 ml/kg·min and increase dose q2–4h until seizures are controlled Doses up to 10 mg/kg·min have been used to control seizures	– Clomethiazole adsorbs to Silastic and PVC tubing. Glass, Teflon and polyethylene tubing should be used – Central line only – 72 h – Increased secretions, allergic reactions, tachycardia, hypotension
* **Diazepam emulsion** 5 mg/ml (Diazemuls)	10 mg D5W only (0.2 mg/ml) or undiluted	0.5 ml/kg·h	0.1 mg/kg·h	Titrate dose to clinical response	– Peripheral or central line – Max. concentration 0.2 mg/ml diluted in D5W – 24 h – Diazemuls may also be infused undiluted via syringe pump – Antidote is flumazenil 0.01–0.025 mg/kg IV prn – Ref. [8, 9]
Dobutamine 12.5 mg/ml pH 2.5–5 **	15 mg/kg D5W, NS	1 ml/h	5 µg/kg·min	2–20 µg/kg·min	– Central venous line preferred – Pink discoloration acceptable – Max. concentration 10 mg/ml – 72 h – Ref. [6, 11, 12]
Dopamine 40 mg/ml pH 2.5–4.5 **	15 mg/kg D5W, NS For children > 20 kg, dilute to half strength	1 ml/h	5 µg/kg·min	2–20 µg/kg·min	– Central venous line only – Avoid extravasation – For infiltration notify doctor immediately re phentolamine protocol – Do not use discolored solutions – Max. concentration 5 mg/ml – 72 h – ref. [6, 11, 12]
Epinephrine (adrenaline) 1:1000 1 mg/ml pH 2.5–5 **	0.3 mg/kg D5W, NS	1 ml/h	0.1 µg/kg·min	0.05–2 µg/kg·min	– Central venous line preferred – Avoid extravasation – Do not use discolored solutions – Max. concentration 500 µg/ml – 72 h – Ref. [11, 12]

Epoprostenol—see prostacyclin

The dilution and dosage recommendations for these drugs do not apply to neonates.
** *For children weighing < 5 kg, more concentrate solutions (2×, 4×) may be used; for children weighing > 20 kg, less concentrated solutions may be used.*

Drug	Dilution (mg or ml to total of 50 ml IV fluid) or special instructions	Infusion rate	Dose delivered	Dose range	Comments
Esmolol 100 mg/10 ml pH 4.5–5.5	100 mg/10 ml vial is ready for use Use undiluted solution	0.6 ml/kg·h	100 μg/kg·min	50–200 μg/kg·min	– Loading dose 500 μg/kg·min over 1 min – Max. concentration is 10 mg/ml (i.e. undiluted) – 72 h – Incompatible with sodium bicarbonate – Ref. [31]
****Fentanyl** 0.05 mg/ml pH 4–7.5	0.05 mg/kg D5W, NS	1 ml/h	1 μg/kg·h	1–4 μg/kg·h	– Loading dose 1–2 μg/kg IV over 1–3 min – Peripheral or central line – Max. concentration 50 μg/ml – Monitor for respiratory depression in nonventilated patients – Antidote is naloxone 0.01–0.1 mg/kg IV prn – 72 h – Ref. [11, 12]
Frusemide—see furosemide					
* **Furosemide** (frusemide) 10 mg/ml pH 8.5–9.3	25 mg/kg D5W, NS	1 ml/h	0.5 mg/kg·h	0.1–1 mg/kg·h	– Peripheral or central line – Do not use discolored solutions – Max. concentration 10 mg/ml – Furosemide is an alkaline drug and does not mix well with catecholamines, e.g. dopamine, epinephrine – 72 h – Ref. [10]
Glyceryl trinitrate—see nitroglycerin					
Heparin 1000 units/ml pH 5–7.5	1000 units/kg D5W, NS	1 ml/h	20 units/kg·h	15–25 units/kg·h individualized based on PTT results (see heparin page 574)	– Loading dose 75 units/kg IV once – Peripheral or central line – Max. concentration 400 units/ml – 72 h – Ref. [6, 12]
Insulin (regular) 100 units/ml pH 7–7.8	5 units NS, 0.45% saline, D5W	1 ml/kg·h	0.1 unit/kg·h	0.05–0.1 unit/kg·h based on serum glucose concentrations	– Only regular insulin is given IV – Preflush tubing with 25–50 ml insulin solution – Peripheral or central line – Max. concentration 5 units/ml
Isoprenaline—see isoproterenol					
****Isoproterenol** (isoprenaline) 0.2 mg/ml pH 3.5–4.5	Chronotrope/ inotrope: 0.075 mg/kg	1 ml/h	0.025 μg/kg·min	0.025–0.1 μg/kg·min	– Peripheral or central line – Discard solution if it darkens or a precipitate is present – Max. concentration 0.2 mg/ml – 72 h
	Bronchodilator: 0.3 mg/kg D5W	1 ml/h	0.1 μg/kg·min	0.1–1.0 μg/kg·min	– Ref. [12, 14]

*The dilution and dosage recommendations for these drugs do not apply to neonates.
** For children weighing < 5 kg, more concentrate solutions (2×, 4×) may be used; for children weighing > 20 kg, less concentrated solutions may be used.

Drug	Dilution (mg or ml to total of 50 ml IV fluid) or special instructions	Infusion rate	Dose delivered	Dose range	Comments
* **Ketamine** 50 mg/ml	30 mg/kg D5W, NS	2 ml/h	20 μg/kg·min	20–40 μg/kg·min	– Watch airway closely – Peripheral line – Max. concentration 50 mg/ml – Ref. [12]
Labetalol 5 mg/ml pH 3–4	50 mg D5W or NS Note—mix 100 mg to total 100 ml IV fluid	1 ml/kg·h	1 mg/kg·h	1–3 mg/kg·h	– Peripheral or central line – Incompatible with NaHCO₃ – Max. concentration 5 mg/ml undiluted – 72 h – Ref. [15, 16]
Lidocaine (lignocaine) 20 mg/ml pH 5–7	< 30 kg: 30 mg/kg D5W	1 ml/h	10 μg/kg·min	20–50 μg/kg·min therapeutic range of lidocaine is 4.5–21 μmol/l	– Loading dose 1 mg/kg q10min prn up to 5 mg/kg – Peripheral or central line – Max. concentration 20 mg/ml – Incompatible with phenytoin and NaHCO₃ – 72 h – Ref. [7, 12]
	> 30 kg: use 2% injection undiluted	0.03 ml/kg·min	10 μg/kg·min	(as above)	
Lignocaine—see lidocaine					
** **Midazolam** 5 mg/ml pH 3–3.6	3 mg/kg D5W, NS	1 ml/h	1 μg/kg·min	0.5–6 μg/kg·min Neonates: 0.5 μg/kg·min	– Use midazolam cautiously and avoid load dose in patients after open heart surgery, septic shock or meningococcemia – Loading dose for neonates is 0.05 mg/kg IV over 15 min – For other patients, loading dose is 0.05–0.1 mg/kg IV over 3 min – Peripheral or central line – Max. concentration is 5 mg/ml – 72 h – Antidote is flumazenil 0.01–0.025 mg/kg IV prn – Ref. [17]
milrinone 1 mg/ml pH: 3.2–4	0.75 mg/kg D5W, NS	1 mL/hr	0.25 mcg/kg/min	0.25–0.75 mcg/kg/min	– Incompatible with furosemide – Peripheral or central line – Loading dose is 50 mcg/kg over 10–15 minutes – Max. concentration 1 mg/ml (undiluted)
** **Morphine** 10 mg/ml pH 2.5–6	0.5 mg/kg D5W, NS	1 ml/h	10 μg/kg·h	Postoperative analgesia/sedation 10–40 μg/kg·h Neonates (< 1 month): dose is 5–20 μg/kg·h Burn patients may require higher doses, e.g. 400 μg/kg·h	– Peripheral or central line – Max. concentration 10 mg/ml – Monitor for respiratory depression in nonventilated patients – Antidote is naloxone 0.01–0.1 mg/kg IV prn – Incompatible with furosemide (frusemide) and NaHCO₃ – 72 h – Ref. [12, 18]

*The dilution and dosage recommendations for these drugs do not apply to neonates.
** For children weighing < 5 kg, more concentrate solutions (2×, 4×) may be used; for children weighing > 20 kg, less concentrated solutions may be used.

Drug	Dilution (mg or ml to total of 50 ml IV fluid) or special instructions	Infusion rate	Dose delivered	Dose range	Comments
**Nitroglycerin (glyceryl trinitrate) 5 mg/ml pH 3–6.5	3 mg/kg D5W, NS For children over 15 kg, dilute to ½ strength	1 ml/h	1 μg/kg·min	0.5–10 μg/kg·min	– Peripheral or central line – Administer via syringe pump with non-PVC tubing – Max. concentration 1 mg/ml – 72 h – Ref. [12]
**Nitroprusside 50 mg/vial pH 3.5–6	3 mg/kg D5W only	1 ml/h	1 μg/kg·min	0.5–8 μg/kg·min *Neonates:* begin at 0.25–0.5 μg/kg·min to max. 6 μg/kg·min Keep thiocyanate < 0.8 mmol/l	– Check thiocyanate levels in high-dose (> 4 μg/kg·min) prolonged (> 48 h) use or renal failure – Do not admix – Peripheral or central line – Protect infusion solution and tubing from light with aluminium foil – Max. concentration 5 mg/ml – 24 h – Ref. [12]
Noradrenaline—see norepinephrine					
Norepinephrine (noradrenaline) 1 mg (base) per ml pH 3–4.5	0.3 mg/kg D5W only Do not mix in NS For children > 20 kg, dilute to half strength	1 ml/h	0.1 μg/kg·min	0.02–0.1 μg/kg·min titrate to maintain blood pressure	– Do not mix in NS or use if solution turns brown – Central venous line only, avoid extravasation – For infiltration, notify doctor immediately re phentolamine protocol – Incompatible with alkalis – Max. concentration 0.5 mg/ml – Dose and calculations in terms of norepinephrine base, i.e: 1 mg base 2 mg bitartrate – 24 h – Ref. [20]
Paraldehyde (100%) 1 g/ml	2.5 ml (to make 5% dilution) NS, D5W	0.4 ml/kg·h	20 mg/kg·h	5–20 mg/kg·h	– Do not admix – Protect infusion from light – Change IV administration set and solution q8h – Discard solution if it has a brown color or a sharp odor of acetic acid – Max. concentration is 5% – 8 h – Peripheral or central line – Ref. [6, 12]
Procainamide 100 mg/ml pH 4–6	60 mg/kg NS only	1 ml/h	20 μg/kg·min	*Children:* 20–80 μg/kg·min Monitoring levels of procainamide recommended *Range:* procainamide 15–37 μmol/L	– Peripheral or central line – Must be diluted prior to use – Load in children: 3–6 mg/kg per dose (max. 100 mg) dilute IV over 5 min, q5–10min to max. 15 mg/kg (hypotension) – 72 h – Ref. [19]

** For children weighing < 5 kg, more concentrate solutions (2×, 4 ×) may be used; for children weighing > 20 kg, less concentrated solutions may be used.

Drug	Dilution (mg or ml to total of 50 ml IV fluid) or special instructions	Infusion rate	Dose delivered	Dose range	Comments
Propofol 200 mg/20 ml inj premixed in soybean oil emulsion	Administer undiluted or dilute in D5W to a concentration no less than 2 mg/ml		5 μg/kg·min	ICU sedation: start at 5–10 μg/kg·min and titrate q5min to 20–60 μg/kg·min Maintenance of anesthesia: 100–250 μg/kg·min	− Strict aseptic technique required − Shake well before opening ampoules − Discard open ampoules immediately − Change IV set q12h − For short use or intermittent use only
Prostacyclin (Epoprostenal) 0.5 mg and 1.5 mg vials for reconstitution with specific sterile diluent	Dissolve the contents of one vial in 50 ml of diluent Do not further dilute in other IV fluids Reconstituted solution is kept at 2–8°C and protected from light		2 ng/kg·min	1–5 ng/kg·min	− Systemic hypotension, bradycardia, flushing, nausea, vomiting, headache − Central venous line only − Infuse in special diluent − Keep infusion solution at 2–8°C − Discard after 24 h
Prostaglandin E$_1$ (alprostadil) 500 μg/ml pH 4.3/D5W	Ductal dilatation/ pulmonary vasodilation: 0.15 mg/kg (150 μg/kg) D5W, D10W	1 ml/h	0.05 μg/kg·min NB. for ductal dilation start at 0.05 μg/kg·min and titrate	0.01–0.2 μg/kg·min	− Incompatible with NaHCO$_3$ − Peripheral or central line (central line preferred for concentration > 10 μg/ml) − Max. concentration 20 μg/ml − Compatible with NaCl, KCl (concentration of 2 mmol/ 100 ml) − 24 h − Ref. [1]
* **Salbutamol** 0.5 mg/ml pH 3.5	May run full strength (25 mg/ 50 ml) or diluted with D5W	0.12 ml/kg·h	1 μg/kg·min	1–10 μg/kg·min	− Peripheral or central line − May use undiluted or diluted to half strength or less − Max. concentration 0.5 mg/ml − 72 h − Ref. [12]
Sodium bicarbonate 1 mEq/ml 1 mmol/ml pH 7.4–8.5	25 mmol (25 ml) (0.5 mmol/ml, 4.2%) dilute with sterile water for injection	1 ml/kg·h	0.5 mmol/kg·h	Sufficient to control acidosis 0.5–2 mmol/kg·h	− Do not admix − Peripheral or central line (central preferred) − Max. concentration: 1 mmol/ml central line 0.5 mmol/ml peripheral line − 72 h − Ref. [12]

*The dilution and dosage recommendations for these drugs do not apply to neonates.

Drug	Dilution (mg or ml to total of 50 ml IV fluid) or special instructions	Infusion rate	Dose delivered	Dose range	Comments
Streptokinase 250 000 units/vial 750 000 units/vial					
High-dose systemic thrombolytic therapy	50 000 units/kg D5W	1 ml/h	1000 units/kg·h	2000 units/kg·h	– Loading dose 4000 units/kg over 30 min – Reconstitute vial with 5 ml NS by rolling and tilting (avoid shaking); further dilute in NS prior to infusion – Discard solutions containing precipitate – 24 h – Ref. [21, 22]
Low-dose local thrombolytic therapy	2500 units/kg D5W	1 ml/h	50 units/kg·h	50–100 units/kg·h	– Low-dose local infusion – 24 h – Ref. [12]
Sufentanil 0.5 mg/ml inj	0.01 mg/kg in D5W/NS	1 ml/h	0.2 μg/kg·h	0.2–3 μg/kg·h	– For higher doses use double and quadruple strength solutions – Periperhal or central line – Max. concentration 50 μg/ml (undiluted) – Antidote: naloxone 0.01–0.1 mg/kg per dose IV prn – 72 h
Thiopental (thiopentone) 25 mg/ml, 2.5% pH 10–11	200 mg (0.4%) D5W/NS	0.25 ml/kg·h	1 mg/kg·h	1–5 mg/kg·h	– Central line only – Avoid extravasation – Maximum concentration 25 mg/ml (2.5%) – Incompatible with catecholamines – 72 h – Ref. [9]
Urokinase 250 000 units/vial	High-dose systemic thrombolytic therapy 100 000 units/kg D5W or NS (mix sufficient for 24 h D5W or NS only)	2 ml/h	4000 units/kg·h	4000 units/kg·h, increase dose if fibrinolysis is not effected Doses up to 50 000 units/kg·h, have been used	– Loading dose 4000 units/kg per dose IV over 10 min – Reconstitute vial with 5.2 ml sterile water *without preservative*: roll and tilt—do not shake – Use solution immediately after preparation – Discard solution after 24 h after reconstitution of powder
	Low-dose local thrombolytic therapy 10 000 units/kg	ml/h	200 units/kg·h	200 units/kg·h	– Ref. [21, 22, 26, 28]

Drug	Dilution (mg or ml to total of 50 ml IV fluid) or special instructions	Infusion rate	Dose delivered	Dose range	Comments
Vasopressin 20 units/ml pH 2.5–4.5	*Central diabetes insipidus:* 1 unit/kg D5W, NS	1 ml/h	0.0003 unit/ kg·min	0.00003–0.0003 unit/kg·min (0.1–1 ml/h) or begin at 1 ml/h (0.0003 unit/kg·min) and titrate infusion downward as control is achieved	– Central line preferred, peripheral – Max. concentration is 1 unit/ml – Avoid extravasation – Ref. [23]
	Gastrointestinal hemorrhage: 50 units	0.12 ml/kg·h	0.002 unit/ kg·min	0.002–0.01 unit/kg·min *Note*—a higher dose may be required but complications are more frequent	– For upper GI hemorrhage begin therapy with a loading dose of 20 units per 1.73 m², then start infusion – Use only with expert consultation; hemostatic techniques may be indicated – Ref. [26, 27]
Vecuronium 10 mg/vial pH 4	3 mg/kg D5W, NS	1 ml/h	1 µg/kg·min	1–10 µg/kg·min	– Reconstitute with sterile water for infusion to 1 mg/ml – Central or peripheral line – Max. concentration 2 mg/ml – 72 h – Ref. [25]

FURTHER READING

1. British Columbia Drug and Poison Information Centre. Poison management manual. Ottawa. Canadian Pharmaceutical Association; 1984
2. The Hospital for Sick Children. Pharmacy Department, verbal communication; 1993
3. Amiodarone Product Monograph; 1983
4. Bucknall C et al. Intravenous and oral amiodarone for arrhythmias in children. Br Heart J 1986; 56: 278–284
5. Lawless S. et al. Amrinone in neonates and infants after critical surgery. Crit Care Med 1989; 17(8): 751–754
6. Ling E, Mcdougal A, Silvius C. Neonatal drug dosage guidelines, 2nd ed. Vancouver: British Columbia's Children's Hospital; 1990
7. Taketomo C, Hodding J, Kraus P, Pediatric dosage handbook. Cleveland: Lexi-Comp; 1992
8. Pharmacia. Verbal communication through medical information from Mr Bob Dobbs, 1–800–363–6877
9. Trissel L, editor. Handbook on injectable drugs, 6th ed. Bethesda: American Society of Hospital Pharmacists; 1990
10. Singh N. Comparison of continuous versu intermittent furosemide administration in post-operative pediatric cardiac patients. Crit Care Med. 1992; 20(1): 17–21
11. Santieros M et al. Guidelines for continuous infusion medications in the neonatal intensive care area. Ann Pharmacother 1992; 26: 271–274.
12. Infusion guidelines for infants and children. Pediatric Intensive Care Area. Vancouver: British Columbia's Children's Hospital; 1989
13. Disesa V. The rational selection of inotropic drugs in cardiac surgery. J Card Surg 1987; 2: 385–406
14. Levin D, editor. Essentials of pediatric intensive care. A pocket companion. St Louis: Quality Medical Publishing; 1990
15. Farine M, Arbus G. Management of hypertensive emergencies in children. Ped Emerg Care 1989; 5(1): 51–55
16. Bunchman T et al. Intravenously administered labetalol for treatment of hypertension in children. J Pediatr 1992; 120: 140–144
17. Booker, PD et al. Sedation of children requiring artificial ventilation using an infusion of midazolam. Br J Anaesth 1986. 58(10): 1104–1108
18. Cederholm I et al. Long term high dose morphine, ketamine and midazolam infusion in a child with burns. Br J Clin Pharmacol 1990; 30: 901–905
19. Micromedex Inc. 1998; 1: 98
20. Dupuis L, editor. The formulary of the Hospital for Sick Children, Toronto, 1991
21. Strife J L et al. Arterial occlusions in neonates; use of fibrinolytic therapy. Radiology 1988; 166(2) 395–400

22. Delaplane D et al. Urokinase therapy for a catheter related right atrial thrombus. J Pediatr 1982; 100(1): 149–152

23. Ralston C, Butt W. Continuous vasopression replacement in diabetes insipidus. Arch Dis Child 1990; 65: 896–897

24. Tuggle D et al. Intravenous vasopression and gastrointestinal hemorrhage in children. J Ped Surg 1988; 23(7): 627–629

25. Eldadah MK et al. Vecuronium by continuous infusion for neuromuscular blockage in infants and children. Crit Care Med 1989, 17: 989–922

26. Abbott Laboratories. Verbal communication from medical information from Lisa Letourneau, 1993

27. Written communication from Dr E. Hassall, pediatric gastroenterologist, British Columbia's Children's Hospital, Vancouver, 1993

28. Verbal communication from Dr J. A. G. Culham, Department of Radiology, British Columbia's Children's Hospital, Vancouver, 1993.

29. Macnab AJ, Robinson JL, Adderley RJ, D'Orsogna L. Heart block secondary to erythromycin induced carbamazepine toxicity Pediatr 1987; 80: 951–953

30. Tashihiro I et al. Thrombolytic therapy for femoral artery thrombosis after pediatric cardiac catheterization. Am Heart J 1988; 115: 633–639

31. Ryan A, Andrew M. Failure of thrombolytic therapy in four children with extensive thromboses. AJDC 1992; 146: 187–193

32. Cuneo BF et al. Pharmacodynamics and pharmaco-kinetics of esmolol, a short-acting β-blocking agent, in children. Pediatr Cardiol 1994; 15: 296–301

33. Laneau S, Evangelista JK, Pizzi AM et al. Proarrythmia associated with cisapride in children Pediatr 1998; 101: 1053–1056

7.3   Reference data and formulae

Henry Hui and Andrew J. Macnab

Normal values*

Blood chemistry	Age range	SI unit value	Non SI unit value
Anion gap $(Na + K)–(Cl + CO_2)$		12–20 mmol/L	mEq/L
Na		135–145 mmol/L	mEq/L
K	0–5 yr	3.5–5.5 mmol/L	mEq/L
	> 5 yr	3.5–5.0 mmol/L	mEq/L
Cl		95–107 mmol/L	mEq/L
HCO_3 (total CO_2)	0–5 yr	18–26 mmol/L	mEq/L
	> 6 yr	23–24 mmol/L	mEq/L
Ca	0–1 yr	1.87–2.5 mmol/L	7.5–10.0 mg/dl
	1–11 yr	2.2–2.5 mmol/L	8.8–10.0 mg/dl
	> 11 yr	2.2–2.67 mmol/L	8.8–10.7 mg/dl
Ca (ionized) normalized to pH 7.40	1–5 days	0.9–1.3 mmol/L	3.6–5.4 mg/dl
	> 5 days	1.1–1.3 mmol/L	4.4–5.4 mg/dl
Mg	0–2 mo	0.66–0.95 mmol/L	1.6–2.3 mg/dl
	3 mo–12 yr	0.78–1.03 mmol/L	1.9–2.5 mg/dl
	> 13 yr	0.74–1.00 mmol/L	1.8–2.4 mg/dl
PO_4	1–5 days	1.55–2.65 mmol/L	4.8–8.2 mg/dl
	6 days–1 yr	1.29–2.58 mmol/L	4.0–8.0 mg/dl
	> 1–13 yr	1.20–1.80 mmol/L	3.7–5.6 mg/dl
	14–16 yr	0.95–1.75 mmol/L	2.9–5.4 mg/dl
Glucose (random)	Newborn (term) day 1	2.2–5.6 mmol/L	40–100 mg/dl
	Child	3.3–7.0 mmol/L	60–125 mg/dl
Urea	Newborn (term)	0.7–6.7 mmol/L	2–19 mg/dl (BUN)
	6 days–1 yr	1.8–8.2 mmol/L	5–23 mg/dl
	> 1 yr–13 yr	2.1–6.4 mmol/L	6–18 mg/dl
	> 14 yr	2.9–7.5 mmol/L	8–21 mg/dl
Creatinine	Newborn (term)	30–125 μmol/L	0.3–1.35 mg/dl
	6 days–1 yr	10–90 μmol/L	0.1–1.0 mg/dl
	1–9 yr	10–60 μmol/L	0.1–0.7 mg/dl
	10–14 yr	40–110 μmol/L	0.4–1.2 mg/dl
Osmolality		285–295 mmol/kg	mOsm/kg
Ammonia	Newborn	42–155 μmol/L	59–217 μg/dl
	Child	9–33 μmol/L	13–46 μg/dl

Blood chemistry	Age range	SI unit value	Non SI unit value
Bilirubin	Newborn (term)		
unconjugated	day 2–5	35–205 μmol/L	2.0–12 mg/dl
conjugated	Child	< 2.0 μmol/L	< 0.1 mg/dl
unconjugated	Child	3–17 μmol/L	0.2–1.0 mg/dl
Alkaline phosphatase	0–1 yr	110–320 units/L	IU/L
(NB variable with age	> 1–9 yr	145–420 units/L	
and gender)	10–15 yr (males)	130–525 units/L	
	(females)	70–230 units/L	
Creatine kinase (total)	1–3 yr	60–305 units/L	IU/L
(NB variable with age	4–6 yr	75–230 units/L	
and gender)	> 7 yr (males)	60–370 units/L	
	(females)	60–295 units/L	
Lactate dehydrogenase	1–5 days	934–2150 units/L	IU/L
(LDH) (NB some	1–6 yr	500–900 units/L	
variation with gender	> 7 yr	400–700 units/L	
> 10 years)			
Aspartate	1–5 days	35–140 units/L	IU/L
Aminotransferase	6 days–3 yr	20–60 units/L	
(AST/SGOT)	4–15 yr	15–40 units/L	
Alanine	0–3 yr	6–50 units/L	IU/L
Aminotransferase	> 4 yr	10–40 units/L	
(ALT/SGOT)			
Protein (total)	0–3 yr	54–70 g/L	5.4–7.0 g/dl
	4–6 yr	59–78 g/L	5.9–7.8 g/dl
	> 7 yr	62–86 g/L	6.2–8.6 g/dl
Albumin	0–5 days	26–36 g/L	2.6–3.6 g/dl
	6 days–3 yr	34–42 g/L	3.4–4.2 g/dl
	4–6 yr	35–52 g/L	3.5–5.2 g/dl
	> 7 yr	37–56 g/L	3.7–5.6 g/dl
Amylase	0–6 mo	0–20 units/L	IU/L
	6 mo–1 yr	5–50 units/L	
	> 1 yr	30–100 units/L	
Lactate (NB arterial sample	0–16 yr	0.5–2.2 mmol/L	4.5–20 mg/dl
values are about 60% less			
than venous levels)			
Urate (uric acid)	0–1 yr	115–470 μmol/L	1.9–7.9 mg/dl
(NB values lower in females	> 1–9 yr	105–295 μmol/L	1.8–4.9 mg/dl
> 10 yr)	10–11 yr	135–320 μmol/L	2.3–5.4 mg/dl
	12–13 yr	160–400 μmol/L	2.7–6.7 mg/dl
	14–15 yr	140–465 μmol/L	2.4–7.8 mg/dl

Urine

Volume	Infant	0.5 ml/kg·hr	
	Child	1.0 ml/kg·hr	

Blood chemistry	Age range	SI unit value	Non SI unit value
Urine (cont.)			
Specific gravity	Newborn and infants	< 1.012	
	Child	1.001–1.035	
Osmolality		50–1200 mmol/kg	mOsm/kg urine water
pH (NB varies with diet)		4.5–8.0	

Blood gases (arterial)			
pH	Newborn 2–5 days	7.30–7.49	
	Child	7.35–7.45	
PaO_2	Newborn 2–5 days	> 8 kPa	> 60 mmHg
	Child	> 9.9 kPa	> 74 mmHg
$PaCO_2$	Newborn 2–5 days	4.4–5.2 kPa	33–39 mmHg
	Child < 2 yr	3.47–5.47 kPa	26–41 mmHg
	Child > 3 yr	4.67–6 kPa	35–45 mmHg
Bicarbonate	Newborn 2–5 days	19–29 mmol/L	mEq/L
(calculated)	Child < 2 yr	17–24 mmol/L	
	Child > 3 yr	18–27 mmol/L	

Hematology			
Hemoglobin	Birth	140–240 g/L	14–24 g/dl
	1 mo	110–170 g/L	11–17 g/dl
	1 yr	110–150 g/L	11–15 g/dl
	9–13 yr	130–155 g/L	13–15.5 g/dl
Hematocrit	Birth	0.44–0.64	44–64%
	14–90 days	0.35–0.49	35–49%
	0.5–1 yr	0.3–0.4	30–40%
	4–10 yr	0.31–0.43	31–43%
Platelets		150–450×10^9/L	$(\times 1000)$ mm^3
White blood cells	Newborn	9–30×10^9/L	$(\times 1000)$ mm^3
(WBC)	3–12 mo	5–15×10^9/L	
total leukocytes	2–5 yr	5–12×10^9/L	
	6–10 yr	4–10×10^9/L	

WBC *differential*		polymorphs/ neutrophils	band cells	lymphocytes
	Newborn	6–26×10^9/L	0–4.5×10^9/L	2–11×10^9/L
	3–12 mo	1.5–8.5	0	4–10.5
	2–5 yr	1.5–8.5	0	2–8
	6–10 yr	1.5–8.0	0	1.5–7

Values for guidance only – based on reference data from: British Columbia's Children's Hospital Laboratory handbook, Lexi Comp Inc., Hudson 1992 and Residents Handbook of Neonatology, 2nd ed. Perlman M, Kirpalani H, Moore A. (eds) St. Louis: B C Decker Inc, 1999. Local reference ranges should be used whenever possible due to variation in methodology and standardization.

Vital signs for age

Age	Resting heart rate (beats/min)	Resting blood pressure (mmHg) Boys	Girls	Resting respiratory rate (breaths/min)
Newborn	120 ± 25	70/50 ± 10/10	70/50 ± 10/10	45 ± 15
1–6 months	140 ± 30	95/50 ± 10/10	90/50 ± 10/10	40 ± 10
1 year	120 ± 20	95/55 ± 10/10	95/50 ± 10/10	35 ± 10
2 years	110 ± 30	95/60 ± 10/10	95/60 ± 10/10	35 ± 5
4 years	100 ± 35	90/55 ± 10/10	90/55 ± 10/10	25 ± 8
6 years	95 ± 25	95/60 ± 10/10	95/60 ± 10/10	22 ± 7
8 years	90 ± 25	100/60 ± 10/10	100/60 ± 10/10	22 ± 7
10 years	80 ± 20	100/65 ± 10/10	100/65 ± 10/10	22 ± 7
12 years	75 ± 20	105/65 ± 10/10	110/70 ± 10/10	20 ± 5
14 years	70 ± 20	110/65 ± 10/10	110/70 ± 10/10	20 ± 5

Source: Adapted from Report of the Second Task Force on Blood Pressure Control in Children – 1987. Pediatrics 79: 1, 1987; J. Liebman. Tables of Normal Standards. In J. Liebman, R. Plonsey, and P.C. Gillette (eds.), Pediatric Electrocardiography. Baltimore: Williams and Wilkins, 1982; W.W. Waring. The History and Physical Examination. In E.L. Kendig and V. Chernick, Disorders of the Respiratory Tract (4th ed.). Philadelphia: Saunders.

From: Baldwin GA (ed). Handbook of Pediatric Emergencies, 2nd ed. Boston: Little, Brown; 1994.

RESPIRATORY PATTERNS

Type	Description	Picture
Normal	Regular rhythm; rate normal for age	
Tachypnea	Regular rhythm; rate greater than normal	
Bradypnea	Regular rhythm; rate less than normal	
Apnea	Absence of breathing	
Periodic	Irregular pattern with short periods of apnea normal in newborns	
Cheyne–Stokes	Gradual increase in rate and depth followed by apnea	
Biot's	Faster and deeper than normal with periods of apnea, consistent depth	
Kussmaul's	Faster and deeper than normal, usually sounds labored	
Apneustic	Prolonged gasping inspiration and short expiration	
Agonal	Deep, gasping respirations preceding death	
Paradoxical	Abdominal muscles move in opposition to chest movements; see-saw movements	

From Brown PA, Blayney F, Brown CA, Gregg-Evans K, editors. Pediatric Intensive Care Nursing. Rockville, MA: Aspen Publishers; 1989.

BLOOD PRESSURE

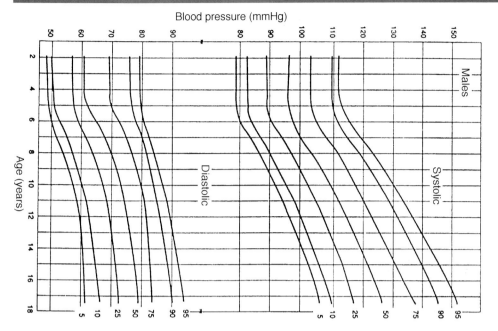

Percentiles for blood pressure: males (seated). From Baldwin GA, editor. Handbook of pediatric emergencies, 2nd ed. Boston: Little, Brown; 1994.

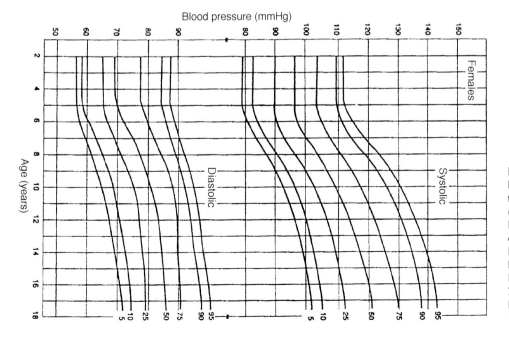

Percentiles for blood pressure: females (seated). From Baldwin GA, editor. Handbook of Pediatric Emergencies. 2nd ed. Boston: Little, Brown; 1994.

FORMULAE

MAINTENANCE FLUIDS

(Requirement for normal hydration/ homeostasis)

Weight (kg)	Fluid requirement (ml/kg·h)	(ml/kg per 24 h)	IV infusion rate (ml/kg·h)
0–10	4 ml/kg for each of first 10 kg	100	4
10–20	+ 2 ml/kg for each of next 10 kg	+50	+2
> 20	+1 ml/kg for each further kg	+20	+1

Insensible water loss

Insensible water loss is about 1/3 maintenance or 400 ml/m2 per day.

BLOOD VOLUME

- Child: 65 ml/kg
- Newborn: 85 ml/kg
- Premature: 95 ml/kg

INOTROPE CONTINUOUS INFUSION

6 × weight (kg) = mg of inotrope to be placed in 100 ml of IV solution
then infusion rate in ml/h = µg/kg·min of inotrope

MEAN ARTERIAL BLOOD PRESSURE

$$MABP = \frac{SAP + 2 \times DAP}{3}$$

where SAP is systolic arterial pressure and DAP is diastolic arterial pressure

CEREBRAL PERFUSION PRESSURE

CPP = MABP – DSP (ICP, ITP, CVP)

where CPP is the cerebral perfusion pressure, MABP is the mean arterial blood pressure, DSP is the downstream pressure, ICP is the intracranial pressure, ITP is the intrathoracic pressure, and CVP is the central venous pressure.

ELECTROLYTES AND OSMOLARITY

Serum osmolarity

serum osmolarity (mOsm) = 2 × serum Na + serum glucose + blood urea nitrogen

if unit mg/L rather than mmol/L, then divide glucose by 18, and divide nitrogen by 28

Fractional excretion of sodium

$$FE_{Na} = \frac{urine\ Na \times serum\ Cr \times 100\%}{urine\ Cr \times serum\ Na}$$

Glomerular filtration rate

$$GFR = \frac{urine\ Cr \times 24\ h\ urine\ output}{serum\ Cr \times 24 \times 60}$$

OXYGEN EQUATIONS

$$Oxygen\ extraction = \frac{(Ca_{O_2} - Cv_{O_2})}{Ca_{O_2}} \quad (normal\ about\ 0.25)$$

Oxygen delivery $D_{O_2} = Ca_{O_2}$ × cardiac output (normal 1000 ml/min)

Oxygen consumption $V_{O_2} = (Ca_{O_2} - Cv_{O_2})$ × cardiac output (normal 250 ml/min)
Cardiac output = $V_{O_2} / (Ca_{O_2} - Cv_{O_2})$

Fick's equation

where Ca_{O_2} is the arterial oxygen content, Cv_{O_2} is the mixed venous oxygen content, and Cc_{O_2} is the pulmonary capillary oxygen content (calculated from the alveolar gas equation).

Alveolar gas equation

$$Pa_{O_2} = (P_B - P_{svp\ water}) \times FI_{O_2} - Pa_{CO_2}/R$$
where $P_{svp\ water}$ is the saturated vapour pressure of water ($= 47$) and R is the respiratory quotient (about 0.8)

Oxygen content

$$(ml/dl\ blood) = 1.36 \times Hb \times Sa_{O_2} + 0.003 \times Pa_{O_2}$$
where Hb is the hemoglobin concentration in blood (g/dl)

Cardiac output

$$= \frac{stroke\ volume\ (SV) \times heart\ rate\ (HR)}{cardiac\ output}$$

Shunt equation

$$shunted\ blood\ flow\ Q_s = (Cc_{O_2} - Ca_{O_2})$$
$$systemic\ blood\ flow\ Q_t = (Cc_{O_2} - Cv_{O_2})$$

Oxygen gradient

$$A\text{-}a\ gradient = PA_{O_2} - Pa_{O_2}$$

Oxygen ratio (PF ratio)

$$oxygen\ ratio = Pa_{O_2} / FI_{O_2}$$

Oxygenation index

$$oxygenation\ index =$$
$$\frac{Mean\ airway\ pressure\ (cm\ water) \times \%\ inspired\ oxygen}{Post\text{-}ductal\ Pa_{O_2}\ (mmHg)}$$

PRESSURES

Central venous pressure 1–5 mmHg (mean)
Left atrial pressure 5–10 mmHg (mean)
Right atrial pressure 1–5 mmHg (mean)

Pulmonary arterial blood pressure 15–30 mmHg (systolic), 5–10 mmHg (diastolic)
Intracranial pressure < 15 mmHg
Cerebral perfusion pressure 40–50 mmHg

MISCELLANEOUS

Weight of child in kg
(1–10 years) = 2 × (age in years + 4)

Size of endotracheal tube in mm =

$$\frac{age\ (years)}{4} + 4$$

OR

$$\frac{age\ (years) + 16}{4}$$

BODY SURFACE AREA

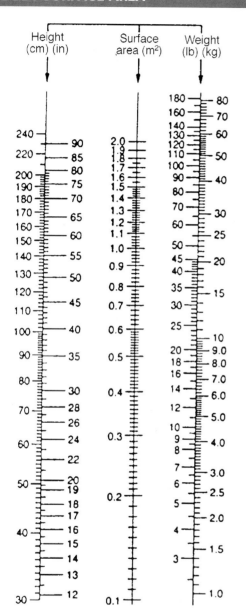

Nomogram showing the relationship between height, weight and surface area. To use the nomogram, a straight line joining the child's height and weight indicates the body surface area at the point of intersection with the center line (modified from data of E. Boyd). Reproduced with permission from Seear M, editor. The Pocket Pediatrician. Cambridge University Press; 1996.

CARDIAC CHANGES FROM BIRTH TO 16 YEARS

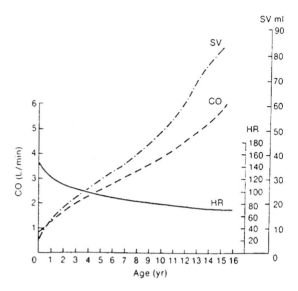

Changes in cardiac output (CO), heart rate (HR), and stroke volume (SV) from birth to 16 years. From Rudolph, AM. Congenital diseases of the heart. Copyright © 1974 by Mosby Year Book Medical Publishers, Inc., Chicago.

DIABETIC KETOACIDOSIS PROTOCOL[a]

Establish diagnosis: blood glucose (BG) $\geq$ 12 mmol/L ($\geq$ 200 mg/dl), ketonuria, capillary pH $\leq$ 7.35.[b]

1. Measure body weight (BW) in kilograms .... (1) _____ kg
2. Establish extent of dehydration (BP, tears, urine output, skin turgor) as ml/kg[c] using the formula below:

	infants:		children:
• mild:	5% = 50 ml/kg	n	3% = 30 ml/kg
• moderate:	10% = 100 ml/kg	n	6% = 60 ml/kg
• severe:	15% = 150 ml/kg	n	9% = 90 ml/kg .... (2) _____ ml/kg

3. Calculate total free water deficit: multiply (1) × (2) .... (3) _____ ml
4. Give 0.9% saline fluid push **only if patient is orthostatic or 'shocky'**[d]
   recommended amount: 10–20 ml/kg BW over 1–2 h.. (4) _____ ml
5. Calculate remainder of free water deficit after fluid push: subtract (4) from (3) ... (5) _____ ml
6. Calculate maintenance fluid requirements for the next **48h**:[e]

      200 ml/kg for the first 10 kg BW
   + 100 ml/kg for the next 10 kg BW
   +   40 ml/kg for the rest of BW .... (6) _____ ml/**48 h**

7. Calculate total amount of fluid still to be given over 48 h: add (5) and (6) ...... (7) _____ ml/**48 h**
8. Calculate hourly rate of fluid replacement: divide (7) by 48 .... (8) _____ ml/h
9. Make up and start a regular human insulin drip at 0.1 unit/kg·h:[f]

   • no bolus necessary
   • piggyback with IV fluids
   • put 50 units insulin in 500 ml 0.9% saline, 25 units in 250 ml, etc.
   • run at 1 ml/kg·h .... (9) _____ ml/h

10. Adjust fluid replacement rate for insulin drip rate: subtract (9) from (8) ...... (10) _____ ml/h
11. Determine type of fluid to use as replacement:

    • sodium:
      – patient's Na$^+$ > 145 mmol/L (> 145 mEq/L): use 0.9% saline
      – patient's Na$^+$ $\leq$ 145 mmol/L ($\leq$ 145 mEq/L): use 0.45% saline

Notes and rationale

[a]Please note that this protocol is designed as an algorithm for treating the majority of cases of DKA in infants, children and adolescents. It cannot replace careful clinical observation and judgment in treating this potentially very serious condition. If you have problems related to the management of DKA or diabetes, a pediatric endocrinologist should be consulted.
[b]Mild hyperglycemia, even with ketonuria and mild acidosis, can often be managed without IV fluids or IV insulin, particularly in the older child or known diabetic patient who is not vomiting or seriously dehydrated.
[c]Rapid, deep mouth-breathing (Kussmaul respiration) often dries out the oral mucosa, which makes the child appear more dehydrated than is the case. The other clinical signs noted above are more accurate.
[d]Large fluid boluses are potentially dangerous[k] and should be administered slowly and with caution, unless the patient is in shock. Only very rarely will a fluid bolus larger than 30–40 ml/kg be required to maintain perfusion.
[e]Since most patients develop DKA over days, slow metabolic repair is generally safest. Overhydration may contribute to cerebral edema.[k] None the less, DKA in children often resolves in less than 48 h.
[f]This relatively high dose of insulin is chosen to inhibit ketogenesis and gluconeogenesis and should be maintained.
   When the patient's BG begins to fall, dextrose is added to the IV fluid in a concentration sufficient to keep the BG in the 10–15 mmol/L (200–250 mg/dl) range. This allows for a buffer against hypoglycemia and a too-rapid fall in the osmolarity.
[g]To correct the serum Na$^+$ for hyperglycemia, add 0.3 mmol/L (1.6 mEq/L) Na$^+$ for every 1.0 mmol/L glucose above 5 mmol/L (100 mg/dl). As the hyperglycemia resolves, the serum Na$^+$ should normally rise; failure of this to occur could indicate excess free water administration. A high uncorrected serum Na$^+$ in the face of hyperglycemia indicates severe dehydration and hyperosmolarity. Such patients should be rehydrated with extreme caution, using fluids with higher osmolar content (e.g. 0.9% saline)

- potassium:
  - patient not urinating: add no K^+
  - patient urinating: add KCl 20–40 mmol/L (mEq/L)[h]
  - may give K^+ as half chloride—half phosphate for the first 8 h[i]
- dextrose:
  - patient's BG > 15 mmol/L (< 250 mg/dl): add no dextrose
  - patient's BG ≤ 15 mmol/L (≤ 250 mg/dl): add 5.0–12.5% dextrose
  - aim to keep BG about 10–15 mmol/L (200–250 mg/dl) without changing insulin rate[f]
- bicarbonate: $NaHCO_3$ is **not** recommended, regardless of pH[j]

12. Start replacement fluid type determined in (11) at rate determined in (10).
13. Close neurological observation and frequent rousing of the child with fingerpokes to detect any changes consistent with cerebral edema. Severe headache, change in sensorium or in BP, dilated pupils, bradycardia, posturing and incontinence are signs of impending deterioration. Rapid intervention (intubation, mild hyperventilation, mannitol bolus 1g/kg BW IV) is imperative.[k]
14. Follow laboratory parameters:

- follow BG by meter every 30–60 min: **does the child respond to the finger prick?**
- follow Na^+, K^+, Cl^-, HCO_3^-, capillary pH every 2–4 h[f,g,h]
- follow Ca^{2+} and P_i if giving phosphate[i]
- check all urine for glucose and ketones

15. Reevaluate appropriateness of replacement fluid type frequently, anticipating the need to add or increase K^+, dextrose, etc.

[h]Serum K^+ levels are usually normal at diagnosis and fall precipitously with treatment. An IV fluid K^+ concentration of 20–40 mmol/L (20–40 mEq/L) is usually required to keep the serum K^+ > 3.0 mmol/L (3.0 mEq/L). Oral/nasogastric KCl boluses (0.5–1 mmol/kg (0.5–1 mEq/kg BW) may also be administered.
[i]While there is no proven benefit to replacing phosphate, it has the theoretical advantage of repleting the severe phosphate deficit of DKA and ameliorating the hyperchloremia which inevitably occurs during DKA treatment. If phosphate is given, however, then serum calcium and phosphate levels should be monitored closely.
[j]The acidosis of DKA is due to both ketone bodies and lactic acid, and it resolves with fluid and insulin replacement. There is no proven benefit to giving $NaHCO_3$, but it does have a number of deleterious effects, including hypokalemia, metabolic alkalosis, and delayed clearance of ketones. Its use in DKA is **not recommended**, regardless of the patient's pH.
[k]Subclinical brain swelling is common in children with DKA. Cerebral edema accounts for more than half of the 1–5% mortality rate of DKA in children. At highest risk are newly diagnosed diabetics, those aged < 5 years, and those with pH < 7.1. The etiology of cerebral edma remains unclear, but overhydration has been implicated in several studies.
   Resuscitation is successful in only 50% of cases. Most experts suggest limiting fluids to < 4 L/m² body surface area, or to < 2.5n maintenance fluid rate, in the first 24 h.

Modified with permission from Metzger D, Kitson H, Endocrinology and Diabetes Unit, British Columbia's Children's Hospital, Vancouver

TETANUS PROPHYLAXIS

Immunization status (doses)	Clean minor wounds, burns		Tetanus-prone wounds, burns	
Children age 7 yr and over	**TD**	**TIG**	**TD**	**TIG**
Uncertain	Yes	No	Yes	Yes
0–1	Yes	No	Yes	Yes
2	Yes	No	Yes	No[a]
3 or more	No[b]	No	No[c]	No
Children under age 7 yr	**DTP (0.5 ml IM)**	**TIG (250 U IM)**	**DTP (0.5 ml IM)**	**TIG (250 U IM)**
Unknown or less than 3 doses	Yes[d]	No	Yes[d]	Yes
Three or more doses	No[e]	No	No[f]	No

Key: TD, tetanus, diphtheria; TIG, tetanus immunoglobulin; DTP, diphtheria, tetanus, pertussis.
[a]Yes if wound or burn more than 24 hours old.
[b]Yes if more than 10 years since last dose.
[c]Yes if more than 5 years since last dose.
[d]The primary immunization series should be completed.
[e]Yes, if the routine immunization schedule has lapsed (i.e. to make up for missed dose).
[f]Yes, if the routine immunization schedule has lapsed, or if more than 5 years has elapsed since the last dose of tetanus toxoid.
Note: TD should be given if DPT is contraindicated. Acetaminophen (paracetamol) should be given with the dose of DPT, 10 mg/kg PO.

From Baldwin, GA, editor. Handbook of Pediatric Emergencies. 2nd ed. Boston: Little, Brown; 1994.

GROWTH PERCENTILES

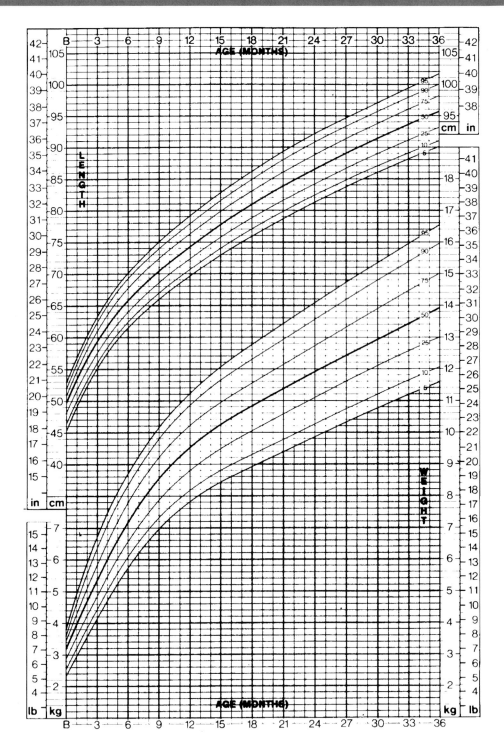

Girls: birth to 36 months

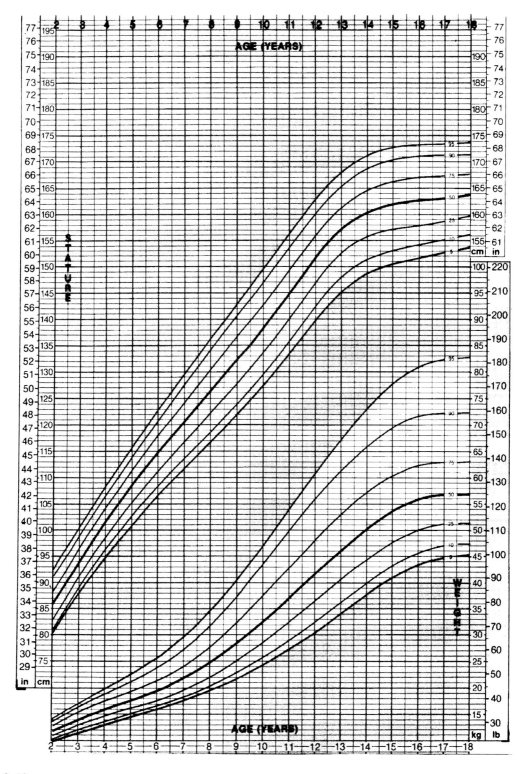

Girls: 2–18 years

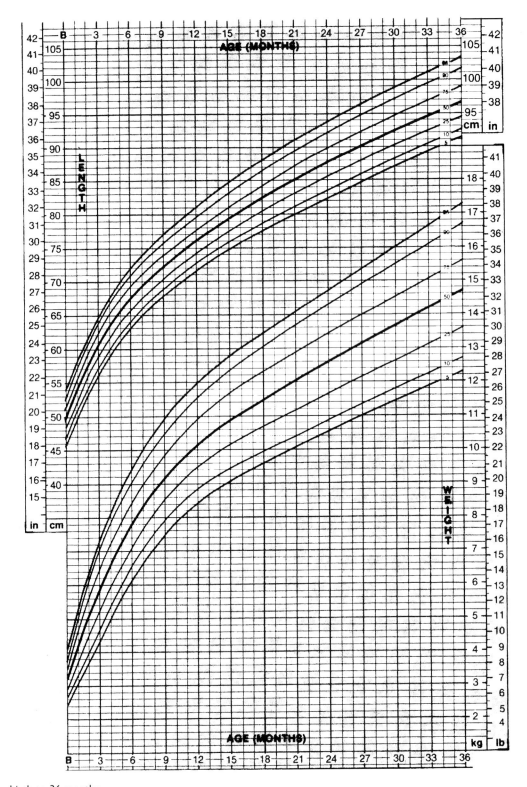

Boys: birth to 36 months

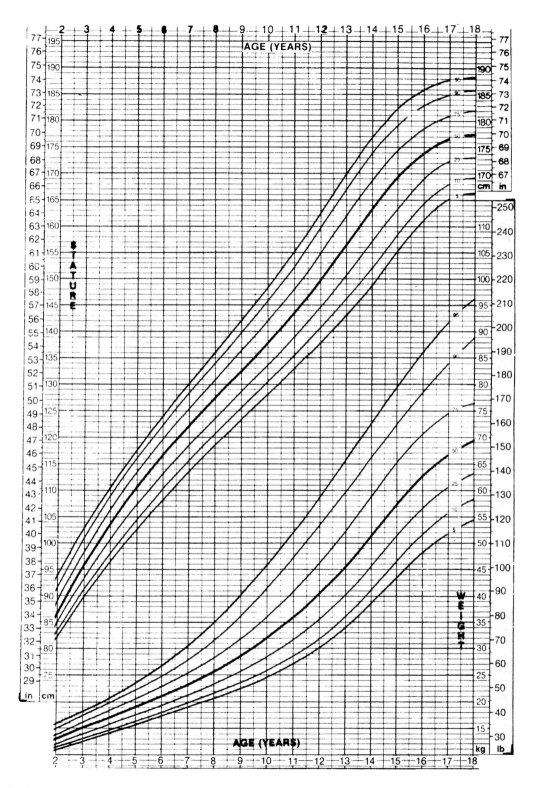

Boys: 2–18 years

7.4 Accidental exposure guidelines re HIV

Andrew J. Macnab

GOAL

To reduce the risk of transmission of human immunodeficiency virus (HIV) in persons accidentally exposed to blood or body fluids.

DEFINITIONS

1. Accidental exposure to HIV: an event where blood or other potentially infectious body fluid inadvertently comes into contact with nonintact skin, mucous membranes, or subcutaneous tissue (via percutaneous injury).
2. Infectious: source known to be HIV-positive or at high risk of being HIV-positive (if source unknown, consider infectious).
3. Definition of persons at high risk for HIV:
   - injection drug users
   - men who have sex with men
   - persons who have had multiple transfusions of blood or blood products, e.g. hemophiliacs prior to November 1985
   - sexual partners of any of the above and of persons known to be HIV-positive
4. Nonintact skin:
   - healing wound (< 3 days old)
   - skin lesion causing disruption of the epidermis
5. Infectious body fluids (capable of transmitting HIV):
   - blood
   - semen; CSF; amniotic, pleural, pericardial, peritoneal and synovial fluids; inflammatory exudates
   - breast milk
   - any body fluid visibly contaminated with blood
   - tissue or organs
6. Noninfectious body fluids (unless bloody) (not implicated in the transmission of HIV unless bloody): stool, urine, tears, saliva, nasal secretions, vomitus

PROCEDURES FOR ASSESSMENT AND MANAGEMENT OF EXPOSURES

Persons accidentally exposed to blood or body fluid should be referred to the nearest health care provider (often an emergency department) capable of providing assessment of infection and management of exposures, risk, counseling, testing, therapy and follow-up. If antiretroviral therapy is indicated, it is most effective if initiated within 2 hours of exposure.

ASSESSMENT OF INFECTION RISK

Infectivity of the source

If
(I) material to which exposure has occurred is a potentially infectious body fluid capable of transmitting HIV (see definition 5)
and
(IIa) source is known to be HIV-positive or at a high risk for HIV infection (see definition 3) or is unknown or refuses testing (unknown sources or persons refusing testing are considered HIV-positive)
or
(IIb) source person's HIV status is unkown but source person consents to testing: consider positive until results of testing are available, unless extremely low risk that source is HIV-positive.

Sources with a previous negative HIV test who have continued to engage in high-risk behavior in the 12 weeks before the test (window period) or any time since the most recent test must be considered HIV-positive.

Whenever possible the source should be HIV-tested (see below). When the results of HIV testing are known, these risk assessments should be reevaluated.

> Assuming the exposed person is HIV-negative, if the answers to I and IIA or IIB are positive, use the table of assessment of the risk of HIV transmission to determine the risk of transmission and the need for chemoprophylaxis

---

Higher risk of transmission (I, IIA or B positive)

Types of exposure

Percutaneous exposure to blood with *either*:

- exposure to blood in the event of deep injury (IM) *or*
- needle recently in source's artery or vein *or*
- visible blood on sharp device *or*
- injection of source's blood *or*
- exposure to high-titer HIV (e.g. source with acute retroviral illness or end-stage AIDS)

Recommendation

Recommend strongly:
zidovudine (ZDV) 200 mg tid + lamivudine (3TC) 150 mg bid
Consult with local expert (e.g. center of excellence) as soon as possible

- test source if possible
- counseling
- baseline HIV test with repeat testing 6, 12, 24 weeks and 1 year after exposure
- arrange for follow-up with physician as soon as possible to arrange continuing antiretroviral therapy if prescribed
- if high-risk exposure, refer to an HIV consultant (see note 1)

Note 1—If the source patient is known to be on antiretroviral therapy, contact the local expert or pharmacy to discuss a prophylactic regimen based on the possibility of drug resistance in the source. However, use the starter kit immediately while making these arrangements.

Moderate risk of transmission (I, IIA or B positive)

Types of exposure

1. Percutaneous exposure to fluid visibly contaminated with blood, other potentially infectious body fluid, or tissue
2. Mucous membrane or nonintact skin exposure to blood or fluid visibly contaminated with blood or other potentially infectious body fluids, or tissue
3. Bites, if there is one of the following:
   - blood in the mouth of the biter
   - blood in the wound of the person bitten
   - high titer of HIV in biter

Recommendation

Recommend:
zidovudine (ZDV) 200 mg tid + lamivudine (3TC) 150 mg bid

- test source, if possible
- offer counseling and HIV testing to exposed person
- baseline HIV test with repeat testing 6, 12, 24 weeks and 1 year after exposure
- arrange for follow-up with physician as soon as possible to continue antiretroviral therapy if prescribed (see note 1)

Negligible risk of transmission (I, IIA or B *not* positive)

Types of exposure

1. Percutaneous, mucous membrane or skin exposure to noninfectious body fluid
2. Intact skin exposure to blood, fluid visibly contaminated with blood, or other potentially infectious body fluid, or tissue
3. Bites other than those with characteristics noted in the moderate risk category

Recommendation

No antiretrovirals recommended:
- in exceptional circumstances antiretroviral therapy might be offered
- offer counseling clarifying the negligible risk of HIV infection and advise on risk prevention (i.e. preventing recurrences of exposure incident)

RISK OF HIV TRANSMISSION AND RECOMMENDATIONS FOR CHEMOPROPHYLAXIS

Dosages for children

Recommended antiretroviral chemoprophylaxis is for a total of 28 days:

- children > 40 kg: ZDV 200 mg tid + 3TC 150 mg bid
- children < 40 kg: ZDV 5 mg/kg tid (max. 600 mg daily) + 3TC 4 mg/kg bid (max. 300 mg daily)

Note—

1. Children < 40 kg and able to swallow capsules and tablets: calculate dose to nearest 100 mg for ZDV (each capsule is 100 mg and should not be divided) and nearest 75 mg for 3TC (half tablet).
2. Children < 40 kg and unable to swallow capsules or tablets: a liquid suspension is available for both drugs. Suspension strength is 10 mg/ml.
3. Any questions on initiation of therapy should be referred to a local expert.

MANAGEMENT OF EXPOSURES

Counseling

Counsel all exposed persons. Initial counseling should concentrate on the rationale for or against initiating antiretroviral therapy and reducing potential risks of HIV transmission from exposed person to others (practicing safe sex, refraining from blood or organ donation, etc.).

Repeat counseling on follow-up with family physician or other qualified counselor as anxiety may limit comprehension in the emergency setting. This should include more in-depth counseling concerning pretest and post-test issues and emotional support for this critical incident.

The following are general guidelines for initial counseling, with the accompanying scientific rationale:

Confidentiality

Confidentiality of test results is often a major concern for persons tested for HIV. Provide assurance that all test results will be treated in a strictly confidential manner. If requested, send their sample to the laboratory without personal identifying information.

Risk of HIV infection after exposure

The average risk of HIV transmission after accidental percutaneous exposure to infected blood or body fluids is estimated to be 0.25%. This figure was derived from metaanalysis of 21 prospective studies examining the risk of HIV transmission following accidental percutaneous exposures in occupational settings. Previous studies had estimated this risk to be 0.4%.

The same metaanalysis found the risk of HIV transmission following mucocutaneous exposure to be 0.1%. Previously, this risk had been estimated to be 0.3%.

These figures represent only an average risk; the risk to an individual may be higher depending on the presence of other risk factors. Factors that increase the risk of HIV transmission include:

- high viral load in the source (source in seroconversion illness or late AIDS disease)
- depth of wound
- volume of blood
- gauge of needle in needlestick exposures (larger-bore needles carry greater risk because of the larger volume of blood exposure)

Reasons for taking antiretroviral therapy

Some persons may be reluctant to accept antiretroviral therapy after a seemingly minor event. Explain that:

- if HIV transmission occurs, it will almost certainly lead to AIDS, which is a fatal disease; drug therapy taken soon after exposure may prevent infection
- recent evidence shows that antiretroviral therapy can reduce the risk of transmission of HIV by 86%; two or more drugs may be used to provide increased protection and to overcome the risk of the source virus being resistant to one drug

- if antiretroviral drugs are taken and HIV infection still occurs, the early use of antiretrovirals may favorably alter the course of the infection
- antiretroviral drugs taken for 1 month will have no long-term side-effects

What is zidovudine?

Zidovudine (ZDV) is an antiretroviral drug also known as azidothymidine (AZT). It works by stopping the virus from replicating. It is commonly used in the treatment of AIDS and HIV infection. It also has a beneficial effect in people with HIV infection who have not yet developed AIDS.

What is lamivudine?

Lamivudine (3TC) is also an antiretroviral drug which has been used extensively in the treatment of AIDS and HIV infection. It appears to be synergistic with zidovudine. This drug is a highly effective short-term therapy for HIV, but resistance develops rapidly; in the short-term setting resistance is not an issue, particularly if 3TC is used with zidovudine.

Evidence that ZDV can prevent HIV transmission

A recent multinational case-control study of HIV seroconversion in health care workers after percutaneous exposure to HIV-infected blood has been conducted by the Needlestick Surveillance Group, CDC, Atlanta. Health care workers who had an occupational (work-related) exposure to HIV-positive blood (i.e. the source was known or determined to be HIV-positive after testing) were divided into cases (those who seroconverted to HIV) and controls (those who did not seroconvert). A robust statistical analysis using logistic regression of many possible risk factors for seroconversion determined that *not* getting zidovudine chemoprophylaxis after percutaneous exposure was a definite risk factor for HIV transmission. Zidovudine reduced the risk of HIV transmission by a factor of five, i.e. the risk was reduced by 80%.

Possible side-effects of antiretroviral drugs

In the past, there was much concern about the possible toxicity of ZDV treatment. A recent study of ZDV use in uninfected infants born to HIV-infected mothers demonstrated that these concerns were not justified. In the study, 151 infants received ZDV for 6 weeks and 123 received placebo. The infants were followed for at least 60 weeks. There were no differences between the groups growth, immunological parameters or neurodevelopment. Short-term toxicity was limited to mild anemia which resolved on its own.

A recent multinational case-control study of HIV seroconversion in health care workers given high doses of zidovudine after exposure for 28 days and followed up for a mean of 30 weeks examined the risk of toxicity. None stopped taking zidovudine for objective toxicity but 35% stopped for subjective toxicity, i.e. fatigue, nausea, headache. This toxicity is less with the present recommended dose of zidovudine.

Lamivudine (3TC) is very well tolerated in short-term therapy and side-effects are rare. Reversible decreased white blood cell count is the most common side-effect. Tingling of the hands and feet (peripheral neuropathy) is very unlikely to occur with 1 month of treatment.

How long before exposed persons can be reasonably sure that they have not been infected?

The vast majority of persons infected will seroconvert within 3 months of infection. Testing for HIV is recommended at the time of exposure, and at 6 weeks, 12 weeks, and 6 months after the exposure. It is recommended that all those who take antiretroviral therapy should be tested again 12 months after exposure because antiretroviral therapy may delay the appearance of the infection.

Note—seroconversion after 12 weeks is uncommon and after 24 weeks extremely unlikely. However, for insurance and compensation purposes it is recommended that late testing be done.

Precautions to avoid transmission to others

While awaiting the test results (3 months to be reasonably sure), the exposed person should take the following precautions to prevent potential HIV transmission to others:

- abstain from sexual intercourse or use a latex condom with a nonpetroleum lubricant at all times during intercourse

- do not donate blood, plasma, organs, tissue or sperm
- do not share toothbrushes, razors, needles or other implements which may be contaminated with blood or body fluids
- do not become pregnant
- breastfeeding should be discontinued whether or not antiretrovirals are taken. This is to prevent HIV transmission to the child if the mother becomes infected. The risk of transmission through breastfeeding is high for women who seroconvert while breastfeeding. Breast milk can be pumped and discarded and nursing can be resumed if the source is found to be HIV-negative

Laboratory testing of source person

1. Ascertain identity of source, if possible.
2. If the source has no risk factors for HIV and has been HIV tested in the preceding 2 months (insurance, etc.) this can be accepted as evidence of HIV seronegativity. However, if the source is engaged in high-risk HIV transmission activities before or after the negative test, HIV serology should be repeated. If there is any suggestion of exposure in the preceding 12 weeks (seroconversion window period) P24 antigen can be requested on the laboratory requisition. However, a negative P24 test does not exclude the possibility that the source is in the seroconversion window period, and expert advice should be sought.
3. Obtain consent for HIV testing of source. The source person should not be tested without consent. Explain to the source that the exposed person will be informed of the result of the HIV test. If the source person is apprehensive about testing, expert counseling should be sought from the local HIV/AIDS expert.
4. Test for HIV if consent given. Testing may be done under a pseudonym or using non-nominal identifiers, as long as these can be traced appropriately.

If specimens are drawn from the source they should be clearly identified as coming from an accidental exposure episode so that they will be dealt with promptly by the laboratory. If the necessity for rapid turnaround is indicated on the requisition there can be a 24–48 h turnaround. Otherwise, the turnaround may be as long as 3 weeks. Direct communication with the laboratory is desirable

5. Ensure appropriate follow-up for the source person according to the test results.
6. If the exposed person is a health care worker in an institution and the source is a patient of that institution or known to the institution, the source's HIV status can be disclosed to the exposed health care worker. This information will fall within the appropriate confidentiality guidelines of the institution.

Antiretroviral therapy

Timing

Initiate antiretroviral therapy as soon as possible after exposure, preferably within 2 hours of exposure, to offer the best chance of preventing HIV transmission.

Antiretroviral therapy should be initiated for eligible exposed persons even if they present later. Many exposed persons in the community do not report the incident for a day or two. It is possible that while use after 96 hours may not prevent HIV transmission, it *may* favorably alter the subsequent disease in the exposed person, with the later onset of advanced disease. Therefore, there is no absolute cut-off time for the initiation of therapy. If uncertain about whether to initiate antiretroviral therapy, consult the local HIV/AIDS expert.

Contraindications to antiretroviral therapy

Avoid or use with extreme caution in:

- persons with chronic renal insufficiency (creatinine more than three times normal), hepatic insufficiency, or bone marrow dyscrasia

- persons treated with myelosuppressive, nephrotoxic or hepatotoxic drugs in the 2 weeks prior to starting antiretroviral therapy

Zidovudine is not contraindicated in pregnancy. It has not been shown to produce fetal malformations when taken after 14 weeks of gestation. The observed proportion of birth defects among infants of women who received ZDV therapy during the first trimester of pegnancy, when the fetus is most sensitive to teratogens, was 2%. This does not differ from the expected incidence of birth defects in all pregnancies (3%). However, the risks versus benefits of use in women less than 14 weeks pregnant should be considered on an individual basis. At this time, there are no data about the safety of other antiretroviral drugs in pregnancy.

If the source is known to be HIV-positive on antiretroviral therapy and the exposed person is pregnant, contact the local HIV/AIDS expert IMMEDIATELY.

Pretreatment laboratory evaluation

No laboratory evaluation is required prior to initiation of the antiretroviral therapy starter kit unless the exposed person is suspected of having hematologic or hepatic disease.

Persons continuing therapy after the starter kit should have a baseline CBC at once, after 2 weeks, and after 4 weeks of therapy.

Drug dosage

- ZDV 200 mg three times a day while awake plus lamivudine (3TC) 150 mg twice a day; continue treatment for 4 weeks
- two drugs are recommended because in many areas strains of HIV are relatively resistant to zidovudine; check your local situation

In the event of higher-risk exposure, additional (e.g. Indinavir) or different antiretroviral therapy may be appropriate.

> A starter kit is intended to provide 5 days of therapy while more detailed assessment of the risk of transmission can occur. The exposed person should see their family physician or designated follow-up physician as soon as possible after the initiation of the starter kit to determine the need for a full 28 days of therapy. Many exposed persons will not require 28 days of therapy, but this decision should be made in consultation with their physician

Availability of drugs

Starter kits with a 5-day course of ZDV-3TC combination antiretrovirals should be kept in the emergency departments of larger hospitals. In hospitals without emergency departments, the kits can be kept in night pharmacy cupboards.

Recommendations for postexposure HIV chemoprophylaxis in children

The risk of children being infected with HIV from accidental needlestick injuries, biting, or sexual assaults is very low. No evidence showing that antiretroviral therapy will decrease the risk of infection in children who sustain needlestick injuries or sexual assault is available. Data that are available refer to the lower risk of perinatal transmission and lowered risk of transmission in exposed health care workers with zidovudine prophylaxis. Antiretroviral agents should be considered for children where the exposure is likely to have resulted in a transfer of potentially infectious body fluid to the recipient. In children this would most commonly occur from blood or semen from a youth or adult who is known to be HIV-positive or could potentially be HIV-positive.

Accidental needlestick injuries in children will usually occur from moderate-risk exposures. Chemoprophylaxis may not be effective in preventing transmission if more than 96 hours has elapsed since the injury. Hepatitis B prophylaxis is recommended for all needlestick exposures in children.

Chemoprophylaxis for HIV should only be considered for human bites in children that result in the skin being broken and when bleeding has occurred and there is blood in the mouth of the biter. The risk of HIV infection is negligible in bites from children. Chemoprophylaxis may not be effective in preventing transmission if more than

96 hours has elapsed since the injury. Should a child bite an HIV-positive person prophylaxis may be considered if there is blood in the mouth of the child and there are areas of nonintact mucosa.

Chemoprophylaxis for HIV should be considered for children sustaining sexual assault resulting in vaginal or anal penetration. Chemo- prophylaxis may not be effective in preventing transmission if more than 96 hours has elapsed since the assault.

Follow-up

Follow-up is required for all persons receiving antiretroviral therapy and those having had a high- or moderate-risk exposure to HIV. Follow-up should be done by the exposed person's family physician. If this is not possible, identify a designated physician or center for follow-up.

Test HIV serology of exposed person according to the following schedule:

- as soon as possible after exposure (copy results to family physician or follow-up agency)
- 6 weeks after exposure
- 12 weeks after exposure
- 24 weeks after exposure
- 1 year after exposure if antiretroviral therapy has been given

Note—seroconversion after 12 weeks is uncommon and after 24 weeks extremely unlikely. However, for insurance and compensation purposes it is recommended that late testing be done.

These guidelines are modified and reproduced with permission from the BC Centre for Excellence in HIV/AIDS, Vancouver.

Index